Treatment of Rheumatoid Arthritis

Treatment of Rheumatoid Arthritis

Edited by **Mary Kellar**

hayle medical

New York

Published by Hayle Medical,
30 West, 37th Street, Suite 612,
New York, NY 10018, USA
www.haylemedical.com

Treatment of Rheumatoid Arthritis
Edited by Mary Kellar

International Standard Book Number: 978-1-63241-374-1 (Hardback)

Printed in China.

Contents

Preface

Rheumatoid Arthritis (RA) is a chronic progressive disease. The aim of this book is to present updated, interesting, and thought-provoking outlooks on several aspects of research regarding available and potential treatments for rheumatoid arthritis. This book consists of state-of-the-art information contributed by veteran researchers in the field of rheumatology from across the planet. It intends to serve as a valuable reference and source of potential fields of investigation for research scientists engaged in the field of rheumatoid arthritis and other inflammatory arthropathies.

This book is the end result of constructive efforts and intensive research done by experts in this field. The aim of this book is to enlighten the readers with recent information in this area of research. The information provided in this profound book would serve as a valuable reference to students and researchers in this field.

At the end, I would like to thank all the authors for devoting their precious time and providing their valuable contribution to this book. I would also like to express my gratitude to my fellow colleagues who encouraged me throughout the process.

Editor

Part 1

DMARDs (Disease Modifying Anti-Rheumatic Drugs) and NSAIDs (Non-Steroidal Anti-Inflammatory Drugs)

1

Novel Formulation Approaches for Dermal and Transdermal Delivery of Non-Steroidal Anti-Inflammatory Drugs

Alper Okyar[1], Yıldız Özsoy[2] and Sevgi Güngör[2]
[1]Istanbul University Faculty of Pharmacy Department of Pharmacology, Beyazıt- Istanbul
[2]Istanbul University Faculty of Pharmacy Department of Pharmaceutical Technology, Beyazıt- Istanbul, Turkey

1. Introduction

Non-steroidal anti-inflammatory drugs (NSAIDs) are among the most frequently prescribed drug groups. These drugs are used dermally or systemically in treatment of various rheumatic diseases, including rheumatoid arthritis (RA), as well as for osteoarthritis, low back pain and some joint diseases. The mechanism of action of NSAIDs is reversible inhibition of the cyclooxygenase enzyme (COX) and decreasing the synthesis of prostaglandins (Lionberger 2010; Massey 2010). However, these drugs lead to unfavorable effects specifically on the stomach as a result of inhibition of prostaglandins (PGs), which play a role in protection of the gastric mucosa, in systemic administration. The severity of these unfavorable side effects may range from a simple ailment like dyspepsia to peptic ulcer and gastrointestinal hemorrhage. Furthermore, the acidic character of NSAIDs may lead to local irritation and lesions on the gastrointestinal mucosa. Therefore, some NSAIDs are administered percutaneously and transdermally to achieve local or systemic effect as an alternative to oral and parenteral administration (Heyneman et al., 2000; Hooper et al., 2004). In dermal administration, the drug substances have to pass the *stratum corneum (SC)* layer to reach lower layers of the skin and/or to enter systemic circulation. In this context, formulation of the product may play a key role for penetration and absorption of the active ingredient (Lee & Maibach, 2006). Several formulation approaches for cutaneous administration of NSAIDs have been employed. The conventional pharmaceutical forms particularly used for dermal administration to achieve local effect are gels, creams and ointments (Williams, 2003). Furthermore, studies on novel drug delivery systems are available for transdermal administration of NSAIDs. These new approaches include liquid crystals, nano/micro emulsions, liposomes, solid lipid particles and patches. These systems are used to enhance cutaneous passage of drugs into systemic circulation and to target different layers of the skin (Guy, 2010; Santos et al., 2008; El Maghraby et al., 2008; Ceve, 2004). Different approaches have been performed to enhance cutaneous passage of drugs with the objective of overcoming the low skin permeability (Guy, 2010; Tromer & Neubert,

2006). The most frequently used approach is to include penetration enhancers in formulations. In addition to penetration enhancers, there are studies available in which physical methods such as iontophoresis is used in improving of skin delivery of drugs (Guy, 1996; Benson, 2005; Williams, 2003).

The chapter deals with the classification and mechanisms of action of NSAIDs used in treatment of various rheumatic diseases as well as for osteoarthritis, low back pain and some joint diseases. The advantages of skin delivery of NSAIDs to target affected tissues and/or to achieve systemic effect are also emphasized. In particular, recent studies in which novel drug delivery systems were developed for dermal and transdermal administration of NSAIDs are summarized.

2. Non-steroidal anti-inflammatory drugs (NSAIDs)

2.1 General view and classification of NSAIDs

NSAIDs are used for chronic inflammatory conditions such as rheumatoid arthritis and osteoarthritis, posttraumatic conditions (e.g. distortion, contusion), for relieving mild to moderate pain of varied origin, reducing fever, as well as for preventing local inflammation such as gout (Hinz & Brune, 2008; Lionberger et al., 2011; Patrono & Rocca, 2009). NSAIDs are employed in systemic as well as local dosage forms particularly for musculoskeletal pain and patients with inflammatory joint disorders. NSAIDs possess antipyretic effect in addition to analgesic-anti-inflammatory actions. NSAIDs may be responsible for side effects such as acute renal failure, undesirable central nervous effects, e.g. dizziness, allergic reactions and fluid retention in the body. Beside some side effects of NSAIDs mentioned before, NSAIDs lead to unfavorable effects on the stomach as a result of inhibition of prostaglandins, which play a role in protection of the gastric mucosa, in systemic administration e.g. oral, parenteral. The severity of this unfavorable gastrointestinal side effect may range from a simple ailment like dyspepsia to gastric bleeding potentially resulting in admission to hospital, necessitating surgery or even resulting in death (Hooper et al., 2004). Furthermore, the acidic character of NSAIDs may lead to local irritation, and lesions on the gastrointestinal mucosa are known as NSAIDs gastropathy (Heynemann et al., 2000). Within the past 20 years many COX inhibitors were removed for undesired drug effects shortly after entering the market e.g. benoxaprofen and isoxicam (Brune et al., 2010). Therefore, some NSAIDs are administered percutaneously to achieve local or systemic effect as an alternative to oral and parenteral administration (Heyneman et al., 2000; Hooper et al., 2004). NSAIDs are classified by their chemical structures as shown in Table 1.

2.2 Mechanism of anti-inflammatory effect of NSAIDs

NSAIDs usually act through decreasing reactions of inflammation that is accompanied with pain. It is known that prostaglandin (PG) derivatives, that are formed from arachidonic acid through COX enzyme, play an important role in formation of inflammation, and that the PGE_1 and PGE_2 levels are increased in the synovial fluid in patients with rheumatoid arthritis. All NSAIDs inhibit the COX enzyme and act through decreasing the synthesis of PGE_2, PGD_2, $PGF_{2\alpha}$, PGI_2 and thromboxane A2 (TxA_2) and prostacycline (Lionberger et al., 2010; Massey et al., 2010). Two isoforms of COX (COX-1 and COX-2) were identified and

Salicylates	Para-aminophenol derivatives	Pyrazolone derivatives	Phenylpropionic acid derivatives	Phenylacetic acid derivatives	Indoleacetic acid derivatives	Fenamic acid derivatives	Oxicams	Other drugs	COX-2 selective NSAIDs
Acetylsalicylic acid	Acetaminophen	Aminopyrine	Ibuprofen	Diclofenac	Indomethacin	Mefenamic acid	Piroxicam	Proquazone	Etodolac
Diflunisal		Metamizole	Ketoprofen	Nabumeton	Acemetasin	Flufenamic acid	Tenoxicam	Azapropazone	Meloxicam
Sodium salicylate		Phenylbutazone	Phenoprofen	Fenclofenac	Tolmetin	Etofenamate	Lornoxicam	Methotrimeprazine	Nimesulide
Salicylic acid		Oxyphenbutazone	Flurbiprofen	Alclofenac	Ketorolac	Tolfenamic acid	Isoxicam	Benzydamine	Selecoxib
Salicylamide		Propyphenazone	Indoprofen	Felbinac	Sulindac	Meclofenamate		Nabumetone	Rofecoxib
		Amidopyrine	Naproxen	Bufexamac		Niflumic acid		Etofenamate	Etoricoxib
			Fenbufen	Aceclofenac					Lumiracoxib
			Zomepirac						Parecoxib
			Dexibuprofen						Valdecoxib
			Dexketoprofen						
			Oxaprozin						
			Tiaprofenic acid						
			Suprofen						

Table 1. Classification of NSAIDs according to chemical structure (Heynemann et al., 2000; Hadgraft et al., 2000; Marnett, 2009).

studies of their regulation and sites of expression led to the hypothesis that it is the molecular target for the anti-inflammatory and analgesic effects of NSAIDs. COX-1 is important for production of gastric mucus and maintenance of renal blood flow. On the other hand, COX-2 is induced by several cytokines, growing factors and endotoxins and plays a role in the inflammatory process observed at the site of inflammation. Nonselective NSAIDs inhibit both COX-1 and COX-2, and the current hypothesis is that COX-2 inhibition is responsible for the anti-inflammatory effects of NSAIDs, whereas COX-1 inhibition is responsible for some other undesired side effects, in particular for gastrointestinal toxicity. Therefore selective inhibition of COX-2 may prevent undesirable gastrointestinal effects of NSAIDs. The discovery and clinical development of selective COX-2 inhibitors (COXIBs) were achieved in the early 1990s. COXIBs have anti-inflammatory effects without side effects on the stomach as compared to traditional NSAIDs. However, these new NSAIDs also possess some side effects, since inhibition of COX-2 affects kidney function and blood pressure and possibly other physiological parameters (Brune & Hinz, 2004; Marnett, 2009; Patrono & Rocco, 2009; Mitchell et al., 1994). Rofecoxib and valdecoxib was withdrawn from the market due to serious cardiovascular side effects, and lumiracoxib was removed from several markets for serious liver toxicity unrelated to COX-2 inhibition. Celecoxib has been marketed in the United States, and celecoxib and etoricoxib was marketed in Europe (Hinz & Brune, 2008).

2.3 Physicochemical properties of NSAIDs

Table 2 demonstrates the open chemical formulas and physicochemical properties of NSAIDs, which have dermal and transdermal commercial preparations and of the molecules which are potential candidates in this group.

The physiochemical properties of drugs are important in dermal and transdermal administration (Potts and Francoeur, 1991; Kalia et al., 1998; Prausnitz & Langer, 2008). The ideal candidate drugs have the following properties: water-solubility (> 1 mg/ml), lipophilicity (log P= 1-3), low molecular weight (< 500 Dalton) and low melting temperature (< 200°C) (Guy, 2007). As can be seen in Table 2, all drugs are under 400 Dalton. The Log P values, which indicate lipophilic characteristics of pharmaceuticals, vary between 2.0 and 3.8 except for flurbiprofen, etofenamate and lumiracoxib. In other words, they have medium lipophilicity. Other NSAIDs except meloxicam and tenoxicam have a melting point under <200°C. Due to these physicochemical properties, NSAIDs are ideal molecules for dermal administration. As a matter of fact, dermal/transdermal commercial preparations of most of NSAIDs are available in pharmacies. Studies on development of skin delivery systems of other molecules are in progress.

3. Dermal and transdermal administration of NSAIDs

3.1 Skin transport

Human skin is the largest organ in our body with its size about 1.8-2.0 m^2. It is a well-engineered organ that protects organism against environmental factors and regulates heat and water loss from the body. It is also easily accessible due to its large surface area. Therefore, it offers an ideal application site to deliver therapeutic agents for both local and systemic actions. The skin consists of three main layers; the epidermis, the dermis, and the hypodermis. In particular, *stratum corneum* (SC), the outermost layer of epidermis is formed by dead and keratinized cells, and thus it is a unique barrier to passage of drugs through the skin (Williams, 2003).The drug substances from dermal or transdermal formulations have to pass through the SC layer to reach lower layers of the skin and/or to enter systemic circulation. The physicochemical characteristics of drug molecules and the types of the formulations are an effective factor in both dermal and transdermal delivery (Hadgraft, 1999). The drugs pass through the skin via three different routes, which are transcellular, intercellular and/or transappendageal (shunt) routes (sweat glands, hair follicles, sebaceous glands) (Williams, 2003).

3.2 The superiorities and limitations of dermal and transdermal delivery

There are two pharmacological approaches in dermal administration of drugs, which are dermal and transdermal. In dermal administration, the applied formulation ensures localization of drugs in dermal layers. In transdermal administration, the drugs reach the dermis of skin via carrier systems and then go into systemic circulation (Williams, 2003).
In dermal administration, the access of drugs to systemic circulation is prevented or minimized. Therefore, the systemic adverse effects of drugs are avoided. The advantages of transdermal administration include high patient compatibility with treatment, ability to discontinue treatment any time necessary, delivery of drug to organism at a controlled rate, ensuring fixed plasma drug level and eliminating the hepatic first-pass effect (Guy, 1996).
NSAIDs administered dermally and transdermally penetrate slowly and in small quantities into the systemic circulation. These approaches also prevent high local drug levels in the alimentary tract and direct toxicity of NSAIDs e.g. vomiting, dyspepsia. Systemic administration of NSAIDs may cause drug-drug interactions. NSAIDs cause fluid retention in the body and may decrease efficacy of antihypertensive agents. Furthermore, dermal and transdermal formulations have better patient compliance (non-invasiveness) and they can be self-administered (Guy, 1996; Taner & Marks, 2008; Heynemann et al., 2000). It was reported that the use of dermal NSAIDs may have led to a reduction in the total daily dosage of systemic NSAIDs. This would cause an increment in side effects of NSAIDs in long term treatment (Sift Carter et al., 1997). Finally, dermally applied NSAIDs have a superior safety profile to oral formulations. Adverse effects secondary to dermal NSAID application occur in approximately 10 to 15% of patients and are primarily cutaneous in nature (rash and pruritus at the site of application (Heynemann et al., 2000)). NSAI drug concentration should reach therapeutic level in the synovial tissue, synovial fluid and intra-articular tissues during dermal application of NSAIDs. There are a number of factors that influence skin absorption of drugs. The greatest challenge for dermal penetration is SC, the uppermost layer of the skin, which as mentioned previously is the rate limiting step for epidermal drug transport. Therefore several formulation approaches are developed to improve its impermeability characteristics.

3.3 Overcoming the barrier properties of the skin

Several chemical and physical approaches are used to overcome the barrier property of the skin in dermal and transdermal administration of drugs. The most frequently used approach is to include chemical penetration enhancers in formulations. Recently, physical

Substance	Chemical Formula	Molecular Weight (g/mol)	Predicted Log P	Melting Point	Predicted aqueous solubility (μg/ml)	pKa	References
Benzydamine	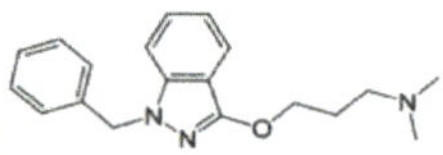	309,4	3.71	160° (bp)	-	9,27	Avdeef et al., 1998. Quane et al.,1998
Bufexamac	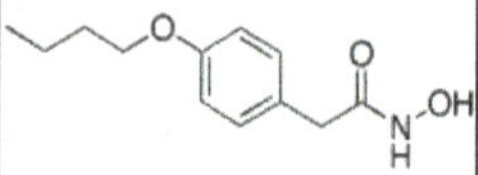	223,3	2,43	154°C	110 μg/ml	9,24	Hadgraft et al., 2000
Celecoxib	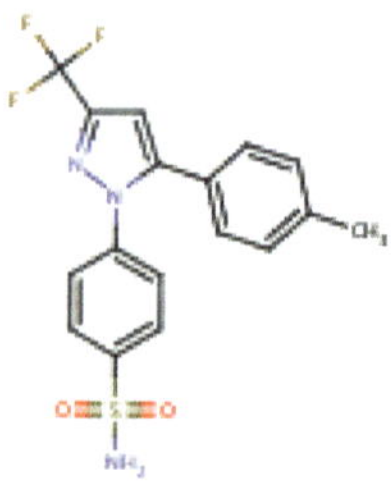	381,4	3,5	157-158°C	3,3 μg/ml	11.1	http://www.drugbank.ca
Diclofenac	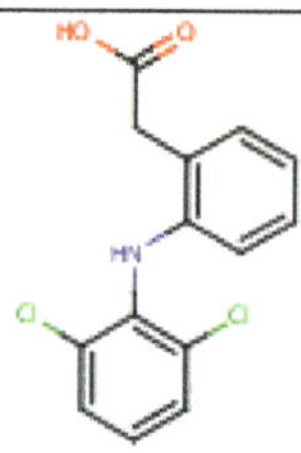	296,1	3,28	157°C	12 μg/ml	4,18	Hadgraft et al., 2000
Etodolac	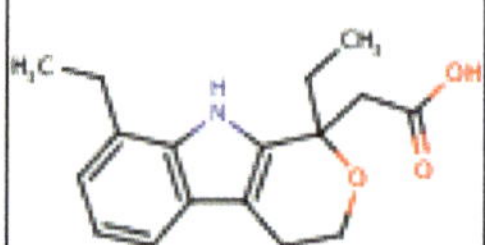	287,4	2,5	145°C	16 μg/ml	4,65	http://www.drugbank.ca
Flurbiprofen	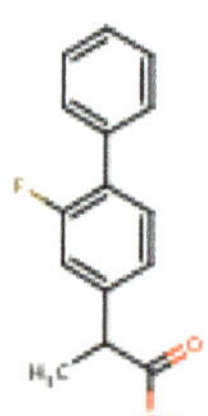	224,3	4,12	110,5°C	2,7 μg/ml	4,14	Hadgraft et al., 2000

Table 2. Chemical formulas and physicochemical properties of NSAIDs.

Substance	Chemical Formula	Molecular Weight (g/mol)	Predicted Log P	Melting Point	Predicted aqueous solubility (µg/ml)	pKa	References
Etofenamate	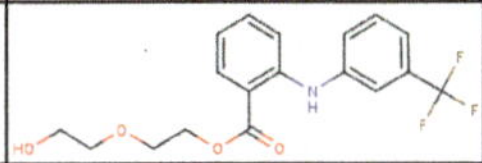	369,3	4.99	130–135°C (bp)	Practically insoluble in water	-	http://www.chembase.com
Felbinac	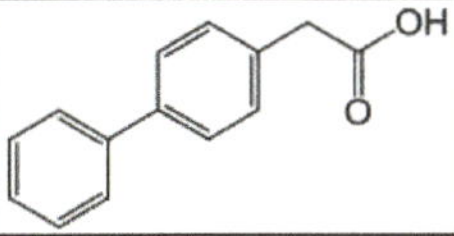	212,2	3,26	164°C	8 µg/ml	4.3	Pygall et al., 2009
Ibuprofen	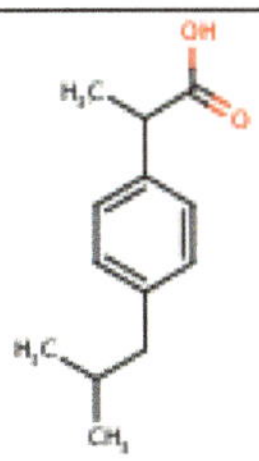	206,3	3,72	76°C	14 µg/ml	4,41	Hadgraft et al., 2000
Indomethacin	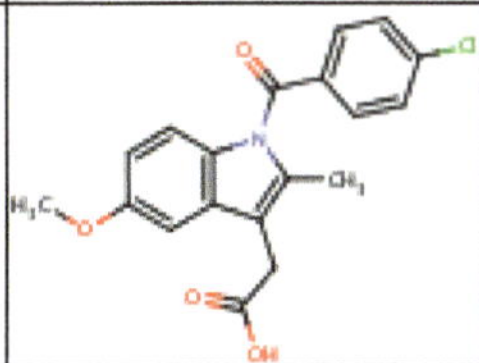	357,8	3,10	155°C	25 µg/ml	4,18	Hadgraft et al., 2000
Ketoprofen	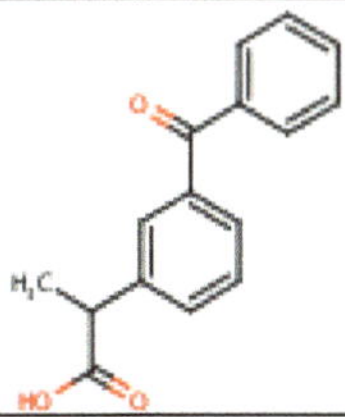	254,3	2,81	94°C	150 µg/ml	4,23	Hadgraft et al., 2000
Ketorolac	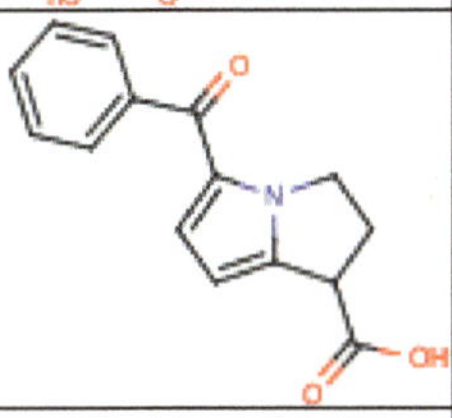	255,3	2,1	165-167°C (tromethamine salt)	25 mg/mL (tromethamine salt)	3,5	http://www.drugbank.ca
Lumiracoxib	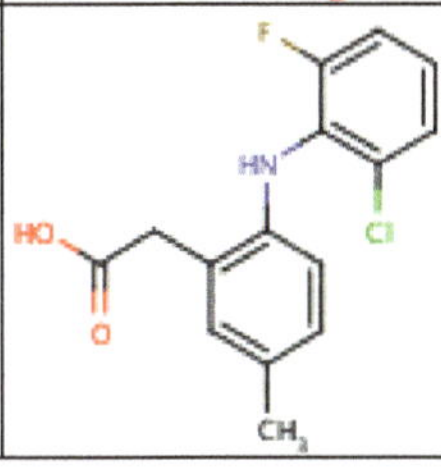	293,7	4,56	139-141°C	5,49 µg/ml	15,87	http://www.drugbank.ca

Table 2. Continued.

Substance	Chemical Formula	Molecular Weight (g/mol)	Predicted Log P	Melting Point	Predicted aqueous solubility (µg/ml)	pKa	References
Meloxicam	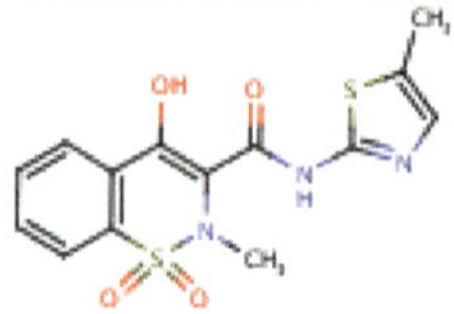	351,4	1,9	242 - 250°C	7,15 µg/ml	4,08	http://www.drugbank.ca
Naproxen	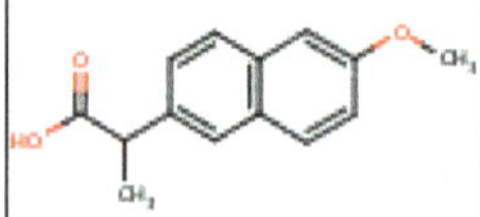	230,3	3,00	155,3°C	23 µg/ml	4,4	Hadgraft et al., 2000
Nimesulide	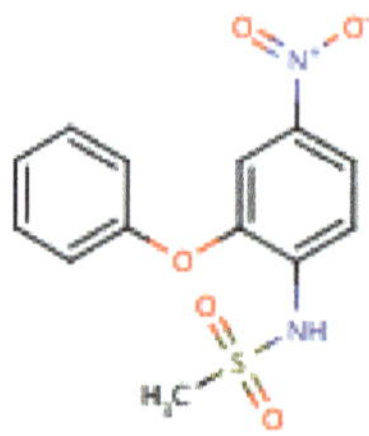	308,3	2,56 1,79	143-144°C	18,2 µg/ml	6,46	http://www.drugbank.ca
Oxyphen-butazone	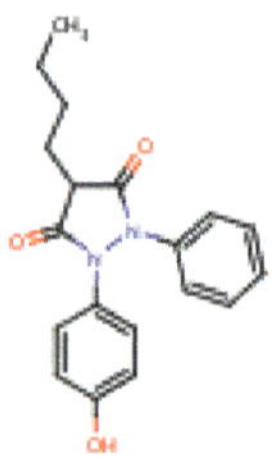	324,4	2,79 3,83	96°C	256 µg/ml	9,29	http://www.drugbank.ca
Piroxicam	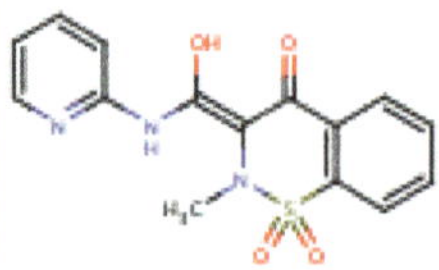	331,4	1,46	199°C	870 µg/ml	13,92	Hadgraft et al., 2000
Suprofen	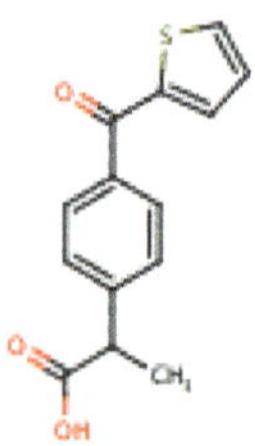	260,3	3,16 3,53	124,3°C	42,2 µg/ml	3,91	http://www.drugbank.ca

Table 2. Continued.

Substance	Chemical Formula	Molecular Weight (g/mol)	Predicted Log P	Melting Point	Predicted aqueous solubility (µg/ml)	pKa	References
Salicylic acid	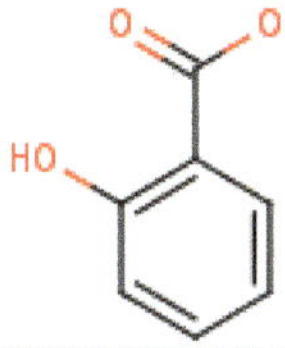	138,1	2,4	158°C	2,24 g/mL	2,97	http://www.drugbank.ca
Tenoxicam	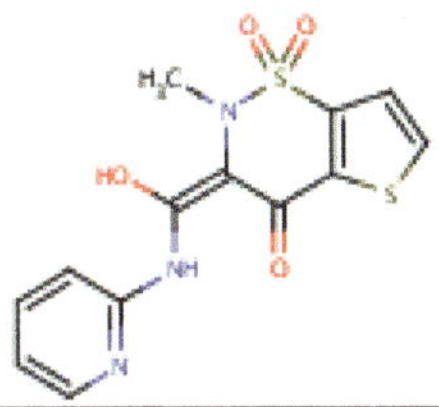	337,4	1,82 1,22	211°C	277 µg/ml	13,63	http://www.drugbank.ca
Tiaprofenic acid	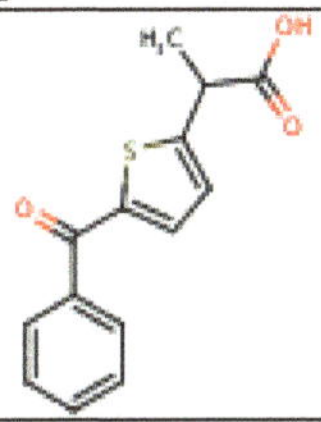	260,3	2,42	96°C	450 µg/ml	4,05	Hadgraft et al., 2000
Valdecoxib	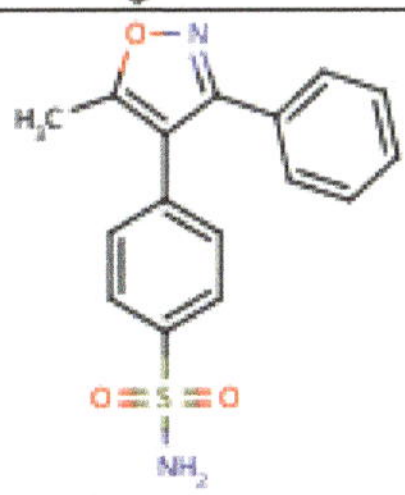	314,4	3,32 2,82	162-164°C	34,8 µg/ml	9,4	http://www.drugbank.ca

Table 2. Continued.

methods such as iontophoresis that enhance penetration of drug molecules through the skin are applied (Mitragotri et al., 2000; Tao & Desai, 2003). Furthermore, vesicular carriers, microemulsions, lipidic and polymeric particulate carrier systems ensure dermal administration of drugs by dermal targeting and enterance of drugs into systemic circulation (Neubert, 2011; Benson, 2005).

3.3.1 Chemical enhancers

Chemical penetration enhancers reversibly change the structure of the skin to improve the flux of drugs through the skin. The mechanism of action of penetration enhancers is explained by Lipid-Protein-Partition (LPP) Theory (Williams & Barry, 1991). According to this theory, penetration enhancers i) disrupt the lipid structure in intercellular domain of SC, or ii) denature or change the conformation of keratin in the intracellular domain and/or iii) improve drug partition to SC and thus establish a drug reservoir in SC to act (Williams &

NSAIDs	Enhancers	Results	Refs
Diclofenac	Oleic acid(OA)/ d-limonene	Addition of the mixture of oleic acid/d-limonene as enhancer into diclofenac sodium formulations has been found to be effective for the dermal and subdermal injuries.	Escribano et al., 2003
Diclofenac	Dimethyl sulfoxide (DMSO)	Dermal administration of diclofenac containing DMSO vehicle has been found to be effective for knee osteoarthritis, and has showed better tolerability than oral diclefenac.	Simon et al., 2009
Etodolac	terpenes	Gel containing anethol increased absorption of etodolac (1,5-fold) significantly in excised rat skin, as compared to control gel.	Taş et al., 2007
Flurbiprofen (nitro ester)	Transcutol®/(OA) lauroglycol isopropyl myristate (IPM)	The efficacy and safety of dermal nitro ester of flurbiprofen was shown with lipophilic ointment containing chemical enhancers.	Minghetti et al., 2003
Flurbiprofen	Turpentine oil	The bioavailability of transdermal patch formulation flurbiprofen containing turpentine oil has been shown to increase 5.56 times with respect to its oral administration.	Charoo et al., 2008
Flurbiprofen	l-menthol/ethanol	Flurbiprofen gel containing ethanol (25%) and l-menthol (3%) has showed high in vivo absorption rate in rabbits.	Morimoto et al., 2000
Flurbiprofen	Linoleic acid (LA)/ /linolenic acid (LNA)/(OA) Palmitic acid (PA)	Fatty acids (PA, OA, LA, and LNA) extracted from Botryococcus braunii was found effective enhancers to improve the skin delivery flurbiprofen.	Fang et al., 2004
Ibuprofen	Ethanol	The flux of ibuprofen was increased by the ethanol (>10-fold flux enhacement) across silicone membrane and human skin.	Watkinson et al., 2009
Ibuprofen	Propylene glycol (PG)	PG and (PG: water) systems has increased the fluxes of ibuprofen due the increase in skin partition of ibuprofen.	Watkinson et al., 2008
Ketorolac	DMSO/d-limonene eucalyptus oil/ Transcutol®	Eucalyptus oil has showed the highest permeation enhancer effect for the transdermal delivery of ketorolac across rat skin.	Amrish & Kumar, 2009
Ketorolac trometamol	IPM/ Brij 92	Dermal formulations of ketorolac trometamol containing Brij 92 exhibited less gastric side effect and higher anti-inflammatory effect than that of containing IPM.	El-Setouhy & El-Ashmony, 2009
Lumiracoxib	OA	Oleic acid (10%) has increased the flux of lumiracoxib through skin and its retention in viable epidermis.	Moreira et al., 2010

NSAIDs	Enhancers	Results	Refs
Meloxicam	N-methyl pyrrolidone (NMP)	Meloxicam gel containing NMP as a solubilizer exhibited significant higher anti-inflammatory in rats compared to commercial gel formulation.	Bachhav & Patravale, 2010
Nimesulide	OA/ Transcutol®	Oleic acid (3%) in the presence of Transcutol® (30%) has led to a significant increase in permeation of drug across the skin.	Gungor & Bergisadi, 2004
Piroxicam	Lauric acid /OA/LA/LNA	All enhancers showed similar extent of permeation, which was 3-fold higher than that of without enhancer administration.	Santoyo & Ygartua, 2000
Tenoxicam	OA/LA/oleyl alcohol	The highest tenoxicam flux was obtained by the addition of fatty acids at 3% concentration to PG.	Gwak & Chun, 2002
Tiaprofenic acid	terpenes	Gel containing d-limonene increased absorption of tiaprofenic acid (6-fold) significantly in excised pig skin, as compared to control gel.	Okyar et al., 2008
Tiaprofenic acid	terpenes	Gel containing d-limonene increased absorption of tiaprofenic acid (6-fold) significantly in excised rat skin. Gel with d-limonene increased tiaprofenic acid skin absorption of 10-fold in vivo in rats, as compared to control gel.	Okyar et al., 2010

Table 3. Effect of chemical penetration enhancers to increase skin permeation of NSAIDs.

Barry, 2004; Thong HY et al., 2007). Co-solvents such as alcohols, oil alcohols, propylene glycol, diethyleneglycol monoethylether (Transcutol®), and compounds like fatty acids terpenes, Azone®, dimethylsulfoxide (DMSO), pyrrolidones, urea and surfactants are frequently included in dermal/transdermal formulations as penetration enhancers (Williams & Barry, 2004; Mohammed et al., 2007). Table 3 summarizes the penetration enhancers to improve passage of NSAIDs through the skin and the results obtained.

3.3.2 Physical enhancement

Iontophoresis is one of the most frequently used physical methods in improving dermal penetration of drugs. Iontophoresis enhances dermal penetration of drug molecules by applying low levels of electrical currents (0,5 mA/cm^2) (Marro et al., 2002). Unlike passive diffusion-based transdermal administration, particularly, iontophoresis ensures dermal penetration of polar and charged drug molecules in high amounts loaded (Kalia et al., 1998; Sieg & Wascotte, 2009).

There are studies investigating whether the iontophoresis technique enhanced dermal penetration of NSAIDs. Curdy et al. (2001) dermally administered a commercial gel formulation containing piroxicam, and studied dermal penetration of piroxicam by using both passive and iontophoresis method. They found that application of low electric current enhanced uptake of piroxicam to SC layer. Moreover, a high piroxicam concentration was obtained in the SC, live epidermis and dermis with the iontophoresis application. Mathy and coworkers studied the percutaneous penetration of flurbiprofen on hairless rats (Mathy et al., 2005). They investigated the flurbiprofen concentrations in the dermal and subcutaneous tissue following administration of iontophoresis. The data obtained demonstrated that application of iontophoresis ensured delivery of flurbiprofen at a high input rate to the dermis and underlying tissues at significant amounts, while maintaining low plasma exposure.

4. Conventional formulations and novel approaches in dermal and transdermal delivery of NSAIDs

Conventional dosage forms of NSAIDs which are commercially available and and possible novel carrier systems of NSAIDs to improve their dermal and transdermal delivery are summarized in Fig.

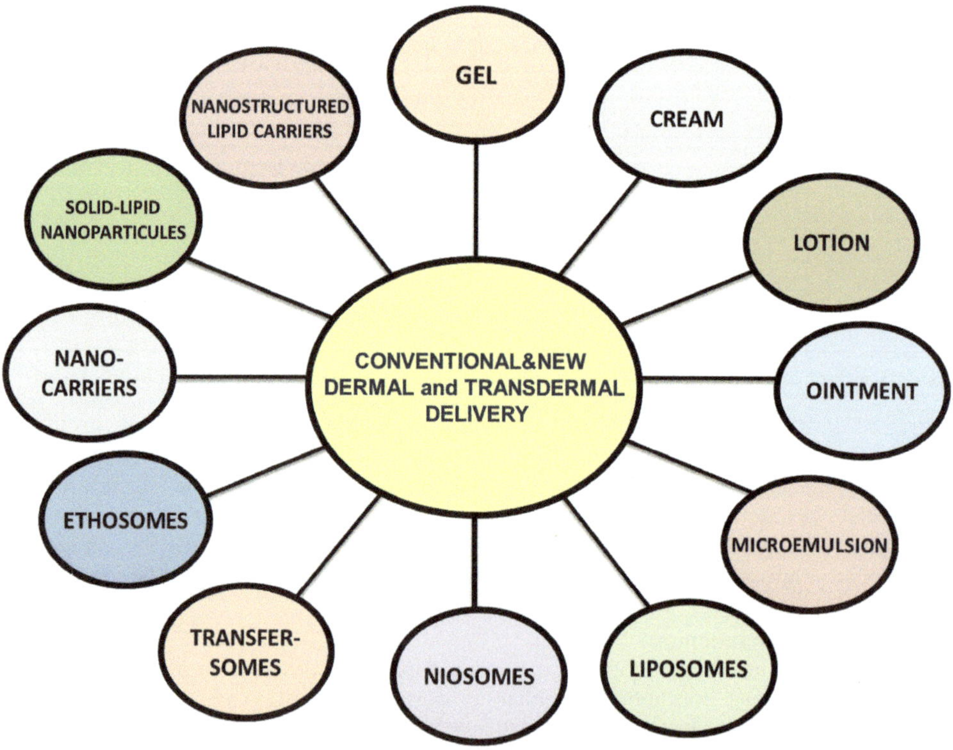

Fig. 1. Schematic representation of the novel and conventional dermal drug delivery systems.

4.1 Conventional formulations

The classical dosage forms of NSAIDs for dermal use that are commercially available are usually gels, creams, ointments and lotions. Table 4 gives a list of NSAIDs which have commercial dermal preparations.

NSAIDs	Formulation type
Benzydamine	Gel, cream
Felbinac	Gel
Bufexamac	Cream, ointment, lotion, emulgel
Diclofenac epolamine	Patch
Diclofenac sodium	Gel, spray gel
Diclofenac potassium	Gel
Diclofenac diethylammonium	Gel, emulgel
Etofenamate	Gel, cream
Ibuprofen	Gel, cream
Ketoprofen	Gel
Naproxen	Gel
Nimesulide	Gel
Piroxicam	Gel
Salicylic acid	Cream, ointment, lotion

Table 4. Commerical dermal formulations of NSAIDs (Micromedex, electronic version, Rx MediaPharma 2011).

4.1.1 Gels

They are two-component semi-solid drug carriers that contain high levels of fluid and viscosity enhancing agents. Polar solvents such as water and alcohol are used in the liquid phase. They contain appropriate viscosity enhancers depending on the physicochemical properties of drug molecule and its compatibility with the vehicle. Simple gels are prepared with a natural polymer, such as carrageen, pectin or sodium alginate, or semi-synthetic stabilizers like cellulose derivatives or synthetic stabilizers like Carbomers (Williams, 2003). As can be seen on Table 3, gel formulations of most of NSAIDs are commercially available because gels are easy to administer, forming a thin film coating on the skin and ensuring rapid action without giving an oily feeling. They are preferred by patients due to these advantages. Besides they are cost-efficient since formulation inputs are less, and they are preferred by manufacturers. Although there are not commercially available dermal formulations of NSAIDs there are studies on development of gel-type formulation of tiaprofenic acid (Okyar et al., 2008 and 2010), meloxicam (Martinez et al., 2007; Jain & Pathak, 2010; Gupta et al., 2002), aceclofenac (Dua et al., 2010) and flurbiprofen (Minghetti et al., 2003; Pandey et al., 2009).

4.1.2 Ointments, creams and lotions

Ointments are semi-solid preparations administered on the skin. Their formulations contain high levels of oil. Typically they have an occlusive action on the skin, and are used for dry lesions. Creams have an emulsion structure although they are defined as semi-solid carrier systems. Emulsions are systems consisting of two phases containing water and oil, where one is disperse in the other. Creams are more acceptable for patients as they have lower viscosity than ointments and are less oily. Lotions are creams with less viscosity (Williams, 2003). There are cream and/or ointment-type preparations of benzydamine bufexamac, etofenamate, ibuprofen and salicylic acid that are commercially available. Lotion-type preparations of bufexamac and salicylic acid are used in treatments (Table 4).

4.2 Novel formulation approaches for improving skin delivery of NSAIDs

4.2.1 Micromemulsions

Microemulsions are transparent liquid dispersions with a droplet size of 20-200 nm. Their formulations include four fundamental components, which are water, oil, surfactant and co-surfactant. The advantages of microemulsions include enhancing solubility of drugs, thermodynamic stability, ease of preparation and low costs (Neubert, 2011). Microemulsions have recently attracted attention in enhancing dermal permeation of lypophilic drugs as well as hydrophilic drugs. The oils and surfactants included in the composition of microemulsions also act as penetration enhancers. Besides, the composition of formulation and the internal structure of phases enhance diffusion of the drug inside the carrier and improve the partition of drug to SC (Kogan & Garti, 2006). The most important disadvantage of microemulsions is potential risk of skin irritation due to their high content of surfactants. Kantarcı et al. (2007) prepared microemulsion formulations containing diclofenac sodium, and optimized it in with vitro tests. The irritant effect of formulations was investigated on healthy volunteers, and their safety was demonstrated. In another study, lecithin microemulsions of ketoprofen were developed (Paolino et al., 2002). Permeation of drug from microemulsion formulation was compared to the conventional dermal ketoprofen formulation. In this study performed with healthy volunteers, it was demonstrated that ketoprofen microemulsions enhanced the permeation of drug and has good skin tolerability (Amrish & Kumar, 2009). Dalmora et al. (2001) administered microemulsions loaded with piroxicam to rats in vivo, and demonstrated that dermal anti-inflammatory effect was extended, and inflammation inhibition lasted for nine days following single-dose administration. In vivo anti-inflammatory activity study has also demonstrated that microemulsions containing flurbiprofen performed better than conventional gel formulation (Ambade et al., 2008). In another study, nano/submicron emulsions of flurbiprofen were suggested as dermal carriers (Fang et al., 2004).

4.2.2 Vesicular carriers

Vesicular systems such as liposomes, niosomes and transfersomes have been developed for optimization of dermal penetration of drugs and particularly for dermal targeting. Vesicular systems have the advantages of controlling release rate of the active ingredient and to ensure localization of dermally administered drugs in dermal layers. Besides, transdermal administration of vesicular systems helps to carry drug molecules into systemic circulation (El Sayed et al., 2007; Ceve, 2004).

4.2.2.1 Liposomes

Liposomes are described as lipidic vesicles containing water. Cholesterol and phospholipids or amphiphilic ingredients of these compounds are typically used as lipids. Liposomes can capture hydrophilic molecules or contain lipophilic molecules in their membranes. Some liposomes can be adsorbed in the skin surface or may go into fusion. Fusion of liposomes may increase the drag force required for permeation of the molecule and facilitate dermal penetration of the drug. However, fusion of liposomes on the skin surface does not apply for macromolecular drugs. Another mechanism is penetration of liposomes to SC before fusion with SC lipids and releasing the drug there. With this mechanism, particularly the drug in liposomes that are dermally administered can be localized in different layers of the skin (El Magraby et al., 2008; Williams, 2003).

Mezei & Gulasekharam (1980) used liposomes as "dermal drug carrier system" for the first time. However, liposomes are localized in the outermost layer of the skin (SC). Therefore, it is advantageous in cases where retaining drug in SC is desirable. It does not seem possible with these systems to penetrate the drug to deeper tissues of the skin or into systemic circulation. Therefore, it is rather preferred to increase dermal moisture for cosmetic purposes (El Magraby et al., 2008; Williams, 2003).

4.2.2.2 Niosomes

Niosomes are liposomes prepared with non-ionic surfactants. Dermal penetration of niosomes depend on i) potential penetration-enhancing activity of surfactants in its content, ii) penetration of the vesicle to SC, iii) accumulation of vesicle on the skin surface and/or increasing thermodynamic activity of the drug on the skin surface. These mechanisms depend on the physicochemical properties of the drug, the vesicle and the lipids used (Choi & Maibach, 2005; Williams, 2003). Niosomes are the vesicular systems that are most studies in dermal and transdermal formulations of NSAIDs. This is because niosomes prevent transepidermal water loss, and they act on the lipid structure in the intracellular domain with the effect of high amount of surfactant in their content and overcome the barrier characteristic of the SC layer.

It has been observed that dermal retention and dermal penetration of the drug was enhanced with dermally administered noisome formulation of nimesulid. Besides, it has been determined that the noisome formulation has a faster anti-inflammatory activity than the commercial gel formulation (Shahiwala & Misra, 2002). Manosroi et al. (2008) obtained a higher flux of the drug in SC and deeper dermal tissues (live epidermis and dermis) with elastic noisome formulations loaded with diclophenac diethylammonium. Niosome-like vesicles consisting of hydrated mixtures of cholesterol and non-ionic surfactants are defined as "proniosomes" (Alsarra et al., 2005; Ammar et al., 2011). Alsarra et al. (2005) demonstrated that proniosomes of ketorolac improves permeation of the drug and shortens its lag time. In another study, formulations of proniosome were developed for transdermal delivery of tenoxicam. It has been stressed that proniosome formulation loaded with tenoxicam had higher anti-inflammatory and analgesic effect than the commercially available tenoxicam tablets (Ammar et al., 2011).

4.2.2.3 Transfersomes

Transfersomes are defined as elastic vesicles that can be highly deformed. They are the first generation of elastic vesicles that contain phospholipids and an edge activator. Classical liposomes have a diameter varying from 200 to 400 nm, which is too large to pass through SC. However, transfersomes reach deeper dermal tissues and even the systemic circulation with their elasticity and highly deformable structure (Benson, 2009). It has been demonstrated that as classical liposomes cannot be deformed in the same way, transfersomes ensure higher skin permeation than liposomes in an in vitro comparison of skin permeation of transfersomes and liposomes loaded with meloxicam (Duangjit et al.,

2011). In the same study, the structure of the skip was studied after administration of transfersomes, and it has been found that the structure of lipids in SC was disrupted.

4.2.2.4 Ethosomes

Ethosomes contain phospholipids like classical liposomes; however, they also contain high levels of alcohol. It has also been demonstrated that its components can reach deeper layers of the skin or enter into systemic circulation. Action mechanisms of these carriers in improving permeation is explained by their alcohol content as penetration enhancers as well as disruption of intercellular lipid structure of SC by the phospholipids in their content (Godin & Touitou, 2003; Williams, 2003). Barupal et al. (2010) prepared ethosomes to investigate dermal administration of aceclofenac. They demonstrated that ethosomes have a high drug loading capacity and a good stability.

4.2.3 Nano carriers (Solid lipid nanoparticles-SLN, nanostructured lipid carriers-NLC, and nanocapsules)

It is observed that SLN and NLC formulations have been developed in the last decade for their desirable properties in terms of transdermal administration. SLN are water-in-oil emulsions containing solids as oil phase, and are prepared from solid lipids or from blends of these lipids. NLCs are new generation lipid particles, which have been developed to overcome certain disadvantages of SLNs, such as limited drug loading capacity, gellification risk and drug leakage due to lipid polymorphism during storage. NLCs contain mixtures of different solid lipids blended with liquid oils. The most important advantage of these carriers is their low risk of toxicity. Small size of lipid particles ensures close contact with SC, and may enhance dermal penetration of drug.

Polymeric nanoparticles are also prepared from biologically degradable or non-degradable polymers. The ability of polymeric particles to improve penetration of drugs and their dermal/transdermal applications to target accumulation in different layers of the skin are studied. However, dermal/transdermal administration of polymeric particles have been less studied than lipidic particles. Table 5 summarizes the studies in the literature on nano-carriers of NSAIDs that are dermally and transdermally administered.

4.2.4 Transdermal patches

Transdermal patches are drug carriers that contain an adhesive layer and ensure access of drugs to systemic circulation with controlled release rate. Additionally, the adhesive layer provides a firm contact for the drug to the skin. In general, transdermal patches are classified into two main groups by their methods of formulation, which are membrane-type (reservoir type) and matrix-type. In the former formulation, drug is contained in the adhesive and the drug release rate is controlled by the membrane. In the latter, drug molecules are dispersed or dissolved in polymer matrix. In cases where the matrix is not self-adhesive, a special adhesive layer is added. In transdermal patches, formulation components should be compatible with the skin, and they should be chemically stable and appropriate for use in combination (Padula et al., 2007; Vasilev et al., 2001; Williams, 2003). Among NSAIDs, adhesive types of transdermal patch formulations of meloxicam have been developed and evaluated in vitro/in vivo (Ah et al., 2010). In vivo anti-inflammatory activity of the formulation was compared to the piroxicam patch using adjuvant arthritis model. In conclusion, the meloxicam patch had a better anti-inflammatory effect. In another study, pharmacokinetic data obtained with dermally administered ketoprofen patch was compared to the data of gel formulation. The obtained plasma level of ketoprofen was demonstrated to be higher than the gel formulation (Mazieres, 2005).

NSAIDs	Nano carrier	Results	Refs
Celecoxib	NLC based gel	Gel formulations of celecoxib prepared with NLC exhibited fasted drug input and sustained anti-inflammatory activity up to 24 h.	Joshi & Patravale, 2008
Flufenamic acid	Poly(lactide-co-glycolide) nanoparticles	Nanoencapsulation of flufenamic acid has significantly increased drug transport and accumulation in the skin.	Luengo et al., 2006
Flurbiprofen	NLC	NLC formulation of flurbiprofen was led to the increase in drug permeation with respect to its conventional solution.	Gonzales-Mira et al., 2011
Flurbiprofen	SLN	SLN dispersion and gel formulation showed a sustained drug release over 24 h period.	Jain et al., 2005
Indomethacin	NLC	Prolonged in vivo anti-inflammatory activity of indomethacin was observed with NLC hydrogels compared to its aqueous solution and hydro-alcoholic gel.	Ricci et al., 2005
Indomethacin	Nanocapsule	Transdermal delivery of indomethacin with poly n-butylcyanoacrylate nanocapsules was improved with respect to conventional gel formulation.	Miyazaki et al., 2003
Ketoprofen	SLN	Ketoprofen loaded SLN formulations showed a prologed anti-inflammatory effect compared to its solution.	Puglia et al., 2008
Ketorolac	NLC	NLC formulation of ketorolac exhibited a sustained drug release pattern due to form a drug reservoir into skin. **requires rewriting**	Puglia et al., 2006
Nimesulide	Nanocapsule /nanoemulsion / nanospheres	Nimesulide-loaded nanocarriers formulated in hydrophilic gels exhibited good physico-chemical properties for its dermal administration.	Alves et al., 2005
Nimesulide	Nanocapsule /nanoemulsion / nanospheres	Following the application of gel formulations of nimesulide based on nanocarriers was detected viable epidermis compared to conventional gel formulations.	Alves et al., 2005

Table 5. Studies on the development of nanocarriers of NSAIDs to improve their skin permeability.

5. Conclusions

During the last two decades, skin has been shown to be a suitable delivery site for drugs that are formulated dermally. Researchers have been trying to overcome gastrointestinal side effects by dermal and transdermal delivery of NSAIDs. Dermal administration of

NSAIDs enables local drug delivery to diseased tissues and obtains high drug concentration in the application site. Dermal application seems to offer an alternative application route for preventing systemic side effects of NSAIDs. However, SC is a highly effective barrier and challenging for absorption of drugs through skin and drugs may not accumulate properly in the target tissues. The most popular strategy is to include chemical enhancers into dermal and transdermal formulations to enhance skin delivery of drugs. However, it is difficult to choose a penetration enhancer, and to date no penetration enhancer has been proven to be ideal. Another approach to improve skin permeation is to develop novel drug carrier systems of NSAIDs, in addition to the conventional dosage forms. Microemulsions and nano carriers are the most frequently preferred carrier systems for NSAIDs. These new carrier systems ensure drug permeation to deeper layers of the skin and reach the synovial fluid. These new drug delivery approaches are jointly aiming at minimizing drug dose, diverting drugs to the target tissue, and enhancing efficacy in patients. The findings seem to be promising and it can be anticipated that the commercial novel carrier systems, providing localization of drugs in viable epidermis and dermis layers of skin, could come into the market. Thus, by employing these novel systems we may achieve a critical leap forward in the safe administration of NSAIDs.

6. References

Ah, YC.; Choi, JK., Choi YK., Ki, HM. & Bae JH. (2010) A novel transdermal patch incorporating meloxicam: in vitro and in vivo characterization. *Int J Pharm*, Vol. 385, pp. 12-19.

Ambade, KW.; Jadhav, SL., Gambhire, MN., Kurmi, SD. & Kadam, VJ. et al. (2008). Formulation and evaluation of flurbiprofen microemulsion. *Curr Drug Deliv*, Vol. 5, No.1, pp. 32-41.

Ammar, HO.; Ghorab, M., El-Nahhas, SA. & Higazy, IM. (2011). Proniosomes as a carrier system for transdermal delivery of tenoxicam. *Int J Pharm*, Vol. 405, pp. 142-152.

Amrish, C. & Kumar, SP. (2009). Transdermal delivery of ketorolac. *Yakagaku Zasshi*, Vol. 129, No. 3, pp. 373-379.

Alsarra IA.; Bosela, AA., Ahmed, SM. & Mahrous, GM. (2005). Proniososomes as a drug carrier for transdermal delivery of ketorolac. *Eur J Pharm Biopharm*, Vol. 59, pp. 485-490.

Alves, PM.; Pohlmann, AR. & Guterres, SS. (2005). Semisolid dermal formulations containing nimesulide-loaded nanocapsules, nanospheres or nanoemulsion: development and rheological characterization. *Pharmazie*, Vol. 60, No.12, pp. 900-904.

Avdeef, A. (1998) pH-metric solubility. 1. Solubility-pH profiles from bjerrum plots. Gibbs buffer and pK_a in the solid state. *Pharm Pharmacol Commun*, Vol. 4, pp. 165–178.

Bachhav, Y & Patravale, V. (2010). Formulation of meloxicam gel for topical application: in vitro and in vivo evaluation. *Acta Pharm*, Vol. 60, pp. 153-163.

Barupal AK,.; Gupta, V. & Ramteke, S. (2010). Preparation and characterization of ethosomes for dermal delivery of aceclofenac. *Indian J Pharm Sci*, Vol. 72, No.5, pp. 582-586.

Benson, HA. (2005). Transdermal drug delivery: Penetration enhancement techniques. *Curr Drug Deliv,* Vol. 2, pp. 23-33

Benson, HA. (2009). Elastic liposomes for dermal and transdermal drug delivery. *Curr Drug Deliv,* Vol. 6, No.3, pp. 217-226.

Brune, K. & Hinz, B. (2004). The discovery and development of anti-inflammatory drugs. *Arthritis Rheum,* Vol. 50, pp. 2391–2399.

Brune K.; Renner, B. & Hinz, B. (2010). Using pharmacokinetic principles to optimize pain therapy. *Nat Rev Rheumatol,* Vol. 6, No 10, pp. 589-598.

Cevc, G. (2004). Lipid vesicles and other colloids as drug carriers on the skin. *Adv Drug Deliv Rev,* Vol. 56, pp. 675-711.

Charoo, NA.; Shamser, AA., Kohli, K., Pillai, K. & Rahman, Z. (2008). Improvement in bioavailability of transdermally applied flurbiprofen using tulsi (*Ocimum sanctum*) and turpentine oil. *Colloids Surfaces B Bionterface,* Vol. 65, pp. 300-307.

Choi, MJ. & Maibach, I. (2005). Liposomes and niosomes as drug delivery systems. *Skin Pharmacol Physiol,* Vol. 18, pp. 209-219.

Curdy, C.; Kalia, Y., Naik, A. & Guy, RH. (2001). Piroxicam delivery into human stratum corneum in vivo: iontophoresis versus passive diffusion. *J Control Release,* Vol. 76, pp. 73-79.

Dalmora, ME.; Dalmora, SE. & Oliveira, AG. (2001). Inclusion complex of piroxicam with beta-cyclodextrine and incorporation in cationic microemulsion. In vitro drug release and in vivo dermal anti-inflammatory effect. *Int J Pharm,* Vol. 222, pp. 45-55.

Dua, K.; Pabreja, K. & Ramana, M. (2010). Aceclofenac dermal dosage forms: In vitro and in vivo characterization. *Acta Pharm,* Vol. 60, pp. 467-478.

Duangjit, S.; Opanasopit, P., Rojanarata, T. & Ngawhirunpat, T. (2011). Characterization and in vitro skin permeation of meloxicam-loaded liposomes versus transferosomes. *J Drug Deliv,* DOI: 10.1155/2011/418316.

El Maghraby, GM.; Barry, BW. & Willams, AC. (2008). Liposomes and skin: from drug delivery to model membranes. *Eur J Pharm Sci,* Vol. 34, pp. 203-222.

El-Setouhy, DA. & El-Ashmony, SM. (2010). Ketorolac trometamol dermal formulations: release behaviour, physical characterization, skin permeation, efficacy and gastric safety. *J Pharm Pharmacol,* Vol. 62, No. 1, pp. 25-34.

Elsayed, MA.; Abdullah, OY., Naggar, VF. & Khalafallah, NM. (2007). Lipid vesicles for skin delivery of drugs: Reviewing three decades of research. *Int J Pharm,* Vol. 332, pp. 1-16.

Escribano, E.; Cristina, C., Queralt, J., Obach, R. & Domenech, J. (2003). Assessment of diclofenac permeation with different formula. *Eur J Pharm Sci,* Vol. 19, pp. 203-129.

Fang JY.; Leu, LY., Chang, CC., Lin, CH. & Tsai, YH. (2004). Lipid nano/submicron emulsions as vehicles for dermal flurbiprofen delivery. *Drug Deliv,* Vol. 11, No. 2, pp. 97-105.

Gonzalez-Mira E.; Nikolic, S., Garcia, ML., Egea, MA. &Souto EB., et al. (2011). Potential use of nanostructured lipid carriers for dermal delivery of flurbiprofen. *J Pharm Sci,* Vol. 100, pp. 242-251.

Godin, B. & Touitou, E. (2003). Ethosomes: new prospects in transdermal delivery. *Crit Rev Ther Drug Carrier Syst,* Vol. 20, No. 1, pp. 63-102.

Gupta SK.; Bansal, P., Bhardwaj, RK., Jaiswal, J. & Velpandian, T. (2002). Comparison of analgesic and anti-inflammatory activity of meloxicam gel with diclofenac and piroxicam gels in animal models: Pharmacokinetic parameters after dermal application. *Skin Pharmacol Appl Skin Physiol*, Vol. 15, pp. 105-111.

Guy, RH. (1996). Current status and future prospects of transdermal drug delivery. *Pharm Res*, Vol.13, pp. 1765-1769.

Guy, RH. (2007). Transdermal science and technology- an update. *Drug Deliv System*, Vol. 22, No. 4, pp. 442-449.

Guy, RH. (2010). Transdermal Drug Delivery. In: *Drug Delivery, Handbook of Experimental Pharmacology*, M. Schäfer- Korting (Ed.), pp.399-410, Springer Verlag, ISBN: 978-3-642-00477-3-13, Berlin, Germany.

Güngör, S. & Bergisadi, N. (2004). Effect of penetration enhancers on in vitro percutaneous penetration of nimesulide through rat skin. *Pharmazie*, Vol. 59, pp. 39-41.

Gwak, HS. & Chun, IK. (2002). Effect of vehicles and penetration enhancers on the in vitro percutaneous absorption of tenoxicam through hairless mouse skin. *Int J Pharm*, Vol. 236, pp. 57-64.

Hadgraft, J. (1999). Passive enhancement strategies in dermal and transdermal drug delivery. *Int J Pharm*, Vol. 184, pp. 1-6.

Hadgraft, J.; Plesis, J. & du Goosen, C. (2000). The selection of non-steroidal anti-inflammatory agents for dermal delivery. *Int J Pharm*, Vol. 207, pp. 31-37.

Heyneman, CA.; Lawless-Liday, C., Wall, GC. (2000). Oral versus dermal NSAIDs in rheumatic diseases. *Drugs*, Vol. 60, No. 3, pp. 555–574.

Hinz, B. & Brune, K. (2008). Can drug removals involving cyclooxygenase-2 inhibitors be avoided? A plea for human pharmacology. *Trends Pharmacol Sci*, Vol. 29, No.8, pp. 391-397.

Hooper L.; Brown, TJ., Elliott, R., Payne, K., Roberts, C., et al. (2004). The effectiveness of five strategies for the prevention of gastrointestinal toxicity induced by nonsteroidal anti-inflammatory drugs: systematic review. *Brit Med J*, Vol. 329, pp. 948.

http://www.drugbank.ca/drugs/DB00482, 25.07.2011.

http://www.chembase.com, 25.07.2011.

Joshi, M. & Patravale, V. (2008). Nanostructured lipid carrier based gel of celecoxib. *Int J Pharm*, Vol. 346, pp. 124-132.

Jain, SK.; Chourasia, MK., Masuriha, R., Soni, V. & Jain, A. et al. (2005). Solid lipid nanoparticles bearing flurbiprofen for transdermal delivery. *Drug Deliv*, Vol. 12, No. 4, pp. 207-215.

Jain, D. & Pathak, K. (2010). Design, characterization, and evaluation of meloxicam gel prepared by suspension and solution polymerization using solubility parameter as the basis for development. *AAPS PharmSciTech*, Vol. 11, No. 1, pp. 133- 142.

Kalia, YN.; Pirot, F., Potts, RO. & Guy, RH. (1998). Ion mobility across human stratum corneum in vivo. *J Pharm Sci*, Vol. 87, No. 12, pp. 1508-1511.

Kantarcı, G.; Özgüney, I., Karasulu, Y., Arzık, S. & Güneri, T. (2007). Comparison of different water/oil microemulsions containing diclofenac sodium: preparation, characterization, release rate, and skin irritation studies. *AAPS PharmSciTech*, Vol. 8, No. 4, pp. E91.

Kogan, A & Garti N. (2006). Microemulsions as transdermal drug delivery vehicles. *Adv Colloid Interfac*, Vol. 123-126, pp. 369-385.

Lee, CM. & Maibach, HI. (2006) Deep percutaneous penetration into muscles and joints. *J Pharm Sci*, Vol. 95, No. 7, pp. 1405- 1412.

Lionberger, DR. & Brennan, MJ. (2010). Dermal nonsteroidal anti-inflammatory drugs for the treatment of pain due to soft tissue injury: diclofenac epolamine dermal patch. *J Pain Res*, Vol. 3, pp. 223-233.

Lionberger, DR.; Joussellin, E., Lanzarotti, A., Yanchick, J. & Magelli, M. (2011). Diclofenac epolamine dermal patch relieves pain associated with ankle sprain. *J Pain Res*, Vol. 4, pp. 47-53.

Luengo J.; Weiss, B., Schneider, M., Ehlers, A. & Stracke, F. et al. (2006). Influence of nanoencapsulation on human skin transport of flufenamic acid. *Skin Pharmacol Physiol*, Vol. 19, No.4, pp. 190-197.

Manosroi A.; Jantrawut, P. & Manosroi, J. (2008). Anti-inflammatory activity of gel containing novel elastic niosomes entrapped with diclofenac diethylammonium. *Int J Pharm*, Vol. 360, pp. 156-163.

Marnett, LJ. (2009). The COXIB experience: a look in the rearview mirror. *Annu Rev Pharmacol Toxicol*, Vol. 49, pp. 265-290.

Marro D.; Kalia, YN., Delgado-Charro, MB. & Guy, RH. (2002). Optimizing iontophoretic drug delivery: identification and distribution of the charge-carrying species. *Pharm Res*, Vol. 18, No. 12, pp. 1709-1713.

Martinez, R.; Gallardo, J., de Benavides, M., Lopez-Duran, G. & Lara, G. (2007). Rheological behaviour of gels and meloxicam release. *Int J Pharm*, Vol. 333, pp. 17-23.

Massey, T.; Derry, S., Moore, RA. & McQuay, HJ. (2010). Dermal NSAIDs for acute pain in adults. *Cochrane Database Syst Rev*, Vol. 16, Issue: 6, Art. No: CD007402.

Mathy, FX; Lombry, C., Verbeeck, RK. & Preat, V. (2005). Study of the percutaneous penetration of flurbiprofen by cutaneous and subcutaneous microdialysis after iontophoretic delivery in rat. *J Pharm Sci*, Vol. 94, No.1, 144-152.

Mazieres, B. (2005). Dermal ketoprofen patch. *Drugs*, Vol. 6, No. 6, pp. 337-334.

Mezei, M. & Gulasekharam, V. (1980). Liposomes--a selective drug delivery system for the topical route of administration. Lotion dosage form. *Life Sci*, Vol. 26, No. 18, pp. 1473-1477.

MICROMEDEX® 1.0, Electronic version, Thomson Reuters, 25.07.2011, Available from http://www.thomsonhc.com/home/dispatch.

Minghetti, P.; Casiraghi, A., Cilurzo, F., Tosi, L. & Montanari, L., et al. (2003). Formulation study and anti-inflammatory efficacy of dermal semi-solids containing a nitro ester of flurbiprofen. *Skin Pharmacol Appl Skin Pharmacol*, Vol. 16, No. 2, pp. 91-99.

Mitchell, JA.; Akarasereenont, P., Thiemermann, C., Flower, RJ. & Vane JR. (1994). Selectivity of nonsteroidal anti-inflammatory drugs as inhibitors of constitutive and inducible cyclooxygenase, *Proc Natl Acad Sci USA*, Vol. 90, pp. 11693-11697.

Mitragotri, S.; Farrell, J., Tang, H., Terahara, T., Kost, J. & Langer, R. (2000). Determination of threshold energy dose for ultrasound-induced transdermal drug transport. *J Control Release*, Vol. 63, No. 1-2, pp. 41-52.

Miyazaki S.; Takahashi, A., Kubo, W., Bachynsky, J. & Löebenberg, R. (2003). Poly n-butylcyanoacrylate (PNBCA) nanocapsules as a carrier for NSAIDs: in vitro release and in vivo skin penetration. *J Pharm Pharm Sci*, Vol. 6, No. 2, pp. 238-245.

Mohammed A.; Ahad, A., Sultana, Y. & Ali, A. (2007). *Drug Discovery Today*, Vol. 12, pp. 23-24.

Moreira, TS.; de Sousa, VP. & Pierre, MB. (2010). A novel transdermal delivery system for the anti-inflammatory lumiracoxib: influence of oleic acid on in vitro percutaneous absorption and in vivo potential cutaneous irritation. *AAPS PharmSciTech*, Vol. 11, No. 2, pp. 621-629.

Morimoto Y, Hayashi T, Kawabata S, Seki T & Sugibayashi K. (2000). Effect of l-menthol-ethanol-water system on the systemic absorption of flurbiprofen after repeated dermal applications in rabbits. *Biol Pharm Bull*, Vol. 23, No. 10, pp. 1254-1257.

Neubert, RHH. (2011). Potentials of new nanocarriers for dermal and transdermal drug delivery. *Eur J Pharm Biopharm*, Vol. 77, pp. 1-2.

Okyar A.; Yıldız, A., Aksu, B., Çınar, C., Özsoy, Y. & Baktır, G. (2008). Effect of terpenes as penetration enhancers on percutaneous penetration of tiaprofenic acid through pig skin. *Acta Pharmaceutica Sciencia*, Vol. 50, No. 3, pp. 247-256.

Okyar A.; Nuriyev, M., Yıldız, A., Pala-Kara, Z., Özturk, N. & Kaptan, E. (2010). The effect of terpenes on percutaneous absorption of tiaprofenic acid gel. *Arch Pharm Res*, Vol. 33, No. 11, pp. 1781-1788.

Padula, C.; Nicoll, S., Aversa, V., Colombo, P., Falson F., et al. (2007). Bioadhesive ve film for dermal and transdermal drug delivery. *Eur J Dermatol*, Vol. 17, No. 4, pp. 309-312.

Paolino, D.; Ventura, CA., Nisticò, S., Puglisi, G. & Fresta, M. (2002). Lecithin microemulsions for the topical administration of ketoprofen: percutaneous adsorption through human skin and in vivo human skin tolerability. *Int J Pharm*, Vol. 244, No. 1-2, pp. 21-31.

Patrono, C. & Rocca, B. (2009). Non-steroidal anti-inflammatory drugs: past, present and future. *Pharmacol Res*, Vol. 59, No. 5, pp. 285-289.

Potts, RO. & Francoeur, ML. (1991). The influence of stratum corneum morphology on water permeability. *J Invest Dermatol*, Vol. 96, No. 4, pp. 495-499.

Prausnitz, MR. & Langer, R. (2008). Transdermal drug delivery. *Nat Biotechnol*, Vol. 26, pp. 1261-1268.

Puglia, C.; Blasi, P., Rizza, L., Schoubben, A., Bonina, F. et al. (2008). Lipid nanoparticles for prolonged dermal delivery: an in vitro and in vivo investigation. *Int J Pharm*, Vol. 357, No. 1-2, pp. 295-304.

Puglia C.; Filosa, R., Peduto, A., de Caprariis, P. & Rizza, L. et al. (2006). Evaluation of alternative strategies to optimize ketorolac transdermal delivery. *AAPS PharmSciTech, Vol.* 7, No. 3, pp. E1.

Pygall, SR.; Kujawinski, S., Timmins, P. & Melia, CD. (2009). Mechanisms of drug release in citrate buffered HPMC matrices. *Int J Pharm* Vol. 370, No. 1-2, pp. 110-120.

Quane, PA.; Graham, GG. & Ziegler, JB. (1998). Pharmacology of benzydamine. *Inflammopharmacology*, Vol. 6, pp. 95-107.

Ricci, M.; Puglia, C., Bonina, F., Di Giovanni, C., Giovagnoli, S & Rossi, C. (2005). Evaluation of indomethacin percutaneous absorption from nanostructured lipid carriers (NLC): in vitro and in vivo studies. *J Pharm Sci,* Vol. 94, No. 5, pp. 1149-1159.

Rx MediaPharma Interaktif Ilac Bilgi Kaynagi. (2011). L. Üstünes (Ed.), Gemas, Izmir-Turkey.

Santos P.; Watkinson, AC., Hadgraft, J. & Lane, ME. (2008). Application of microemulsions in dermal and transdermal drug delivery. *Skin Pharmacol Physiol,* Vol. 21, pp. 246-259.

Santoyo, S. & Ygartua, P. (2000). Effect of skin pretreatment with fatty acids on percutaneous absorption and skin retention of piroxicam after its topical application. *Eur J Pharm Biopharm,* Vol. 50, No. 2, pp. 245-250.

Shahiwala, A. & Misra, A. (2002). Studies in dermal application of nisomally entrapped nimesulid. *J Pharm Pharmaceut Sci,* Vol. 5, No. 3, pp. 220-225.

Sieg, A. & Wascotte, V. (2009). Diagnostic and therapeutic applications of iontophoresis. *J Drug Target,* Vol. 17, No. 9, pp. 690-700.

Simon LS, Grierson LM, Naseer Z, Bookman AAM & Shainhouse JZ. (2009). Efficacy and safety of dermal diclofenac containing dimethyl sulfoxide (DMSO) compared with those of dermal placebo, DMSO vehicle and oral diclofenac for knee osteoarthritis. *Pain,* Vol. 143, pp. 238-245.

Sift Carter, R.; Ebner, D., Brenner, D. & Bruppacher, R. (1997). Use of dermal NSAIDs in patients receiving systemic NSAID treatment: a pharmacy-based study in Germany. *J Clin Epidemiol,* Vol. 50, pp. 217-218.

Taner, T. & Marks, R. (2008). Delivering drugs by the transdermal route: review and comment. *Skin Res Technol,* Vol. 14, pp. 249-260.

Tao, SL. & Desai, TA. (2003). Microfabricated drug delivery systems: from particles to pores. *Adv Drug Deliv Rev,* Vol. 55, No. 3, pp. 315-328.

Taş C.; Özkan, Y., Okyar, A. & Savaşer, A. (2007). In vitro and ex vivo permeation studies of etodolac from hydrophilic gels and effect of terpenes as enhancers. *Drug Deliv,* Vol. 14, No. 7, pp. 453-459.

Thong, HY.; Zhai, H. & Maibach, HI. (2007). Percutaneous penetraration enhancers: an overview. *Skin Pharmacol Physiol,* Vol. 20, pp. 272-282.

Tromer, H. & Neubert, RHH. (2006). Overcoming the stratum corneum: the modulation of skin penetration. *Skin Pharmacol Physiol,* Vol. 19, pp. 106-121.

Vasilev, AE.; Krasnyuk, II., Ravikumar, S. & Tokhmakhchi, VN. (2001). Drug synthesis methods and manufacturing technology. Transdermal therapeutic systems for controlled drug release. *Khimiko-Farmatsevicheskii Zhurnal,* Vol. 35, No. 11, pp. 29-42.

Watkinson, RM.; Herkenne, C., Guy, RH., Hadgraft, J. & Oliveira, G., et al. (2009). Influence of ethanol on the solubility, ionization and permeation charactheristics of ibuprofen in silicone and human skin. *Skin Pharmacol Physiol,* Vol. 22, pp. 15-21.

Watkinson, RM.; Guy, RH., Oliveira, G., Hadgraft. J. & Lane, ME. (2008). Optimization of cosolvent concentration for dermal drug delivery III – Influence of lipophilic vehicles of ibuprofen permeation. *Skin Pharmacol Physiol,* Vol. 24, pp. 22-26.

Williams, A. (2003). Transdermal and dermal drug delivery: From theory to clinical practice. London, Pharmaceutical Press. ISBN 0-85369-489-3.

Williams, AC. & Barry, BW. (2004). Penetration enhancers. *Adv Drug Deliv Rev*, Vol. 56, pp. 603-618.

2

The Clinical Role of Glucocorticoids in the Management of Rheumatoid Arthritis

Hussein Al-Mossawi and John R. Kirwan
Academic Rheumatology Unit, Bristol Royal Infirmary, Bristol UK

1. Introduction

In 1949 Hench & Kendall published the first report of a treatment that was to revolutionise the management of rheumatoid arthritis (RA) (Hench & Kendall, 1949) and indeed, much of medicine. Their work was based on the observation that RA seemed to improve in patients who were pregnant or jaundiced. The adrenal cortex extract they used contained the hormone 17-hydroxy-11-dehydrocorticosterone, and they set the scene for the use of glucocorticoid (GC) therapy in the management of RA. In the 62 years since that seminal publication, our knowledge of the mechanisms of action of GC has increased markedly. The extent of GC use has ebbed and flowed because of concerns about adverse effects and in the light of the subsequent discovery of new anti rheumatic agents, but nevertheless the role of GC in the clinic has endured and around 10 million new prescriptions for oral GC are written each year in the USA alone (Schäcke et al, 2002)

In recent years the importance of GC in preventing long term joint erosions has been confirmed (Kirwan et al., 1995). Today they are seen as an important "disease modifying" agent in their own right and are recommended by the UK National Institute for Health and Clinical Excellence (NICE) for the early treatment of rheumatoid arthritis (Rudolph, 2009). Moreover, they remain an effective clinical tool for achieving short term control of disease flares especially in high doses administered intravenously. Their use in intra-articular injections is also a mainstay for targeting disease flares in particular joints and thus GC continue to form an important part of the therapeutic armoury of rheumatological practice (van Vollenhoven, 2009).

The main clinical problem associated with the use of GC is the numerous adverse effects. The most serious of these include the development of glucose resistance or in some instances type 2 diabetes. Other important adverse effects include hypertension, osteoporosis, skin changes, sleep disturbance, weight gain and changes to body fat distribution (Schäcke et al., 2002). This wide spectrum of actions reflects the many physiological roles of endogenous GC.

As our knowledge of the action of GC increases, we can begin to tackle the two key challenges that lie ahead. Firstly, how can the benefits of these drugs be utilised while minimising their many adverse effects. Secondly, is it possible to identify a distinct subset of patients with inflammatory disorders who are resistant to GC. Apart from RA, clinical GC resistance can be found in a range of inflammatory conditions including asthma, inflammatory bowel disease and uveitis (Barnes & Adcock, 2009). GC-resistant disease is the cause of considerable morbidity, as affected individuals are subject both to the adverse sequelae of on-going inflammation, and the systemic adverse effects of GC. The mechanisms underlying this phenomenon are becoming more apparent and understanding and overcoming GC resistance in a subset of RA patients may offer further insight into the pathophysiology of RA itself.

2. Glucocorticoid use in rheumatoid arthritis

GC are still widely used in the management of RA and between 25-75% of patients with RA are treated more or less continuously with GC (Johannes et al., 2010). They are used in high doses (including intra-articular injection which provides a high dose to the synovium) to rapidly control acute disease flares. Moreover, the anti-inflammatory effects of lower dose GC can also be beneficial for a large number of patients especially when starting standard disease modifying anti-rheumatioc drugs (DMARDs) which often take weeks to months to have their full effect. Whether this anti-inflammatory effect persists in the long term over and above that achieved by standard DMARDs is a matter of debate.

The most recently confirmed role of GC is their use in preventing long term joint erosions as measured through radiological progression. In the last 10-15 years this observation (Kirwan et al., 2007) has put GC firmly back on the map as effective disease modifying agents in their own right.

2.1 High dose short term therapy

The use of high dose GC therapy to control life threatening complications of rheumatic diseases such as rheumatoid vasculitis is widespread. Intravenous methyprednisolone is often used in "pulsed therapy" at doses of around 1000mg. At these doses all GC receptors are saturated and there are undoubtedly non-genomic effects as discussed later in this chapter (Tyrrell & Baxter, 1995).

The necessity of such high doses in clinical practice remains a matter for debate due to the lack of large randomized controlled trials in rheumatoid arthritis which specifically address this question. The practice has been inherited largely from success in managing life threatening systemic lupus erythematosus and from transplant rejection rescue. In the clinical setting however, such doses seem to be successful and this success is captured in small non controlled and retrospective trials (Jacobs et al., 2001; Weusten et al., 1993). These small trials also demonstrate that short term pulsed therapy is relatively safe but there remains the concern over significant infection from profound immunosupression. A review by Badsha et al in 2003 suggested that lower (but still high) doses may be just as effective (Badsha & Edwards, 2003).

2.2 Anti-Inflammatory effects of low dose therapy

GC therapy is often initiated shortly after diagnosis in RA usually in combination with disease modifying agents. Many patients find GC to be very effective in controlling their symptoms and continue the therapy long term. A recent Cochrane review confirmed the effectiveness of low dose (<15mg per day) GC therapy compared to traditional NSAIDs and placebo. It analysed 10 studies with 320 patients and the overall results showed an improvement in all parameters with GC therapy. These included pain scales, joint scores, morning stiffness, fatigue and improvement in acute phase reactant levels (Criswell et al., 2000; Gotzsche & Johansen, 2004). The therapeutic benefit is much greater than that of other anti-inflammatory treatments, with an effect size of about 1.25. However, these results do not seem to be sustained in most patients after 6 to 12 months. In practice some patients are unable to completely come off GC therapy as they experience a recurrence of symptoms.

2.3 Role of low dose glucocorticoids in prevention of joint erosions

The first report of the disease modifying effects of long term low dose glucocorticoids was in 1995. The Arthritis and Rheumatism Council Low Dose Glucocorticoid Study was a double blind placebo controlled trial which studied the effects of 7.5mg of prednisolone (in addition to standard therapy for RA) on radiographic joint erosions. The results showed a significant benefit in the prednsiolone group but no statistically significant difference in adverse events between treatment and placebo (Kirwan et al., 1995). This observation again confirms that low dose GC is relatively safe in clinical practice and in this case the risk versus harm balance clearly falls in favour of treatment with GC.

There are now 14 randomised controlled trials included in a Cochrane meta-analysis (Kirwan et al., 2007) which concludes that low dose GC therapy in addition to standard therapy in rheumatoid arthritis significantly reduces the rate of joint erosions (Fig 1). The doses needed to achieve these effects are modest and hence associated with less adverse effects. Even in studies of patients not taking other conventional DMARDs alongside GC, the average reduction in the rate of joint progression was 70%.

Review: Effects of glucocorticoids on radiological progression in rheumatoid arthritis
Comparison: 01 Glucocorticoids vs comparator
Outcome: 01 Erosions at 1 year as proportion of maximum score

Study or sub-category	Glucocorticoids N	Glucocorticoids Mean (SD)	Comparator N	Comparator Mean (SD)	Weight %	SMD (random) 95% CI
Empire 1957	35	6.00(8.28)	31	10.00(11.69)	5.53	-0.39 [-0.88, 0.09]
Joint 1960	41	4.88(10.03)	35	14.29(16.37)	5.96	-0.70 [-1.16, -0.23]
Harris 1983	18	1.85(7.86)	16	8.33(14.91)	3.11	-0.54 [-1.23, 0.15]
Kirwan 1995	49	0.93(18.15)	54	8.84(22.34)	7.74	-0.38 [-0.77, 0.01]
Schaardenburg 1995	26	1.50(2.27)	24	1.92(2.63)	4.48	-0.17 [-0.72, 0.39]
van Gestel 1995	1	0.00(0.00)	1	0.00(0.00)		Not estimable
Boers 1997	70	1.57(2.36)	65	2.93(3.04)	9.24	-0.50 [-0.84, -0.16]
Hansen 1999	42	1.29(3.85)	34	2.43(7.28)	6.21	-0.20 [-0.65, 0.25]
van Everdingen 2002	39	2.14(3.48)	35	3.93(3.92)	6.00	-0.48 [-0.94, -0.02]
Capell 2004	59	15.10(15.08)	55	12.60(1.47)	8.39	0.23 [-0.14, 0.60]
Suponitskaia 2004	20	3.43(10.29)	20	4.93(12.00)	3.71	-0.13 [-0.75, 0.49]
Choy 2005	32	-0.42(5.28)	30	1.97(5.48)	5.25	-0.44 [-0.94, 0.07]
Goekoop 2005	121	0.32(0.68)	115	1.25(2.93)	12.89	-0.44 [-0.70, -0.18]
Svensson 2005	101	0.29(0.57)	112	0.86(1.43)	12.14	-0.51 [-0.79, -0.24]
Wassenberg 2005	68	0.42(1.37)	72	1.68(2.42)	9.35	-0.63 [-0.97, -0.29]
Total (95% CI)	722		699		100.00	-0.39 [-0.52, -0.26]

Test for heterogeneity: Chi² = 18.03, df = 13 (P = 0.16), I² = 27.9%
Test for overall effect: Z = 5.96 (P < 0.00001)

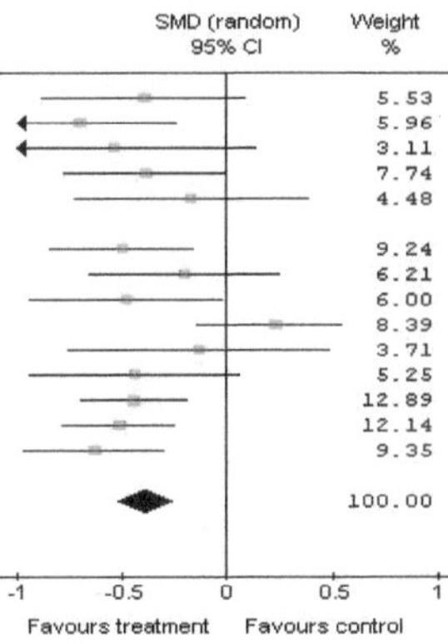

Fig. 1. Summary of data from Cochrane meta-analysis (Kirwan et al., 2007)

Subsequent analysis of longer term follow up data from some of these studies shows that the anti-erosive effects of GC persist several years after the treatment has been discontinued (Fig 2). In particular the data from the COBRA trial which compared sulphasalazine alone with combination sulphasalazine, methotrexate and a tapering dose of prednisolone showed anti-erosive benefits at 5 years in the GC group, long after the GC had been discontinued (Landew et al., 2002). The Uterecht trial (Johannes et al., 2006) which looked at the effects of 10mg prednisolone in a DMARD naïve group of patients also demonstrated a significant reduction in radiological joint progression at 2 years which was sustained at 5 years (2 years after discontinuation of the prednisolone). This continued benefit of GC in preventing joint erosions long after their anti-inflammatory benefits have subsided is noteworthy. There is increasingly an appreciation in the literature for several simultaneous pathogenic processes taking place in the RA joint. In particular joint erosions and synovitis seem to be two distinct processes and their apparent dissociation in the case of GC therapy is therefore not surprising (Kirwan, 2004).

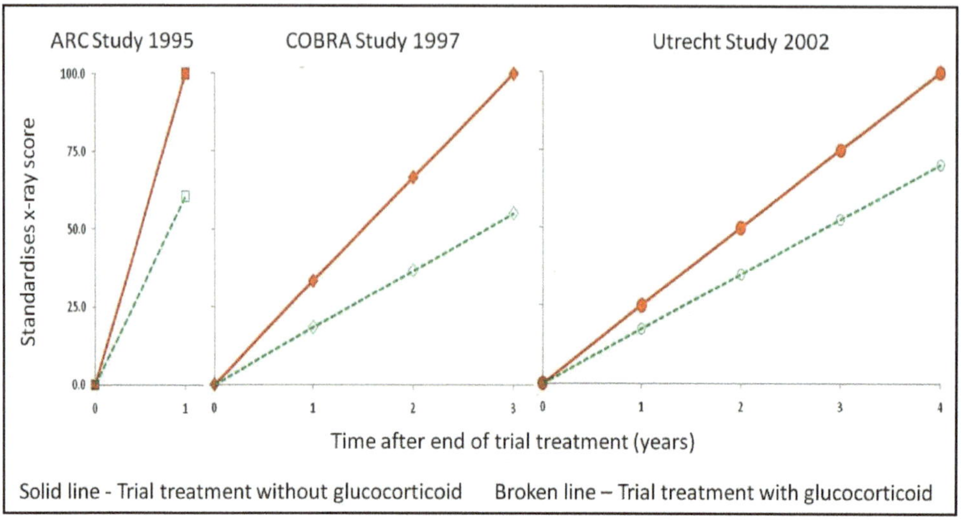

Fig. 2. X-ray progression after stopping trial therapy

2.4 Adverse effects of glucocorticoids in rheumatology practice

In 2007 Hoes et al published the EULAR evidence-based recommendations on the management of systemic GC therapy in rheumatic diseases (Hoes et al., 2007). The table of their key recommendations is reproduced below (Fig 3) but as part of their review process they quantified the incidence of reported adverse events in the glucocorticoid treated arms from 18 studies which included 963 patients taking 30mg or less of prednisolone (or equivalent) for the treatment of rheumatic diseases. The average dose across all studies was 8mg of prednisolone and the mean duration of follow up was 19.6 months. The results (Fig 4) are reported as adverse events per 100 patient years and provide an overview of the types of adverse events reported in GC use at these doses. (Not all these will actually be attributable to GC).

An important point to note when considering cardiovascular and osteoporotic fracture risk in the context of GC use is the underlying risk posed by the inflammatory disease itself. It has been shown that chronic inflammatory conditions are associated with an increased fracture risk and bone mineral density loss (Cooper et al., 1995; Staa et al., 2006; Hoff et al., 2007). Moreover, the increased cardiovascular risks associated RA and other inflammatory conditions are now very well established (Peters et al., 2010). Clearly the relationship between the beneficial effects of GC in controlling inflammation which, drives adverse events in these settings, and the GC contributions to the above risks are quite complex.

Proposition	Strength of Recommendation (0-100 VAS)
The adverse effects of GC therapy should be considered and discussed with the patient before GC therapy is started	92
• This advice should be reinforced by giving information regarding GC management	93
• If GC are to be used for a more prolonged period of time, a "glucocorticoid card" is to be issued to every patient, with the date of commencement of treatment, the initial dosage and the subsequent reductions and maintenance regimens	79
Initial dose, dose reduction and long-term dosing depend on the underlying rheumatic disease, disease activity, risk factors and individual responsiveness of the patient	86
• Timing may be important, with respect to the circadian rhythm of both the disease and the natural secretion of GC	57
When it is decided to start GC treatment, comorbidities and risk factors for adverse effects should be evaluated and treated where indicated; these include hypertension, diabetes, peptic ulcer, recent fractures, presence of cataract or glaucoma, presence of (chronic) infections, dyslipidaemia and comedication with non-steroidal anti inflammatory drugs	92
For prolonged treatment, the GC dosage should be kept to a minimum, and a GC taper should be attempted in case of remission or low disease activity; the reasons to continue GC therapy should be regularly checked	86
During treatment, patients should be monitored for body weight, blood pressure, peripheral oedema, cardiac insufficiency, serum lipids, blood and/or urine glucose and ocular pressure depending on individual patient's risk, GC dose and duration	93
If a patient is started on prednisone >7.5 mg daily and continues on prednisone for more than 3 months, calcium and vitamin D supplementation should be prescribed	100
• Antiresorptive therapy with bisphosphonates to reduce the risk of GC-induced osteoporosis should be based on risk factors, including bone-mineral density measurement	93
Patients treated with GC and concomitant non-steroidal anti-inflammatory drugs should be given appropriate gastro-protective medication, such as proton pump inhibitors or misoprostol, or alternatively could switch to a cyclo-oxygenase-2 selective inhibitor	93
All patients on GC therapy for longer than 1 month, who will undergo surgery, need perioperative management with adequate GC replacement to overcome potential adrenal Insufficiency	93
GC during pregnancy have no additional risk for mother and child	87
Children receiving GC should be checked regularly for linear growth and considered for growth-hormone replacement in case of growth impairment	93

Fig. 3. Summary of EULAR recommendations for the use of GC in rheumatological practice. (VAS=visual analogue score)

Indeed a cohort study examining the interaction between GC therapy and cardiovascular risk in RA showed GC therapy to be associated with an increased risk only if patients were rheumatoid factor (RF) positive (Davis et al., 2007). In fact in RF negative patients GC were not associated with increased risk regardless of the cumulative dose and indeed showed a trend towards being protective.

Type of Adverse Event	**Median:(25th-75th percentiles) AEs per 100 patient years**
Cardovascular (dyslipidemia, oedema, hypertension, heart failure)	15 (3-28)
Infectious (viral, bacterial, skin infections)	15 (3-15)
Gastrointestinal (peptic ulcer, pancreatitis)	10 (4-20)
Psychological and behavioural (minor mood disturbance, psychosis)	9 (2-236)
Endocrine and metabolic (glucose intolerance, diabetes, fat redistribution)	7 (3-34)
Dermatological (cutaneous atrophy, acne, hirsutism, alopecia)	5 (2-80)
Musculoskeletal (osteoporosis, osteonecrosis, myopathy)	4 (3-9)
Ophthalmological (glaucoma, cataract)	4 (0-5)

Fig. 4. Reported adverse events in GC treated patients with rheumatological diseases.

In summary, GC are widely used in the management of RA and rheumatologists have over 60 years experience in their use. At low doses they act as to reduce the symptoms of RA in the first 6 to 12 months but in addition, their use early in the disease process substantially slows the progression of joint destruction and results in less disability in the long term. Remarkably this joint protective effect seems to be sustained years after GC are discontinued and for this reason GC can both be considered to be true "disease modifying" anti-rheumatic drugs (Bijlsma et al., 2010) and to have some kind of effect on the underlying long term disease process. At higher doses they are effective in treating severe and life threatening flares of disease. Adverse effects remain a significant problem but in the balance of risk versus benefit, GC (especially at lower doses) can be considered relatively safe. The summary of the EULAR recommendations in GC use are reproduced below and are a useful tool for clinicians to refer to in their daily practice.

3. Mechanism of action of GC

A better understanding of the mechanisms of GC action is crucial for understanding how to utilise these drugs more effectively in the clinical setting while minimising their adverse effects. In general terms the mechanisms of action can be divided into genomic and non-genomic. The genomic actions of GC are medicated through gene transcription and take hours to days to occur while the non-genomic actions are more rapid (Fig 5).

3.1 Genomic mechanisms

GC have a lipophilic structure and low molecular mass. They therefore pass easily through the cell membrane and exert their effects mainly through binding with the glucocorticoid receptor (GCR) in the cytoplasm (Rhen & Cidlowski, 2005). There are two isoforms of the GCR, α and β. GCR-α is the biologically active form of the receptor and mediates the intracellular effects of GC. GCR-β is an alternativley spliced form which may act as dominant neagtive inhibitor of GC action (Lewis-Tuffin, 2006). Over expression of GCR-β may be implictaed in GC resistance as will be discussed later in this chapter.

The GCR-α in the cytoplasm is associated with various heat shock proteins (HSPs) including HSP40, HSP56, HSP 70 and HSP90 (McLaughlin & Jackson, 2002) which are released when the receptor binds to GC After binding, the complex translocates to the neucleus where it exerts its effects on gene transcription (Davies et al., 2002). At the neucleus GCRs homodimerise and bind to GC response elements (GREs) in the promoter region of the target genes and lead to activation or inhbition of gene transcription. In addition the DNA bound GCR can also directly bind transcription co-activator molecules and exert further actions this way (Barnes, 2006).

In activated inflammatory cells there is an additional route for GC action. This is because inflammatory stimuli ultimately lead to the activation of neuclear factor κB (NFκB) which binds to specific κB recognition sites on promoter regions of inflammatory genes in addition to coactivators such as cyclic AMP response element binding protein (CBP). The coactivators cause acetylation of core histones which leads to their unravelling and opens up the genes for transcription. Activated GCRs and the HSPs that are released when the GC binds to the receptor inhibit this effect directly by binding the coactivators and recruiting histone deacetylase (HDAC) 2 which inhibits acetylation (Rhen & Cidlowski, 2005). GC also switch on the transcription of certain genes including mitogen-activated protein (MAP) kinase phosphatase 1 (MKP1) hence inhibiting the MAP kinase pathway which is involved in proinflammatory gene transcription (Clark, 2003). The existence of this pathway has led to a search for ways of enhancing this GC effect, which would apply only in activated inflammatory cells and would therefore not be relevant to other body tissues, and hence would not contribute to adverse effects.

3.2 Non-genomic mechanisms

Some of the effects of GC occur within minutes of their administration especially at high intravenous doses (Croxtall et al., 2000). The mechanisms involved in mediating this rapid action are non-genomic as they are transcription independent. So far three such non-genomic actions of GC have been described. The first involved the observation of the rapid reversal by dexamethasone of epidermal growth factor-stimulated activation of phospholipase A2. It is thought that this effect is medicated by chaperone molecules such as Src which are rapidly released from the GCR-GC complex on ligation (Croxtall et al., 2000).

Non-specific non-genomic effects are seen at very high doses of GC therapy and are thought to be due the saturation of all available GCRs in the cells at doses above 100mg perdnisolone or equivalent (Tyrrell & Baxter, 1995). At these doses it is thought that GC molecules dissolve into the membranes and alter proton leak hence influencing membrane transport (Buttgereit & Scheffold, 2002).

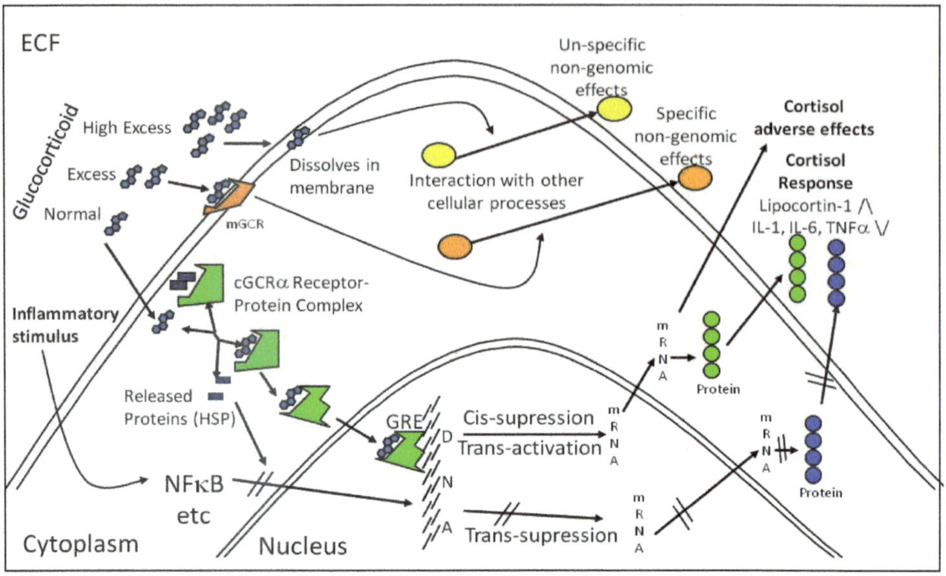

Fig. 5. Cellular action of glucocorticoids

It is now thought that GC also have specific non-genomic effects that are mediated through membrane bound GCRs which are found in small numbers on human peripheral blood mononuclear cells (Bartholome et al., 2004). Moreover, stimulation of these cells in vitro by lipopolyscaharide (LPS) increases the percentage of membrane GCR expressing monocytes indicating an active upregulation of this process (Bartholome et al., 2004). Interestingly in patients with RA who have an activated immune system, the percentage memebrane GCR expressing monocytes is increased, in keeping with the in-vitro observations. These membrane expressed receptors are thought to be variants of the classical cytoplasmic GCRs (Löwenberg et al., 2007) and have recently been shown to also interact with the MAP kinase pathway (Strehl et al., 2011) Moreover, the engagement of these receptors is thought to inhibit T cell signalling by acting through downstream TCR associated signalling proteins lymphocyte-specific tyrosine kinase (LCK) and FYN oncogene (Lowenberg et al., 2006). It is possible that memberane glucocorticoid receptors will prove to have therapeutic implications.

3.3 Understanding adverse effects of GC therapy

The functions of endogenous GC are numerous. It is estimated that GC influence the transcription of ~1% of the entire genome and 20% of genes expressed on human leukocytes through their direct effects on transcription and their interaction with coactivators and transcription factors (Galon et al., 2002; Goulding & Flower, 2001). These include effects on metabolism, homeostasis and immune function. Most of the therapeutic effects are mediated via repression of gene activation in pro-inflammatory pathways. However, only certain adverse effects result from repression of gene transcription such as suppression of the hypothalamic-pituitary-adrenal axis while others are mediated via activation of gene transcription as is the case with diabetes. In some instances such as osteoporosis, there may be a complex interaction between gene activation and repression and the exact mechanism remains unclear in many cases (Schäcke et al., 2002) (Fig 6).

Adverse Effect	Primary Targeted Molecule	Mechanism [X= Confirmed, (X)= Possible]		
		DNA Dependent		DNA Independent
		Activation	Repression	Repression
Skin atrophy	Type I collagen			(X)
	Type II collagen		(X)	(X)
	Tenscin C		(X)	(X)
	Sulfated glycosaminoglycans		(X)	(X)
Wound healing	Pro-inflmmatory genes			X
Osteoporosis	Osteoblast/osteocyte apoptosis	X		
	OPG-L	X		
	OPG		(X)	(X)
	Osteocalcin		X	
	Type I collagen			(X)
Muscle atrophy	Glutamine synthetase	(X)		
	Ubiquitin-proteasome pathway	(X)		
Glaucoma	TIGR/MYOC gene product	X		
	Fibronectin	(X)		
	Type IV collagen	(X)		
	Type I collagen	(X)		
Psychiatric	$5HT_{1A}$ receptor			X
HPA suppression	CRH			X
	POMC/ACTH		X	
Diabetes Mellitus	TAT	X		
	AAT	X		
	G6Pase	X		
	PEPCK	X		
Hypertension	αENAC	X		
	sgk	X		

Fig. 6. Adverse effect associated proteins: regulation by GC and mechanisms. Reproduced from Schäcke et al, Pharmacology and therapeutics 96 (2002) 23-43

GC have a mixture of genomic and non-genomic therapeutic effects depending on the dosage used. Broadly speaking genomic effects occur at lower doses while non-genomic effects become relevant at higher doses with the combined effect of the two mechanisms accounting for the total effect of GC therapy (Fig 7). This has implications for therapeutics as at the lower doses not all the mechanisms are activated therefore the adverse effect profile may significantly differ. In essence low dose GC therapy is a very different treatment compared to high dose therapy both in terms of therapeutic effects and safety (Kirwan & Power, 2007).

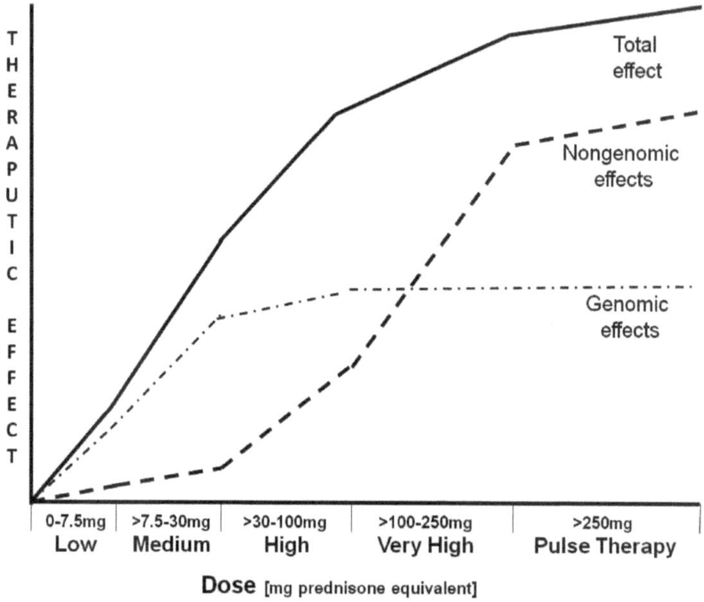

Fig. 7. Contribution of genomic and non genomic therapeutic effects of GC action is dose dependent.

4. New drug development in glucocorticoid therapy

There are several exciting developments in the world of GC therapy which aim to maintain the now well described benefits of this class of drugs whilst minimising adverse events. A better understanding of the mechanisms involved in GC action has made this goal a realistic one and there are already new licensed drugs on the market which are available for use in rheumatological practice. Broadly speaking there are two research strategies which are being pursued. The first approach aims to develop new GC analogues which can selectively reduce inflammation while minimising adverse effects (Kirwan & Power, 2007). This class of drugs are known as selective glucocorticoid receptor agonists or SEGRAs. This approach is based on the notion that the majority of therapeutic GC effects are due to the repression of gene transcription while the majority of the adverse effects are due to gene activation. Dissociating these two actions of GC is an attractive goal. The second approach utilises the improved understanding of the circadian HPA axis and its interaction with the inflammatory pathways and aims to develop new GC therapies that are better targeted to augment the natural diurnal variation.

4.1 SEGRAs

Dissociating the beneficial and adverse effects of GC was suggested over 10 years ago but has so far proved largely elusive. The first such compound was RU24858 which was described in 1997 by Vayssiere et al (Vayssière et al., 1997). Despite showing initial promise in dissociation of GC mediated gene activation and repression, the in-vivo effects were more disappointing and the drug did not make it into clinical trials (Belvisi et al., 2001). Other drugs such as A276575 have again shown promise but fared little better (Lin et al., 2002). The only SEGRA in clinical trials at the moment is ZK 245186 which is in Phase III trials for topical use post cateract surgery after initial results from animal models showed promise (Proksch et al., 2011). The Pahse II trail was concluded at the end of 2010 but results have not yet been released. The struggle to take SEGRAs from the bench to the bedside has been quite disappointing but not entirely surprising given the sheer number of biological mechanisms influenced by GC in vivo.

4.2 Modified release glucocorticoids

Modelling of the diurnal variation of the HPA axis and its effects on the secretion of systemic inflammatory cytokines in RA has been a novel approach which has yielded positive results. The cytokine IL-6 has been unequivocally shown to have a diurnal variation which causes an increase in serum concentrations during the night, before the natural increase in serum cortisol, and which reaches a peak at the time of morning waking (Perry et al., 2009). This has opened the door for the development of a modified release form of GC tablet which is taken at night and releases the active ingredients in the early hours of the morning (approximately 2 am) in order to target the peak in IL-6 levels (Kirwan, 2011). The rationale behind this approach suggests that better targeting of glucocorticoids within the HPA axis may produce better efficacy hence allowing clinicians to use smaller doses of GC. Indeed a multi-centre RCT comparing a modified release GC preparation with the equivalent prednisolone dose showed significant improvements in the duration of early morning stiffness in RA (Buttgereit et al., 2008). Interestingly, a recent study by Clarke et al. (Fig 8), which measured overnight cortisol concentrations as well as IL-6 in RA patients treated with modified release GC, showed the normal pre-treatment cortisol response to be suppressed in active RA and this suppression was reversed using the correctly timed modified release therapy with a corresponding decrease in IL-6 levels and clinical symptoms (Clarke et al., 2011).

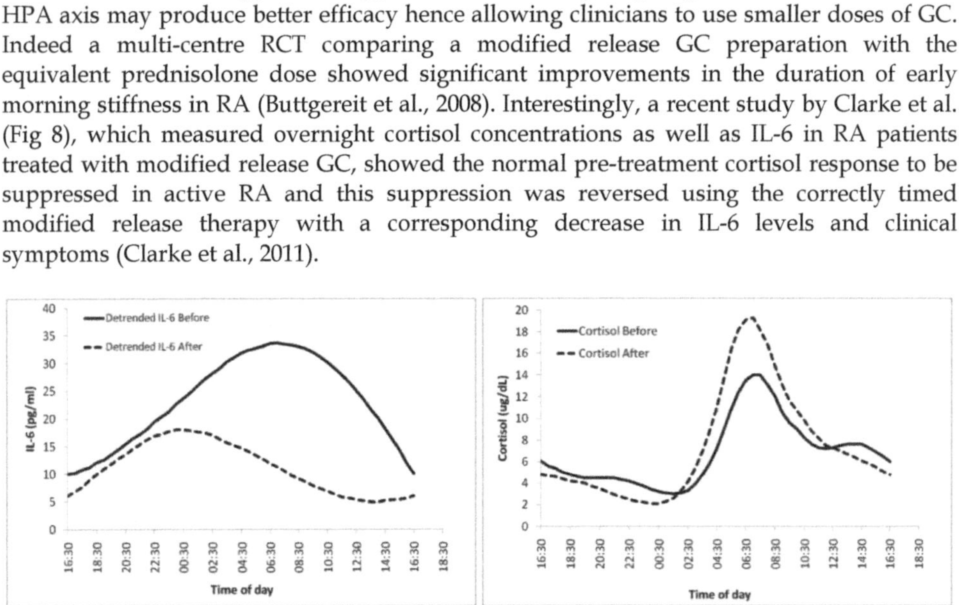

Fig. 8. Effects of modified release GC on 24 hour diurnal variation of systemic IL-6 and cortisol in RA patients

4.3 Other therapeutic advances

Another interesting approach in the use of GC has been their use in combination with drugs that can amplify their intracellular effects at low doses. One approach looked at a preparation which combines low dose prednisolone in combination with dipyridamole (Kvien et al., 2008). This combination seemed to enhance the ability of GC to suppress the pro-inflammatory NFκB pathway (as mentioned in section 3.1) while sparing the gene-transcription element of GC action which is associated with adverse effects. Other novel strategies involve targeting of the GC to the site of inflammation by encapsulating them in long-circulating liposomes (Schiffelers et al., 2006). This approach has shown promise in animal models of inflammatory arthritis but clinical studies are still lacking. These advances represent a potential new dawn for the use of GC in rheumatoid arthritis and have implications for a number of other inflammatory diseases.

5. Glucocorticoid resistance

5.1 The problem of glucocorticoid resistance

GC resistance has been observed in the clinical setting for a long time and represents a challenge for clinicians as treatment requires larger doses of GC associated with an increased risk of adverse events. GC resistance may occur in a quarter to a third of RA patients. The emergence of this subgroup was first reported in a paper by Van Schaardenburg et al in 1995 (Van Schaardenburg et al., 1995). This study looked at elderly onset RA patients treated with oral prednisolone and a 30% discontinuation rate due to lack of efficacy was reported. Further confirmation of this phenomenon came in a study by Sliwinska-Stanczyk et al (Sliwinska-Stanczyk et al., 2007) who showed a 25% resistance rate in their 44 patients who had moderately active RA and who were not taking other disease modifying agents. This group went on to show that clinical GC resistance seemed to correlate with a failure of GC to adequately suppress in vitro peripheral blood mononuclear cell (PBMC) proliferation in the affected individuals.

The problem of GC-resistance is not unique to RA and has been observed in a range of inflammatory conditions including ulcerative colitis (UC), asthma and uveitis (Creed & Probert, 2007; Lee et al., 2009; Sousa et al., 2000; Barnes & Adcock, 2009). The proportion of 25-33% GC resistance seems to be preserved across the various diseases and the possible mechanisms underlying this are explored in the following sections.

5.2 Genetic and acquired glucoccorticoid resistance

There is a rare but well described familial or sporadic mutation of the GCR gene which results in GC resistance. This leads to activation of the HPA axis and compensatory elevations in circulating adrenocorticotropic hormone (ACTH) and cortisol. Patients with this disorder can develop adrenal hyperplasia as a result of the excess ACTH. Subsequent increase in mineralocorticoid and androgen release leads to a broad clinical spectrum whose manifestations depend on the severity of the disorder (Charmandari et al., 2008). This group of patients represents only a very small minority of GC resistance cases whilst acquired GC resistance in inflammatory conditions is quite common. In the last 10 years, more research effort has been focused on the problem of acquired GC resistance and several competing theories behind the underlying mechanism have emerged.

5.3 Glucocrticoid receptor β expression

GCR-β is an alternatively spliced form of the GC receptor and its over-expression has been linked with GC resistance in asthma, RA and inflammatory bowel disease (Hamid et al., 1999; Sousa et al., 2000; Kozaci et al., 2007; Orii et al., 2002). GCR-β does not bind GC and in fact its natural ligand (if it has one) remains unknown (Lewis-Tuffin, 2006). However, it does compete with GCR-α for the GRE binding sites on DNA, thus acting as a dominant negative inhibitor. Another anti-GC mechanism may be the disruption of active GCR-α translocation to the nucleus since the down regulation of GCR-β in the alveolar macrophages of patients with asthma leads to enhanced GCR-α localization and a greater response to GC. Moreover, it has been shown that various pro-inflammatory cytokines can up regulate the expression of GCR-β and this may explain why patients seem to develop clinical GC resistance with worsening of their inflammatory disease (Webster et al., 2001).

5.4 Defects in histone acetylation

The role of defective histone acetylation in acquired GC resistance has emerged principally from studies on patients with asthma and chronic obstructive pulmonary disease (COPD).

As described previously, inflammatory stimuli ultimately lead to the activation of NFκB which binds to specific κB recognition sites on the promoter regions of inflammatory genes in addition coactivators which cause acetylation of core histones. This leads to their unravelling and opens up the genes for transcription. Activated GCRs inhibit this effect directly by binding the coactivators and recruiting histone deacetylase (HDAC) 2 which reverses the acetylation (Rhen & Cidlowski, 2005). GCRs themselves become acetylated upon ligand binding to allow them to bind GREs and can be targeted directly by HDAC2.

HDAC2 activity has been shown to be reduced in alveolar macrophages of GC resistant asthma patients and patients with COPD (Ito et al., 2005; Hew et al., 2006). This reduced activity is thought to be secondary to the oxidative stress resulting from smoking (Rahman & Adcock, 2006). Smoking and obesity, both causes of oxaditive stress, are both risk factors for developing rheumatoid arthritis (Symmons et al., 1997). In COPD it has been shown that low dose oral theophylline can reverse GC resistance by restoring HDAC2 activity (Ito et al., 2005). This effect is independent of phosphodiesterase inhibition and is mediated via the selective inhibition phospho-inositide-3-kinase-δ (PI3Kδ). This is an enzyme which is activated by oxidative stress in patients with COPD (To et al., 2010). This pathway has not been studied in rheumatoid arthritis and presents a novel way of reversing GC resistance.

5.5 T Helper-17 cells and glucocorticoid resistance

T helper (Th) cells differentiate into distinct phenotypes under the influence of the inflammatory cytokine milieu which is largely dictated by cytokines released from monocyte derived macrophages. IL-17 producing T-helper cells (TH-17 cells) have recently been identified as a distinct pro-inflammatory T-helper subset and their role in various autoimmune processes including RA (Kirkham et al., 2006), multiple sclerosis (Matusevicius et al., 1999), psoriasis and inflammatory bowel disease (Duerr, 2006) is becoming more apparent. They seem to have a reciprocal relationship with regulatory IL-10 secreting T helper cells (McGeachy, 2007) and drive an inflammatory response which is dominated by neutrophils (Miossec et al., 2009). There is increasing evidence to suggest they play a role in GC resistance in a variety of inflammatory diseases.

The earliest reports of TH-17 cell involvement in GC resistance emerged from the asthma research community. McKinley et al. showed in a mouse model of asthma that naive T cells which were polarized to the TH-17 phenotype during differentiation (by adding IL-23, IL-6 and TGF-β in vitro) were less sensitive to dexamethasone compared to cells which differentiated to the TH-2 phenotype (McKinley et al., 2008). Subsequent work has shown an expanded TH-17 subset within PBMC cultures of patients with UC and uveitis (Lee et al., 2009; Lee et al., 2007). The data from the uveitis and UC studies seems to suggest that the TH-17 phenotype is inherently GC resistant when tested using in-vitro stimulation assays. It seems that their number is expanded in patients with clinical GC resistance.

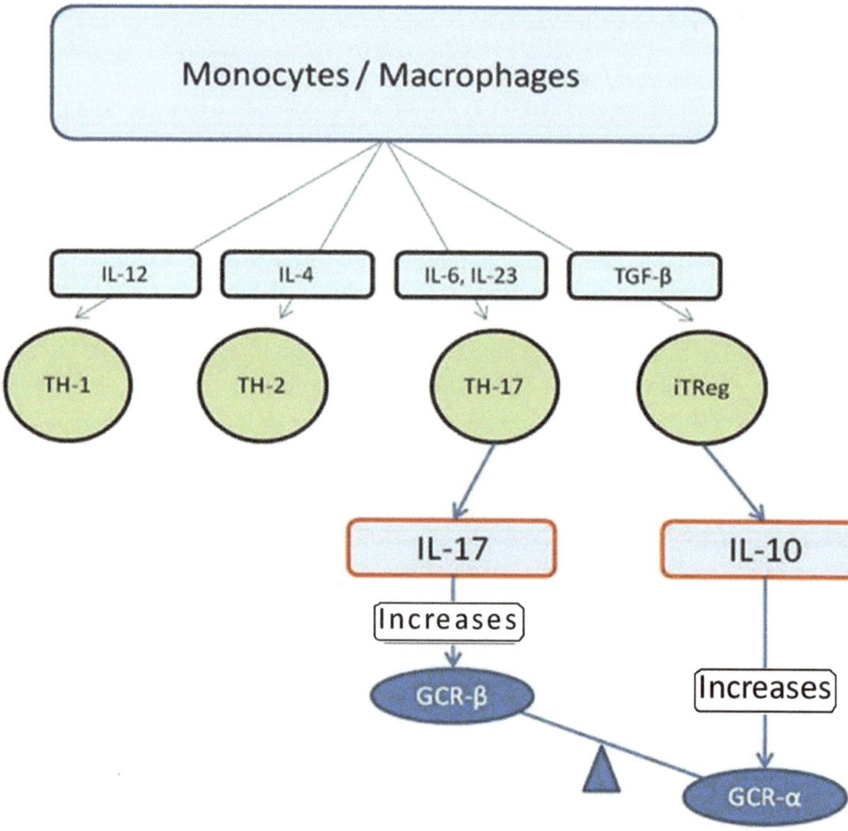

Fig. 9. The proposed model for GC resistance. Monocyte derived macrophages influence T helper cell phenotype differentiation through various cytokines. The balance of pro-inflammatory TH-17 cells and induced regulatory iTRegs alters the balance of IL-17, which increases GCR-β expression and hence reduces response to GC, and IL-10, which increases GCR-α expression and hence increases responsiveness to GC. The balance between these cytokines determines the balance between GC resistance and GC responsiveness.

Other work in this area has shown higher levels of IL-17 mRNA in the bronchial biopsies of asthmatic patients compared to controls with increased expression of GCR-β in response to IL-17. Dexamethasone was unable to decrease IL-17 induced IL-6 expression in these asthmatic patients (Vazquez-Tello et al., 2010). Conversely, the synthetic GC dexamethasone (Dex) normally induces the anti-inflammatory cytokine IL-10 in Th cells, and a deficiency in IL-10 up regulation in response to GC has been demonstrated in GC-resistant asthma (Xystrakis, 2005). Importantly IL-10 has been shown to enhance expression of GCR-α (Xystrakis, 2005). Very little work has been carried out in this field in the context of RA but these findings suggest that a disturbed balance of T cell derived cytokines may be causing GC resistance by altering the balance of GCR subtype expression.

5.6 A unifying model for glucocorticoid resistance

The emerging concept is that the human GC-resistant phenotype is disease independent, and observations of immune responses in GC-resistant individuals across medical specialities strongly supports this (Barnes & Adcock 2009; Schewitz et al., 2009; Norman & Hearing, 2002). Moreover, the data suggests that T helper cell responses in GC-resistant individuals are biased against IL-10 and in favour of IL-17. Importantly, there is also evidence that such a cytokine profile may be instrumental in regulating the ratio of glucocorticoid receptor (GCR) isoforms. IL-10 has been shown to enhance expression of GCR-α (Xystrakis, 2005), which augments GC-responses (Lewis-Tuffin, 2006), and IL-17 upregulates the level of GCR-β (Vazquez-Tello et al., 2010), which attenuates GC-responses. Consistent with this, PBMCs from GC-resistant patients with RA express higher levels of GCR-β (Kozaci et al., 2007) as do bronchoalveolar lavage washings from patients with GC-resistant asthma (Vazquez-Tello et al., 2010). As mentioned earlier, monocyte derived macrophages and dendritic cells have a huge influence on T helper phenotype differentiation and their precise role in this model requires further research. Macrophages may well be the master regulators of this GC-resistant phenotype through their influencing of the T helper cells (Fig 9).

It is interesting to note that there seems to be no resistance to the action of GC in terms of adverse effects. The most likely reason for this is that adverse effects are predominantly mediated by the excess activation of the transcription pathways which mediate the physiological role of GC action. Therefore administered exogenous GC potentially acts on all cells while the anti-inflammatory effects of GC are only mediated via their action on activated pro-inflammatory cells. Thus if these pro-inflammatory cells become GC resistant, GC resistant inflammation will occur alongside GC mediated adverse events. One key weakness of this model is that it does not take into account the important findings relating to histone acetylation which Barnes and colleagues have elucidated over the last 20 years and it would be interesting to study the effects of T helper derived cytokines on HDAC2 expression.

6. Conclusions

Glucocorticoids have become an even more important therapeutic intervention in rheumatoid arthritis both for the control of acute disease flares and for the long term prevention of joint erosions. A better understanding of their mechanisms of action has begun to address the two key challenges which limit their use: developing better targeted GCs which achieve clinical benefit while minimising adverse effects, and reversing GC resistance. There is likely to be progress on both fronts over the next few years.

7. References

Badsha, Humeira, and Christopher J. Edwards. 2003. Intravenous pulses of methylprednisolone for systemic lupus erythematosus. *Seminars in Arthritis and Rheumatism* 32, no. 6 (June): 370-377. doi:53/sarh.2002.50003.

Barnes, P. J, and I. M Adcock. 2009. Glucocorticoid resistance in inflammatory diseases. *The Lancet* 373, no. 9678: 1905–1917.

Barnes, P. J. 2006. Corticosteroid effects on cell signalling. *European Respiratory Journal* 27, no. 2 (February 1): 413 -426. doi:10.1183/09031936.06.00125404.

Bartholome, Burkhard, Cornelia M Spies, Timo Gaber, Sebastian Schuchmann, Timea Berki, Désirée Kunkel, Maren Bienert, et al. 2004. Membrane glucocorticoid receptors (mGCR) are expressed in normal human peripheral blood mononuclear cells and up-regulated after in vitro stimulation and in patients with rheumatoid arthritis. *The FASEB Journal: Official Publication of the Federation of American Societies for Experimental Biology* 18, no. 1 (January): 70-80. doi:10.1096/fj.03-0328com.

Belvisi, Maria G., Sharon L. Wicks, Clifford H. Battram, Stephen E. W. Bottoms, Jane E. Redford, Paul Woodman, Thomas J. Brown, Stephen E. Webber, and Martyn L. Foster. 2001. Therapeutic Benefit of a Dissociated Glucocorticoid and the Relevance of In Vitro Separation of Transrepression from Transactivation Activity. *The Journal of Immunology* 166, no. 3 (February 1): 1975 -1982.

Bijlsma, Johannes W.J., Marlies C. Van Der Goes, Jos N. Hoes, Johannes W.G. Jacobs, Frank Buttgereit, and John Kirwan. 2010. Low-dose glucocorticoid therapy in rheumatoid arthritis: an obligatory therapy. *Annals of the New York Academy of Sciences* 1193, no. 1 (4): 123-126. doi:10.1111/j.1749-6632.2009.05342.x.

Buttgereit, Frank, Gisela Doering, Achim Schaeffler, Stephan Witte, Stanislaw Sierakowski, Erika Gromnica-Ihle, Slawomir Jeka, Klaus Krueger, Jacek Szechinski, and Rieke Alten. 2008. Efficacy of modified-release versus standard prednisone to reduce duration of morning stiffness of the joints in rheumatoid arthritis (CAPRA-1): a double-blind, randomised controlled trial. *The Lancet* 371, no. 9608 (January 19): 205-214. doi:10.1016/S0140-6736(08)60132-4.

Buttgereit, Frank, and Alexander Scheffold. 2002. Rapid glucocorticoid effects on immune cells. *Steroids* 67, no. 6 (May): 529-534.

Charmandari, Evangelia, Tomoshige Kino, Takamasa Ichijo, and George P. Chrousos. 2008. Generalized Glucocorticoid Resistance: Clinical Aspects, Molecular Mechanisms, and Implications of a Rare Genetic Disorder. *Journal of Clinical Endocrinology & Metabolism* 93, no. 5 (May 1): 1563 -1572. doi:10.1210/jc.2008-0040.

Clark, AR. 2003. MAP kinase phosphatase 1: a novel mediator of biological effects of glucocorticoids? *J Endocrinol* 178, no. 1 (July 1): 5-12. doi:10.1677/joe.0.1780005.

Clarke, Lynsey L, David S Jessop, Linda P Hunt, Rainer H Straub, Mark G Perry, and John R Kirwan. 2011. Alleviation of morning joint stiffness by low-dose prednisone in rheumatoid arthritis is associated with circadian changes in IL-6 and cortisol.

International Journal of Clinical Rheumatology 6, no. 2 (4): 241-249. doi:10.2217/ijr.11.12.

Cooper, C, C Coupland, and M Mitchell. 1995. Rheumatoid arthritis, corticosteroid therapy and hip fracture. *Annals of the Rheumatic Diseases* 54, no. 1 (January 1): 49 -52. doi:10.1136/ard.54.1.49.

Creed, T. J., and C. S. J. Probert. 2007. Review article: steroid resistance in inflammatory bowel disease - mechanisms and therapeutic strategies. *Alimentary Pharmacology & Therapeutics* 25, no. 2 (1): 111-122. doi:10.1111/j.1365-2036.2006.03156.x.

Criswell, LA, KG Saag, H. B. Sems, and others. 2000. Moderate-term, low dose corticosteroids for rheumatoid arthritis. *Cohchrane Database Syst Rev* 2: CD001158.

Croxtall, Jamie D, Qam Choudhury, and Rod J Flower. 2000. Glucocorticoids act within minutes to inhibit recruitment of signalling factors to activated EGF receptors through a receptor-dependent, transcription-independent mechanism. *British Journal of Pharmacology* 130, no. 2 (5): 289-298. doi:10.1038/sj.bjp.0703272.

Davies, Todd H., Yang-Min Ning, and Edwin R. Sánchez. 2002. A New First Step in Activation of Steroid Receptors. *Journal of Biological Chemistry* 277, no. 7 (February 15): 4597 -4600. doi:10.1074/jbc.C100531200.

Davis, John M., Hilal Maradit Kremers, Cynthia S. Crowson, Paulo J. Nicola, Karla V. Ballman, Terry M. Therneau, Véronique L. Roger, and Sherine E. Gabriel. 2007. Glucocorticoids and cardiovascular events in rheumatoid arthritis: A population-based cohort study. *Arthritis & Rheumatism* 56, no. 3 (3): 820-830. doi:10.1002/art.22418.

Duerr, R. H. 2006. A genome-wide association study identifies IL23R as an inflammatory bowel disease gene. *Science* 314: 1461-1463. doi:10.1126/science.1135245.

Galon, J, D Franchimont, N Hiroi, G Frey, A Boettener, M Ehrhart-Bornstein, J J O'shea, G P Chrousos, and S R Bornstein. 2002. Gene profiling reveals unknown enhancing and suppressive actions of glucocorticoids on immune cells. *The FASEB Journal* 16, no. 1 (January 1): 61 -71. doi:10.1096/fj.01-0245com.

Gotzsche, P C, and H K Johansen. 2004. Short-term low-dose corticosteroids vs placebo and nonsteroidal antiinflammatory drugs in rheumatoid arthritis. *Cochrane Database of Systematic Reviews (Online)*, no. 3: CD000189. doi:10.1002/14651858.CD000189.pub2.

Goulding, Nicolas J., and Rod J. Flower. 2001. *Glucocorticoids*. Birkhäuser, May 11.

Hamid, Q, S E Wenzel, P J Hauk, A Tsicopoulos, B Wallaert, J Lafitte, G P Chrousos, S J Szefler, and D Y M Leung. 1999. Increased Glucocorticoid Receptor beta in Airway Cells of Glucocorticoid-insensitive Asthma. *Am. J. Respir. Crit. Care Med.* 159, no. 5 (May 1): 1600-1604.

Hench, P S, and E C Kendall. 1949. The effect of a hormone of the adrenal cortex (17-hydroxy-11-dehydrocorticosterone; compound E) and of pituitary adrenocorticotropic hormone on rheumatoid arthritis. *Mayo Clinic Proceedings. Mayo Clinic* 24, no. 8 (April 13): 181-197.

Hew, Mark, Pankaj Bhavsar, Alfons Torrego, Sally Meah, Nadia Khorasani, Peter J. Barnes, Ian Adcock, Kian Fan Chung, and for the National Heart Lung and Blood Institute's Severe Asthma Research Program. 2006. Relative Corticosteroid Insensitivity of Peripheral Blood Mononuclear Cells in Severe Asthma. *Am. J. Respir. Crit. Care Med.* 174, no. 2 (July 15): 134-141. doi:10.1164/rccm.200512-1930OC.

Hoes, J N, J W G Jacobs, M Boers, D Boumpas, F Buttgereit, N Caeyers, E H Choy, et al. 2007. EULAR evidence-based recommendations on the management of systemic glucocorticoid therapy in rheumatic diseases. *Annals of the Rheumatic Diseases* 66, no. 12 (December 1): 1560 -1567. doi:10.1136/ard.2007.072157.

Hoff, M., G. Haugeberg, and T. K Kvien. 2007. Hand bone loss as an outcome measure in established rheumatoid arthritis: 2-year observational study comparing cortical and total bone loss. *Arthritis research and therapy* 9, no. 4: 81.

Ito, K., M. Ito, W. M Elliott, B. Cosio, G. Caramori, O. M Kon, A. Barczyk, et al. 2005. *Decreased histone deacetylase activity in chronic obstructive pulmonary disease*. Vol. 352. 19.

Jacobs, J W G, R Geenen, A W M Evers, C H M van Jaarsveld, F W Kraaimaat, and J W J Bijlsma. 2001. Short term effects of corticosteroid pulse treatment on disease activity and the wellbeing of patients with active rheumatoid arthritis. *Annals of the Rheumatic Diseases* 60, no. 1 (January 1): 61 -64. doi:10.1136/ard.60.1.61.

Jacobs, Johannes W. G., Amalia A. Van Everdingen, Suzan M. M. Verstappen, and Johannes W. J. Bijlsma. 2006. Followup radiographic data on patients with rheumatoid arthritis who participated in a two-year trial of prednisone therapy or placebo. *Arthritis & Rheumatism* 54, no. 5 (5): 1422-1428. doi:10.1002/art.21809.

Kirkham, Bruce W., Marissa N. Lassere, John P. Edmonds, Katherine M. Juhasz, Paul A. Bird, C. Soon Lee, Ron Shnier, and Ian J. Portek. 2006. Synovial membrane cytokine expression is predictive of joint damage progression in rheumatoid arthritis: A two-year prospective study (the DAMAGE study cohort). *Arthritis & Rheumatism* 54, no. 4 (4): 1122-1131. doi:10.1002/art.21749.

Kirwan, J. R, and The Arthritis and Rheumatism Council Low-dose Glucocorticoid Study Group. 1995. The effect of glucocorticoids on joint destruction in rheumatoid arthritis. *New England Journal of Medicine* 333, no. 3: 142.

Kirwan, John, and Lynsey Power. 2007. Glucocorticoids: action and new therapeutic insights in rheumatoid arthritis. *Current Opinion in Rheumatology* 19, no. 3 (5): 233-237. doi:10.1097/BOR.0b013e3280d6471a.

Kirwan, John R, Johannes WJ Bijlsma, Maarten Boers, and Beverley Shea. 2007. Effects of glucocorticoids on radiological progression in rheumatoid arthritis. In *Cochrane Database of Systematic Reviews*, ed. Issue 1. Art. No.: CD006356. DOI: 0.1002/14651858.CD006356.

Kirwan, John R. 2004. The synovium in rheumatoid arthritis: Evidence for (at least) two pathologies. *Arthritis & Rheumatism* 50, no. 1 (1): 1-4. doi:10.1002/art.11496.

Kirwan, John Richard. 2011. Targeting the time of day for glucocorticoid delivery in rheumatoid arthritis. *International Journal of Clinical Rheumatology* 6, no. 3 (6): 273-279. doi:10.2217/ijr.11.23.

Kozaci, D. L., Y. Chernajovsky, and I. C. Chikanza. 2007. The differential expression of corticosteroid receptor isoforms in corticosteroid-resistant and -sensitive patients with rheumatoid arthritis. *Rheumatology* 46, no. 4 (April 1): 579 -585. doi:10.1093/rheumatology/kel276.

Kvien, T K, E Fjeld, B Slatkowsky-Christensen, M Nichols, Y Zhang, A Prøven, K Mikkelsen, Ø Palm, A A Borisy, and J Lessem. 2008. Efficacy and safety of a novel synergistic drug candidate, CRx-102, in hand osteoarthritis. *Annals of the Rheumatic Diseases* 67, no. 7 (July 1): 942 -948. doi:10.1136/ard.2007.074401.

Landew, Robert B. M., Maarten Boers, Arco C. Verhoeven, Rene Westhovens, Mart A. F. J. van de Laar, Harry M. Markusse, J. Christiaan van Denderen, et al. 2002. COBRA combination therapy in patients with early rheumatoid arthritis: Long-term structural benefits of a brief intervention. *Arthritis & Rheumatism* 46, no. 2 (2): 347-356. doi:10.1002/art.10083.

Lauren P. Schewitz, Richard W. J. Lee, Colin M. Dayan, and Andrew D. Dick. 2009. Glucocorticoids and the emerging importance of T cell subsets in steroid refractory diseases. Review-article. February 17. http://informahealthcare.com/doi/abs/10.1080/08923970802334848.

Lee, Richard W. J., Thomas J. Creed, Lauren P. Schewitz, Paul V. Newcomb, Lindsay B. Nicholson, Andrew D. Dick, and Colin M. Dayan. 2007. CD4+CD25int T Cells in Inflammatory Diseases Refractory to Treatment with Glucocorticoids. *The Journal of Immunology* 179, no. 11 (December 1): 7941 -7948.

Lee, Richard W. J., Lauren P. Schewitz, Lindsay B. Nicholson, Colin M. Dayan, and Andrew D. Dick. 2009. Steroid Refractory CD4+ T Cells in Patients with Sight-Threatening Uveitis. *Investigative Ophthalmology & Visual Science* 50, no. 9: 4273 -4278. doi:10.1167/iovs.08-3152.

Lewis-Tuffin, L. J. 2006. The Physiology of Human Glucocorticoid Receptor beta (hGRbeta) and Glucocorticoid Resistance. *Annals of the New York Academy of Sciences* 1069, no. 1 (6): 1-9. doi:10.1196/annals.1351.001.

Lin, Chun Wel, Masaki Nakane, Mike Stashko, Doug Falls, Jane Kuk, Loan Miller, Ruth Huang, et al. 2002. trans-Activation and Repression Properties of the Novel Nonsteroid Glucocorticoid Receptor Ligand 2,5-Dihydro-9-hydroxy-10-methoxy-2,2,4-trimethyl-5-(1-methylcyclohexen-3-y1)-1H-[1]benzopyrano[3,4-f]quinoline (A276575) and Its Four Stereoisomers. *Molecular Pharmacology* 62, no. 2: 297 -303. doi:10.1124/mol.62.2.297.

Löwenberg, M., A. P Verhaar, G. R van den Brink, and D. W Hommes. 2007. Glucocorticoid signaling: a nongenomic mechanism for T-cell immunosuppression. *Trends in molecular medicine* 13, no. 4: 158–163.

Löwenberg, Mark, Auke P Verhaar, Joyce Bilderbeek, Jan van Marle, Frank Buttgereit, Maikel P Peppelenbosch, Sander J van Deventer, and Daniel W Hommes. 2006. Glucocorticoids cause rapid dissociation of a T-cell-receptor-associated protein complex containing LCK and FYN. *EMBO Rep* 7, no. 10 (October): 1023-1029. doi:10.1038/sj.embor.7400775.

Matusevicius, D, P Kivisäkk, B He, N Kostulas, V Özenci, S Fredrikson, and H Link. 1999. Interleukin-17 mRNA expression in blood and CSF mononuclear cells is augmented in multiple sclerosis. *Multiple Sclerosis* 5, no. 2 (April 1): 101 -104. doi:10.1177/135245859900500206.

McGeachy, M. J. 2007. TGF-[bgr] and IL-6 drive the production of IL-17 and IL-10 by T cells and restrain TH-17 cell-mediated pathology. *Nature Immunol.* 8: 1390-1397. doi:10.1038/ni1539.

McKinley, Laura, John F. Alcorn, Alanna Peterson, Rachel B. DuPont, Shernaaz Kapadia, Alison Logar, Adam Henry, et al. 2008. TH17 Cells Mediate Steroid-Resistant Airway Inflammation and Airway Hyperresponsiveness in Mice. *J Immunol* 181, no. 6 (September 15): 4089-4097.

McLaughlin, Stephen H., and Sophie E. Jackson. 2002. Folding and stability of the ligand-binding domain of the glucocorticoid receptor. *Protein Science* 11, no. 8 (8): 1926-1936. doi:10.1110/ps.5000102.

Miossec, P., T. Korn, and V. K Kuchroo. 2009. Interleukin-17 and type 17 helper T cells. *The New England journal of medicine* 361, no. 9: 888.

Norman, Michael, and Stephen D. Hearing. 2002. Glucocorticoid resistance -- what is known? *Current Opinion in Pharmacology* 2, no. 6 (December 1): 723-729. doi:10.1016/S1471-4892(02)00232-1.

Orii, F., T. Ashida, M. Nomura, A. Maemoto, T. Fujiki, T. Ayabe, S. Imai, Y. Saitoh, and Y. Kohgo. 2002. Quantitative analysis for human glucocorticoid receptor [alpha]/[beta] mRNA in IBD* 1. *Biochemical and biophysical research communications* 296, no. 5: 1286–1294.

Perry, M G, J R Kirwan, D S Jessop, and L P Hunt. 2009. Overnight variations in cortisol, interleukin 6, tumour necrosis factor α and other cytokines in people with rheumatoid arthritis. *Annals of the Rheumatic Diseases* 68, no. 1 (January 1): 63 -68. doi:10.1136/ard.2007.086561.

Peters, M J L, D P M Symmons, D McCarey, B A C Dijkmans, P Nicola, T K Kvien, I B McInnes, et al. 2010. EULAR evidence-based recommendations for cardiovascular risk management in patients with rheumatoid arthritis and other forms of inflammatory arthritis. *Annals of the Rheumatic Diseases* 69, no. 2 (February 1): 325 -331. doi:10.1136/ard.2009.113696.

Proksch, Joel, Ezra Lowe, and Keith Ward. 2011. Ocular Pharmacokinetics of Mapracorat, a Novel, Selective Glucocorticoid Receptor Agonist, in Rabbits and Monkeys. *Drug Metabolism and Disposition* (March 25). doi:10.1124/dmd.111.039099. http://dmd.aspetjournals.org/content/early/2011/03/25/dmd.111.039099.abstract.

Rahman, I., and I. M. Adcock. 2006. Oxidative stress and redox regulation of lung inflammation in COPD. *European Respiratory Journal* 28, no. 1 (July 1): 219 -242. doi:10.1183/09031936.06.00053805.

Rhen, T., and J. A Cidlowski. 2005. Antiinflammatory action of glucocorticoids–new mechanisms for old drugs. *New England Journal of Medicine* 353, no. 16: 1711.

Rudolph, Michael. 2009. NICE: The management of rheumatoid arthritis in adults. National Institute for Clinical Excellence.

Schäcke, H., W. D Döcke, and K. Asadullah. 2002. Mechanisms involved in the side effects of glucocorticoids. *Pharmacology & therapeutics* 96, no. 1: 23–43.

Schiffelers, Raymond M., Manuela Banciu, Josbert M. Metselaar, and Gert Storm. 2006. Therapeutic Application of Long-Circulating Liposomal Glucocorticoids in Auto-Immune Diseases and Cancer. *Journal of Liposome Research* 16, no. 3 (9): 185-194. doi:10.1080/08982100600851029.

Sliwinska-Stanczyk, P., J. Pazdur, M. Ziolkowska, J. Jaworski, E. Kaminska-Tchorzewska, and J. K. Lacki. 2007. The effect of methylprednisolone on proliferation of PBMCs obtained from steroid-sensitive and steroid-resistant rheumatoid arthritis patients. *Scandinavian Journal of Rheumatology* 36, no. 3 (1): 167-171. doi:10.1080/03009740601154111.

Sousa, A R, S J Lane, J A Cidlowski, D Z Staynov, and T H Lee. 2000. Glucocorticoid resistance in asthma is associated with elevated in vivo expression of the glucocorticoid receptor beta-isoform. *The Journal of Allergy and Clinical Immunology* 105, no. 5 (May): 943-950. doi:10.1067/mai.2000.106486.

Staa, T. P. Van, P. Geusens, J. W. J. Bijlsma, H. G. M. Leufkens, and C. Cooper. 2006. Clinical assessment of the long-term risk of fracture in patients with rheumatoid arthritis. *Arthritis & Rheumatism* 54, no. 10 (10): 3104-3112. doi:10.1002/art.22117.

Strehl, Cindy, Timo Gaber, Mark Löwenberg, Daniel W Hommes, Auke P Verhaar, Saskia Schellmann, Martin Hahne, et al. 2011. Membrane-Bound Glucocorticoid Receptor: Origin And Functional Activity Ofthe Membrane-Bound Glucocorticoid Receptor. *Arthritis and Rheumatism* In Press.

Symmons, Deborah P. M., Clare R. Bankhead, Beverley J. Harrison, Paul Brennan, Alan J. Silman, Elizabeth M. Barrett, and David G. I. Scott. 1997. Blood transfusion, smoking, and obesity as risk factors for the development of rheumatoid arthritis. Results from a primary care-based incident case-control study in Norfolk, England. *Arthritis & Rheumatism* 40, no. 11 (11): 1955-1961. doi:10.1002/art.1780401106.

To, Y., K. Ito, Y. Kizawa, M. Failla, M. Ito, T. Kusama, W. M. Elliott, J. C. Hogg, I. M. Adcock, and P. J. Barnes. 2010. Targeting Phosphoinositide-3-Kinase- with Theophylline Reverses Corticosteroid Insensitivity in Chronic Obstructive Pulmonary Disease. *American Journal of Respiratory and Critical Care Medicine* 182, no. 7 (3): 897-904. doi:10.1164/rccm.200906-0937OC.

Tyrrell, J. B., and J. D. Baxter. 1995. Glucocorticoid therapy. *Endocrinology and metabolism. 3rd ed. New York: McGraw-Hill* 859.

Van Schaardenburg, Dirkjan, Roelf Valkema, Ben A. C. Dijkmans, Socrates Papapoulos, Aeilko H. Zwinderman, K. Hubert Han, Ernest K. J. Pauwels, and Ferdinand C. Breedveld. 1995. Prednisone treatment of elderly-onset rheumatoid arthritis. *Arthritis & Rheumatism* 38, no. 3 (3): 334-342. doi:10.1002/art.1780380307.

Vayssière, Béatrice M., Sonia Dupont, Agnès Choquart, Francis Petit, Teresa Garcia, Christian Marchandeau, Hinrich Gronemeyer, and Michèle Resche-Rigon. 1997. Synthetic Glucocorticoids That Dissociate Transactivation and AP-1 Transrepression Exhibit Antiinflammatory Activity in Vivo. *Molecular Endocrinology* 11, no. 9: 1245 -1255. doi:10.1210/me.11.9.1245.

Vazquez-Tello, A., A. Semlali, J. Chakir, J. G. Martin, D. Y. Leung, D. H. Eidelman, and Q. Hamid. 2010. Induction of glucocorticoid receptor-β expression in epithelial cells of asthmatic airways by T-helper type 17 cytokines. *Clinical & Experimental Allergy* 40, no. 9 (6): 1312-1322. doi:10.1111/j.1365-2222.2010.03544.x.

van Vollenhoven, Ronald F. 2009. Treatment of rheumatoid arthritis: state of the art 2009. *Nature Reviews Rheumatology* 5, no. 10 (10): 531-541. doi:10.1038/nrrheum.2009.182.

Webster, Jeffrey C., Robert H. Oakley, Christine M. Jewell, and John A. Cidlowski. 2001. Proinflammatory cytokines regulate human glucocorticoid receptor gene expression and lead to the accumulation of the dominant negative β isoform: A mechanism for the generation of glucocorticoid resistance. *Proceedings of the National Academy of Sciences* 98, no. 12 (June 5): 6865 -6870. doi:10.1073/pnas.121455098.

Weusten, Bas L.A.M., Johannes W.G. Jacobs, and Johannes W.J. Bijlsma. 1993. Corticosteroid pulse therapy in active rheumatoid arthritis. *Seminars in Arthritis and Rheumatism* 23, no. 3 (December): 183-192. doi:16/S0049-0172(05)80039-3.

Xystrakis, E. 2005. Reversing the defective induction of IL-10-secreting regulatory T cells in glucocorticoid-resistant asthma patients. *Journal of Clinical Investigation* 116, no. 1 (12): 146-155. doi:10.1172/JCI21759.

Part 2

Biologics

3

Mycobacterial Infections Associated with TNF-α Inhibitors

Sarah K. Brode and Theodore K. Marras
University of Toronto
Canada

1. Introduction

Tumor necrosis factor (TNF) is a proinflammatory cytokine involved in the pathogenesis of rheumatoid arthritis and other chronic inflammatory diseases. TNF also plays a critical role in host responses to intracellular pathogens and in granuloma formation and maintenance. The TNF-α inhibitors are a class of highly effective, targeted anti-inflammatory medications in widespread use for the treatment of rheumatoid arthritis. However, evidence has accumulated since the introduction of the TNF-antagonists that they are also associated with an increased risk of granulomatous infections, including tuberculosis and non-tuberculous mycobacterial (NTM) infections.

This chapter will review the literature on the role of TNF in response to mycobacterial infection, the various TNF-α inhibitors and their biological differences, and the indications for TNF-α inhibitors in the treatment of rheumatoid arthritis. We will also review the literature to date on the risk of tuberculosis associated with rheumatoid arthritis and TNF-antagonist therapy. We will discuss the clinical evaluation and treatment of latent tuberculosis infection in the setting of proposed TNF-antagonist therapy, as well as the presentation and treatment of active tuberculosis. We will review the current literature on the risk of NTM disease associated with TNF-α inhibitor therapy, as well as the presentation, treatment, and prevention of NTM disease in this setting.

2. TNF and TNF-α inhibitors

2.1 TNF biology

TNF is produced primarily by activated monocytes/macrophages, T- and B-lymphocytes, and natural killer cells. It is made as a transmembrate protein (tmTNF), which is then cleaved to a soluble form (sTNF). Three monomers then associate to form trimeric TNF, which is biologically active. This trimeric TNF binds to cell-surface receptors TNFR1 and TNFR2. Both TNFR1 and TNFR2 can signal pro-inflammatory pathways and anti-apoptotic pathways. TNFR1 can also signal via death domain caspase-dependent pathways to induce apoptosis.

TNF plays a major role in the initial host response to infection. With respect to tuberculosis, TNF is involved in macrophage activation; it increases the phagocytic capacity of the macrophage and enhances its killing of intracellular bacteria, via the generation of reactive nitrogen and oxygen species (Bekker et al. 2001). TNF also stimulates macrophages and T-lymphocytes to produce chemokines, and induces the expression of vascular adhesion molecules (Roach et al. 2002). These activities recruit immune cells and promote a focused accumulation of cells at the site of infection, which sequesters the mycobacteria and prevents their dissemination. This focused accumulation of cells is known as the granuloma, and TNF is involved in both the formation of the granuloma and the maintenance of its integrity. In TNF-deficient mice infected with *M. tuberculosis*, granuloma formation is delayed and malorganized. Treating chronically tuberculosis-infected mice (which are used as a model to simulate latent tuberculosis infection in humans) with a TNF-neutralizing antibody results in an increased bacillary load, compromised granuloma structure, and shortened survival (Mohan et al. 2001).

TNF therefore plays a critical role in the host response to mycobacterial infection, via its role in macrophage activation, cell recruitment, granuloma formation, and maintenance.

2.2 TNF-α inhibitors

There are currently four anti-TNF monoclonal antibodies in clinical use for the treatment of rheumatoid arthritis; infliximab, adalimumab, golimumab, and certolizumab pegol. Infliximab is a chimeric monoclonal antibody containing a human immunoglobulin (Ig)G1 constant region and a murine variable region. Adalimumab and golimumab both contain human IgG1 constant and variable regions. Certolizumab pegol is a pegylated, humanised monoclonal anti-TNF Fab′ (fragment, antigen binding) fragment. Infliximab is administered by intravenous infusion. Adalimumab, certotolizumab and golimumab are administered by subcutaneous injection, usually every other week.

Etanercept is a soluble TNF receptor; the only one of its kind in clinical use. It is comprised of two extracellular domains of human TNFR2 fused to the Fc (fragment, crystallizable) fragment of human IgG1. It binds trimeric TNF and lymphotoxin. It is administered by subcutaneous injection, usually once or twice per week.

All of the TNF-antagonists are approved for use in rheumatoid arthritis. They are also variably in use for the treatment of other chronic inflammatory conditions, including psoriatic arthritis, plaque psoriasis, ankylosing spondylitis, Crohn's disease, and ulcerative colitis.

There are several notable differences between the various TNF inhibitors. Firstly, peak blood levels of infliximab are several times greater than those of etanercept and adalimumab (Wallis 2008). The clinical implication of this difference is unclear, however, given that the infection risk with adalimumab seems similar to that of infliximab (see below). Also, the various TNF-antagonists may bind soluble TNF (sTNF) with different affinities, but results are conflicting; one study has shown that etanercept binds sTNF with less affinity than infliximab (Scallon et al. 2002), whereas another study has shown the opposite (Nesbitt et al. 2006 as cited in Wallis 2008). Additionally, the anti-TNF monoclonal antibodies inhibit T-cell activation and cytokine expression (other than TNF), whereas etanercept has little or no effect in these systems (Saliu et al. 2006).

The differential binding of the TNF antagonists for transmembrane TNF (tmTNF) may partially explain differences in clinical efficacy and possibly infection risk. Infliximab binds transmembrane TNF (tmTNF) with more affinity than etanercept, and inhibits tmTNF-mediated cellular activation more effectively (Scallon et al. 2002). Additionally, some studies have shown that the anti-TNF antibodies can cross-link tmTNF and thereby induce apoptosis in TNF-expressing T cells, whereas etanercept lacks this activity (Wallis 2008). This induction of apoptosis may play a role in their efficacy in Crohn's disease, where defective apoptosis in gut lymphocytes is believed to be a major feature in the pathogenesis of the disease (Wallis 2008).

However, the clinical importance of tmTNF-mediated apoptosis is still a matter of debate, as highlighted by the activity of certolizumab pegol. Certolizumab cannot crosslink tmTNF nor participate in complement activation given its monovalent structure and lack of Fc. It therefore cannot induce apoptosis in TNF-expressing cells. However, it appears to be effective in the treatment of Crohn's disease (Sandborn et al. 2007), and does appear to increase the risk of tuberculosis (see below). This implies that the induction of cell death may be less important in the mechanism of action of these medications than other properties (Wallis 2008). Nonetheless, several animal experiments have shown that selective inhibition of sTNF (and not tmTNF) may be beneficial in reducing infection risks. For instance, one study showed that inhibition of both sTNF and tmTNF protected from clinical signs of inflammation in a murine model of rheumatoid arthritis, yet increased the risk of reactivation of latent tuberculosis, and increased susceptibility of infection to *Listeria monocytogenes* (Spohn et al. 2007). However, specific inhibition of sTNF, while sparing tmTNF was still effective in reducing inflammation, yet did not increase the risk of infection with these pathogens.

2.3 TNF-α inhibitor therapy in rheumatoid arthritis

The first randomized controlled clinical trial of a TNF antagonist was published in 1994; this study showed a significant improvement in signs and symptoms of rheumatoid arthritis compared with placebo (Elliott et al. 1994). There have since been numerous clinical trials demonstrating the efficacy of all five TNF antagonists in rheumatoid arthritis, in various endpoints including signs and symptoms, health-related quality of life, and delayed progression of joint damage (Saag et al. 2008). TNF-antagonists given alone are not significantly better than methotrexate in controlling rheumatoid arthritis signs and symptoms, but they do result in a significant improvement compared with traditional DMARDs when given *together* with methotrexate in patients who do not completely respond to DMARD therapy. Therefore, treatment with TNF- antagonists in combination with methotrexate or other DMARDs is recommended in most guidelines for rheumatoid arthritis patients who partially respond to at least one DMARD including methotrexate (Saag et al. 2008).

The American College of Rheumatology also recommends the use of TNF antagonists in combination with methotrexate in DMARD-naive patients with early rheumatoid arthritis (disease duration of less than 3 months) who have high disease activity and markers of poor prognosis (Saag et al. 2008). However, the European League against Rheumatism recommends initial treatment with methotrexate alone in early rheumatoid arthritis because of a favourable benefit to risk ratio, given that better outcomes with early combination therapy are seen mainly in a subset of patients with severe disease (Combe et al. 2007).

To date, there have not been any randomized clinical trials comparing the efficacy of the different TNF-α inhibitors.

3. Tuberculosis in the setting of TNF-α inhibitors

3.1 The risk of tuberculosis associated with rheumatoid arthritis

Patients with autoimmune rheumatic diseases, including systemic lupus erythematosus and rheumatoid arthritis, are at higher risk of infections, including tuberculosis. This increased risk is thought to be related to the immune disturbances caused by the disease itself, as well as to treatment with immunosuppressive drugs. Several studies have looked at the risk of tuberculosis associated with rheumatoid arthritis.

In Quebec, Canada, one retrospective cohort study of 24,282 patients with rheumatoid arthritis identified 50 cases of tuberculosis from 1992 to 2003 (Brassard et al. 2009). The standardized incidence rate was 45.8 cases per 100,000 person-years of follow-up. This rate is much higher than the incidence of tuberculosis in the general population of Quebec, of 4.2 cases per 100,000 person-years. This translates to a standardized incidence ratio of 10.9 (95% confidence interval [CI] 7.9–15.0). Using a nested-case control design, they found that some of the increased risk may be explained by the use of non-biologic DMARDs; the adjusted relative risk of tuberculosis was 2.4 (95%CI 1.1–5.4) with corticosteroid use and 3.0 (95%CI 1.6–5.8) with other nonbiologic DMARD use (including methotrexate, leflunamide, and others).

These results are in stark contrast to an American study (Wolfe et al. 2004) which prospectively followed 10,782 patients with rheumatoid arthritis from 1998 to 1999 with surveys. They only identified one case of tuberculosis, translating to a rate of 6.2 cases per 100,000 patients. This rate is *not* increased compared with the rate in the general US population. However, this study may have underestimated the rate of tuberculosis in rheumatoid arthritis, owing to decreased study participation of foreign-born and minority populations.

In Asia, one prospective Japanese study identified 4 cases of tuberculosis in 5544 patients with rheumatoid arthritis followed for 1 year (Yamada et al. 2006). The age-adjusted incidence of tuberculosis was 42.4 per 100,000 patients, and the relative risk for tuberculosis was 3.21 (95%CI 1.21-8.55) compared with the general Japanese population. They also found a much higher risk of tuberculosis in men compared with women. One retrospective Korean study of 1285 rheumatoid arthritis patients found 9 cases of tuberculosis from 2001 to 2005, resulting in a rate of 257 per 100,000 person-years of follow-up (Seong et al. 2007). This rate was 8.9 times higher than the rate in the general Korean population (95%CI 4.6–17.2).

A report from Spain (Carmona et al. 2003) studied a cohort of 788 patients with rheumatoid arthritis over 10 years, and found 7 cases of tuberculosis, yielding a mean annual incidence (1990–2000) of 134 per 100,000 patients. The incidence risk ratio of pulmonary tuberculosis in patients with rheumatoid arthritis compared to the general Spanish population was 3.68 (95%CI 2.36–5.92). A Swedish study examined a cohort of rheumatoid arthritis patients from 1999 to 2001 and looked at the risk of hospitalization for tuberculosis (Askling et al. 2005). They found that rheumatoid arthritis patients were at a two-fold increased risk of being hospitalized for tuberculosis compared with the general population (relative risk 2.0, 95%CI 1.2-3.4).

In summary, several observational studies from different countries around the world have shown that patients with rheumatoid arthritis are at increased risk of tuberculosis. This increased risk is independent of TNF-α inhibitors, but may be due to other disease modifying drugs, and possibly to the disease itself. The magnitude of the relative risk ranges between 2 and 11. Only one study, which was from the United States, showed no increased risk of tuberculosis in rheumatoid arthritis patients compared with the general population.

3.2 The risk of tuberculosis associated with TNF-α inhibitors

Studies estimating the risk of tuberculosis associated with TNF-α inhibitors face many challenges. For one, tuberculosis rates are relatively low in North America and Europe, and they may vary significantly by country, ethnicity of the individual, and underlying medical condition. Also, patients with rheumatoid arthritis and other rheumatic diseases may be treated with several different disease modifying medications, in addition to TNF-α inhibitors, which may also increase the risk of tuberculosis. Additionally, when studying the risk associated with a particular drug, it is unclear if the risk is increased only during active drug treatment, or if there is a carry-over effect when the patient is no longer taking the medication but is still at risk. Also, the rate of active tuberculosis is affected by the rate of screening and treatment for latent tuberculosis infection, which may vary based on local practice.

Despite these challenges, a large number of observational studies from all over the world have been conducted examining this issue. The methods of data collection have varied from retrospective voluntary reporting to prospective national registries. The results are also variably reported; some report rates of tuberculosis per number of people treated with drug, while others report rates per number of people treated *per time*, and time may be time on drug or time at risk or follow-up time. The major studies examining the risk of tuberculosis associated with TNF-α inhibitors will be reviewed below, and are summarized in Table 1.

Study (first author, year)	Country	Type of study	TB incidence rate per 100,000 person-years			Rate ratio I:A:E	Rate ratio compared with RA
			Infliximab	Adalimumab	Etanercept		
FDA AERS (Wallis, 2004)	USA	Cases voluntarily reported	54*	--	28*	1.9:N/A:1	--
PharMetrics (Brassard, 2006)	USA	Search of pharmacy database	--	--	--	--	1.5
NDB (Wolfe, 2004)	USA	Data from registry	52.5	--	0	N/A	10$^{\infty}$
RATIO (Tubach, 2009)	France	Data from registry	187.5	215.0	9.3	20.1:23.1:1	--
RABBIT (Listing, 2005)	Germany	Data from registry	310	--	0	N/A	--
GEARSPR (Fonseca, 2006)	Portugal	Data from registry	1754*	2339*	300*	5.8:7.8:1.0	--
BIOBADASER (Gomez-Reino 2007)	Spain	Data from registry	383	176	114	3.4:1.5:1	2.4
BIOBADASER (Gomez-Reino 2003)	Spain	Data from registry	1503	--	0	N/A	15.8
ARTIS (Askling, 2005)	Sweden	Data from registry	145	--	80	1.8:N/A:1	4.0
BSRBR (Dixon, 2010)	UK	Data from registry	123	217	53	2.2:4.2:1	--
Single centre cohort (Seong, 2007)	Korea	Retrospective chart review	2558	--	0	N/A	30.1

TB: tuberculosis; I:A:E: infliximab:adalimumab: etanercept relative risk; RA:rheumatoid arthritis, *:cases per 100,000 treated persons; --: not reported; N/A: not applicable; ∞: for inflixmab only

Table 1. Major studies reporting tuberculosis risk in patients treated with TNF-α antagonists

Several studies have been published estimating the incidence of tuberculosis associated with TNF inhibitors in North America. In 2004, Wallis *et al.* reported rates of tuberculosis and other granulomatous infections associated with infliximab and etanercept (Wallis et al. 2004). The cases were voluntarily reported to the United States Food and Drug Administration (FDA) Adverse Events Reporting System (AERS) from January 1998 to September 2002. A correction was published soon after (Wallis et al. 2004), which removed erroneously included tuberculosis cases from Europe. This study published a tuberculosis rate of 54 per 100,000 treated persons associated with infliximab, and 28 per 100,000 persons treated with etancercept. Infliximab was therefore associated with a two-fold increased risk compared with etanercept. Their overall tuberculosis rate was 41 per 100,000 persons.
Wolfe *et al.* published a study in 2004 that looked at rates of tuberculosis in patients with rheumatoid arthritis registered in the National Data Bank (NDB) of Rheumatic Disease in the United States (Wolfe et al. 2004). They prospectively collected data on rheumatoid arthritis patients treated with infliximab and etanercept over a 30-month period, from January 2000 to June 2002. They identified 4 cases of tuberculosis, all in patients treated with infliximab; this translates to a rate of 62 per 100,000 infliximab-treated persons.
Brassard *et al.* published a study in 2006 that used medical and pharmaceutical claims data to determine rates of tuberculosis in American patients with rheumatoid arthritis (Brassard et al. 2006). A nested case-control design was used to estimate the risk of tuberculosis associated with disease modifying anti-rheumatic drugs (DMARDs), including infliximab and etanercept. They identified 357 cases of tuberculosis, 51 of which were associated with anti-TNF agents. This translates to a tuberculosis rate of 257 per 100,000 person-years of follow-up associated with anti-TNF agents. The tuberculosis risk was higher with infliximab than with etanercept (adjusted rate ratio 1.6 vs 1.2). However, cases of latent tuberculosis infection may have been misclassified as active disease (Mines & Novelli 2007). Indeed, the tuberculosis rate in the entire rheumatoid arthritis cohort was much higher than expected.
The incidence of tuberculosis in the United States in the general population in 1999 was 6.4 per 100,000 persons. The incidence in rheumatoid arthritis patients during the same year was 6.2 per 100,000 persons (Wolfe et al. 2004). The rates reported in these studies are therefore many times higher than these background rates (see Table 1).
National registries of biological agents have been established in many European countries to collect data on the long-term effects of these medications. Studies using these registries have consistently shown increased risks of tuberculosis associated with TNF-α inhibitors. The first was from the BIOBADASER (Spanish Registry of Adverse Events of Biological Therapies in Rheumatic Diseases) registry (Gomez-Reino et al. 2003). This study published mostly prospectively collected data on rates of tuberculosis in patients with rheumatic diseases being treated with infliximab or etanercept in Spain from 1999 to 2002. They reported 17 cases of tuberculosis in patients receiving infliximab, 15 of whom had rheumatoid arthritis. There were no cases of tuberculosis in patients treated with etanercept. The tuberculosis incidence in patients receiving infliximab was 1,893 per 100,000 patients in 2000 and 1,113 cases per 100,000 patients in 2001. The risk ratio of tuberculosis in patients treated with infliximab compared to the background rate in Spain was 90.1 (95%CI 58.8-146.0) in 2000 and 53.0 (95%CI 34.5-89.0) in 2001. The risk ratio of tuberculosis in infliximab-treated rheumatoid arthritis patients vs. rheumatoid arthritis patients not exposed to therapy was 19.9 (95%CI 16.2-24.8) in 2000 and 11.7 (95%CI 9.5-14.6) in 2001.
A follow-up study using the same registry was published in 2007 (Gomez-Reino et al. 2007). This study prospectively collected data on patients in Spain treated with infliximab,

etanercept, and adalimumab from March 2002 (after national guidelines on screening and treatment of latent tuberculosis infection were introduced) to January 2006. They had 15 cases of tuberculosis translating to an incidence of 172 per 100,000 patient-years. The risk ratio compared with the general population was 7 (95%CI 3-13), and the risk ratio compared to Spanish rheumatoid arthritis patients was 2.4, which was not statistically significantly increased. There appeared to be differential risks posed by the three TNF-α inhibitors, with the risk seemingly highest with infliximab, but the differences were not statistically significant.

A prospective French study using the RATIO (French Research Axed on Tolerance of Biotherapies) registry identified 69 cases of tuberculosis from 2004 to 2006 in patients treated with infliximab, etanercept, or adalimumab (Tubach et al. 2009). The tuberculosis incidence rate was 117 per 100,000 person-years (adjusted for sex and age), which is 12.2 times greater than the incidence of tuberculosis in the general French population. Most of this risk seemed to be caused by infliximab (standardized incidence ratio (SIR) = 18.6, 95%CI 13.4-25.8) and adalimumb (SIR = 29.3, 95%CI 20.3-42.4), rather than etanercept (SIR=1.8, 95%CI 0.7-4.3). A Portugese registry, GEARSPR (Grupo de Estudos de Artrite Reumato´ ide da Sociedade Portuguesa de Reumatologia), also found that the risk of tuberculosis posed by infliximab and adalimumab was much higher than that posed by etanercept (Fonseca et al. 2006). They reported 13 cases of tuberculosis between 1999 to 2005 in patients exposed to anti-TNF therapy. The risk of tuberculosis with adalimumab and infliximab was 8-fold and 6-fold higher, respectively, than that with etanercept.

Recently, a prospective observational study from the United Kingdom using the BSRBR registry (The British Society for Rheumatology Biologics Register) identified 40 cases of tuberculosis in patients on TNF-α inhibitors from 2001 to 2008 (Dixon et al. 2010). This resulted in a tuberculosis rate of 118 per 100,000 person-years at risk, which is 8 times higher than the general UK population. Again, the risk of tuberculosis was greater with the monoclonal antibiodies than the soluble TNF receptor. Specificially, the rate of tuberculosis associated with adalimumab was 144 per 100,000 person-years on therapy, that with infliximab was 136 per 100,000 person-years, and the rate with etancercept was 39 per 100,000 person-years. The adjusted incidence rate ratio compared with etancercept was 3.1 for infliximab and 4.2 for adalimumab.

Smaller registries from Sweden and Germany have also reported an increased risk of tuberculosis in association with TNF-α inhibitors. The Swedish registry ARTIS (Anti-Rheumatic Treatment in Sweden) identified 15 cases of tuberculosis, with an incidence of 118 per 100,000 person-years treated (Askling et al. 2005). Rheumatoid arthritis patients treated with TNF antagonists had a 4-fold increased risk of tuberculosis compared with rheumatoid arthritis patients not treated with TNF antagonists. The risk was 2-fold higher with infliximab versus etanercept. The German registry RABBIT (Rheumatoid Arthritis-Observation of Biologic Therapy) identified 1 case of tuberculosis in a patient on infliximab; there were no cases in patients on etanercept (Listing et al. 2005).

An important Asian study describing rates of tuberculosis amongst patients on TNF-α inhibitors comes from Korea (Seong et al. 2007). This publication reports retrospective data collected at one medical centre in Seoul between 2001 and 2005. They reviewed the records of 90 patients treated with infliximab and 103 patients treated with etancercept; they identified 2 cases of tuberculosis amongst infliximab-treated patients, and none with etanercept. The rate of tuberculosis with infliximab was 2558 per 100,000 person-years of follow-up, this was 30.1-fold higher than the risk of tuberculosis in the general Korean population, and was also higher than the risk of tuberculosis in Korean patients with rheumatoid arthritis.

In summary, this large body of epidemiological evidence confirms an increased risk of tuberculosis associated with TNF-α inhibitors, above national background rates and above rates in patients with rheumatoid arthritis. The risk of tuberculosis associated with TNF-inhibitors appears to be between 1.5 and 30 times greater than the risk associated with rheumatoid arthritis alone. Unfortunately, limitations of the available data make more precise estimates of risk impossible.

The risk of tuberculosis differs amongst the various TNF-α inhibitors. The monoclonal antibodies infliximab and adalimumab portend more risk than the soluble TNF receptor etanercept (see Table 1 for relative risk estimates). Additionally, the time from initiation of treatment to onset of tuberculosis seems to be shorter with infliximab than etanercept. The FDA AERS study showed that median time from initiation of TNF-anatgonist therapy to presentation of tuberculosis was 17 weeks for infliximab versus 48 weeks for etanercept (Wallis et al. 2004); the Pharmetics study reported 17 weeks for infliximab and 79 weeks for etanercept (Brassard et al. 2006). The BSRBR reported a median time to tuberculosis diagnosis from the start of anti-TNF therapy of 13.4 months for etanercept, 5.5 months for infliximab, and 18.5 months for adalimumab (Dixon et al. 2010). Their results are somewhat surprising given the longer median onset time with adalimumab, which would be expected to behave similarly to infliximab. However, the RATIO study showed similar tuberculosis onset times for infliximab and adalimumab, with the onset time being longer with etanercept (Tubach et al. 2009). The reason for the difference in risk and time to development of tuberculosis amongst the drugs of this class is not known, but may be related to different pharmacokinetic properties of the drugs, differential binding of soluble and transmembrance receptors, and differential effects on immune cell function and death, as described in section 2.2.

There has been little published to date on the risk of tuberculosis associated with the newer drugs certolizumab pegol and golimumab. However, two phase III placebo-controlled trials of certolizumab in patients with rheumatoid arthritis (RAPID 1 and 2) each reported 5 cases of active tuberculosis in the certolizumab arms, and none in the placebo arms (Keystone et al. 2008; Smolen et al. 2009), suggesting an increased risk.

3.3 Diagnostic testing for latent tuberculosis infection

In areas of low tuberculosis prevalence and transmission, most active tuberculosis cases associated with TNF-antagonists are thought to be related to progression of latent infection acquired in higher prevalence regions or time periods. It is therefore felt that the most effective way of preventing active tuberculosis is to identify and treat latent tuberculosis infections before the initiation of anti-TNF-α therapy. National guidelines or statements have been published by several countries providing recommendations in this regard; the major English language guidelines are summarized in Table 2. These statements provide significantly different recommendations in a number of areas. Recently, a European consensus statement has been published by the TBNET group on this matter, which provides its own recommendations (Solovic et al. 2010).

The traditional method used to identify latent tuberculosis infection is the tuberculin skin test. This test elicits a cell-mediated, delayed hypersensitivity reaction after the volar aspect of the forearm is intradermally injected with purified protein derivative (PPD), a sterile extract derived from *M. tuberculosis*. The site of injection is observed within 48 to 72 hours; the largest diameter of the induration transverse to the long axis of the arm is recorded in millimetres. The test is positive if the induration is above a pre-specified size; the size cutoff for positivity varies depending upon the positive predictive value of the test.

Country (reference)	TST	TST: One or two step	Positive TST	IGRA	Criteria for LTBI treatment	LTBI treatment*
USA (Centers for Disease et al. 2004)	All	One	5 mm if IS, 10 mm if increased risk, 15 mm if low risk	No	TST+, TST- if clinical or epidemiological risks	9H
France (Salmon et al. 2002)	All	One	10 mm	No	TST+, previous TB inadequately treated, CXR lesions >1 cm³ not treated	2RZ or 3RH or 9H
Germany (Diel et al. 2009)†	Only in certain circumstances¶	One	5 mm	Yes	IGRA+, abnormal CXR consistent with TB inadequately treated, history of exposure not treated	9H or 4R
Ireland (Kavanagh et al. 2008)	All	One	5 mm if IS, others 10 mm	No	TST+	9H or 4R or 4RH
Portugal (Fonseca et al. 2006)†	All	Two	5 mm	No	TST+, consider in TST-	9H
Spain (Carmona et al. 2005)	All	Two	5 mm	No	TST+, previous TB inadequately treated, abnormal CXR consistent with TB inadequately treated	9H
Switzerland (Beglinger et al. 2007)	No	N/A	N/A	Yes	IGRA+, abnormal CXR consistent with past TB inadequately treated, history of exposure not treated	9H or 4R
UK (British Thoracic Society Standards of Care 2005)	All	One	5 mm if no BCG, 15 mm if BCG	No	TST+, previous TB or abnormal CXR inadequately treated, IS patients with epidemiologic risk	6H or 3RH
TBNET (Solovic et al. 2010)	Only if no history of BCG	One	10 mm	Yes	TST+ or IGRA+	9-12H or 3RH

TST: tuberculin skin test; IGRA: interferon gamma release assay; LTBI: latent tuberculosis infection; IS: immunosuppressed; mm: millimetres; BCG: Bacille Calmette-Guérin vaccination; H: isoniazid; R: rifampin; Z: pyrazinamide; ¶: TST should be given only if a discrepancy exists between strong epidemiological evidence of prior TB exposure and negative IGRA; *: the number is the number of months of latent TB treatment; †: English abstract only.

The LTBI treatment regimen of rifampin and pyrazinamide for 2 months, presented in the French recommendations of 2002, is generally not a recommended regimen because of high rates of severe hepatotoxicity (Centers for Disease et al. 2001).

Table 2. Published recommendations on identification and treatment of latent tuberculosis infection in the setting of TNF-α inhibitor therapy (Modified from Solovic et al. 2010)

Tuberculin skin testing does not distinguish between persistent *M. tuberculosis* infection and immunological memory of a previous infection that has been eradicated. Additionally, tuberculin skin test responses may be falsely positive in individuals who have been previously vaccinated with Bacille Calmette-Guerin (BCG) or who have nontuberculous mycobacterial infections, as the PPD contains antigens that are shared amongst many mycobacterial species. However, the BCG vaccine is less likely to be the cause of a positive test in adulthood if it is administered before 1 year of age (Menzies & Vissandjee 1992).

Tuberculin skin test responses are decreased in rheumatoid arthritis (Ponce de Leon et al. 2005), likely due to the use of immunosuppressive medications, but also possibly secondary to the disease itself. For this reason, some experts recommend reducing the size threshold for positivity in these patients (for example, to 5 mm) and/or repeated testing (boosting) 7-10 days after a negative test (the two step skin test). These strategies may increase the sensitivity of the test, but reduce the specificity.

More recently, tests that measure the cell-mediated reaction to *M. tuberculosis* antigens *in vitro* have been developed and implemented in clinical practice. With these tests, peripheral blood cells are stimulated with specific *M. tuberculosis* antigens; T-cells previously sensitized to *M. tuberculosis* antigens then recognize them upon re-exposure and secrete a variety of cytokines, including interferon gamma. The tests measure release of interferon gamma, and are therefore termed interferon gamma release assays (IGRAs). One type of IGRA incubates peripheral blood mononuclear cells with *M. tuberculosis* antigens and measures the percentage of T-cells releasing interferon gamma via an enzyme-linked immunospot (ELISPOT) assay; this is commercially available as the T-SPOT.*TB* (Oxford Immunotec). In the other available test, whole blood is incubated with *M.tuberculosis* antigens and the amount of inteferon gamma released into the supernatant is measured using an enzyme-linked immunosorbent assay (ELISA); this is the Quantiferon-TB Gold In-Tube (Cellestis). The major advantage of IGRAs over tuberculin skin tests is an increased specificity. This feature is derived from the fact that the stimulating antigens used in IGRAs are not found in Bacille Calmette-Guérin (BCG) vaccine nor in most non-tuberculous mycobacterial species. Therefore, IGRAs are less likely to produce a false-positive test in individuals with previous BCG vaccination or NTM infection (Pai et al. 2008).

A question of particular relevance in the population of patients with rheumatic diseases is whether interferon gamma release assays have increased sensitivity compared with the tuberculin skin test, as patients with rheumatic diseases are known to have a reduced response to the tuberculin skin test. Calculating the sensitivy (and specificity) of IGRAs is challenging, because of the lack of a ‚gold standard' for the diagnosis of latent tuberculosis infection. Nonetheless, a number of such studies have been performed, as has a meta-analysis (Pai et al. 2008). The results are inconsistent. The sensitivity seems to depend on the individual's level of immunosuppression and the IGRA test used, as the ELISPOT-based assay has been shown to be more sensitive in immunocompromised patients than the ELISA-based test (Pai et al. 2008; Solovic et al. 2010).

A number of observational studies have been conducted to evaluate the clinical use of IGRAs as an alternative to the tuberculin skin test in identifying latent tuberculosis infection in patients with chronic inflammatory conditions. These studies have been compiled and reviewed by the TBNET group (Solovic et al. 2010). To summarize, they found that the results of IGRAs and tuberculin skin tests correlate poorly. However, correlation is best in areas with low tuberculosis prevalence and low rates of individuals with previous BCG vaccination. IGRAs are more frequently positive than tuberculin skin tests in unvaccinated populations, suggesting that IGRAs are more sensitive than tuberculin skin tests in patients with chronic inflammatory conditions. Addtionally, positive IGRAs seem to be more closely associated with risk factors for latent tuberculosis infection, implying that they are more specific than the tuberculin skin test in this setting (Solovic et al. 2010).

Despite this emerging evidence supporting the clinical utility of IGRAs, to date no studies have been conducted examining the positive predictive value of IGRA responses for the developent of tuberculosis in patients treated with TNF-α inhibitors. Additionally, some studies have shown discordant results between tuberculin skin tests and IGRAs, which are as yet unexplained. Concern regarding the increased cost of IGRAs above that of the tuberculin skin test has also hindered their universal acceptance.

Most national guidelines, other than those from Germany and Switzerland, currently recommend the tuberculin skin test as the diagnostic tool of choice for latent tuberculosis infection prior to TNF-α inhibitor therapy. The European TBNET consensus guidelines endorse the IGRA, but suggest the tuberculin skin test as an alternative in patients not previously BCG-vaccinated. Guidelines also vary in how the tuberculin skin test should be administered; some suggest a one-step skin test while others suggest boosting. The TBNET consensus guidelines do not recommend the two-step approach, because of limited evidence of increased sensitivity but considerable evidence of reduced specificity. Controversy also exists in the interpretation of the tuberculin skin test in this setting. Some guidelines suggest a reduced cut-off of 5 mm in order to increase sensitivity, while others suggest 10 or 15 mm.

3.4 Clinical evaluation and treatment of latent tuberculosis infection

Given the strong epidemiological evidence confirming an increased risk of reactivation of tuberculosis in patients receiving TNF-α inhibitors, all patients should be screened for latent tuberculosis infection prior to the initiation of TNF-antagonists; active tuberculosis infection should also be ruled out. The clinical evaluation should include the following: a history to assess for previous active tuberculosis, previous tuberculosis therapy, known exposure to active tuberculosis, a history of residing in a high prevalence area, and symptoms of active tuberculosis; a chest radiograph, to assess for features of previous or current active tuberculosis; and either a tuberculin skin test or IGRA. Any patient suspected of having active tuberculosis based on symptoms and/or chest radiographic abnormalities such as infiltrates, cavities, pleural effusion, or mediastinal lymphadenopathy should be thoroughly investigated to rule out active disease prior to initiation of anti-TNF-α therapy. This work-up should include sputum microscopy for acid-fast bacilli and culture and/or aspiration or biopsy of extrapulmonary sites. Patients with confirmed active tuberculosis should be promptly treated based upon local guidelines and the patient's *M. tuberculosis* drug susceptibility results. Initiation of TNF-α inhibitor therapy should be delayed; most would recommend initiation of TNF-antagonist therapy only after a full course of treatment has been completed.

If there is no suspicion of active tuberculosis infection, the clinician must decide if the patient has a latent tuberculosis infection and requires prophylactic chemotherapy. The decision to treat a patient for latent tuberculosis infection should be based upon the entire clinical evaluation; local guidelines should be used to assist in defining those patients who require preventive chemotherapy (table 2) prior to the initiation of TNF-α inhibitor therapy. Although etancercept has been shown to carry a much lower risk of causing progression of

latent tuberculosis infection to active disease than the monoclonal antibodies, current guidelines universally recommend tuberculosis prophylaxis prior to *all* TNF-α inhibitors.
There has only been one study conducted which examined the effectiveness of preventive chemotherapy for latent tuberculosis infection prior to the initiation of TNF-antagonists (Carmona et al. 2005). This observational study came from Spain, where national recommendations were released in early 2002 that suggested patients be screened for latent tuberculosis infection with a chest x-ray and two-step tuberculin skin test using a 5 mm threshold, before the initiation of TNF-antagonist therapy. Patients diagnosed with latent tuberculosis infection were to receive 9 months of isoniazid therapy, and at least 1 month was to have been completed before starting a TNF-α inhibitor (infliximab, etanercept, or adalimumab). Tuberculosis rates in their biologics registry prior to the release of the recommendations were compared with those afterwards. They found a 78% reduction (incidence risk ratio 0.22, 95%CI 0.03-0.88) in rates of active tuberculosis after implementation of the recommendations. Additionally, there were no cases of serious liver toxicity amongst the 324 patients on isoniazid therapy for latent tuberculosis infection.
Based on this study and several large studies published decades ago (Comstock et al. 1979; Anonymous 1982), many national guidelines recommend isoniazid therapy for a duration of 9 months for the treatment of latent tuberculosis infection, both in general and prior to TNF-antagonist therapy. However, some national guidelines recommend other validated but less effective regimens, including 6 months of isoniazid, 3-4 months of rifampicin plus isoniazid, and 4 months of rifampicin. The French guidelines are unique in recommending 4 months of rifampicin plus pyrazinamide as a potential regimen; this combination has been avoided by others because of a risk of severe hepatotoxicity (Centers for Disease et al. 2001).
The duration of therapy required before starting anti-TNF-α therapy is also not well established, and national guidelines also vary in this regard. Most guidelines suggest a 1 month delay, but some suggest that no delay is necessary, while others suggest completion of prophylaxis before starting TNF-antagonists.

3.5 The presentation and treatment of active tuberculosis

In areas of low tuberculosis prevalence, active tuberculosis most commonly develops due to reactivation of latent infection. However, there may also be an increased risk of primary progression to active disease of newly acquired tuberculosis in patients on TNF-α inhibitors who have high-risk exposures. Several cases of this have been described (Arend et al. 2007; Wallis et al. 2009) .
The presentation of active tuberculosis in patients on TNF-α inhibitors appears to differ from classically described tuberculosis. When associated with TNF-α inhibitors, tuberculosis is more likely to be extra-pulmonary and more likely to be disseminated at presentation. One report looked at the patterns of disease in 70 cases of infliximab-associated tuberculosis. They found that 56% had extrapulmonary tuberculosis, and 24% had disseminated disease (Keane et al. 2001). In contrast, in cases of tuberculosis not associated with HIV infection, about 18% are extrapulmonary and less than 2% are disseminated (Rieder et al. 1990). Another series described the clinical characteristics of 130 infliximab-associated tuberculosis cases reported to the U.S. Food and Drug Administration, and found that 45% had extrapulmonary tuberculosis and 23% had disseminated disease (Raval et al. 2007).
When tuberculosis is diagnosed, prompt treatment should be initiated. Treatment regimens should be based upon local guidelines and the patient's *M. tuberculosis* drug susceptibility

results. Most recommend that TNF-α inhibitor therapy be discontinued, at least temporarily. However, discontinuation of anti-TNF therapy may be associated with a paradoxical worsening of tuberculosis disease. This is felt to be similar to the immune reconstitution syndrome seen in HIV-infected persons who are treated with anti-retroviral therapy. When occuring in the setting of TNF-inhibitor withdrawal, the paradoxical reaction is believed to be due to recovery of TNF-dependent inflammation. The largest series describing such cases retrospectively reviewed charts of patients who developed infliximab-associated tuberculosis from 1999 to 2003 in three Spanish medical centres. They found six cases of tuberculosis, four (67%) of which were associated with a paradoxical reaction (Garcia Vidal et al. 2005). Others have described this paradoxical reaction in association with infliximab withdrawal (Belknap et al. 2005; Arend et al. 2007), etanercept withdrawal (Winthrop et al. 2008), and adalimumab withdrawal (Wallis et al. 2009).

The optimal treatment of the paradoxial reaction is currently unknown. Some recommend corticosteroid therapy (Garcia-Vidal et al. 2009) given favorable results in HIV-infected patients. Other case reports have described the successful re-institution of TNF-antagonist therapy to treat severe tuberculosis paradoxical reactions (Blackmore et al. 2008; Wallis et al. 2009).

Despite these case reports of paradoxical reactions associated with withdrawal of anti-TNF therapy, most experts believe that this phenomenon is relatively uncommon, and that discontinuation of TNF-α inhibitors upon diagnosis of active tuberculosis is advisable. The optimal timing of re-institution of TNF-α inhibitors is unknown, but many experts suggest completing a full course of anti-tuberculosis treatment before re-starting TNF-inhibitors (Solovic et al. 2010).

4. Nontuberculous mycobacterial infections in the setting of TNF-α inhibitors

Nontuberculous mycobacteria (NTM) include species of mycobacteria other than those belonging to the *Mycobacterium tuberculosis* complex and *M. leprae*. They are a large group of ubiquitous environmental organisms that can cause pulmonary and extrapulmonary infections. Pulmonary NTM disease is often associated with underlying structural lung disease, including chronic obstructive pulmonary disease and bronchiectasis. In many other cases, there is no obvious underlying lung disease or overt immune incompetence. The relative proportions of NTM lung disease patients with and without underlying lung disease probably varies by population, but it appears that the majority of cases occur without demonstrable predisposing factors. NTM organisms may be isolated from the sputum in the absence of clinically relevant disease, and thus the diagnosis of pulmonary NTM disease rests on the presence of multiple positive cultures, and clinical (symptoms and radiology) data (Griffith et al. 2007). Extrapulmonary NTM disease is less common than lung disease, and may manifest as a localized infection of lymph nodes, skin, soft tissue, or bone, or may be disseminated. It is diagnosed when biopsy specimens of the involved organ(s) culture the causative organism, or, in the case of disseminated disease, with positive blood cultures (Griffith et al. 2007).

4.1 The risk of NTM disease associated with TNF-α inhibitors

Given the known role of tumor necrosis factor (TNF) in granuloma formation and maintenance, it is likely that TNF-α inhibitors increase the risk of all granulomatous infections, including NTM infection. However, in comparion to tuberculosis, relatively little has been published on this association. NTM infection is more difficult to study than tuberculosis, since the diagnosis is more complex as it relies on clinical data in addition to positive cultures. Additionally, in many jurisdictions, NTM isolation and NTM disease are not reportable to public health authorities.

Most literature associating NTM disease with TNF-α inhibitors has been in the form of case reports; a broad range of different NTM species infecting different body sites have been described in association with infliximab, adalimumab, and etanercept therapy (van Ingen et al. 2008). However, incidence studies are scarce. In 2004, Wallis *et al.* reported rates of granulomatous infections in persons treated with infliximab and etanercept. The cases were voluntarily reported to the United States Food and Drug Administration (FDA) Adverse Events Reporting System (AERS) from January 1998 to September 2002. A correction was published soon after (Wallis et al. 2004), which removed erroneously included cases from Europe. This study identified 29 cases of unspecified NTM infections, which translates to a rate of 17 per 100,000 treated persons (Wallis et al. 2004). This is much higher than the background incidence of 4 cases per 100,000 persons, reported in the United States in 1996 (Centers for Disease et al. 1996).

An updated study of the same Medwatch database, extending the time period to 2007, reported 105 confirmed or probable cases of NTM infection associated with TNF-α inhibitors (Winthrop et al. 2009). These cases were most frequently associated with infliximab (n = 73, 69%), followed by etanercept (n = 25, 24%), and then adalimumab (n = 7, 7%). Unfortunately, they did not have information regarding drug exposure, and so were unable to calculate rates of infection.

Interestingly, the original report of the US FDA Medwatch data found that the incidence of NTM infection was significantly lower than the incidence of tuberculosis in patients on TNF-α inhibitors (Wallis et al. 2004). However, a more recent report, based on a survey of infectious disease physicians in the United States, found the opposite; there were more cases of NTM infection than tuberculosis infection associated with TNF-α inhibitors in the United States (32 vs. 17 cases) (Winthrop et al. 2008). This finding is not unexpected, given the low prevalence of tuberculosis in the United States, and the widespread belief that rates of NTM disease are increasing (Griffith et al. 2007), but it highlights the fact that NTM disease is an underrecognized but important complication of TNF-antagonist therapy.

4.2 The presentation, treatment, and prevention of NTM disease associated with TNF-α inhibitors

Similar to tuberculosis, in the setting of TNF-α inhibitor therapy, extra-pulmonary and disseminated NTM disease appear to be more common. In the 2009 report of the US FDA Medwatch data, 56% of the confirmed or probable NTM cases were pulmonary, and 44% were extrapulmonary; 26% involved skin or soft tissue, 9% bone or joint, and 8% were disseminated (Winthrop et al. 2009). In contrast, in the United States during the period from 1993 through 1996, the NTM isolates reported by state public health laboratories were divided as follows; 75% were pulmonary, 5% were from blood, 2% from skin/soft tissue, and 0.4% from lymph node isolates (Centers for Disease et al. 1996).

Patients with rheumatoid arthritis, however, may be more likely than those with other indications for TNF-antagonist therapy to have pulmonary NTM disease. The US FDA Medwatch study showed that compared with patients with extrapulmonary NTM disease, patients with pulmonary NTM disease were 3.6 times more likely to have underlying rheumatoid arthritis (95%CI 1.5–8.8) (Winthrop et al. 2009). There are several possible reasons for this. For one, rheumatoid lung disease, which can include bronchiolitis and bronchiectasis, occurs in about 10% of people with rheumatoid arthritis, and can predispose to NTM disease (Winthrop et al. 2009). Also, rheumatoid arthritis and NTM lung disease have similar epidemiologic risk profiles, as both occur more commonly in elderly women (Winthrop et al. 2009). Additionally, rheumatoid arthritis is more common in the elderly, who may have comorbidities predisposing to NTM lung disease, such as chronic obstructive pulmonary disease.

NTM disease is associated with a high level of morbidity and mortality when it develops on TNF-α inhibitor therapy. In the report from Winthrop et al., 61% of patients with NTM infections were hospitalized, and 9% died (Winthrop et al. 2009).

A broad range of different NTM species have been described in association with TNF-α inhibitors, including those of high and low pathogenicity (van Ingen et al. 2008). In the US Medwatch study, *M. Avium* was the most common etiologic organism reported (49%), followed by rapidly growing mycobacteria (19%), and *M. marinum* (8%) (Winthrop et al. 2009).

NTM disease seems to occur after many months of TNF-α inhibitor therapy. The report of the US FDA Medwatch data showed that the median time between TNF-α inhibitor start date and infection diagnosis was 43 weeks for infliximab (range 2-200 weeks), 35 weeks for etanercept (range 0-288 weeks), and 18 weeks for adalimumab (range 4–94 weeks) (Winthrop et al. 2009). This group therefore surmised that most cases represent newly acquired infection. However, given the natural course of pulmonary NTM disease, which typically is insidious in onset and slowly progressive, the possibility exists that some patients had undiagnosed pulmonary NTM disease before starting TNF-antagonist therapy.

The experience of treating NTM disease in the setting of TNF-α inhibitor therapy is limited. Anti-TNF-α therapy should likely be held for an unknown duration. However, one case report described a paradoxical worsening of NTM disease after withdrawal of infliximab (Salvana et al. 2007), similar to the paradoxical reaction sometimes seen with tuberculosis; the clinician should be aware of this complication. Treatment of NTM disease is complicated because different regimens exist for the different NTM species. Futhermore, prolonged antimicrobial therapy is required and results are often disappointing; expert consultation should always be sought.

The best approach to screening and prevention of NTM disease prior to initiation of TNF-α inhibitor therapy is unknown. Unlike tuberculosis, there is no evidence of a latent phase in NTM disease. Additionally, screening is complicated by the possibility of NTM colonization without active disease, and the ongoing environmental inoculation that is likely present. However, given the insidious nature of NTM disease and its slow progression, unrecognized NTM disease may be present in some patients prior to starting TNF-antagonist therapy. Screening for such patients should be considered. Screening should include chest radiography, which must be done for all patients prior to starting TNF-α inhibitors to screen for tuberculosis. However, chest radiographs are not sensitive for detecting bronchiectasis or other parenchymal abnormalities associated with pulmonary NTM disease. Computerized tomography (CT) should therefore be considered in patients suspected of predisposing pulmonary diseases, including those with chronic unexplained cough. If chest CT is suggestive of possible NTM disease, sputum or bronchoscopy specimens should be cultured to rule out active NTM disease prior to initiation of TNF-antagonist therapy (van Ingen et al. 2008; Winthrop et al. 2009).

During therapy with TNF-α inhibitors, patients should be regularly assessed to rule out active infections. With respect to NTM disease, repeated sputum cultures during therapy should be considered in the setting of chest symptoms or co-morbid pulmonary disease, as well as chest radiography or CT scans. Extrapulmonary disease should be thoroughly investigated, and biopsy specimens should be stained for acid-fast bacilli and cultured for mycobacteria (van Ingen et al. 2008).

5. Conclusion

The TNF-α inhibitors, including the four currently available anti-TNF monoclonal antibodies and the soluble TNF receptor, have revolutionized the treatment of rheumatoid arthritis and other chronic inflammatory diseases since their introduction over a decade ago. However, their use is associated with an increased risk of granulomatous infections, including tuberculosis and NTM disease. The biological basis of this infection risk is the critical role played by TNF in the host response to mycobacterial infection, via its role in macrophage activation, cell recruitment, and granuloma formation and maintenance.

The magnitude of the risk of tuberculosis associated with TNF-antagonist therapy appears to be between 1.5 and 30 times above the risk associated with rheumatoid arthritis alone. The risk of tuberculosis differs amongst the various TNF-α inhibitors; the monoclonal antibodies portend more risk and are associated with a shorter tuberculosis onset time than the soluble TNF receptor. These differences may be related to different pharmacokinetic properties of the drugs, differential binding of soluble and transmembrance receptors, and differential effects on immune cell function and death.

All patients should be clinically evaluated for latent tuberculosis infection prior to the initiation of TNF-α inhibitor therapy. This evaluation should include a history, chest radiograph, and either a tuberculin skin test or an IGRA. IGRAs appear to be more specific for latent tuberculosis infection than tuberculin skin tests; they may also be more sensitive but this has not been definitively established. Most national guidelines recommend the tuberculin skin test as the diagnostic tool of choice for latent tuberculosis infection in this setting. The treatment of latent tuberculosis infection prior to the initiation of TNF-α inhibitors has proven benefit. Isoniazid therapy for a duration of 9 months is the most commonly recommended regimen, although some national guidelines recommend other regimens. The duration of therapy required before starting anti-TNF-α therapy is not well established.

The presentation of active tuberculosis in patients on TNF-α inhibitors is different from classically described tuberculosis; it is more likely to be extra-pulmonary and more likely to be disseminated at presentation. Discontinuation of anti-TNF-α therapy may be associated with a paradoxical worsening of tuberculosis disease, but discontinuation of therapy is still recommended in most guidelines.

NTM disease is an under recognized but important complication of TNF-antagonist therapy. Some research has suggested that NTM disease may be more common than tuberculosis in the setting of TNF-α inhibitor therapy, however the magnitude of the risk of NTM disease in this setting is unknown. NTM disease is associated with a high level of morbidity and mortality when it develops on TNF-α inhibitor therapy and may have atypical presentations. The best approach to screening and prevention of NTM disease prior to initiation of TNF-α inhibitor therapy is unknown.

Future research should include prospective studies establishing the magnitude of the risk of NTM disease with TNF-α inhibitor therapy; such studies may guide development of preventive strategies. Prospective studies estimating the positive predictive value of IGRA responses compared with tuberculin skin test responses for the developent of tuberculosis in patients treated with TNF-α inhibitors are also needed. Reports on treatment and outcomes of tuberculosis and NTM disease in the setting of TNF-α inhibitor therapy are also necessary.

6. References

Anonymous (1982). Efficacy of various durations of isoniazid preventive therapy for tuberculosis: five years of follow-up in the IUAT trial. International Union Against Tuberculosis Committee on Prophylaxis. *Bulletin of the World Health Organization,* Vol. 60, No. 4, pp. 555-64.

Arend, S. M., Leyten, E. M. S., Franken, W. P. J., Huisman, E. M. & van Dissel, J. T. (2007). A patient with de novo tuberculosis during anti-tumor necrosis factor-alpha therapy illustrating diagnostic pitfalls and paradoxical response to treatment. *Clinical Infectious Diseases,* Vol. 45, No. 11, (Dec 1), pp. 1470-5.

Askling, J., Fored, C. M., Brandt, L., Baecklund, E., Bertilsson, L., Coster, L., Geborek, P., Jacobsson, L. T., Lindblad, S., Lysholm, J., Rantapaa-Dahlqvist, S., Saxne, T., Romanus, V., Klareskog, L. & Feltelius, N. (2005). Risk and case characteristics of tuberculosis in rheumatoid arthritis associated with tumor necrosis factor antagonists in Sweden. *Arthritis & Rheumatism,* Vol. 52, No. 7, (Jul), pp. 1986-92.

Beglinger, C., Dudler, J., Mottet, C., Nicod, L., Seibold, F., Villiger, P. M. & Zellweger, J.-P. (2007). Screening for tuberculosis infection before the initiation of an anti-TNF-alpha therapy. *Swiss Medical Weekly,* Vol. 137, No. 43-44, (Nov 3), pp. 620-2.

Bekker, L. G., Freeman, S., Murray, P. J., Ryffel, B. & Kaplan, G. (2001). TNF-alpha controls intracellular mycobacterial growth by both inducible nitric oxide synthase-dependent and inducible nitric oxide synthase-independent pathways. *Journal of Immunology,* Vol. 166, No. 11, (Jun 1), pp. 6728-34.

Belknap, R., Reves, R. & Burman, W. (2005). Immune reconstitution to Mycobacterium tuberculosis after discontinuing infliximab. *International Journal of Tuberculosis & Lung Disease,* Vol. 9, No. 9, (Sep), pp. 1057-8.

Blackmore, T. K., Manning, L., Taylor, W. J. & Wallis, R. S. (2008). Therapeutic use of infliximab in tuberculosis to control severe paradoxical reaction of the brain and lymph nodes. *Clinical Infectious Diseases,* Vol. 47, No. 10, (Nov 15), pp. e83-5.

Brassard, P., Kezouh, A. & Suissa, S. (2006). Antirheumatic drugs and the risk of tuberculosis. *Clinical Infectious Diseases,* Vol. 43, No. 6, (Sep 15), pp. 717-22.

Brassard, P., Lowe, A.-M., Bernatsky, S., Kezouh, A. & Suissa, S. (2009). Rheumatoid arthritis, its treatments, and the risk of tuberculosis in Quebec, Canada. *Arthritis & Rheumatism,* Vol. 61, No. 3, (Mar 15), pp. 300-4.

British Thoracic Society Standards of Care, C. (2005). BTS recommendations for assessing risk and for managing Mycobacterium tuberculosis infection and disease in patients due to start anti-TNF-alpha treatment. *Thorax,* Vol. 60, No. 10, (Oct), pp. 800-5.

Carmona, L., Gomez-Reino, J. J., Rodriguez-Valverde, V., Montero, D., Pascual-Gomez, E., Mola, E. M., Carreno, L. & Figueroa, M. (2005). Effectiveness of recommendations to prevent reactivation of latent tuberculosis infection in patients treated with tumor necrosis factor antagonists. *Arthritis & Rheumatism,* Vol. 52, No. 6, (Jun), pp. 1766-72.

Carmona, L., Hernandez-Garcia, C., Vadillo, C., Pato, E., Balsa, A., Gonzalez-Alvaro, I., Belmonte, M. A., Tena, X. & Sanmarti, R. (2003). Increased risk of tuberculosis in patients with rheumatoid arthritis. *Journal of Rheumatology,* Vol. 30, No. 7, (Jul), pp. 1436-9.

Centers for Disease, Control & Prevention (1996). Nontuberculous Mycobacteria Reported to the Public Health Laboratory Information System by State Public Health Laboratories United States, 1993-1996, cdc.gov/ncidod/dastlr/mycobacteriology.htm (no longer available).

Centers for Disease, Control & Prevention (2001). Update: Fatal and severe liver injuries associated with rifampin and pyrazinamide for latent tuberculosis infection, and revisions in American Thoracic Society/CDC recommendations--United States, 2001. *MMWR - Morbidity & Mortality Weekly Report,* Vol. 50, No. 34, (Aug 31), pp. 733-5.

Centers for Disease, Control & Prevention (2004). Tuberculosis associated with blocking agents against tumor necrosis factor-alpha--California, 2002-2003. *MMWR - Morbidity & Mortality Weekly Report,* Vol. 53, No. 30, (Aug 6), pp. 683-6.

Combe, B., Landewe, R., Lukas, C., Bolosiu, H. D., Breedveld, F., Dougados, M., Emery, P., Ferraccioli, G., Hazes, J. M., Klareskog, L., Machold, K., Martin-Mola, E., Nielsen, H., Silman, A., Smolen, J., Yazici, H. & Hazes, J. M. W. (2007). EULAR recommendations for the management of early arthritis: report of a task force of the European Standing Committee for International Clinical Studies Including Therapeutics (ESCISIT). *Annals of the Rheumatic Diseases,* Vol. 66, No. 1, (Jan), pp. 34-45.

Comstock, G. W., Baum, C. & Snider, D. E., Jr. (1979). Isoniazid prophylaxis among Alaskan Eskimos: a final report of the bethel isoniazid studies. *American Review of Respiratory Disease,* Vol. 119, No. 5, (May), pp. 827-30.

Diel, R., Hauer, B., Loddenkemper, R., Manger, B. & Kruger, K. (2009). [Recommendations for tuberculosis screening before initiation of TNF-alpha-inhibitor treatment in rheumatic diseases]. *Pneumologie,* Vol. 63, No. 6, (Jun), pp. 329-34.

Dixon, W. G., Hyrich, K. L., Watson, K. D., Lunt, M., Galloway, J., Ustianowski, A., Symmons, D. P. M. & Register, B. S. R. B. (2010). Drug-specific risk of tuberculosis in patients with rheumatoid arthritis treated with anti-TNF therapy: results from the British Society for Rheumatology Biologics Register (BSRBR). *Annals of the Rheumatic Diseases,* Vol. 69, No. 3, (Mar), pp. 522-8.

Elliott, M. J., Maini, R. N., Feldmann, M., Kalden, J. R., Antoni, C., Smolen, J. S., Leeb, B., Breedveld, F. C., Macfarlane, J. D., Bijl, H. & et al. (1994). Randomised double-blind comparison of chimeric monoclonal antibody to tumour necrosis factor alpha (cA2) versus placebo in rheumatoid arthritis. *Lancet,* Vol. 344, No. 8930, (Oct 22), pp. 1105-10.

Fonseca, J. E., Canhao, H., Silva, C., Miguel, C., Mediavilla, M. J., Teixeira, A., Castelao, W., Nero, P., Bernardes, M., Bernardo, A., Mariz, E., Godinho, F., Santos, M. J., Bogas, M., Oliveira, M., Saavedra, M. J., Barcelos, A., Cruz, M., Santos, R. A., Mauricio, L., Rodrigues, M., Figueiredo, G., Quintal, A., Patto, J. V., Malcata, A., da Silva, J. C., Araujo, D., Ventura, F., Branco, J. & Queiroz, M. V. (2006). [Tuberculosis in rheumatic patients treated with tumour necrosis factor alpha antagonists: the

Portuguese experience]. *Acta Reumatologica Portuguesa,* Vol. 31, No. 3, (Jul-Sep), pp. 247-53.

Fonseca, J. E., Lucas, H., Canhao, H., Duarte, R., Santos, M. J., Villar, M., Faustino, A. & Raymundo, E. (2006). [Recommendations for the diagnosis and treatment of latent and active tuberculosis in patients with inflammatory joint diseases treated with tumour necrosis factor alpha inhibitors]. *Acta Reumatologica Portuguesa,* Vol. 31, No. 3, (Jul-Sep), pp. 237-45.

Garcia-Vidal, C., Rodriguez-Fernandez, S., Teijon, S., Esteve, M., Rodriguez-Carballeira, M., Lacasa, J. M., Salvador, G. & Garau, J. (2009). Risk factors for opportunistic infections in infliximab-treated patients: the importance of screening in prevention. *European Journal of Clinical Microbiology & Infectious Diseases,* Vol. 28, No. 4, (Apr), pp. 331-7.

Garcia Vidal, C., Rodriguez Fernandez, S., Martinez Lacasa, J., Salavert, M., Vidal, R., Rodriguez Carballeira, M. & Garau, J. (2005). Paradoxical response to antituberculous therapy in infliximab-treated patients with disseminated tuberculosis. *Clinical Infectious Diseases,* Vol. 40, No. 5, (Mar 1), pp. 756-9.

Gomez-Reino, J. J., Carmona, L. & Angel Descalzo, M. (2007). Risk of tuberculosis in patients treated with tumor necrosis factor antagonists due to incomplete prevention of reactivation of latent infection. *Arthritis & Rheumatism,* Vol. 57, No. 5, (Jun 15), pp. 756-61.

Gomez-Reino, J. J., Carmona, L., Valverde, V. R., Mola, E. M. & Montero, M. D. (2003). Treatment of rheumatoid arthritis with tumor necrosis factor inhibitors may predispose to significant increase in tuberculosis risk: a multicenter active-surveillance report. *Arthritis & Rheumatism,* Vol. 48, No. 8, (Aug), pp. 2122-7.

Griffith, D. E., Aksamit, T., Brown-Elliott, B. A., Catanzaro, A., Daley, C., Gordin, F., Holland, S. M., Horsburgh, R., Huitt, G., Iademarco, M. F., Iseman, M., Olivier, K., Ruoss, S., von Reyn, C. F., Wallace, R. J., Jr. & Winthrop, K. (2007). An official ATS/IDSA statement: diagnosis, treatment, and prevention of nontuberculous mycobacterial diseases. *American Journal of Respiratory & Critical Care Medicine,* Vol. 175, No. 4, (Feb 15), pp. 367-416.

Kavanagh, P. M., Gilmartin, J. J., O'Donnell, J. & O'Flanagan, D. (2008). Tumour necrosis factor-alpha and tuberculosis: guidance from the National TB Advisory Committee. *Irish Medical Journal,* Vol. 101, No. 1, (Jan), pp. 6-7.

Keane, J., Gershon, S., Wise, R. P., Mirabile-Levens, E., Kasznica, J., Schwieterman, W. D., Siegel, J. N. & Braun, M. M. (2001). Tuberculosis associated with infliximab, a tumor necrosis factor alpha-neutralizing agent. *New England Journal of Medicine,* Vol. 345, No. 15, (Oct 11), pp. 1098-104.

Keystone, E., Heijde, D. v. d., Mason, D., Jr., Landewe, R., Vollenhoven, R. V., Combe, B., Emery, P., Strand, V., Mease, P., Desai, C. & Pavelka, K. (2008). Certolizumab pegol plus methotrexate is significantly more effective than placebo plus methotrexate in active rheumatoid arthritis: findings of a fifty-two-week, phase III, multicenter, randomized, double-blind, placebo-controlled, parallel-group study.[Erratum appears in Arthritis Rheum. 2009 May;60(5):1249]. *Arthritis & Rheumatism,* Vol. 58, No. 11, (Nov), pp. 3319-29.

Listing, J., Strangfeld, A., Kary, S., Rau, R., von Hinueber, U., Stoyanova-Scholz, M., Gromnica-Ihle, E., Antoni, C., Herzer, P., Kekow, J., Schneider, M. & Zink, A.

(2005). Infections in patients with rheumatoid arthritis treated with biologic agents. *Arthritis & Rheumatism,* Vol. 52, No. 11, (Nov), pp. 3403-12.

Menzies, R. & Vissandjee, B. (1992). Effect of bacille Calmette-Guerin vaccination on tuberculin reactivity. *American Review of Respiratory Disease,* Vol. 145, No. 3, (Mar), pp. 621-5.

Mines, D. & Novelli, L. (2007). Antirheumatic drugs and the risk of tuberculosis. *Clinical Infectious Diseases,* Vol. 44, No. 4, (Feb 15), pp. 619-20; author reply 620-1.

Mohan, V. P., Scanga, C. A., Yu, K., Scott, H. M., Tanaka, K. E., Tsang, E., Tsai, M. M., Flynn, J. L. & Chan, J. (2001). Effects of tumor necrosis factor alpha on host immune response in chronic persistent tuberculosis: possible role for limiting pathology. *Infection & Immunity,* Vol. 69, No. 3, (Mar), pp. 1847-55.

Pai, M., Zwerling, A. & Menzies, D. (2008). Systematic review: T-cell-based assays for the diagnosis of latent tuberculosis infection: an update. *Annals of Internal Medicine,* Vol. 149, No. 3, (Aug 5), pp. 177-84.

Ponce de Leon, D., Acevedo-Vasquez, E., Sanchez-Torres, A., Cucho, M., Alfaro, J., Perich, R., Pastor, C., Harrison, J. & Sanchez-Schwartz, C. (2005). Attenuated response to purified protein derivative in patients with rheumatoid arthritis: study in a population with a high prevalence of tuberculosis. *Annals of the Rheumatic Diseases,* Vol. 64, No. 9, (Sep), pp. 1360-1.

Raval, A., Akhavan-Toyserkani, G., Brinker, A. & Avigan, M. (2007). Brief communication: characteristics of spontaneous cases of tuberculosis associated with infliximab. *Annals of Internal Medicine,* Vol. 147, No. 10, (Nov 20), pp. 699-702.

Rieder, H. L., Snider, D. E., Jr. & Cauthen, G. M. (1990). Extrapulmonary tuberculosis in the United States. *American Review of Respiratory Disease,* Vol. 141, No. 2, (Feb), pp. 347-51.

Roach, D. R., Bean, A. G. D., Demangel, C., France, M. P., Briscoe, H. & Britton, W. J. (2002). TNF regulates chemokine induction essential for cell recruitment, granuloma formation, and clearance of mycobacterial infection. *Journal of Immunology,* Vol. 168, No. 9, (May 1), pp. 4620-7.

Saag, K. G., Teng, G. G., Patkar, N. M., Anuntiyo, J., Finney, C., Curtis, J. R., Paulus, H. E., Mudano, A., Pisu, M., Elkins-Melton, M., Outman, R., Allison, J. J., Suarez Almazor, M., Bridges, S. L., Jr., Chatham, W. W., Hochberg, M., MacLean, C., Mikuls, T., Moreland, L. W., O'Dell, J., Turkiewicz, A. M. & Furst, D. E. (2008). American College of Rheumatology 2008 recommendations for the use of nonbiologic and biologic disease-modifying antirheumatic drugs in rheumatoid arthritis. *Arthritis & Rheumatism,* Vol. 59, No. 6, (Jun 15), pp. 762-84.

Saliu, O. Y., Sofer, C., Stein, D. S., Schwander, S. K. & Wallis, R. S. (2006). Tumor-necrosis-factor blockers: differential effects on mycobacterial immunity. *Journal of Infectious Diseases,* Vol. 194, No. 4, (Aug 15), pp. 486-92.

Salmon, D., GTI & AFSSAPS (2002). Recommendations about the prevention and management of tuberculosis in patients taking infliximab. *Joint, Bone, Spine: Revue du Rhumatisme,* Vol. 69, No. 2, (Mar), pp. 170-2.

Salvana, E. M. T., Cooper, G. S. & Salata, R. A. (2007). Mycobacterium other than tuberculosis (MOTT) infection: an emerging disease in infliximab-treated patients. *Journal of Infection,* Vol. 55, No. 6, (Dec), pp. 484-7.

Sandborn, W. J., Feagan, B. G., Stoinov, S., Honiball, P. J., Rutgeerts, P., Mason, D., Bloomfield, R. & Schreiber, S. (2007). Certolizumab pegol for the treatment of Crohn's disease. *New England Journal of Medicine,* Vol. 357, No. 3, (Jul 19), pp. 228-38.

Scallon, B., Cai, A., Solowski, N., Rosenberg, A., Song, X.-Y., Shealy, D. & Wagner, C. (2002). Binding and functional comparisons of two types of tumor necrosis factor antagonists. *Journal of Pharmacology & Experimental Therapeutics,* Vol. 301, No. 2, (May), pp. 418-26.

Seong, S.-S., Choi, C.-B., Woo, J.-H., Bae, K. W., Joung, C.-L., Uhm, W.-S., Kim, T.-H., Jun, J.-B., Yoo, D.-H., Lee, J.-T. & Bae, S.-C. (2007). Incidence of tuberculosis in Korean patients with rheumatoid arthritis (RA): effects of RA itself and of tumor necrosis factor blockers. *Journal of Rheumatology,* Vol. 34, No. 4, (Apr), pp. 706-11.

Smolen, J., Landewe, R. B., Mease, P., Brzezicki, J., Mason, D., Luijtens, K., van Vollenhoven, R. F., Kavanaugh, A., Schiff, M., Burmester, G. R., Strand, V., Vencovsky, J. & van der Heijde, D. (2009). Efficacy and safety of certolizumab pegol plus methotrexate in active rheumatoid arthritis: the RAPID 2 study. A randomised controlled trial. *Annals of the Rheumatic Diseases,* Vol. 68, No. 6, (Jun), pp. 797-804.

Solovic, I., Sester, M., Gomez-Reino, J. J., Rieder, H. L., Ehlers, S., Milburn, H. J., Kampmann, B., Hellmich, B., Groves, R., Schreiber, S., Wallis, R. S., Sotgiu, G., Scholvinck, E. H., Goletti, D., Zellweger, J. P., Diel, R., Carmona, L., Bartalesi, F., Ravn, P., Bossink, A., Duarte, R., Erkens, C., Clark, J., Migliori, G. B. & Lange, C. (2010). The risk of tuberculosis related to tumour necrosis factor antagonist therapies: a TBNET consensus statement. *European Respiratory Journal,* Vol. 36, No. 5, (Nov), pp. 1185-206.

Spohn, G., Guler, R., Johansen, P., Keller, I., Jacobs, M., Beck, M., Rohner, F., Bauer, M., Dietmeier, K., Kundig, T. M., Jennings, G. T., Brombacher, F. & Bachmann, M. F. (2007). A virus-like particle-based vaccine selectively targeting soluble TNF-alpha protects from arthritis without inducing reactivation of latent tuberculosis. *Journal of Immunology,* Vol. 178, No. 11, (Jun 1), pp. 7450-7.

Tubach, F., Salmon, D., Ravaud, P., Allanore, Y., Goupille, P., Breban, M., Pallot-Prades, B., Pouplin, S., Sacchi, A., Chichemanian, R. M., Bretagne, S., Emilie, D., Lemann, M., Lortholary, O., Mariette, X. & Research Axed on Tolerance of Biotherapies, G. (2009). Risk of tuberculosis is higher with anti-tumor necrosis factor monoclonal antibody therapy than with soluble tumor necrosis factor receptor therapy: The three-year prospective French Research Axed on Tolerance of Biotherapies registry.[Erratum appears in Arthritis Rheum. 2009 Aug;60(8):2540 Note: Lorthololary, O [corrected to Lortholary, O]]. *Arthritis & Rheumatism,* Vol. 60, No. 7, (Jul), pp. 1884-94.

van Ingen, J., Boeree, M. J., Dekhuijzen, P. N. R. & van Soolingen, D. (2008). Mycobacterial disease in patients with rheumatic disease. *Nature Clinical Practice Rheumatology,* Vol. 4, No. 12, (Dec), pp. 649-56.

Wallis, R. S. (2008). Tumour necrosis factor antagonists: structure, function, and tuberculosis risks. *The Lancet Infectious Diseases,* Vol. 8, No. 10, (Oct), pp. 601-11.

Wallis, R. S., Broder, M., Wong, J. & Beenhouwer, D. (2004). Granulomatous infections due to tumor necrosis factor blockade: correction. *Clinical Infectious Diseases,* Vol. 39, No. 8, (Oct 15), pp. 1254-5.

Wallis, R. S., Broder, M. S., Wong, J. Y., Hanson, M. E. & Beenhouwer, D. O. (2004). Granulomatous infectious diseases associated with tumor necrosis factor antagonists. *Clinical Infectious Diseases,* Vol. 38, No. 9, (May 1), pp. 1261-5.

Wallis, R. S., van Vuuren, C. & Potgieter, S. (2009). Adalimumab treatment of life-threatening tuberculosis. *Clinical Infectious Diseases,* Vol. 48, No. 10, (May 15), pp. 1429-32.

Winthrop, K. L., Chang, E., Yamashita, S., Iademarco, M. F., LoBue, P. A., (2009). Nontuberculous mycobacteria infections and anti-tumor necrosis factor-alpha therapy. *Emerging Infectious Diseases,* Vol. 15, No. 10, (Oct), pp. 1556-61.

Winthrop, K. L., Yamashita, S., Beekmann, S. E. & Polgreen, P. M. (2008). Mycobacterial and other serious infections in patients receiving anti-tumor necrosis factor and other newly approved biologic therapies: case finding through the Emerging Infections Network. *Clinical Infectious Diseases,* Vol. 46, No. 11, (Jun 1), pp. 1738-40.

Wolfe, F., Michaud, K., Anderson, J. & Urbansky, K. (2004). Tuberculosis infection in patients with rheumatoid arthritis and the effect of infliximab therapy. *Arthritis & Rheumatism,* Vol. 50, No. 2, (Feb), pp. 372-9.

Yamada, T., Nakajima, A., Inoue, E., Tanaka, E., Hara, M., Tomatsu, T., Kamatani, N. & Yamanaka, H. (2006). Increased risk of tuberculosis in patients with rheumatoid arthritis in Japan. *Annals of the Rheumatic Diseases,* Vol. 65, No. 12, (Dec), pp. 1661-3.

4

Expression of Tumor Necrosis Factor-Alpha (TNF-α), TNF- α Converting Enzyme and Matrix Metalloproteinase-3 in SAPHO Syndrome Synovium - A Rare Case Accompanied by Acrodermatitis Continua of Hallopeau: A Case Report and Review of Anti-TNF- α Therapy

Koichiro Komiya[1], Nobuki Terada[1],
Yoshikazu Mizoguchi[2] and Harumoto Yamada[3]
[1]*Department of Orthopaedic Surgery, Fujita Health University Second Hospital*
[2]*Department of Pathology, Fujita Health University Second Hospital*
[3]*Department of Orthopaedic Surgery, Fujita Health University*
Japan

1. Introduction

Synovitis-acne-pustulosis-hyperostosis-osteitis (SAPHO) syndrome is a rare disorder characterized by osteoarticular and dermatological manifestations. The denotation was first proposed by Chamot et al. in 1987 after investigation of 85 cases (Chamot et al., 1987). The most common site of SAPHO syndrome is the upper anterior chest wall, characterized by predominantly osteosclerotic lesions and hyperostosis. The axial skeleton and peripheral bones can be involved. Peripheral synovitis is also common. Skin manifestations include palmoplantar pustulosis (PPP), severe acne and various patterns of psoriasis.

The pathogenesis of SAPHO syndrome has not been determined. Most of the reported series to date are anecdotal, small or uncontrolled, thus a variety of therapeutic approaches exist. Treatment remains empirical with several drugs including non-steroidal anti-inflammatory drugs (NSAIDs), corticosteroids, antibiotics, disease modifying anti-rheumatic drugs (DMARDs) and/or bisphosphonates (BPs), but results are inconsistent and usually variable.

Recently, some successful experiences with anti-tumor necrosis factor-alpha (TNF-α) agents for refractory cases have been reported (Asmussen, 2003; Ben Abdelghani et al., 2010; Castellvi et al., 2010; Deutschmann et al., 2005; Iqbal & Kolodney, 2005; Kyriazis et al., 2004; Massara et al., 2006; Moll et al., 2008; Olivieri et al., 2002; Sabugo et al., 2008; Wagner et al., 2002; Widmer et al., 2003). The therapeutic strategy was largely originated from that for spondyloarthropathies, because accumulated arguments indicate that SAPHO syndrome can be classified with the inflammatory spondyloarthropathies (Takigawa et al., 2008) and treatment with anti-TNF-α agents is now well established in spondyloarthropathies or rheumatoid arthritis (RA). Chronic proliferative synovitis is one of the most important pathological features in RA, and proliferated synovium is a major source of proinflammatory cytokines and proteinases. TNF-α is a key cytokine, which triggers the inflammatory cascade and stimulates the production of matrix degradable proteinases such as matrix metalloproteinases (MMPs) (Okada, 2005). TNF-α converting enzyme (TACE) processes a membrane form of TNF-α to a soluble form (Moss et al., 1997), and the binding of the latter form to TNF receptors triggers pathological events in RA (Christodoulou & Choi, 2006; Horiuchi et al., 2010; Ohta et al., 2001). Although synovitis is one of the major manifestations of SAPHO syndrome, detailed information on the pathological features is still lacking.

In this chapter, we describe a patient with SAPHO syndrome accompanied by marked knee synovitis and acrodermatitis continua of Hallopeau (ACH) as a skin manifestation. ACH is a rare acropustular eruption, characterized by sterlile pustules, paronychia and atrophic skin changes, onychodystrophy and osteolysis of the distal phalanges of the fingers and toes (Ryan et al., 2009). ACH is considered to be a localized subtype of pustular psoriasis (Yerushalmi et al., 2000) and our report is a first case of ACH as a skin manifestation of SAPHO syndrome. We focused on synovitis, analyzed synovial tissues histopathologically and demonstrated the expression of TNF-α, TACE and MMP-3 in SAPHO syndrome synovium. We also concisely review cases treated with anti-TNF-α agents in the literature and discuss the therapeutic strategy for SAPHO syndrome.

2. Case report

A 76-year-old Japanese man first presented to a neighborhood university hospital in 1993 with subungal pustules, erythema and onychodystrophy on all fingers and toes. A diagnosis of ACH was histologically confirmed at the time. He had been treated with topical corticosteroid and vitamin D3. In January 2006, he presented to our department for the first time with persistent swelling and pain in his left knee. Physical examination showed marked patellar ballottement with local heat. A knee puncture yielded 60mL of yellow cloudy joint fluid, but cultures for bacteria were negative. For other osteoarticular symptoms, moderate lower back and buttock pain existed but no other joint pain, costa-sterno-clavicular joint included, was found. At the time, dermatological symptoms of ACH still remained on all fingers and toes (Figure 1a, b). Laboratory tests showed almost within normal value including indices of inflammation (erythrocyte sedimentation rate 10mm/hour, C-reactive protein level 0.19mg/dL [normal <0.30mg/dL]) and rheumatoid factor was negative. Radiographic study revealed characteristic osteolysis in phalanges of fingers and toes (Figure 1c, d). Magnetic resonance imaging revealed knee synovitis and bone marrow edema at the second lumbar vertebral body (Figure 2), compatible with sterile osteitis.

We made a diagnosis of SAPHO syndrome because the presence of ACH (a variant of pustular psoriasis), knee synovitis, and osteitis of the vertebral body were sufficient to the criteria. The patient was treated with NSAIDs for osteoarticular symptoms and topical treatment for skin lesions.

In October 2007, arthroscopic surgery was performed for knee synovitis. Intra-operative findings showed marked proliferation of villous contoured synovial tissues with rich blood circulation (Figure 3a). Continuous paraffin sections of biopsied synovial tissues were used for histopathological analyses, and standard microscopic study showed hyperplastic synovitis with lymphocytes infiltration and many blood vessels similar to RA (Figure 3b, c, d). Immunohistochemistry revealed the expression of TNF-α (Figure 3e), TACE (Figure 3f)

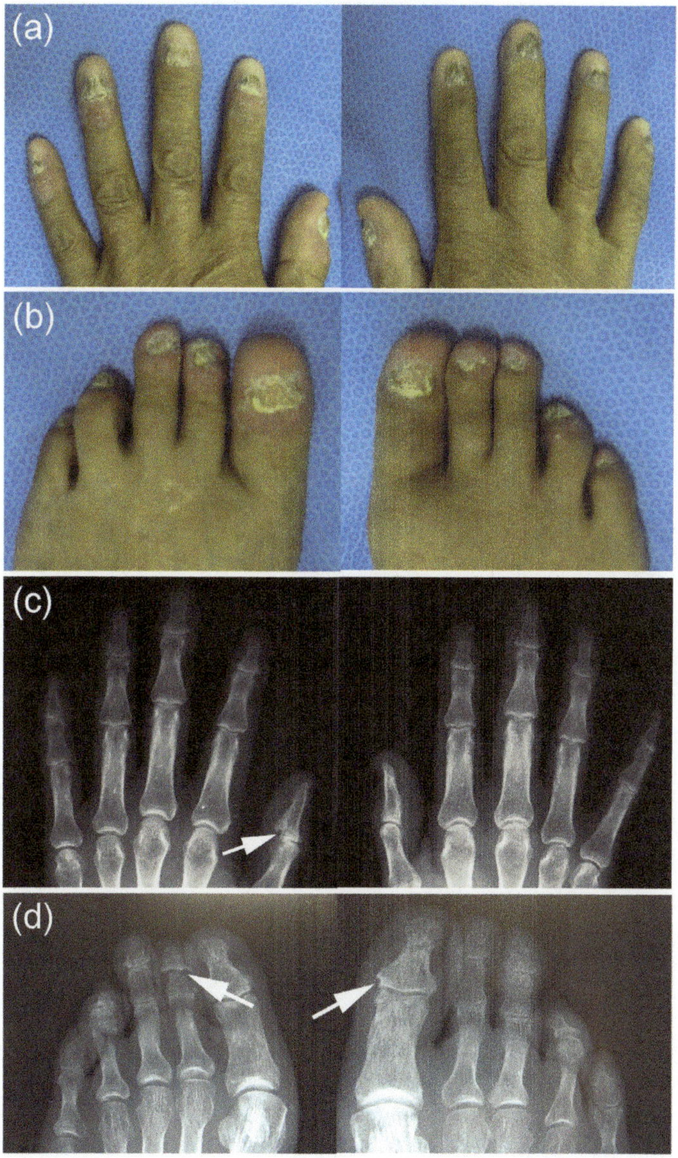

Fig. 1. Clinical findings of fingers (a), toes (b), and radiographs of bilateral fingers (c) and toes (d) in a patient with SAPHO syndrome accompanied by acrodrmatitis continua of Hallopeau. Erythema, pustules and onychodystrophy are present on all fingers and toes, which are compatible with the dermatological features of acrodermatitis continua of Hallopeau (a, b). Characteristic osteolysis of acrodermatitis continua of Hallopeau are observed in phalanges of fingers (c) and toes (d).

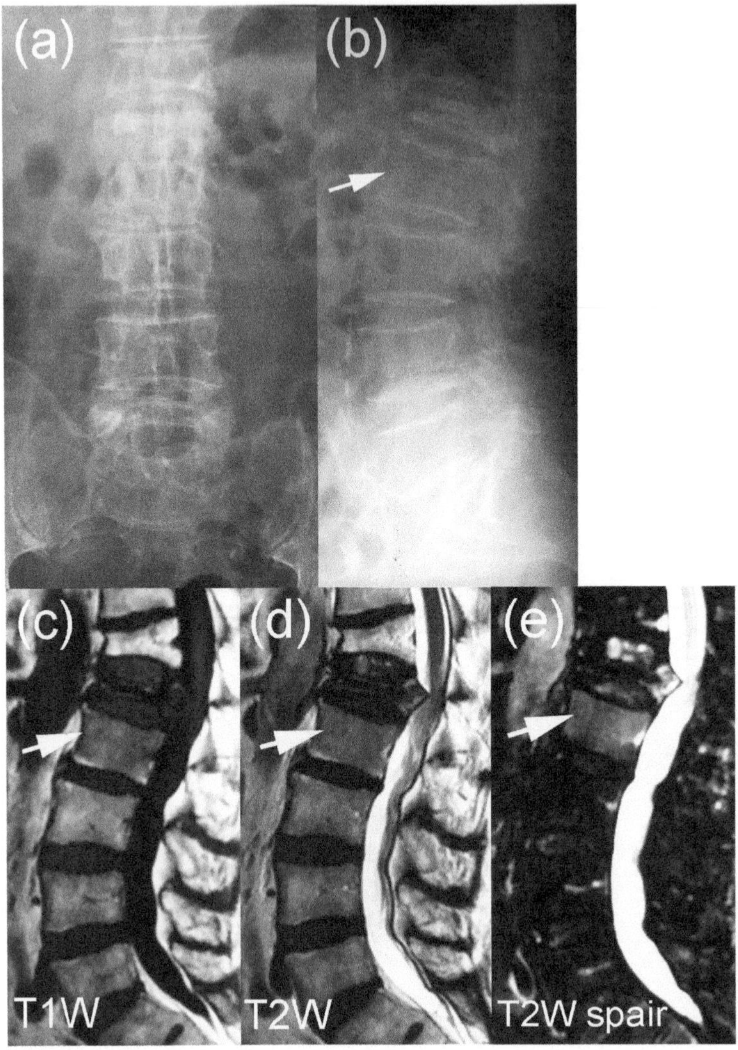

Fig. 2. Radiographic study (a, b) and magnetic resornance imaging (c, d, e) of lumber spine in a patient with SAPHO syndrome accompanied by acrodrmatitis continua of Hallopeau. Bone marrow edema at the second lumbar vertebral body (arrow) is compatible with sterile osteitis.

and MMP-3 (Figure 3g) in synovial cells of the lining layer. TNF-α and TACE were expressed dominantly in CD68 positive synovial cells of the lining and sublining layer, whereas MMP-3 was expressed dominantly in CD68 negative synovial cells of the lining layer (Figure 3e-h). Primary antibodies used for these analyses were polyclonal antibodies for TNF-α (654250; Calbiochem, Germany), TACE (sc-25782; Santa Cruz Biotechnology, USA), monoclonal antibodies for MMP-3 (55-2A2; Daiichi Fine Chemical Co., Japan) and CD68 (M0814; DakoCytomation, Denmark). After arthroscopic synovectomy, his knee symptoms immediately diminished. In 2008, additional administration of alendronate (35

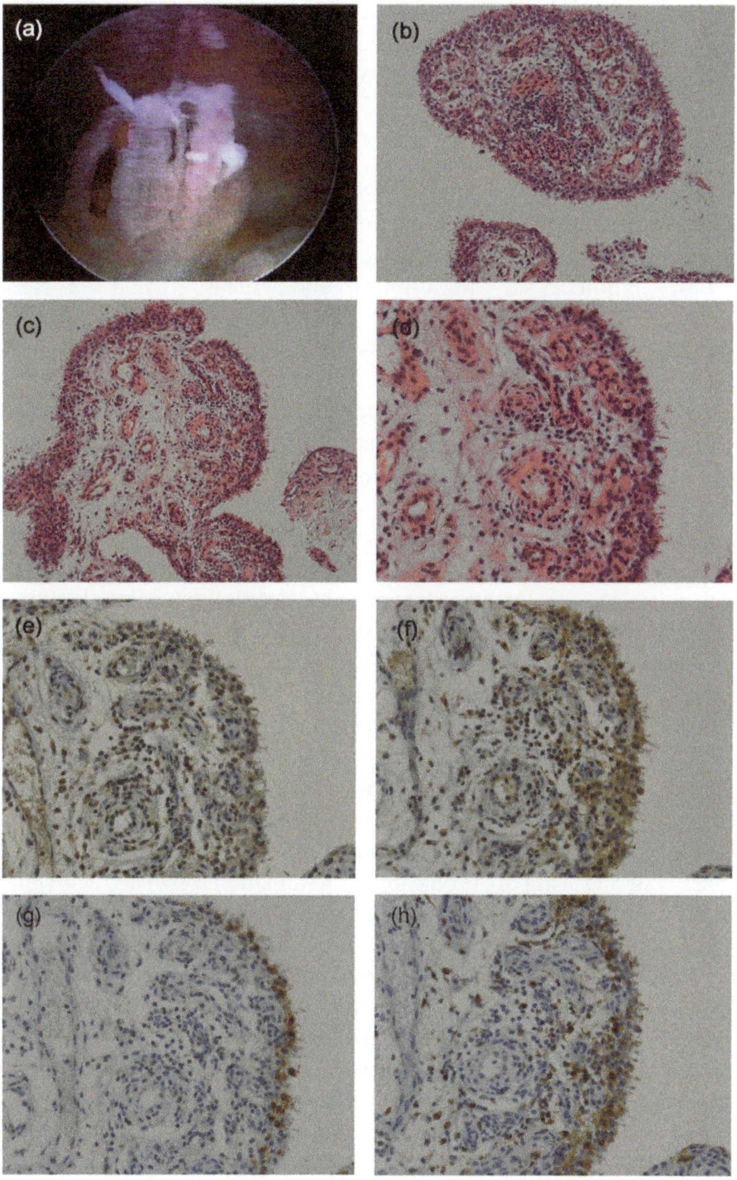

Fig. 3. Macro- and microscopic findings of knee synovitis in a patient with SAPHO syndrome accompanied by acrodrmatitis continua of Hallopeau. Arthroscopy reveals RA like villous contoured synovial tissues with rich blood circulation (a). Continuous paraffin sections (b-h) were stained with hematoxylin and eosin (b-d) or immunostained with antibodies against TNF-α (e), TACE (f), MMP-3 (g), or CD68 (h). Note that hyperplastic synovitis with lymphocytes infiltration, rich blood vessels similar to RA (b, c, d), and TNF-α, TACE and MMP-3 are expressed in synovial lining cells (e-g).

mg/week) was started. In the four year follow-up period, there has been no recurrence of knee synovitis, no exacerbation of dermatological symptoms of ACH, and the patient has had only mild low back pain which have responded to NSAIDs and alendronate.

3. Discussion

In the present case, we investigated the histopathological features of SAPHO syndrome synovitis. Arthroscopic findings showed moderate proliferation of villous contoured synovial tissues with rich blood circulation. Microscopic findings showed hyperplastic synovitis with lymphocytes infiltration and many blood vessels. Further immunohistochemistry showed that TNF-α and TACE were expressed dominantly in CD68 positive macrophage like synovial cells of lining and sublining layer while MMP-3 was expressed dominantly in CD68 negative fibroblast like synovial cells of lining layer. These histopathological features were overlapped with those of RA synovitis. But the extent of each microscopic feature, such as hyperplasticity of lining layers, lymphocytes infiltration and vascular density, seemed to be more marked in RA than SAPHO syndrome. Furthermore, in our previously reported a case of SAPHO syndrome accompanied by marked knee synovitis and PPP as a skin manifestation, the histopathological features of synovitis were also similar to this case (Komiya et al., 2009). Although it is difficult to compare with past cases for lack of reports with detailed histopathological analyses of SAPHO syndrome synovitis, it is speculated that TNF-α may be produced abundantly and well activated by TACE in SAPHO synovitis, and this condition at least partially have a common with RA synovial pathogenesis.

SAPHO syndrome is characterized by the osteoarticular and dermatological symptoms that were compiled by French rheumatologists after a national survey carried in 1987 (Chamot et al., 1987). The acronym SAPHO stands for synovitis, acne, pustulosis, hyperostosis, osteitis (Chamot et al., 1987). As described by Kahn et al. in 1994, three diagnostic criteria characterize SAPHO syndrome: 1) multifocal osteomyelitis with or without skin manifestations; 2) sterlile acute or chronic joint inflammation associated with either pustular psoriasis or palmo-plantar pustulosis, or acne, or hidradenitis; 3) sterlile osteitis in the presence of one of the skin manifestations (Kahn et al., 1993, 1994). According to Kahn, one of the criteria is sufficient for the diagnosis of SAPHO syndrome.

The etiology and prevalence of SAPHO syndrome has not been determined because of the variety in clinical appearance. Although the osteoarticular symptoms of SAPHO syndrome are most commonly observed in the anterior chest wall and the spine, the taxonomic concept of spinal lesions of SAPHO syndrome is still confused and controversial; whether SAPHO synrdome is classified in to seronegative spondyloarthropathy (SNSA) or not (Hayem et al., 1999; Higashi et al., 2005). Accumulated data suggested that SAPHO syndrome can be classified into SNSA; a high prevalence of axial involvement (up to 90%), an increased frequency of positive HLA-B27 (15%), and an association with psoriasis and inflammatory bowel syndrome in 13% of cases (Ben Abdelghani et al., 2010; Kahn et al., 1992). Furthermore, many researchers have supported a link between SAPHO syndrome and SNSA. Maugars reported that 43% and 33% of 19 SAPHO syndrome patients fullfilled the criteria of European Spondylarthropathy Study Group (ESSG) (Dougados et al., 1991) and Amor (Amor et al., 1990), respectively (Maugars et al., 1995). Hukuda et al. reported that

4.7% and 0.3% of Japanese 990 SNSA patients showed PPP and SAPHO syndrome, respectively (Hukuda et al., 2001). Takigawa et al. reported that 23% of 13 SAPHO syndrome patients met the criteria of SNSA regardless of whether ESSG or Amor criteria were used (Takigawa et al, 2008). In their series, if PPP is added as a skin lesion to the criteria of spondyloarthropathy, 100% and 92% of their cases would fullfill the diagnostic criteria of ESSG and Amor, respectively. Sonozaki proposed pustulotic arthro-osteitis is one subtype of SNSA (Sonozaki et al., 1981). Thus Takigawa et al. proposed that SAPHO syndrome, especially spinal lesions related to PPP, should be recognized as a subtype of SNSA (Takigawa et al., 2008).

The treatment of SAPHO syndrome remains empirical. In practice, NSAIDs are applied for osteoarticular symptoms and topical treatment for skin lesions. This first-line treatment is effective in two-thirds of cases (Hayem et al., 1999). In cases not respond to the first-line treatment, the second-line treatment, including glucocorticoids, BPs, and DMARDs such as methotrexate and sulfasalazine, is considered, but results are usually inconsistent and insufficient (Hayem et al., 1999). Recently some successful experiences with anti-TNF-α agents for recalcitrant cases of SAPHO syndrome have been reported (Asmussen, 2003; Ben Abdelghani et al., 2010; Castellvi et al., 2010; Deutschmann et al., 2005; Iqbal & Kolodney, 2005; Kyriazis et al., 2004; Massara et al., 2006; Moll et al., 2008; Olivieri et al., 2002; Sabugo et al., 2008; Wagner et al., 2002; Widmer et al., 2003). This therapeutic strategy was largely originated from that for spondyloarthropathies in which the efficacy and safety of anti-TNF-α therapy is well established (Davis et al., 2003; Mease et al., 2000; Moreland et al., 1999).

TNF-α is a proinflammatory cytokine found in increased concentrations in the joints and skin of patients with RA, pasoriatic arthritis and psoriasis, and plays crucial roles in the pathogenesis of these chronic inflammatory disease (Bradley, 2008; Ettehadi et al., 1994; Feldmann & Maini, 2001; Partsch et al., 1997; Tutrone et al., 2001). In RA synovium, TNF-α is produced abundantly and contribute to the pathogenesis by inducing the production of other proinflammatory cytokines, chemokines, and MMPs (Brennan et al., 1995; Ivashkiv, 1996; MacNaul et al., 1990). TNF-α is generated as a proform called transmembrane TNF-α that is consist of 233 amino acid residues (26kDa) and expressed on TNF-α-producing cells as a homotrimer (Kriegler et al., 1988; Luettiq et al., 1989; Pennica et al., 1984). This transmembrane TNF-α is cleaved between alanine76-valine77 bond by TACE, resulting in the release of soluble TNF-α that is consist of 157 amino acid residues (17kDa). Soluble TNF-α is a homotrimer of 17-kDa cleaved monomers and transmembrane TNF-α also exists as a homotrimer of 26-kDa uncleaved monomers (Tang et al., 1996). Both soluble and transmembrane TNF-α mediate pleiotrophic effects (apoptosis, cell proliferation and cytokine production) through binding to type 1 and type 2 TNF receptors (TNF-R1 and TNF-R2), but transmembrane TNF-α is supposed to mediate its biological activities mainly through TNF-R2 (Bazzoni & Beutler, 1996; Black et al., 1997; Grell et al., 1995; Moss et al., 1997; Vandenabeele et al., 1995). The remaining of cytoplasmic domain of transmembrane TNF-α after cleavage with TACE migrated back into the nucleus of the transmembrane TNF-α-expressing cells and is supposed to mediate cytokine production (Domonkos et al., 2001). It is very interesting that transmembrane TNF-α transmits signals both as a ligand and as a receptor. Differential clinical efficacies of anti-TNF-α agents may be explained by their different action on transmembrane TNF-α-expressing cells (Horiuchi et al., 2010).

TACE plays a crucial role in post-translational regulation of TNF-α. Binding of soluble TNF-α to TNF receptors activate various pathological events including the production of MMPs. TACE is a member of the ADAM (a disintegrin and metalloproteinase) family proteins, which possess characteristics of both cell surface adhesion molecules and proteinases. Some of the ADAM family proteins, including TACE, are considered to be responsible for the proteolytic processing of ectodomain of various cell surface molecules such as cytokines, cytokine receptors, adhesion molecules, and enzymes (Klein & Bischoff, 2011; Okada, 2005; Seals & Courtneidge, 2003). Several studies indicate that TACE levels are elevated in RA joints compared with osteoarthritis or normal articulations, suggesting that abnormal TACE activity contributes to TNF-α action in RA pathogenesis (Ohta et al, 2001). In the present case and in our previously reported case (Komiya et al., 2009), we demonstrated the expression of TNF-α, TACE and MMP-3 in SAPHO syndrome synovitis, thus it is speculated that TACE play roles in the pathogenesis of SAPHO syndrome synovitis through the processing of TNF-α, which triggers a cascade of pathological events through a mechanism similar to RA.

To our knowledge, 26 cases of SAPHO syndrome treated with anti-TNF-α agents (infliximab, etanercept or adalimumab) have been described, all of them showing a sustained response of osteoarticular manifestations (Asmussen, 2003; Ben Abdelghani et al., 2010; Castellvi et al., 2010; Deutschmann et al., 2005; Iqbal & Kolodney., 2005; Kyriazis et al., 2004; Massara et al., 2006; Moll et al., 2008; Olivieri et al., 2002; Sabugo et al., 2008; Wagner et al, 2002; Widmer et al., 2003), but not favorable for cutaneous manifestations in some cases (Ben Abdelghani et al., 2010; Massara et al., 2006). In the 26 previously reported cases in the literature, clinical response was rapid after within 2 infusions of anti-TNF-α agent in most of cases (24/26 cases, 92%). Clinical response was maintained in all cases, and clinical remission, which usually described as no recurrence of osteoarticular pain, was maintained with a follow up 8 to 42 months during treatment. Thus it is considered that the efficacy of anti-TNF-α agents on osteoarticular symptoms is reliable. Whereas, relapse or worsening of the skin lesion after anti-TNF-α therapy was observed in 5/26 cases (19%) (Ben Abdelghani et al., 2010; Massara et al., 2006). ACH, a skin lesion of this case, is a rare chronic pustular eruption of the distal portions of the hands and feet, characterized by sterlile pustules, paronychia and atrophic skin changes, onychodystrophy and osteolysis of the distal phalanges (Puig et al., 2010; Ryan et al., 2009). It is considered by many to be a localized variant of pustular psoriasis. (Kurooka et al., 2010; Yerushalmi et al., 2000). ACH is notoriously difficult to treat, with limited success with numerous agents including topical treatments, photochemotherapy, ciclosporin, methotrexate, retinoids, dapson and tetracyclines (Nikkels et al., 1999). Recently successful treatment of ACH with anti-TNF-α agents have been reported (Ahmad & Rogers, 2007; Bonish et al., 2006; Kazinski et al., 2005; Mang et al., 2004; Ryan et al., 2009). But in some cases of ACH, failed treatment with anti-TNF-α agents have been also reported (Adisen et al., 2007; Thielen et al., 2008; Ryan et al., 2009). In a recent review, 120 patients (with RA, ankylosing spondylitis, psoriasis, Crohn disease, SAPHO syndrome, psoriatic arthritis, and other diagnosis) from the literature who developed pustular lesions during treatment with anti-TNF-α agents were reported (Wollina et al., 2008). Psoriasis (except palmoplantar pustular type) was the most common adverse effect during anti-TNF-α agent treatment (n=73), followed by PPP (n=37). The reasons for these negative or paradoxical effects of anti-TNF-α agents on cutaneous manifestations have not yet been determined. One possible reason is that TNF-α is a pivotal mediator of the activation of neutrophils (Lebwohl, 2003), because in SAPHO syndrome, skin lesions are usually characterized by nuetrophil infiltration similar to those of pustular psoriasis. Another possible reason for deterioration of skin pustules could be activation of *Propionibacterium acnes* with anti TNF-α. *P. acnes* is anaerobic skin saprophyte, which has been strongly implicated in SAPHO syndrome (Perry & Lambert, 2006). Assmann et al. showed positive bacteriological cultures for *P. acnes* in 14 of 21 (67%) patients who had undergone a needle biopsy of ostitis lesions (Assmann et al., 2009). Rozin reported that *P. acnes* was positive in 38/90 cases (42%) in bone lesions in cases of SAPHO syndrome in the literature (Rozin, 2009). Bacterial or viral infections induces rheumatic condition, thus *P.acnes* could be an important pathogen in SAPHO syndrome. Thus, taking into consideration of *P. acnes*, combination of anti-TNF-α agents and antibiotics may prevent the exacerbation of skin lesion.

In cases not respond to the first-line treatment, BPs could be a good therapeutic modality except anti-TNF-α agents. Recently some successful treatments of SAPHO syndrome with BPs have been reported (Amital et al., 2004; Colina et al., 2009; Siau & Laversuch, 2010). BPs are potent inhibitors of osteoclastic bone resorption and are an important therapeutic modality in the management of Paget's disease, multiple myeloma, malignancy-associated hypercalcaemia, bone metastasis and osteoporosis. Not only the effect on bone remodeling, BPs have also an anti-inflammatory effect by suppressing the production of proinflammatory cytokines, such as interleukin (IL)-1, TNF-α, IL-6, and by inhibiting the antigen-presenting capacity of macrophages (de Vries et al., 1982; Pennanen et al., 1995). Amital et al. reported successful treatment with pamidronate in 10 patients with SAPHO syndrome (Amital et al., 2004). Intravenous administration of pamidronate was effective for not only osteoarticular manifestations but also skin lesions (Amital et al., 2004). Oral administration of BPs is also effective in treating SAPHO syndrome (Ichikawa et al., 2009). The modulation ability of BPs for anti-inflammatory cytokines, including TNF-α, could be a reason for their efficacy in several rheumatological conditions, such as ankylosing spondylitis, hypertrophic osteoarthropathy, reflex sympathetic dystrophy, diabetic neuropathic arthropathy and the SAPHO syndrome (de Vries et al., 1982; Garske & Bell, 2002; Guignard et al., 2002; Kubalek et al., 2001; Maksymowych et al., 2002; Marshall et al., 2002; Maugars et al., 1995; Pennanen et al., 1995; Selby et al., 1994). Ben Abdelghani et al. reported five cases not respond to BPs and four of these cases responded to anti-TNF-α therapy (Ben Abdelghani et al., 2010). Thus, anti-TNF-α therapy seems effective even for cases resistant to BPs.

The difficulties in the treatment of SAPHO syndrome are integrated into its complicated, not single, pathogenesis. Our experience support the importance of TNF-α and TACE in the pathogenesis of SAPHO syndrome, but further investigations are clearly needed to elucidate this rare and complicated disorder.

4. Conclusion

We describe a rare case of SAPHO syndrome accompanied by marked knee synovitis and ACH as a skin manifestation. We demonstrated the expression of TNF-α, TACE and MMP-3 in SAPHO syndrome synovium and also shown the similarity between SAPHO syndrome and RA synovitis. These new findings support the recently reported successful treatment of osteoarticular manifestations of SAPHO syndrome with anti-TNF-α agents.

5. References

Adisen, E., Oztas, M., & Gurer, MA. (2007). Lack of efficacy of etanercept in acrodermatitis continua of Hallopeau. *International Jouranal of Dermatology*, Vol.46, No.11, pp. 1205-1207.

Ahmad, K. & Rogers, S. (2007). Two years of experience with etanercept in recalcitrant psoriasis. *The British Journal of Dermatology*, Vol.156, No.5, pp. 1010-1014.

Amital, H., Applbaum, YH., Asmar, S., Daniel, N., & Rubinow, A. (2004). SAPHO syndrome treated with pamidronate: an open-label study of 10 patients. *Rheumatology (Oxford)*, Vo.43, No.5, pp. 658-661.

Amor, B., Dougados, M., & Mijiyawa, M. (1990). Criteria of the classification of spondyloarthropathies. *Revue du Rhumatisme et des Maladies Osteoarticulaires*, Vol.57, No.2, pp. 85-89.

Asmussen, KH. (2003). Successful treatment of SAPHO syndrome with infliximab. A case report [abstract]. *Arthritis and Rheumatism*, Vol.48, S621A.

Assmann, G., Kueck, O., Kirchhoff, T., Rosenthal, H., Voswinkel, J., Pfreundschuh, M., Zeidler, H., & Wagner, AD. (2009). Efficacy of antibiotic therapy for SAPHO syndrome is lost after its discontinuation: interventional study. *Arthritis Research & Therapy*, Vol.11, No.5, R140.

Bazzoni, F. & Beutler, B. (1996). The tumor necrosis factor ligand and receptor families. *The New England Journal of Medicine*, Vol.334, No.26, pp. 1717-1725.

Ben Abdelghani, K., Dran, DG., Gottenberg, JE., Morel, J., Sibilia, J., & Combe, B. (2010). Tumor necrosis factor-alpha blockers in SAPHO syndrome. *The Journal of Rheumatology*, Vol.37, No.8, pp. 1699-1704.

Black, RA., Rauch, CT., Kozlosky, CJ., Peschon, JJ., Slack, JL., Wolfson, MF., Castner, BJ., Stocking, KL., Reddy, P., Srinivasan, S., Nelson, N., Boiani, N., Schooley, KA., Gerhart, M., Davis, R., Fitzner, JN., Johnson, RS., Paxton, RJ., March, CJ., & Cerretti, DP. (1997). A metalloproteinase disintegrin that releases tumor-necrosis factor-alpha from cells. *Nature*, Vol.385, No.6618, pp. 729-733.

Bonish, B., Rashid, RM., & Swan, J. (2006). Etanercept responsive acrodermatitis continua of Hallopeau: Is a pattern developing? *Journal of Drugs in Dermatology*, Vol.5, No.9, pp. 903-904.

Bradley, JR. (2008). TNF-mediated inflammatory disease. *Journal of Pathology*, Vol.214, No.2, pp. 149-160.

Brennan, FM., Maini, RN., & Feldmann, M. (1995). Cytokine expression in chronic inflammatory disease. *British Medical Bulletin*, Vo.51, No.2, pp. 368-384.

Castellvi, I., Bonet, M., Nazarez, JA., & Molina-Hinojosa, JC. (2010). Successful treatment of SAPHO syndrome with adalimumab: a case report. *Clinical Rheumatology*, Vol.29, No.10, pp. 1205-1207.

Chamot, AM., Benhamou, CL., Kahn, MF., Beraneck, L., Kaplan, G., & Prost, A. (1987). Acne-pustulosis-hyperostosis-osteitis syndrome. Results of a national survey. 85

cases. *Revue du Rhumatisme et des Maladies Osteoarticulaires*, Vol.54, No.3, pp. 187-196.

Christodoulou, C. & Choy, EH. (2006). Joint inflammation and cytokine inhibition in rheumatoid arthritis. *Clinical and Experimental Medicine*, Vol.6, No.1, pp. 13-19.

Colina, M., La Corte, R., & Trotta, F. (2009). Sustained remission of SAPHO syndrome with pamidronate: a follow-up of fourteen cases and a review of the literature. *Clinical and Experimental Rheumatology*, Vo.27, No.1, pp. 112-115.

Davis, JC Jr., van der Heijde, D., Braun, J., Dougados, M., Cush, J., Clegg, DO., Kivitz, A., Fleischmann, R., Inman, R., & Tsuji, W.; Enbrel Ankylosing Spondylitis Study Group. (2003). Recombinant human tumor necrosis factor receptor (etanercept) for treating ankylosing spondylitis: a randomized, controlled trial. *Arthritis and Rheumatism*, Vol.48, No.11, pp. 3230-3236.

Deutschmann, A., Mache, CJ., Bodo, K., Zebedin, D., & Ring, E. (2005). Successful treatment of chronic reccurent multifocal osteomyelitis with tumor necrosis factor-blockage. *Pediatrics*, Vol.116, No.5, pp. 1231-1233.

de Vries, E., van der Weij, JP., van der Veen, CJ., van Paassen, HC., Jager, MJ., Sleeboom, HP., Bijvoet, OL., & Cats, A. (1982). In vitro effect of (3-amino-1-hydroxypropylidene)-1, 1-bisphosphonic acid (APD) on the function of mononuclear phagocytes in lymphocyte proliferation. *Immunology*, Vol.47, No.1, pp. 157-163.

Domonkos, A., Udvardy, A., Laszlo, L., Nagy, T., & Duda, E. (2001). Receptor-like properties of the 26 kDa transmembrane form of TNF. *European Cytokine Network*, Vol.12, No.3, pp. 411-419.

Dougados, M., van der Linden, S., Juhlin, R., Huitfeldt, B., Amor, B., Calin, A., Dijkmans, B., Olivieri, I., & Pasero, G. (1991). The European Spondyloarthropathy Study Group preliminary criteria for the classification of spondyloarthropathy. *Arthritis and Rheumatism*, Vol.34, No.10, pp. 1218-1227.

Ettehadi, P., Greaves, MW., Wallach, D., Aderka, D., & Camp, RD. (1994). Elevated tumor necrosis factor-alpha (TNF-alpha) biological activity in psoriatic skin lesions. *Clinical and Experimental Immunology*, Vol.96, No.1, pp. 146-151.

Feldmann, M. & Maini, RN. (2001). Anti-TNF alpha therapy of rheumatoid arthritis: what have we learned? *Annual Review of Immunology*, Vol.19, pp. 163-196.

Garske, LA. & Bell, SC. (2002). Pamidronate results in symptom control of hypertrophic pulmonary osteoarthropathy in cystic fibrosis. *Chest*, Vo.121, No.4, pp. 1363-1366.

Grell, M., Douni, E., Wajant, H., Lohden, M., Clauss, M., Maxeiner, B., Georgopoulos, S., Lesslauer, W., Kollias, G., Pfizenmaier, K., & Scheurich, P. (1995). The transmembrane form of tumor necrosis factor is the prime activating ligand of the 80 kDa tumor necrosis factor receptor. *Cell*, Vol.83, No.5, pp. 793-802.

Guignard, S., Job-Deslandre, C., Sayag-Boukris, V., & Kahan, A. (2002). Pamidronate treatment in SAPHO syndrome. *Joint Bone Spine*, Vol.69, No.4, pp. 392-396.

Hayem, G., Bouchaud-Chabot, A., Benali, K., Roux, S., Palazzo, E., Silbermann-Hoffman, O., & Meyer, O. (1999). SAPHO syndrome: a long-term follow-up study of 120 cases. *Seminars in Arthritis and Rheumatism*, Vol.29, No.3, pp. 159-171.

Higashi, S., Nakamura, T., Tomoda, K., Tsukano, M., Sakaguchi, M., & Kuga, F. (2005). A study of ten Japanese patients with seronegative spondyloarthropathy: a tentative proposal. *Modern Rheumatology*, Vol.15, No.5, pp. 329-335.

Horiuchi, T., Mitoma, H., Harashima, S., Tsukamoto, H., & Shimoda, T. (2010). Transmembrane TNF-α: structure, function and interaction with anti-TNF agents. *Rheumatology (Oxford)*, Vol.49, No.7, pp. 1215-1228.

Hukuda, S., Minami, M., Saito, T., Mitsui, H., Matsui, N., Komatsubara, Y., Makino, H., Shibata, T., Shingu, M., Sakou, T., & Shichikawa, K. (2001). Spondyloarthlopathies in Japan: nationwide questionnaire survey performed by the Japan Ankylosing Spondylitis Society. *The Journal of Rheumatology*, Vol.28, No.3, pp. 554-559.

Ichikawa, J., Sato, E., Haro, H., Ando, T., Maekawa, S., & Hamada, Y. (2009). Successful treatment of SAPHO syndrome with an oral bisphosphonate. *Rheumatology International*, Vol.29, No.6, pp. 713-715.

Iqbal, M. & Kolodney, MS. (2005). Acne fulminans with synovitis-acne-pustulosis-hyperostosis-osteitis (SAPHO) syndrome treated with infliximab. *Journal of the American Academy of Dermatology*, Vo.52, No.5 (Suppl 1), S118-120.

Ivashkiv, LB. (1996). Cytokine expression and cell activation in inflammatory arthritis. *Advances in Immunology*, Vol.63, pp. 337-376.

Kahn, MF., Bouchon, JP., Chamot, AM., & Palazzo, E. (1992). Chronic Enterocolopathies and SAPHO syndrome. 8 cases. *Revue du Rhumatisme et des Maladies Osteoarticulaires*, Vo.59, No.2, pp. 91-94.

Kahn, MF. (1993). Psoriatic arthritis and synovitis, acne, pustulosis, hyperostosis, and osteitis syndrome. *Current Opinion in Rheumatology*, Vol.5, No.4, pp. 428-435.

Kahn, MF. & Kahn, MA. (1994). The SAPHO-syndrome, In: *Psoriatic Arthritis (Baillere's Clinical Rheumatology)*. Wright V. & Helliwell P., Vol.8/2, pp. 333-362, Baillere Tindall, ISBN 0702018201.

Kazinski, K., Joyce, KM., & Hodson, D. (2005). The successful use of etanercept in combination therapy for treatment of acrodermatitis continua of Hallopeau. *Journal of Drugs in Dermatology*, Vol.4, No.3, pp. 360-364.

Klein, T. & Bischoff, R. (2011). Active metalloproteases of the A Disintegrin and Metalloprotease (ADAM) family: biological function and structure. *Journal of Proteome Research*, Vol.10, No.1, pp. 17-33.

Komiya, K., Yamada, H., Terada, N., Mizoguchi, Y., Yamada, M., Suzuki, M., & Kato, S. (2009). Expression of tumor necrosis factor-alpha converting enzyme and matrix metalloproteinase-3 in proliferated synovium in a patient with synovitis-acne-pustulosis-hyperostosis-osteitis syndrome: a case report. *Journal of medical case reports*, 3:9123. (doi: 10.4076/1752-1947-3-9123).

Kriegler, M., Perez, C., DeFay, K., Albert, I., & Lu, SD. (1988). A novel form of TNF/cashectin is a cell surface cytotoxic transmembrane protein: ramifications for the complex physiology of TNF. *Cell*, Vol.53, No.1, pp. 45-53.

Kubalek, I., Fain, O., Paries, J., Kettaneh, A., & Thomas, M. (2001). Treatment of reflex sympathetic dystrophy with pamidronate: 29 cases. *Rheumatology (Oxford)*, Vol.40, No.12, pp. 1394-1397.

Kurooka, S., Tsuruta, D., Hino, M., Yanagihara, S., & Ishii, M. (2010). Acrodermatitis continua of Hallopeau appearing at specific, high leucocyte counts. *The British Journal of Dermatology*, Vol.163, No.2, pp. 428-430.

Kyriazis, NC., Tachoula, AV., & Sfontouris, CI. (2004). Successful treatment of refractory SAPHO syndrome with infliximab [abstract]. *Annals of the Rheumatic Diseases*, Vol.63, 388-9A.

Lebwohl, M. (2003). Psoriasis. *Lancet*, Vol.361, No.9364, pp. 1197-1204.

Luettig, B., Decker, T., & Lohmann-Matthes, ML. (1989). Evidence for the exsistence of two form membrane tumor necrois factor: an integral protein and a molecule attached to its receptor. *Journal of Immunology*, Vol.143, No.12, pp. 4034-4038.

MacNaul, KL., Chartrain, N., Lark, M., Tocci, MJ., & Hutchinson, NI. (1990). Discoordinate expression of stromelysine, collagenase, and tissue inhibitor of metalloproteinases-1 in rheumatoid human synovial fibroblasts. Synergistic effects of interleukin-1 and tumor necrosis factor-alpha on stromelysine expression. *The Journal of Biological Chemistry*, Vol.265, No.28, pp. 17238-17245.

Maksymowych, WP., Jhangri, GS., Fitzgerald, AA., LeClercq, S., Chiu, P., Yan, A., Skeith, KJ., Aaron, SL., Homik, J., Davis, P., Sholter, D., & Russell, AS. (2002). A six-month randomized, controlled, double-blind, dose-response comparison of intravenous pamidronate (60 mg versus 10 mg) in the treatment of nonsteroidal antiinflammatory drug-refractory ankylosing spondylitis. *Arthritis and Rheumatism*, Vol.46, No.3, pp. 766-773.

Mang, R., Ruzicka, T., & Stege, H. (2004). Successful treatment of acrodermatitis Hallopeau by the tumor necrosis factor-alpha inhibitor infliximab (Remicade). *The British Journal of Dermatology*, Vol.150, No.2, pp. 379-380.

Marshall, H., Bromilow, J., Thomas, AL., & Arden, NK. (2002). Pamidronate: a novel treatment for the SAPHO syndrome? *Rheumatolgy (Oxford)*, Vol.41, No.2, pp. 231-233.

Massara, A., Cavazzini, PL., & Trotta, F. (2006). In SAPHO syndrome anti-TNF-alpha therapy may induce persistent amelioration of osteoarticular complaints, but may exacerbate cutaneous manifestations. *Rheumatology*, Vol.45, No.6, pp. 730-733.

Maugars, Y., Berthelot, JM., Ducroux, JM., & Prost, A. (1995). SAPHO syndrome: a followup study of 19 cases with special emphasis on enthesis involvement. *The Journal of Rheumatology*, Vol.22, No.11, pp. 2135-2141.

Mease, PJ., Goffe, BS., Metz, J., VanderStoep, A., Finck, B., & Burge, DJ. (2000). Etanercept in the treatment of psoriatic arthritis and psoriasis: a randomized trial. *Lancet*, Vol.356, No.9227, pp. 385-390.

Moll, C., Hernandez, MV., Canete, JD., Gomez-Puerta, JA., Soriano, A., Collado, A., & Sanmarti, R. (2008). Ilium osteitis as the main manifestation of the SAPHO syndrome: response to infliximab therapy and review of the literature. *Seminars in Arthritis and Rheumatism*, Vol.37, No.5, pp. 299-306.

Moreland, LW., Schiff, MH., Baumgartner, SW., Tindall, EA., Fleischmann, RM., Bulpitt, KJ., Weaver, AL., Keystone, EC., Furst, DE., Mease, PJ., Ruderman, EM., Horwitz, DA., Arkfeld, DG., Garrison, L., Burge, DJ., Blosch, CM., Lange, ML.,

McDonnell, ND., & Weinblatt, ME. (1999). Etanercept therapy in rheumatoid arthritis. A randomized, controlled trial. *Annals of Internal Medicine*, Vol.130, No.6, pp. 478-486.

Moss, ML., Jin, SL., Becherer, JD., Bickett, DM., Burkhart, W., Chen, WJ., Hassler, D., Leesnitzer, MT., McGeehan, G., Milla, M., Moyer, M., Rocque, W., Seaton, T., Schoenen, F., Warner, J., & Willard, D. (1997). Structural features and biochemical properties of TNF-alpha converting enzyme (TACE). *Journal of Neuroimmunology*, Vol.72, No.2, pp. 127-129.

Nikkels, AF., Nikkels-Tassoudji, N., & Pierard, GE. (1999). Breaking the relentless course of Hallopeau's acrodermatitis by dapsone. *European Journal of Dermatology*, Vol.9, No.2, pp. 126-128.

Ohta, S., Harigai, M., Tnaka, M., Kawaguchi, Y., Sugiura, T., Takagi, K., Fukasawa, C., Hara, M., & Kamatani, N. (2001). Tumor necrosis factor-alpha (TNF-alpha) converting enzyme contributes to production of TNF-alpha in synovial tissues from patients with rheumatoid arthritis. *Journal of Rheumatology*, Vol.28, No.8, pp. 1756-1763.

Okada, Y. (2005). Proteinases and matrix degradation, In: *Kelley's Textbook of Rheumatology (7th edition)*, Harris ED Jr., Budd RC., Ruddy S., Genovese MC., Firestein GS., & Sargent JS., pp. 63-81, Elsevier Saunders, ISBN 0721601413, Philadelphia

Olivieri, I., Padula, A., Ciancio, G., Salvarani, C., Niccoli, L., & Cantini, F. (2002). Successful treatment of SAPHO syndrome with infliximab: report of two cases. *Annals of the Rheumatic Diseases*, Vo.61, No.4, pp. 375-376.

Partsch, G., Steiner, G., Leeb, BF., Dunky, A., Broll, H., & Smolen, JS. (1997). Highly increased levels of tumor necrosis factor-alpha and other proinflammatory cytokines in psoriatic arthritis synovial fluid. *Journal of Rheumatology*, Vol.24, No.3, pp. 518-523.

Pennanen, N., Lapinjoki, S., Urtti, A., & Monkkonen, J. (1995). Effect of liposomal and free bisphosphonates on the IL-1beta, IL-6, and TNF alpha secretion from RAW264 cells in vitro. *Pharmaceutical Research*, Vol.12, No.6, pp. 916-922.

Pennica, D., Nedwin, GE., Hayflick, JS., Seeburg, PH., Derynck, R., Palladino, MA., Aggarwal, BB., & Goeddel, DV. (1984). Human tumor necrosis factor: precursor structure, cDNA cloning, expression and homology to lymphotoxin. *Nature*, Vol.312, No.5996, pp. 724-729.

Perry, AL. & Lambert, PA. (2006). Propionibacterium acnes. *Letters in Applied Microbiology*, Vol.42, No.3, pp. 185-188.

Puig, L., Barco, D., Vilarrasa, E., & Alomar, A. (2010). Treatment of acrodermatitis continua of Hallopeau with TNF-blocking agents: case report and review. *Dermatology*, Vol.220, No.2, pp. 154-158.

Rozin, AP. (2009). SAPHO syndrome: Is a range of pathogen-associated rheumatic disease extend? *Arthritis Research & Therapy*, Vol.11, No.6, 131. (doi:10.1186/ar2837), Available from http://arthritis-research.com/content/11/6/131

Ryan, C., Collins, P., Kirby, B., & Rogers, S. (2009). Treatment of acrodermatitis continua of Hallopeau with adalimumab. *The British Journal of Dermatology*, Vol.160, No.1, pp. 203-205.

Sabugo, F., Liberman, C., Niedmann, JP., Soto, L., & Cuchacovich, M. (2008). Infliximab can induce a prolonged clinical remission and a decrease in thyroid hormonal requirements in a patient with SAPHO syndrome and hypothyroidism. *Clinical Rheumatology*, Vol.27, No.4, pp. 533-535.

Seals, DF. & Courtneidge, SA. (2003). The ADAMs family of metalloproteases: multidomain proteins with multiple functions. *Genes and Development*, Vo.17, No.1, pp. 7-30.

Selby, PL., Young, MJ., & Boulton, AJ. (1994). Bisphosphonates: a new treatment for diabetic Charcot neuroarthropathy? *Diabetic Medicine*, Vol.11, No.1, pp. 28-31.

Siau, K. & Laversuch, CJ. (2010). SAPHO syndrome in an adult with ulcerative colitis responsive to intravenous pamidronate: a case report and review of the literature. *Rheumatology International*, Vol.30, No.8, pp. 1085-1088.

Sonozaki, H., Kawashima, M., Hongo, O., Yaoita, H., Ikeno, M., Matsuura, M., Okai, K., & Azuma, A. (1981). Incidence of arthro-osteitis in patients with pustulosis palmaris et plantaris. *Annals of the Rheumatic Disease*, Vol.40, No.6, pp. 554-557.

Takigawa, T., Tanaka, M., Nakanishi, K., Misawa, H., Sugimoto, Y., Takahata, T., Nakahara, H., Nakahara, S., & Ozaki, T. (2008). SAPHO syndrome associated spondylitis. *European Spine Journal*, Vol.17, No.10, pp. 1391-1397.

Tang, P., Hung, M-C., & Klostergaard, J. (1996). Human pro-tumor necrosis factor is a homotrimer. *Biochemistry*, Vol.35, No.25, pp. 8216-8225.

Thielen, AM., Barde, C., Marazza, G., & Saurat, JH. (2008). Long-term control with etanercept (Enbrel) of a severe acrodermatitis continua of Hallopeau refractory to infliximab (Remicade). *Dermatology*, Vol.217, No.2, pp. 137-139.

Tutrone, WD., Kagen, MH., Barbagallo, J., & Weinberg, JM. (2001). Biologic therapy for psoriasis: a brief history, II. *Cutis*, Vol.68, No.6, pp. 367-372.

Vandenabeele, P., Declercq, W., Beyaert, R., & Fiers, W. (1995). Two tumor necrosis factor receptors: structure and function. *Trends in Cell Biology*, Vol.5, No.10, pp. 392-399.

Wagner, AD., Andresen, J., Jendro, MC., Hulsemann, JL., & Zeidler, H. (2002). Sustained response to tumor necrosis factor alpha-blocking agents in two patients with SAPHO syndrome. *Arthritis and Rheumatism*, Vol.46, No.7, pp. 1965-1968.

Widmer, M., Weishaupt, D., Bruhlmann, P., Michel, BA., & Forster, A. (2003). Infliximab in the treatment of SAPHO syndrome: clinical experience and MRI response [abstract]. *Annals of the Rheumatic Diseases*, Vol.62, 250-1A.

Wollina, U., Hansel, G., Koch, A., Schonlebe, J., Kostler, E., & Haroske, G. (2008). Tumor necrosis factor-alpha inhibitor-induced psoriasis or psoriasiform exanthemata: first 120 cases from the literature including a series of six new patients. *American Journal of Clinical Dermatology*, Vol.9, No.1, pp. 1-14.

Yerushalmi, J., Grunwald, MH., Hallel-Halevy, D., Avinoach, I., & Halevy, S. (2000). Chronic pustular eruption of the thumbs. Diagnosis: acrodermatitis continua of Hallopeau (ACH). *Archives of Delmatology*, Vol.136, No.7, pp. 925-930.

5

The Role of Tocilizumab in the Treatment of Rheumatoid Arthritis

Yasuhiko Hirabayashi[1,2]
[1]*Hikarigaoka Spellman Hospital,*
[2]*Graduate School of Medicine, Tohoku University*
Japan

1. Introduction

The characteristic pathophysiology in rheumatoid arthritis (RA) is the destruction of bone and cartilage due to persistent synovitis of unknown etiology. Pro-inflammatory cytokines, including tumor necrosis factor alpha (TNFα), interleukin-1 (IL-1), and interleukin-6 (IL-6), are overproduced in inflamed synovial membranes, and are critically involved in the spread and persistence of the inflammation. IL-6, which was identified as a B-cell stimulatory factor in 1986, is a multifunctional cytokine (Hirano, 2010), and a key mediator in the pathological processes of RA, especially in the activation of immune cells and osteoclasts (Cronstein, 2007). For RA drug therapy, therefore, inhibition of IL-6 signaling is suitable for shutting down both inflammation and bone destruction. Tocilizumab (TCZ) is a humanized monoclonal antibody (human IgG_1 κ subclass) against IL-6 receptor (IL-6R). The data from the recent clinical studies on TCZ suggests that TCZ has several advantages over other anti-rheumatic drugs (Bergman et al., 2010).

2. Pharmacological properties

2.1 Pharmacodynamics

Human IL-6 binds to human IL-6 R with a dissociation constant (Kd) of 5.5 nM, and this low affinity complex subsequently recruits a gp130 molecule to form a high-affinity complex (IL-6/IL-6R/gp130 ternary complex) with a Kd of 50 pM (Hibi et al, 1990). TCZ binds selectively and competitively to both soluble IL-6R (sIL-6R) and membrane bound IL-6R (mIL-6R) with a Kd of 0.71 nM and 2.54 nM, respectively (Japan Pharmacists Education Center, 2008; Mihara et al., 2005). TCZ suppressed the binding of IL-6 (10 ng/mL) to sIL-6R in a dose dependent manner at of a concentration between 0.002 and 4 μg/mL and completely inhibited at concentrations of > 4 μg/mL. Moreover, TCZ was able to dissociate IL-6/sIL-6R preformed complex which was made by mixing IL-6 (200 ng/mL) and sIL-6R (40 ng/mL). The percentage binding of IL-6 to sIL-6R fell in a TCZ concentration-dependent manner, and was less than 10% of the binding seen in the presence of TCZ at concentrations of > 1 μg/mL. On the other hand, the binding of TCZ to sIL-6R rose in a concentration-dependent manner and reached a plateau at 0.1 μg/mL (Mihara et al., 2005). *In vitro,* 100 μg/mL of TCZ completely inhibited cell growth of IL-6 dependent KT-3 cells in the presence of up to 0.32 ng/mL IL-6. Cell growth inhibition by TCZ was dose-dependently decreased by IL-6 at concentrations of > 0.32 ng/mL, and no inhibition of cell growth by TCZ was observed in the presence of 1 μg/mL IL-6 (Australian Government, 2011). *In vivo*, serum levels of IL-6 and sIL-6R markedly increased after TCZ treatment in patients with RA. While free TCZ concentration remains 1 μg/mL or more, serum C-reactive protein (CRP) is normalized, indicating that sIL-6R is saturated with TCZ and IL-6 signaling is completely inhibited (Nishimoto et al., 2008).

2.2 Pharmacokinetic properties

PK data were based on a population PK analysis of 1793 patients with RA who received a 1 hour infusion of TCZ 8mg/kg every 4 weeks for 24 weeks (Frey et al., 2010). The $t_{1/2}$ of TCZ was concentration-dependent. The effective $t_{1/2}$ decreased with decreasing concentrations of TCZ within a dosing interval from 14 days to 8 days. After administration of TCZ, the predicted steady-state the mean area under the concentration-time curve (AUC), maximum concentration (C_{max}), the steady-state volume of distribution, and the trough concentration (C_{min}) values were 35.0 mg·h/mL, 183 μg/mL, 6.4 L, and 9.7 μg/mL, respectively. The Cmin value is 91 fold higher that the Kd of TCZ for the binding at the sIL-6R (Kd is 0.71 nM = 0.10 μg/ml). Therefore, IL-6R was completely occupied even at the end of each 8 mg/kg dosing interval in most of the patients. Age, gender and ethnicity did not affect the PK of TCZ.

TCZ is not excreted via the renal or biliary route. Instead, TCZ is predominantly eliminated via catabolism including degradation in plasma and distribution to tissues. TCZ undergoes biphasic elimination from the circulation. Total clearance is concentration dependent and includes linear at higher TCZ concentrations and non-linear clearance at low TCZ concentration. No formal studies on the effect of renal or hepatic impairment on the PK of TCZ have been conducted. Mild renal impairment (creatinine clearance based on Cockcroft-Gault < 80 ml/min and ≥ 50 ml/min) did not affect the PK of TCZ.

Nor is the clearance of TCZ affected by concomitant use of methotrexate (MTX), nonsteroidal anti-inflammatory drugs (NSAIDs), or corticosteroids. TCZ may normalize the expression of hepatic cytochrome P450 (CYP) isozymes which are suppressed by IL-6 (Oldfield et al., 2009). Therefore, administration or discontinuation of TCZ may affect the serum concentrations of drugs metabolized via CYP3A4, CYP1A2, CYP2C9 or CYP2C19 (e.g., omeprazole, dextromethorphan, atorvastatin, simvastatin, calcium channel blockers, cyclosporine, and warfarin).

3. Therapeutic efficacy

3.1 Clinical studies

In a 12-week, multicenter, randomized, double-blind, placebo-controlled phase I/II study, 164 Japanese patients with refractory RA were randomly administered either placebo, or 4 mg/kg or 8 mg/kg TCZ (Nishimoto et al., 2004). A dose-dependent reduction in the American College of Rheumatology (ACR) 20 response was observed. At 3 months, 78% of patients in the 8 mg/kg group, 57% in the 4 mg/kg group, and 11% in the placebo group achieved an ACR20 response. This study was extended to evaluate the long-term efficacy and safety of TCZ 8 mg/kg monotherapy for five years and designated STREAM (long-term Safety and efficacy of Tocilizumab, an anti-interleukin-6 REceptor monoclonal Antibody, in Monotherapy, in patients with rheumatoid arthritis) (Nishimoto et al., 2009a). A total 143 patients were enrolled, and 94 patients completed 5 years. At 5 years, 84.0%, 69.1%, and

43.6% of the patients achieved ACR20, ACR50, and ACR70 responses, respectively. Remission (the 28-joint disease activity score using erythrocyte sedimentation rate (DAS28ESR) <2.6) was achieved in 55.3% of the patients.

The CHARISMA (the Chugai Humanized Anti-human Recombinant Interleukin-Six Monoclonal Antibody) study was a 16-week, multicenter, randomized, double-blind, placebo-controlled phase II trial in 359 European patients in whom the response to MTX was inadequate (Maini et al., 2006). ACR20 response was achieved by 61% and 63% of patients receiving 4 mg/kg and 8 mg/kg of TCZ as monotherapy, respectively.

There are seven phase III studies (Table 1). SAMURAI (Study of Active controlled Monotherapy Used for Rheumatoid Arthritis, an Interleukin-6 inhibitor) was a randomized, 52-week, multicenter, x-ray reader-blinded, controlled phase III trial to evaluate the ability of TCZ monotherapy to inhibit progression of structural joint damage in patients with RA of <5 years' duration (Nishimoto et al., 2007). A total 306 Japanese patients were randomly assigned to two groups: (i) TCZ 8 mg/kg (n = 158) and (ii) conventional disease-modifying anti-rheumatic drug (DMARD) therapy (n = 148). At week 52, the TCZ group showed statistically less radiographic change in modified Total Sharp Score (mTSS) (mean 2.3) than the DMARD group (mean 6.1). The TCZ group also showed significantly better results than the DMARD group in ACR20, 50, and 70 responses, DAS28ESR, and Modified Health Assessment Questionnaire (MHAQ) scores.

	Population Size (n=)	Subject	Control arm	Primary endpoint	Duration
SAMURAI (Nishimoto et al., 2007)	refractory to DMARDs n=306	TCZ	DMARDs	ACR, DAS28ESR, mHAQ, and mTSS at week 52	52 w
SATORI (Nishimoto et al., 2009b)	refractory to MTX n=125	TCZ+ placebo	MTX+ placebo	ACR at week 24	24 w
RADIATE (Emery et al., 2008)	refractory to anti-TNFs n=498	MTX+ TCZ	MTX+ placebo	ACR at week 24	24 w
OPTION (Smolen et al., 2008)	refractory to MTX n=623	MTX+ TCZ	MTX+ placebo	ACR at week 24	24 w
TOWARD (Genovese et al., 2008)	refractory to DMARDs n=1220	DMARDs+ TCZ	DMARDs+ placebo	ACR at week 24	24 w
AMBITION (Jones et al., 2010)	MTX-naïve or MTX-free for ≥6 months n=673	TCZ	MTX	ACR at week 24	24 w
LITHE (Kremer et al., 2011)	refractory to MTX n=1196	MTX+ TCZ	MTX+ placebo	ACR at week 24; mTSS and HAQ at week 52	2 y

Table 1. Phase III trials of TCZ in patients with RA

SATORI (Study of Active controlled Tocilizumab mOnotherapy for Rheumatoid arthritis patients with an Inadequate response to metotrexate) was a 24-week, multicenter, randomized, double-blind, placebo-controlled phase III trial in patients with RA in whom the response to MTX was inadequate (Nishimoto et al., 2009b). A total 125 Japanese patients were randomly assigned to one of two groups: (i) TCZ 8 mg/kg plus MTX placebo (n = 61) and (ii) TCZ placebo plus MTX (n = 66). At week 24, 25.0% in the MTX group and 80.3% in the TCZ group achieved ACR20 response. Additionally, serum vascular endothelial growth factor (VEGF) levels were significantly decreased by TCZ treatment, but not by MTX treatment.

RADIATE (Research on Actemra Determining efflcacy after Anti-TNF failurEs) was a 24-week, multicenter, randomized, double-blind, placebo-controlled, parallel-group phase III trial to evaluate the efficacy and safety of TCZ in patients with active RA refractory to TNF antagonist therapy (Emery et al., 2008). A total 498 US and Western Europe patients were randomly assigned to three groups: (i) TCZ 8 mg/kg plus MTX (n = 175), (ii) TCZ 4 mg/kg (n = 163) plus MTX, and (iii) TCZ placebo plus MTX (n = 160). ACR20 was achieved at 24 weeks by 50.0%, 30.4% and 10.1% of patients in the 8 mg/kg, 4 mg/kg and control groups, respectively. Patients responded regardless of most recently failed anti-TNF or the number of failed treatments.

OPTION (tOcilizumab Pivotal Trial in methotrexate Inadequate respONders) was a 24-week, multicenter, randomized, double-blind, placebo-controlled phase III trial in patients with active RA in whom the response to MTX was inadequate (Smolen et al., 2008). A total 623 patients from 17 countries were randomly assigned to three groups: (i) TCZ 8 mg/kg plus MTX (n = 205), (ii) TCZ 4 mg/kg (n = 214) plus MTX, and (iii) placebo plus MTX (n = 204). ACR20 achieved at 24 weeks by 59%, 48%, and 26% of patients in the 8 mg/kg, 4 mg/kg and control groups, respectively. Significantly greater numbers of patients receiving TCZ showed ACR50/ACR70 responses or clinical remission (DAS28ESR <2.6) at week 24 than did those receiving placebo. In patients receiving TCZ, there were greater improvements in HAQ-DI score, the Short-Form 36 Health Survey (SF-36), and Functional Assessment of Chronic Illness Therapy (FACIT)-Fatigue assessment indicating that TCZ treatment significantly improves physical and mental function.

TOWARD (Tocilizumab in cOmbination With traditional DMARD therapy) was a 24-week, multicenter, randomized, double-blind, placebo-controlled phase III trial to evaluate the efficacy and safety of TCZ combined with conventional DMARDs in patients with active RA (Genovese et al., 2008). A total 1220 patients from 18 countries were randomly assigned to two groups: (i) TCZ 8 mg/kg plus DMARD (n = 805) and (ii) TCZ placebo plus DMARD therapy (n = 415). ACR20 achieved at 24 weeks 61% for TCZ 8 mg/kg versus 25% for placebo. Similar to the results of OPTION, the TCZ group showed significantly better results than the placebo group in ACR50/ACR70 response, clinical remission rate (DAS28ESR <2.6), HAQ-DI, SF-36 and FACIT-Fatigue assessment.

AMBITION (Actemra versus Methotrexate double-Blind Investigative Trial In mONotherapy) was a 24-week, multicenter, randomized, double-blind, double-dummy, placebo-controlled phase III trial evaluating the efficacy and safety of TCZ monotherapy versus MTX in patients with active RA (Jones et al., 2010). A total of 673 patients from the US, Canada, and Israel were randomly assigned to three groups: (i) MTX (escalating dose regimen: initial dose 7.5 mg/week, increasing to 15 mg/week at week 4 and 20 mg/week at week 8) for 24 weeks (n = 284), (ii) TCZ 8 mg/kg for 24 weeks (n = 288), and (iii) TCZ placebo for 8 weeks then TCZ 8 mg/kg for 16 weeks (n = 101). The intention-to-treat analysis demonstrated that TCZ was better than MTX treatment with a higher ACR20 response (69.9 vs 52.5%; $p<0.001$) and rate of DAS28ESR <2.6 (33.6 vs 12.1%) at week 24. The superiority of TCZ to MTX was observed in the intention-to-treat population from week 2 and throughout this study. The proportion of ACR50 (44%) and ACR70 (28%) responders at week 24 was also statistically superior for TCZ compared with MTX (weighted difference between treatments: 0.12 for ACR50 (95% confidence interval (CI) 0.04 to 0.20; $p = 0.002$); and 0.14 for ACR70 (95% CI 0.07 to 0.22; $p<0.001$). The superiority of TCZ to MTX was also shown in improvement of HAQ-DI at week 24. No significant difference was seen in the incidence of serious adverse events between TCZ treatment (3.8%) and MTX treatment (2.8%) ($p = 0.50$).

LITHE (tociLIzumab safety and THE prevention of structural joint damage) is a 2 (or 3)-year, multicenter, randomized, double-blind, placebo-controlled phase III trial evaluating the ability of TCZ add-on therapy to inhibit progression of structural joint damage and improve physical function in patients with moderate to severe RA who respond inadequately to MTX. A total of 1196 patients from 14 countries were randomly assigned to three groups: (i) placebo plus MTX (n = 393), (ii) TCZ 4 mg/kg plus MTX (n = 399), and (iii) TCZ 8 mg/kg plus MTX (n = 398). Results from year 1 were reported (Kremer et al., 2011). Mean change in the total Genant-modified Sharp score was 0.29 and 0.34 with TCZ 8 mg/kg plus MTX and 4 mg/kg plus MTX, respectively, versus 1.13 with placebo plus MTX ($P <0.0001$). Additionally, the HAQ-DI significantly decreased in the groups of TCZ (8 mg/kg and 4 mg/kg) add-on treatment compared with the group with placebo plus MTX.

3.2 Additional remarks

MTX has the highest efficacy among conventional DMARDs and has been used as an anchor drug in the treatment of RA. The AMBITION study and the SATORI study demonstrated that TCZ monotherapy is superior to MTX monotherapy. Several studies have demonstrated that MTX monotherapy is equivalent or superior to TNF inhibitor monotherapy (Donahue et al., 2008). Comparison of TCZ with abatacept demonstrated that the rate of withdrawal due to no effect in TCZ treatment was lower than that in abatacept treatment (Leffers et al., 2011). A meta-analysis revealed that the effectiveness of TCZ appeared to be greater for ACR70 (Bergman et al., 2010). Thus, TCZ is superior to MTX, TNF inhibitors, and abatacept in the case of monotherapy. The superiority between TCZ monotherapy and TCZ plus MTX treatment has not yet been established. Yamanaka et al. (2011) reported that the improvement of DAS28ESR and HAQ-DI in TCZ plus MTX treatment was better than that in TCZ monotherapy. Nakashima et al. (2010) reported that there was no significant difference in the improvement of DAS28ESR between TCZ monotherapy and TCZ plus MTX treatment. Data from the ACT-RAY study demonstrated that TCZ provided clinical benefit, regardless of whether it was given in combination with MTX or as a monotherapy (Dougados et al., 2011).

4. Safety and tolerability

Infections are the most frequent adverse events during therapy with TCZ and other biologics or DMARDs. In the AMBITION study, TCZ monotherapy was compared with MTX monotherapy (Jones et al., 2010). Infection rates per patient year were similar (TCZ 1.06 vs MTX 1.09). In both groups, nasopharyngitis and upper respiratory tract infection were common. The common serious infections were pneumonia. Neither opportunistic infections nor tuberculosis were reported in the patients receiving TCZ. Similar results were observed in a meta-analysis of TCZ monotherapy in Japanese patients (Nishimoto et al., 2010). Long-term exposure did not increase the incidence of serious infections. TCZ may not increase the risk of de novo infection of tuberculosis. TCZ did not affect the humoral response to influenza vaccination (Tsuru et al., 2008).

Infusion reactions (any adverse event occurring during, or within 24 h after infusion) occurred in 5.6% of patients with TCZ (Jones et al., 2010). The majority occurred during the first two infusions, and no serious infusion reactions were reported. In the meta-analysis of TCZ monotherapy, total 133 infusion reactions were observed in 93 patients (Nishimoto et al., 2010). Most of them occurred within the first four infusions. Headache, increased blood pressure, and pruritus were common. Anaphylactic reactions were observed in 3 patients.

In worldwide Roche clinical trials, the rate of malignancies in patients receiving TCZ was 11.6 events per 1000 patient-years while the rate in the patients receiving synthetic DMARDs was 17.7 events per 1000 patient-years (van Vollenhoven et al., 2010). As it usually takes several years before a malignant neoplasm grows to be clinically recognized after the appearance of the first malignant cell, TCZ may not have been involved in the carcinogenesis of the malignancies found during TCZ treatment to date.

Decreases in the neutrophil count were commonly observed in patients receiving TCZ. In the meta-analysis of TCZ monotherapy, grade 2 (<1500–1000/μL) and grade 3 neutropenia (<1000–500/μL) were observed in 92 (15.3%) and 36 patients (6.0%), respectively (Nishimoto et al., 2010). However, the decreases were not progressive, and neither febrile neutropenia nor agranulocytosis occurred. There was no obvious association between decreases in neutrophils and the occurrence infections. Decreases in the neutrophil are probably due to inhibition of the biological effects of IL-6 on recruitment of neutrophils into peripheral blood, not due to myelosuppression. Transient or intermittent elevations of alanine aminotransferase (ALT) or aspartate aminotransferase (AST) have often been observed in patients receiving TCZ. The incidence of elevations of AST or ALT in patients treated with TCZ monotherapy was no more than that in patients treated with MTX monotherapy (Jones et al., 2010). Prolonged exposure to TCZ therapy did not appear to be associated with an increased likelihood of developing increases in ALT or AST because the numbers of patients developing increased ALT or AST values was highest in the first 6 months of treatment (Australian Government, 2011). Mean total cholesterol (T-cho) rose upon treatment with TCZ, but showed no continuous increase. As high-density lipoprotein (HDL) also increased, the atherogenic index [(T-cho – HDL)/HDL] did not change. Small low-density lipoprotein (LDL), which may be proatherogenic, did not increase with TCZ treatment while both large very low density lipoprotein (VLDL) and small HDL increases were observed (McInnes et al., 2010). Inhibition IL-6 signaling decreases lipoprotein A serum levels which correlate with coronary heart disease (Schultz et al., 2010; Daneshet al., 2000). Treatment with TCZ may not increase the risk of cardiovascular disease.

Gastrointestinal (GI) perforation occurred in 26 cases out of 4009 patients treated with TCZ in worldwide Roche clinical trials (van Vollenhoven et al., 2009). The rate of GI perforations was 2.8 events per 1000 patient-years with TCZ therapy while the rate in patients with RA who were exposed to corticosteroids was 3.9 events per 1000 patient-years. The majority of the patients who experienced GI perforations treated with TCZ were also receiving corticosteroids, NSAIDS, and MTX. GI perforations occur mainly in lower GI tract, and 16 of the 18 patients with colonic perforations had diverticulitis. Prevention of constipation is important not only to reduce the incidence of colonic perforations but also to improve quality of life. A case of multiple ulcers in the small and large intestines during TCZ therapy has been reported (Iwasa et al., 2011). In mice, Il-6 signal is necessary for the development of lamina propria T_H17 cells which may play a role in the maintenance of intestinal mucosal homeostasis (Atarashi et al., 2008). A causal relationship between TCZ and gastrointestinal perforation/ulceration should be addressed in future studies.

Experience with TCZ use in human pregnancy is very limited. Thirty-three pregnancies were reported in 32 patients (19 to 42 years) (Rubbert-Roth et al., 2010). Of the 32 patients, 26 received TCZ + MTX and 6 received TCZ monotherapy or TCZ + DMARD other than MTX. In patients who continued their pregnancies, TCZ and MTX were discontinued when the pregnancy was discovered. Of 11 term deliveries (2 received TCZ monotherapy, 9 received TCZ + MTX), 10 were of healthy newborns. One infant died of ARDS 3 days after emergency cesarean section. It is difficult to evaluate the safety of TCZ during pregnancy from the current data.

In conclusion, clinical trials demonstrated that TCZ was generally well tolerated in patients with active RA. The incidence of adverse events of TCZ monotherapy is no more than that of MTX monotherapy. Also, the risk of adverse events is comparable with that of other biologics and the risk of serious infection may be less than that for TNF inhibitors (Campbell et al, 2011). There was no increase in the frequency of adverse events with long-term treatment with TCZ (Nishimoto et al., 2010).

5. The advantages, and potential advantages, of TCZ

5.1 Synovitis

The characteristic pathophysiology of RA is the destruction of bone and cartilage due to "persistent" synovitis; however, the mechanism of this "persistence" is not yet clear. It is reported that an IL-17A-triggered positive-feedback loop of IL-6 expression is present in fibroblasts (Ogura et al., 2008). Moreover, IL-6 stimulates megakaryocytes to increase platelet counts and induces platelet activation (Oleksowicz et al., 1994; Kaser et al., 2009), while platelet-derived microparticles in turn prominently elicit IL-6, not TNF, from synovial fibroblasts (Boilard et al., 2010). These phenomena may be involved in "persistent" inflammation. TCZ is the only drug that can directly cut these positive-feedback loops.

5.2 Insulin resistance

IL-6 is involved in the pathology of type II diabetes mellitus related insulin resistance (Fève & Bastard, 2009). The expression of IL-6 was markedly increased (up to 15-fold) in human fat cells from insulin-resistant individuals (Rotter et al., 2003). Inhibition of IL-6 signaling affects insulin resistance in a positive way (Schultz et al, 2010). A significant decrease of HbA1c was observed at only 1 month after TCZ treatment (Ogata et al., 2011a). Thus, TCZ may help to resolve insulin RA patients.

5.3 Malignancies

TCZ was originally planned as an anti-myeloma drug because TCZ suppressed growth of the IL-6-dependent myeloma cell line, KPMM2 (Mihara et al., 2005). In fact, in an RA patient with IgA-kappa type multiple myeloma, TCZ not only improved RA symptoms dramatically but also stabilized serum IgA levels for 13 months (Matsuyama et al,. 2011). TCZ decreases the serum levels of VEGF (Nishimoto et al., 2009b). This effect may interfere with the angiogenesis and growth of tumors. For example, the antitumor effect of TCZ for oral squamous cell carcinoma has been reported (Shinriki et al., 2009). Targeting of the IL-6 system may be beneficial in the treatment of malignancies (Hong et al., 2007).

5.4 Mycobacterium infection

The TNFα -/- mice or the IL-6 -/- mice demonstrated that TNF is critical for initiation of the granulomatous response, and IL-6 plays a key role in the granuloma maintenance response (Welsh et al., 2008). Unlike Il-6 -/- mice, TCZ does not completely inactivate the IL-6 system because TCZ works as a competitive inhibitor of IL-6. Moreover, TCZ, unlike TNF inhibitors, does not inhibit *M. tuberculosis* antigen-induced interferon gamma (IFN-γ) production (Ogata et al., 2010b). TNF inhibitors increase the risk of infection or reactivation of *M. tuberculosis* while TCZ does not in clinical practice. Of course, TCZ should not be used in the patients with active mycobacterium infection. However, TCZ may be a candidate for intractable RA patients with mycobacterium infection which is treated. A patient with intractable RA was treated with TCZ without aggravation of *M. avium* infection which had been treated in advance (Nakahara et al., 2010).

5.5 Anemia

IL-6 increases the production of hepcidin, which is an iron-regulatory peptide secreted from liver cells, inhibits the signal transduction of erythropoietin, and causes anemia (Ganz and Nemeth 2009). Therefore, inhibition of IL-6 signaling by TCZ significantly improves anemia caused by chronic inflammation and benefits patients'general physical condition (Song et al., 2010).

5.6 Amyloidosis

Secondary amyloidosis is a life-threatening complication of RA. Mortality, amyloid burden, and renal prognosis significantly correlate with serum amyloid A (SAA) concentration. As amyloid deposits regressed in 60% of patients who had a median SAA concentration of less than 10 μg/ml, normalization of the SAA concentration not only prevents but also treats secondary amyloidosis (Lachmann et al., 2007). TCZ treatment almost completely normalizes the serum SAA level because IL-6 signal is essential for the expression of SAA (Hagihara et al., 2005). Therefore, TCZ is very useful for the treatment of secondary amyloidosis (Sato et al., 2009; Inoue et al., 2010).

5.7 Osteoporosis

IL-6 levels are significantly higher (30 to 1000-fold) in synovial fluid than in sera (Desgeorges et al., 1997), and IL-6 drives osteoclastgenesis (Le Goff et al., 2010). Since osteoclasts are primarily involved in bone resorption, reduction in their number would be anticipated to reduce bone loss. This expectation is supported by the results of Axmann et al (2009) who demonstrated that blockade of IL-6R dose dependently decreased the joint osteoclast count and the number of bone erosions. They concluded that the mechanism for this effect was that blockade of IL-6R negatively affects osteoclast differentiation (Axmann et al., 2009).

6. Improving clinical outcomes

6.1 Strategies for improving clinical outcomes

The response rate and the speed of improvement basically depend on the ratio between the target cytokine and the biological agent which traps the target cytokine. To lessen the amount of the target cytokine, it is very important that any comorbidity (e.g., infectious diseases, lifestyle diseases, etc.) is treated or controlled as well as possible before and during administration of biological agents. This not only stops stimulation of the production of inflammatory cytokines from factors other than RA, but also serves to reduce adverse events, which results in better efficacy and safety. This also directly improves physical function irrespective of disease activity (Radner et al., 2010).

The standard dosage of TCZ for the treatment of RA is 8 mg/kg every 4 weeks. The serum TCZ concentrations 4 weeks after 3 doses are greater than 1 mg/mL, which is an effective dose, in about 80% of patients. However, this means that the serum TCZ concentrations are not sufficiently high in approximately 20% of patients. In these patients, increasing the dosage of TCZ and/or shortening the dosage interval may improve efficacy. Indeed, during clinical trials, it was observed that arthritis improved following the first dose but returned after 3 weeks in several patients. This suggested that the blood level could not be maintained over the 4-week period. I thus decided to give the second dose after an interval of 3 weeks following the first. By doing this, none of the patients suffered repeat deterioration by the time of the second dose in symptoms that had improved following the first, and no additive adverse effects were observed. A shorter dose interval at the start may be thought to be perfectly reasonable in terms of maintaining blood levels of biologics. In practice, this administration method is used for infliximab and abatacept.

6.2 Clinical efficacy and safety in our experience

6.2.1 Patients

The subjects of this analysis were patients who met the 1987 revised criteria for the classification of RA from ACR. Patients were included in the analysis if they started treatment with TCZ for the first time after 16 April 2008 (the date of insurance approval in Japan) (Table 2). This is an extension of a previous study (Hirabayashi et al, 2010). Data were collected until 20 March 2010. More than 23 and 51 weeks had elapsed since the first administration of TCZ in all 101 and in 70 patients, respectively. To reduce adverse events, any comorbidity was treated or controlled as well as possible before giving TCZ. All patients had a thoracic CT scan and were tested for the tuberculin reaction (or QuantiFERON ®), anti-streptolysin O (ASO), anti-streptokinase (ASK), treponema pallidum haemagglutination (TPHA), hepatitis B surface antigen (and anti-hepatitis B core antigen antibody), anti-hepatitis C virus antibody, and β-D-glucan in order to screen for infections. If tooth plaque or caries were present, I arranged for assessment and treatment by a dentist. If chronic rhinorrhea or nasal blockage was seen, the patient was assessed and treated by an otolaryngologist. Patients were asked whether they had hemorrhoids. Patients were required to abstain from smoking.

Among the various therapies being used by the patients in the three months before they received TCZ, infliximab was discontinued at least one month before, adalimumab at least one week before, and etanercept at least 4 days before the new treatment commenced. Salazosulfapyridine, bucillamine, sodium aurothiomalate and mizoribine were discontinued upon initiating TCZ. The patients continued on MTX, tacrolimus and steroids at the same dose levels as before at least until dose 3 of TCZ. Then, MTX and tacrolimus were tapered off until 6 months after. The steroid dose was decreased slowly to avoid steroid withdrawal syndrome. There were no users of auranofin, D-penicillamine, hydroxychloroquine, minocycline or lobenzarit disodium.

Patient Characteristics	
Age, mean ± SD, median (min - max), years	60.6 ± 12.7, 61 (23 – 82)
Male : Female	20 : 81
Duration of disease, mean, years	11.3
Steinbrocker Class (I, II, III, IV) : Stage (I, II, III, IV)	37, 49, 15, 0 : 16, 19, 15, 53
DAS28ESR, mean ± SE	4.60 ± 0.12
Previous medications	No. of patients treated
Prednisolone	71 (mean dosage: 3.9 mg/day)
TNF inhibitors (IFX, ETA, ADA)	11 (8, 2, 1)
MTX	38
Tacrolimus	11
Other DMARDs	48
No DMARDs for 3 months prior to TCZ treatment	20

Table 2. Patient demographics, clinical characteristics, and previous medications at baseline. SD: standard deviation. SE: standard error. 'Previous medications' denotes drugs used in the 3 months before administration of TCZ. IFX: Infliximab, ETA: etanercept, ADA: adalimumab. 'Other DMARDS' were sodium aurothiomalate, bucillamine, salazosulfapyridine, and mizoribine.

6.2.2 Clinical efficacy

The mean DAS28ESR at the start of TCZ treatment in all 101 patients was 4.60 ± 0.12 (mean ± standard error of the mean (SEM)). Mean DAS28ESR had fallen below the remission threshold (<2.6) to 2.20 ± 0.10 after two doses and had further improved to 1.61 ± 0.08 at 23 weeks (intention-to-treat with last observation carried forward (ITT-LOCF)) and 1.50 ± 0.09 at 51 weeks (ITT-LOCF). The clinical response was evaluated using the European League Against Rheumatism (EULAR) response criteria. At 51 weeks (ITT-LOCF), 64 out of 70 patients (91.4%) had achieved remission with treatment response of good in 91.4%, moderate in 7.1% and one case of no response. The no response seen beyond five doses was due to a rise in DAS28ESR associated with a temporary deterioration in symptoms due to factors other than RA and did not represent secondary non-response. To date, no patient has discontinued the treatment due to lack of response.

Next, the patients were classified based on DAS28ESR into a high-activity group at >5.1, a moderate-activity group at 3.2-5.1 and a low-activity group at <3.2. Although mean DAS28ESR had been 5.84 ± 0.13 (n=36) in the high-activity group before treatment with TCZ, this improved rapidly to below the remission threshold to 2.31 ± 0.20 after 3 doses (after 11-12 weeks; Fig. 1a). Mean DAS28ESR further improved to 1.92 ± 0.15 at 23 weeks and 1.66 ± 0.17 at 51 weeks. TCZ proved to be very effective regardless of baseline disease activity. Also, patients were classified based on disease duration into three groups (≥10 years, 2≤~<10, <2). Although mean DAS28ESR had been 4.57 ± 0.21 (n=30) in the ≥10 years group before treatment, this improved rapidly to below the remission threshold to 2.30 ± 0.17 after 2 doses (after 7 weeks; Fig. 1b). Mean DAS28ESR further improved to 1.60 ± 0.14 at 51 weeks. TCZ proved to be effective regardless of disease duration. However, in the ≥10 years group, the number of swelling joints rapidly decreased while the number of joints with tenderness decreased slowly, indicating that inflammation had subsided rapidly but that tenderness at the damaged joints was prolonged.

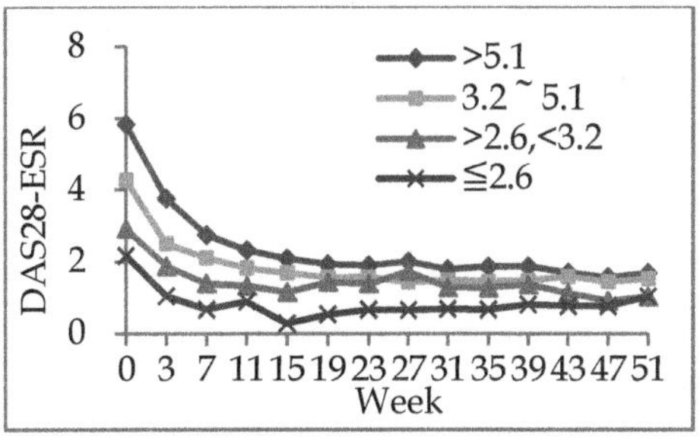

a

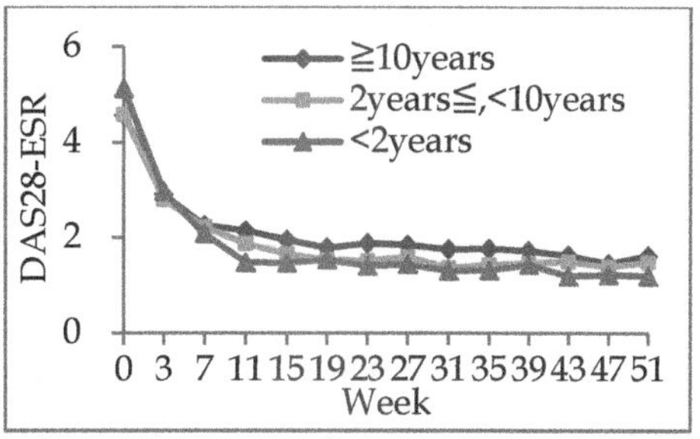

b

Fig. 1. Change in DAS28ESR by disease activity at baseline (a) and by duration of disease (b). Mean values shown. The criteria for exclusion from the analysis set were as follows: (i) autoimmune disease comorbidities except Sjögren's syndrome and Hashimoto's disease, (ii) functional class IV based on the Steinbrocker criteria, (iii) presence of active infection, (iv) pregnancy, (v) drug poisoning, including alcohol, (vi) lymphocyte count £ 500 cells/mL, and (vii) positive serum β-D-glucan. The method of administering TCZ that has received insurance approval in Japan is continuous infusion of a dose of 8 mg/kg over a period of at least 1 hour once every 4 weeks. The interval between infusions was shortened to 3 weeks between the first and second infusions only, and an interval of 4 ± 1 weeks was used thereafter. Treatment was continued unless there were adverse events requiring discontinuation or the patient requested that treatment be stopped.

6.2.3 Safety

A total of 72 adverse events occurred in 64 of the 101 patients and these are listed in Table 3. The adverse events seen during infusion were transient bone pain (back pain, lumbar discomfort and ischial pain). These all appeared a few minutes into infusion and disappeared within a few minutes. Infections were the most frequent adverse events. Nasopharyngitis (common cold) was most frequent among the infections; however, the frequency was similar to that in normal individuals. A total of 10 serious adverse events requiring hospitalization occurred in 8 patients. Three patients developed pneumonia. A 60-year-old woman with old tuberculosis and bronchiectasis as comorbidities showed a slight rise over her previous level of hemosputum, and bacterial pneumonia appeared subsequently. An 80-year-old woman was suspected of having pneumonia due to *Chlamydia pneumoniae*. Both recovered with treatment. A 67-year-old man developed *pneumocystis carinii* pneumonia followed by cytomegalovirus pneumonia and died. MTX was administrated concurrently to only this person due to scleritis suggesting vasculitis. A 68-year-old man had chronic pancreatitis as a comorbidity with several episodes of acute exacerbations before exposure to TCZ. He died of an acute exacerbation of chronic pancreatitis. One patient who died due to cerebellar infarction was elderly, at 82 years of age, and had once suffered strokes in the past. A patient with malignant lymphoma discovered as a left axillary mass underwent PET-CT scan to assess the activity of interstitial pneumonia before being treated with TCZ. Accumulation was picked up in the left axillary lymph nodes. Tiny lymphadenopathy was found at the same site by CT scan. Retrospectively, it may be inferred that the accumulation seen by PET had been the early stages of malignant lymphoma. A patient who had developed colitis probably due to viral infection recovered quickly.

PT (MedDRA Ver13.0)	a	b
Adverse drug reactions		
Bone pain	2	5
Total	2	5
Events possibly related to TCZ		
Nasopharyngitis	13	15
Sinusitis	4	4
Pneumonia*	1	2
Cystitis	3	3
Periodontitis	2	2
Otitis media	3	3
Paronychia	1	1
Infection	1	1
Bronchitis	1	2
Pneumocystis jiroveci Pneumonia*	1	1
Gastroenteritis	1	1
Pneumonia chlamydial*	1	1
Herpes zoster	1	1
Total	33	37

	a	b
Events hardly related to TCZ		
Rhinitis allergic	2	2
Diarrhoea	3	3
Haemorrhoids	2	2
Rash	2	2
Conjunctivitis allergic	1	1
Abdominal pain upper	1	1
Platelet count decreased	1	1
Asthma	1	1
Ileus	1	1
Pancreatitis acute*	1	2
Cough	1	1
Colitis*	1	1
Dizziness	1	1
Total	18	19
Events unrelated to TCZ		
Liver disorder	3	3
WBC count decreased	1	1
Lymphoma*	1	1
Cerebral infarction*	2	2
Hypoglossal nerve disorder	1	1
Toxic skin eruption	1	1
Bowen's disease	1	1
Compression fracture	1	1
Total	11	11

Table 3. Adverse events. *serious adverse events requiring hospitalization, a: No. of patients, b: No. of events. WBC: white blood cell.

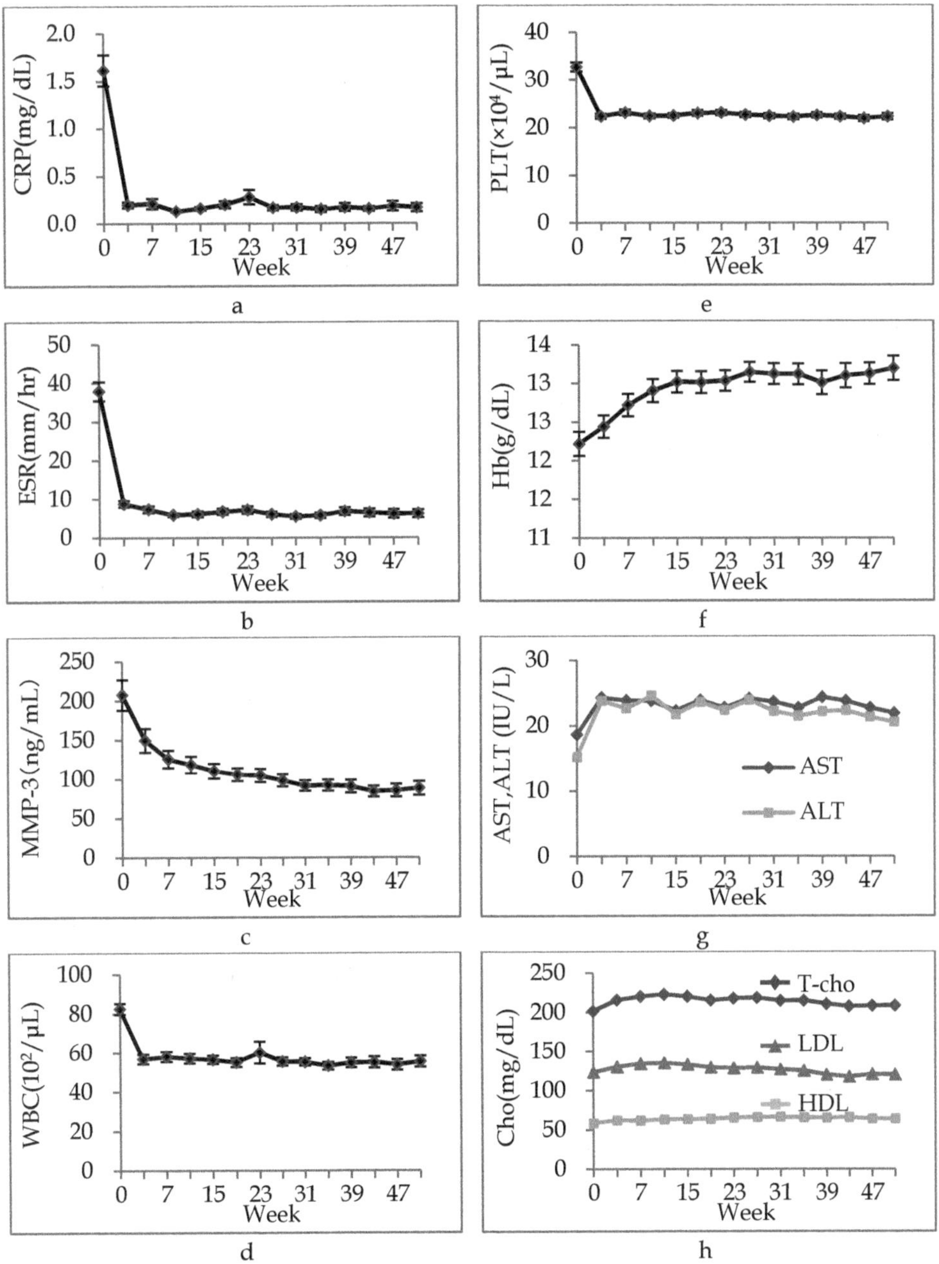

Fig. 2. Change in laboratory findings. a: CRP, b: ESR. c: MMP-3, d: WBC, e: PLT, f: Hb, g: AST and ALT, h: T-cho, HDL, and LDL. Mean values shown. Bars indicate SE.

Changes in laboratory findings are shown in figure 2. CRP virtually normalized in all patients after the first dose of TCZ (1.61 ± 0.16 → 0.20 ± 0.03 mg/dL) (Fig. 2a). Erythrocyte sedimentation rate (ESR) likewise normalized quickly after the first dose (37.9 ± 2.47 → 8.8 ± 0.85 mm/h) (Fig. 2b). Both followed a normal course afterwards as well. The level of matrix metalloproteinase-3 (MMP-3) gradually decreased from 207.7 ng/ml at baseline to 88.4 ± 8.79 ng/ml at 51 weeks (Fig. 2c). The mean leukocyte count was 8260 ± 278 /mL at baseline; however, this decreased to approximately 5500 /mL after the first dose. There was no progressive fall as seen in myelosuppression and no significant increase in infections (Fig. 2d). Likewise, the mean platelet count of 328000 ± 9100 /mL at baseline decreased to approximately 220000 /mL after the first dose (Fig.2e). The hemoglobin (Hb) level rose gradually and anemia improved after treatment with TCZ began (Fig. 2f). Figure 2g shows changes over time in AST and ALT as an index of liver function. Even though abnormal values for AST or ALT were seen, these were transient and all were of grade I based on the National Cancer Institute Common Toxicity Criteria. Mean total T-cho at baseline was 201.7 ± 3.46 mg/dL. Upon treatment with TCZ, it rose to approximately 220 mg/dL and then decreased to 210 mg/dL (Fig. 2h). I provided lifestyle guidance and monitored the clinical course without administering drug treatment at least until dose 3. Several patients whose level nevertheless exceeded 280 mg/dL were treated with a HMG-CoA reductase inhibitor. HDL and LDL at baseline were 58.4 ± 1.55 mg/dL and 123.5 ± 3.08 mg/dL, respectively. HDL rose to approximately 65 mg/dL. LDL transiently rose to approximately 130 mg/dL but returned to baseline thereafter (Fig. 2h). I encountered no laboratory test abnormalities so severe that treatment with TCZ could not continue. TCZ was generally well tolerated, as was observed in clinical trials.

7. Impact of TCZ on the treatment strategy for rheumatoid arthritis

Examination by MRI of RA patients has revealed that in approximately half of the patients, bone destruction in joints had begun within 4 months of the onset of inflammation (McQueen et al., 1998). It is, therefore, important to achieve remission within 4 months of the onset of RA to reduce the chances of bone destruction. In treatment with the conventional DMRADs including MTX and with TNF inhibitors, patients who do not respond or who show insufficient response are often encountered. In these patients, bone destruction often progresses whilst disease activity remains uncontrolled. Medically, there is no reason why MTX or TNF inhibitors must be used initially. Therefore, to achieve tight control, and to reduce the number of such unfortunate patients, TCZ monotherapy is recommended from the beginning in new onset patients because it shows high efficacy and response rates. After tight control is achieved, how long to continue TCZ treatment and what treatment to use after completion of TCZ treatment are topics for future study.

8. References

Atarashi, K, Nishimura, J, Shima, T, Umesaki, Y, Yamamoto, M, Onoue, M, Yagita, H, Ishii, N, Evans, R, Honda, K, & Takeda, K. (2008). ATP drives lamina propria $T_{(H)}17$ cell differentiation. *Nature*, Vol. 455, No. 7214, pp. 808-812, ISSN 0028-0836

Australian Government Department of Health and Ageing. (2011). Australian Public Assessment Report for Tocilizumab. pp. 1-107

Axmann, R, Böhm, C, Krönke, G, Zwerina, J, Smolen, J, & Schett, G. (2009). Inhibition of interleukin-6 receptor directly blocks osteoclast formation in vitro and in vivo. *Arthritis and Rheumatism*, Vol. 60, No. 9, pp. 2747-2756, ISSN 0004-3591

Bergman, G.J, Hochberg, M.C, Boers, M, Wintfeld, N, Kielhorn, A, & Jansen, J.P. (2010). Indirect comparison of tocilizumab and other biologic agents in patients with rheumatoid arthritis and inadequate response to disease-modifying antirheumatic drugs. *Seminars in Arthritis and Rheumatism*, Vol. 39, No. 6, pp. 425-441, ISSN 0049-0172

Boilard, E, Nigrovic, P.A, Larabee, K, Watts, G.F, Coblyn, J.S, Weinblatt, M.E, Massarotti, E.M, Remold-O'Donnell, E, Farndale, R.W, Ware, J, & Lee, D.M. (2010). Platelets amplify inflammation in arthritis via collagen-dependent microparticle production. *Science*, Vol. 327, No. 5965, pp. 580-583, ISSN 0036-8075

Campbell, L, Chen, C, Bhagat, S.S, Parker, R.A, & Östör, A.J. (2011). Risk of adverse events including serious infections in rheumatoid arthritis patients treated with tocilizumab: a systematic literature review and meta-analysis of randomized controlled trials. *Rheumatology (Oxford, England)*, Vol. 50, No. 3, pp. 552-562, ISSN 1462-0324

Cronstein, B.N. (2007). Interleukin-6--a key mediator of systemic and local symptoms in rheumatoid arthritis. *Bulletin of the NYU Hospital for Joint Diseases*, Vol. 65 Suppl 1, pp. S11-S15, ISSN 1936-9719

Danesh, J, Collins, R, & Peto, R. (2000). Lipoprotein(a) and coronary heart disease. Meta-analysis of prospective studies. *Circulation*, Vol. 102, No. 10, pp. 1082-1085, ISSN 0009-7322

Desgeorges, A, Gabay, C, Silacci, P, Novick, D, Roux-Lombard, P, Grau, G, Dayer, J.M, Vischer, T, & Guerne, P.A. (1997). Concentrations and origins of soluble interleukin 6 receptor-alpha in serum and synovial fluid. *Journal of Rheumatology*, Vol. 24, No. 8, pp. 1510-1516, ISSN 0315-162X

Donahue, K.E, Gartlehner, G, Jonas, D.E, Lux, L.J, Thieda, P, Jonas, B.L, Hansen, R.A, Morgan, L.C, & Lohr, K.N. (2008). Systematic review: comparative effectiveness and harms of disease-modifying medications for rheumatoid arthritis. *Annals of Internal Medicine*, Vol. 148, No. 2, pp. 124-134, ISSN 0003-4819

Dougados, M, Huizinga, T, Sheeran, T, Tak, P, Conaghan, P, Navarro-Sarabia, F, Hou, A, Bernasconi, C, & Kissei, K. (2011). Tocilizumab (TCZ) plus methotrexate (MTX) does not have superior clinical efficacy to TCZ alone in RA patients with inadequate response to MTX: 24-week results of the ACT-RAY study. *Annals of the Rheumatic Diseases*, Vol. 70, No. Suppl 3, pp. 73, ISSN 0003-4967

Emery, P, Keystone, E, Tony, H.P, Cantagrel, A, van Vollenhoven, R, Sanchez, A, Alecock, E, Lee, J, & Kremer, J. (2008). IL-6 receptor inhibition with tocilizumab improves treatment outcomes in patients with rheumatoid arthritis refractory to anti-tumour necrosis factor biologicals: results from a 24-week multicentre randomised placebo-controlled trial. *Annals of the Rheumatic Diseases*, Vol. 67, No. 11, pp. 1516-1523, ISSN 0003-4967

Fève, B & Bastard, J.P. (2009). The role of interleukins in insulin resistance and type 2 diabetes mellitus. *Nature Reviews Endocrinology*, Vol. 5, No. 6, pp. 305-311, ISSN 1759-5037

Frey, N, Grange, S, & Woodworth, T. (2010). Population pharmacokinetic analysis of tocilizumab in patients with rheumatoid arthritis. *Journal of Clinical Pharmacology*, Vol. 50, No. 7, pp. 754-766, ISSN 0091-2700

Ganz, T & Nemeth, E. (2009). Iron sequestration and anemia of inflammation. *Seminars in Hematology*, Vol. 46, No. 4, pp. 387-393, ISSN 0037-1963

Genovese, M.C, McKay, J.D, Nasonov, E.L, Mysler, E.F, da Silva, N.A, Alecock, E, Woodworth, T, & Gomez-Reino, J.J. (2008). Interleukin-6 receptor inhibition with tocilizumab reduces disease activity in rheumatoid arthritis with inadequate response to disease-modifying antirheumatic drugs: the tocilizumab in combination with traditional disease-modifying antirheumatic drug therapy study. *Arthritis and Rheumatism*, Vol. 58, No. 10, pp. 2968-2980, ISSN 0004-3591

Hagihara, K, Nishikawa, T, Sugamata, Y, Song, J, Isobe, T, Taga, T, & Yoshizaki, K. (2005). Essential role of STAT3 in cytokine-driven NF-kappaB-mediated serum amyloid A gene expression. *Genes to Cells*, Vol. 10, No. 11, pp. 1051-1063, ISSN 1356-9597

Hibi, M, Murakami, M, Saito, M, Hirano, T, Taga, T, & Kishimoto, T. (1990). Molecular cloning and expression of an IL-6 signal transducer, gp130. *Cell*, Vol. 63, No. 6, pp. 1149-1157, ISSN 0092-8674

Hirabayashi, Y, Ishii, T, & Harigae, H. (2010). Clinical efficacy of tocilizumab in patients with active rheumatoid arthritis in real clinical practice. *Rheumatology International*, Vol. 30, No. 8, pp. 1041-1048, ISSN 0172-8172

Hirano, T. (2010). Interleukin 6 in autoimmune and inflammatory diseases: a personal memoir. *Proceedings of the Japan Academy Series B, Physical and Biological Sciences*, Vol. 86, No. 7, pp. 717-730, ISSN 0386-2208

Hong, D.S, Angelo, L.S, & Kurzrock, R. (2007). Interleukin-6 and its receptor in cancer: implications for translational therapeutics. *Cancer*, Vol. 110, No. 9, pp. 1911-1928, ISSN 0008-543X

Inoue, D, Arima, H, Kawanami, C, Takiuchi, Y, Nagano, S, Kimura, T, Shimoji, S, Mori, M, Tabata, S, Yanagita, S, Matsushita, A, Nagai, K, Imai, Y, & Takahashi, T. (2010). Excellent therapeutic effect of tocilizumab on intestinal amyloid a deposition secondary to active rheumatoid arthritis. *Clinical Rheumatology*, Vol. 29, No. 10, pp. 1195-1197, ISSN 0770-3198

Iwasa, T, Nakamura, K, Ogino, H, Itaba, S, Akiho, H, Okamoto, R, Iboshi, Y, Aso, A, Murao, H, Kanayama, K, Ito, T, & Takayanagi, R. (2011). Multiple ulcers in the small and large intestines occurred during tocilizumab therapy for rheumatoid arthritis. *Endoscopy*, Vol. 43, No. 1, pp. 70-72, ISSN 0013-726X

Japan Pharmacists Education Center. (2008). Tocilizumab. *New Drug Approval Package* No.02, pp. 1-77 (in Japanese)

Jones, G, Sebba, A, Gu, J, Lowenstein, M.B, Calvo, A, Gomez-Reino, J.J, Siri, D.A, Tomsic, M, Alecock, E, Woodworth, T, & Genovese, M.C. (2010). Comparison of tocilizumab monotherapy versus methotrexate monotherapy in patients with moderate to severe rheumatoid arthritis: the AMBITION study. *Annals of the Rheumatic Diseases*, Vol. 69, No. 1, pp. 88-96, ISSN 0003-4967

Kaser, A, Brandacher, G, Steurer, W, Kaser, S, Offner, F.A, Zoller, H, Theurl, I, Widder, W, Molnar, C, Ludwiczek, O, Atkins, M.B, Mier, J.W, & Tilg, H. (2001). Interleukin-6 stimulates thrombopoiesis through thrombopoietin: role in inflammatory thrombocytosis. *Blood*, Vol. 98, No. 9, pp. 2720-2725, ISSN 0006-4971

Kremer, J.M, Blanco, R, Brzosko, M, Burgos-Vargas, R, Halland, A.M, Vernon, E, Ambs, P, & Fleischmann, R. (2011). Tocilizumab inhibits structural joint damage in rheumatoid arthritis patients with inadequate responses to methotrexate: results from the double-blind treatment phase of a randomized placebo-controlled trial of tocilizumab safety and prevention of structural joint damage at one year. *Arthritis and Rheumatism*, Vol. 63, No. 3, pp. 609-621, ISSN 0004-3591

Lachmann, H.J, Goodman, H.J, Gilbertson, J.A, Gallimore, J.R, Sabin, C.A, Gillmore, J.D, & Hawkins, P.N. (2007). Natural history and outcome in systemic AA amyloidosis. *New England Journal of Medicine*, Vol. 356, No. 23, pp. 2361-2371, ISSN 0028-4793

Le Goff, B, Blanchard, F, Berthelot, J.M, Heymann, D, & Maugars, Y. (2010). Role for interleukin-6 in structural joint damage and systemic bone loss in rheumatoid arthritis. *Joint, Bone, Spine*, Vol. 77, No. 3, pp. 201-205, ISSN 1297-319X

Leffers, H.C, Ostergaard, M, Glintborg, B, Krogh, N.S, Foged, H, Tarp, U, Lorenzen, T, Hansen, A, Hansen, M.S, Jacobsen, M.S, Dreyer, L, & Hetland, M.L. (2011). Efficacy of abatacept and tocilizumab in patients with rheumatoid arthritis treated in clinical practice: results from the nationwide Danish DANBIO registry. *Annals of the Rheumatic Diseases*, Vol. 70, No. 7, pp. 1216-1222, ISSN 0003-4967

Maini, R.N, Taylor, P.C, Szechinski, J, Pavelka, K, Bröll, J, Balint, G, Emery, P, Raemen, F, Petersen, J, Smolen, J, Thomson, D, & Kishimoto, T. (2006). Double-blind randomized controlled clinical trial of the interleukin-6 receptor antagonist, tocilizumab, in European patients with rheumatoid arthritis who had an incomplete response to methotrexate. *Arthritis and Rheumatism*, Vol. 54, No. 9, pp. 2817-2829, ISSN 0004-3591

Matsuyama, Y, Nagashima, T, Honne, K, Kamata, Y, Iwamoto, M, Okazaki, H, Sato, K, Ozawa, K, & Minota, S. (2011). Successful Treatment of a Patient with Rheumatoid Arthritis and IgA-Kappa Multiple Myeloma with Tocilizumab. *Naika Internal Medicine*, Vol. 50, No. 6, pp. 639-642,

McInnes, I.B, Lee, J.S, Wu, W, Giles, J.T, Bathon, J.M, Salmon, J.E, & Beaulieu, A.D. (2010). Lipid and inflammation parameters: a translational, randomized placebo-controlled study to evaluate effects of tocilizumab: the MEASURE study. *Arthritis and Rheumatism*, Vol. 62, No. Suppl 10, pp. 1441, ISSN 0004-3591

McQueen, F.M, Stewart, N, Crabbe, J, Robinson, E, Yeoman, S, Tan, P.L, & McLean, L. (1998). Magnetic resonance imaging of the wrist in early rheumatoid arthritis reveals a high prevalence of erosions at four months after symptom onset. *Annals of the Rheumatic Diseases*, Vol. 57, No. 6, pp. 350-356, ISSN 0003-4967

Mihara, M, Kasutani, K, Okazaki, M, Nakamura, A, Kawai, S, Sugimoto, M, Matsumoto, Y, & Ohsugi, Y. (2005). Tocilizumab inhibits signal transduction mediated by both mIL-6R and sIL-6R, but not by the receptors of other members of IL-6 cytokine family. *International Immunopharmacology*, Vol. 5, No. 12, pp. 1731-1740, ISSN 1567-5769

Mihara, M, Shiina, M, Nishimoto, N, Yoshizaki, K, Kishimoto, T, & Akamatsu, K. (2004). Anti-interleukin 6 receptor antibody inhibits murine AA-amyloidosis. *Journal of Rheumatology*, Vol. 31, No. 6, pp. 1132-1138, ISSN 0315-162X

Nakahara, H, Kamide, Y, Hamano, Y, Hosokawa, T, Nishide, M, Lin, Y, Kawamoto, K, Fusama, M, Higa, S, Kuroiwa, T, Igarashi, T, Kuritani, T, & Maeda, K. (2011). A case report of a patient with rheumatoid arthritis complicated with Mycobacterium avium during tocilizumab treatment. *Mod Rheumatol*, ISSN 1439-7609

Nakashima, Y, Kondo, M, Harada, H, Horiuchi, T, Ishinishi, T, Jojima, H, Kuroda, K, Miyahara, H, Nagamine, R, Nakashima, H, Otsuka, T, Saikawa, I, Shono, E, Suematsu, E, Tsuru, T, Wada, K, & Iwamoto, Y. (2010). Clinical evaluation of tocilizumab for patients with active rheumatoid arthritis refractory to anti-TNF biologics: tocilizumab in combination with methotrexate. *Mod Rheumatol*, Vol. 20, No. 4, pp. 343-352, ISSN 1439-7609

Nishimoto, N, Yoshizaki, K, Miyasaka, N, Yamamoto, K, Kawai, S, Takeuchi, T, Hashimoto, J, Azuma, J, & Kishimoto, T. (2004). Treatment of rheumatoid arthritis with humanized anti-interleukin-6 receptor antibody: a multicenter, double-blind, placebo-controlled trial. *Arthritis and Rheumatism*, Vol. 50, No. 6, pp. 1761-1769, ISSN 0004-3591

Nishimoto, N, Hashimoto, J, Miyasaka, N, Yamamoto, K, Kawai, S, Takeuchi, T, Murata, N, van der Heijde, D, & Kishimoto, T. (2007). Study of active controlled monotherapy used for rheumatoid arthritis, an IL-6 inhibitor (SAMURAI): evidence of clinical and radiographic benefit from an x ray reader-blinded randomised controlled trial of tocilizumab. *Annals of the Rheumatic Diseases*, Vol. 66, No. 9, pp. 1162-1167, ISSN 0003-4967

Nishimoto, N, Terao, K, Mima, T, Nakahara, H, Takagi, N, & Kakehi, T. (2008). Mechanisms and pathologic significances in increase in serum interleukin-6 (IL-6) and soluble IL-6 receptor after administration of an anti-IL-6 receptor antibody, tocilizumab, in patients with rheumatoid arthritis and Castleman disease. *Blood*, Vol. 112, No. 10, pp. 3959-3964, ISSN 0006-4971

Nishimoto, N, Miyasaka, N, Yamamoto, K, Kawai, S, Takeuchi, T, & Azuma, J. (2009a). Long-term safety and efficacy of tocilizumab, an anti-IL-6 receptor monoclonal antibody, in monotherapy, in patients with rheumatoid arthritis (the STREAM study): evidence of safety and efficacy in a 5-year extension study. *Annals of the Rheumatic Diseases*, Vol. 68, No. 10, pp. 1580-1584, ISSN 0003-4967

Nishimoto, N, Miyasaka, N, Yamamoto, K, Kawai, S, Takeuchi, T, Azuma, J, & Kishimoto, T. (2009b). Study of active controlled tocilizumab monotherapy for rheumatoid arthritis patients with an inadequate response to methotrexate (SATORI): significant reduction in disease activity and serum vascular endothelial growth factor by IL-6 receptor inhibition therapy. *Mod Rheumatol*, Vol. 19, No. 1, pp. 12-19,

Nishimoto, N, Ito, K, & Takagi, N. (2010). Safety and efficacy profiles of tocilizumab monotherapy in Japanese patients with rheumatoid arthritis: meta-analysis of six initial trials and five long-term extensions. *Mod Rheumatol*, Vol. 20, No. 3, pp. 222-232, ISSN 1439-7609

Ogata, A, Morishima, A, Hirano, T, Hishitani, Y, Hagihara, K, Shima, Y, Narazaki, M, & Tanaka, T. (2010a). Improvement of HbA1c during treatment with humanised anti-interleukin 6 receptor antibody, tocilizumab. *Annals of the Rheumatic Diseases*, Vol. 70, No. 6, pp. 1164-1165, ISSN 0003-4967

Ogata, A, Mori, M, Hashimoto, S, Yano, Y, Fujikawa, T, Kawai, M, Kuwahara, Y, Hirano, T, Arimitsu, J, Hagihara, K, Shima, Y, Narazaki, M, Yokota, S, Kishimoto, T, Kawase, I, & Tanaka, T. (2010b). Minimal influence of tocilizumab on IFN-gamma synthesis by tuberculosis antigens. *Mod Rheumatol*, Vol. 20, No. 2, pp. 130-133, ISSN 1439-7609

Ogura, H, Murakami, M, Okuyama, Y, Tsuruoka, M, Kitabayashi, C, Kanamoto, M, Nishihara, M, Iwakura, Y, & Hirano, T. (2008). Interleukin-17 promotes autoimmunity by triggering a positive-feedback loop via interleukin-6 induction. *Immunity*, Vol. 29, No. 4, pp. 628-636, ISSN 1074-7613

Oldfield, V, Dhillon, S, & Plosker, G.L. (2009). Tocilizumab: a review of its use in the management of rheumatoid arthritis. *Drugs*, Vol. 69, No. 5, pp. 609-632, ISSN 0012-6667

Oleksowicz, L, Mrowiec, Z, Zuckerman, D, Isaacs, R, Dutcher, J, & Puszkin, E. (1994). Platelet activation induced by interleukin-6: evidence for a mechanism involving arachidonic acid metabolism. *Thrombosis and Haemostasis*, Vol. 72, No. 2, pp. 302-308, ISSN 0340-6245

Radner, H, Smolen, J.S, & Aletaha, D. (2010). Impact of comorbidity on physical function in patients with rheumatoid arthritis. *Annals of the Rheumatic Diseases*, Vol. 69, No. 3, pp. 536-541, ISSN 0003-4967

Rotter, V, Nagaev, I, & Smith, U. (2003). Interleukin-6 (IL-6) induces insulin resistance in 3T3-L1 adipocytes and is, like IL-8 and tumor necrosis factor-alpha, overexpressed in human fat cells from insulin-resistant subjects. *Journal of Biological Chemistry*, Vol. 278, No. 46, pp. 45777-45784, ISSN 0021-9258

Rubbert-Roth, A, Goupille, P.M, Moosavi, S, & Hou, A. (2010). First experiences with pregnancies in RA patients receiving tocilizumab (TCZ) therapy. *Arthritis and Rheumatism*, Vol. 62, No. Suppl 10, pp. 384, ISSN 0004-3591

Sato, H, Sakai, T, Sugaya, T, Otaki, Y, Aoki, K, Ishii, K, Horizono, H, Otani, H, Abe, A, Yamada, N, Ishikawa, H, Nakazono, K, Murasawa, A, & Gejyo, F. (2009). Tocilizumab dramatically ameliorated life-threatening diarrhea due to secondary amyloidosis associated with rheumatoid arthritis. *Clinical Rheumatology*, Vol. 28, No. 9, pp. 1113-1116, ISSN 0770-3198

Schultz, O, Oberhauser, F, Saech, J, Rubbert-Roth, A, Hahn, M, Krone, W, & Laudes, M. (2010). Effects of inhibition of interleukin-6 signalling on insulin sensitivity and lipoprotein (a) levels in human subjects with rheumatoid diseases. *PLoS One*, Vol. 5, No. 12, pp. e14328ISSN 1932-6203

Shinriki, S, Jono, H, Ota, K, Ueda, M, Kudo, M, Ota, T, Oike, Y, Endo, M, Ibusuki, M, Hiraki, A, Nakayama, H, Yoshitake, Y, Shinohara, M, & Ando, Y. (2009). Humanized anti-interleukin-6 receptor antibody suppresses tumor angiogenesis and in vivo growth of human oral squamous cell carcinoma. *Clinical Cancer Research*, Vol. 15, No. 17, pp. 5426-5434, ISSN 1078-0432

Smolen, J.S, Beaulieu, A, Rubbert-Roth, A, Ramos-Remus, C, Rovensky, J, Alecock, E, Woodworth, T, & Alten, R. (2008). Effect of interleukin-6 receptor inhibition with tocilizumab in patients with rheumatoid arthritis (OPTION study): a double-blind, placebo-controlled, randomised trial. *Lancet*, Vol. 371, No. 9617, pp. 987-997, ISSN 0099-5355

Song, S.N, Tomosugi, N, Kawabata, H, Ishikawa, T, Nishikawa, T, & Yoshizaki, K. (2010). Down-regulation of hepcidin resulting from long-term treatment with an anti-IL-6 receptor antibody (tocilizumab) improves anemia of inflammation in multicentric Castleman disease. *Blood*, Vol. 116, No. 18, pp. 3627-3634, ISSN 0006-4971

Tsuru, T, Suzaki, M, Yoshio, N, Mima, T, Nakashima, H, Amamoto, T, Aoki, C, Uchino, A, Terao, K, Kakehi, T, & Nishimoto, N. (2008). Immune response to influenza vaccine in patients during the treatment with tocilizumab - comparison with conventional DMARDs and TNF inhibitors. *Annals of the Rheumatic Diseases*, Vol. 67, No. Suppl II, pp. 339, ISSN 0003-4967

van Vollenhoven, R.F, Keystone, E.C, Furie, R, Blesch, A, Wang, C, & Curtis, J.R. (2009). Gastrointestinal safety in patients with rheumatoid arthritis treated with tocilizumab: data from Roche clinical trials. *Arthritis and Rheumatism*, Vol. 60, No. Suppl 10, pp. 1613, ISSN 0004-3591

van Vollenhoven, R.F, Scali, J, Curtis, J.R, Krasnow, J, Vernon, E, & Alten, R. (2010). Safety of tocilizumab in patients with rheumatoid arthritis: analysis of median of 2.6 years of treatment in long-term extension studies. *Annals of the Rheumatic Diseases*, Vol. 69, No. Suppl 3, pp. 544, ISSN 0003-4967

Welsh, K.J, Abbott, A.N, Hwang, S.A, Indrigo, J, Armitige, L.Y, Blackburn, M.R, Hunter, R.L, & Actor, J.K. (2008). A role for tumour necrosis factor-alpha, complement C5 and interleukin-6 in the initiation and development of the mycobacterial cord factor trehalose 6,6'-dimycolate induced granulomatous response. *Microbiology*, Vol. 154, No. Pt 6, pp. 1813-1824, ISSN 1350-0872

Yamanaka, H, Nishimoto, N, Inoue, E, Hara, M, Tomatsu, T, & Kamatani, N. (2007). Incidence of malignancies in Japanese Rheumatoid arthritis patients treated with tocilizumab in comparison to those in an observational cohort of Japanese patients and a Japanese population database. *Annals of the Rheumatic Diseases*, Vol. 66, No. Suppl II, pp. 122ISSN 0003-4967

Yamanaka, H, Tanaka, Y, Inoue, E, Hoshi, D, Momohara, S, Hanami, K, Yunoue, N, Saito, K, Amano, K, Kameda, H, & Takeuchi, T. (2011). Efficacy and tolerability of tocilizumab in rheumatoid arthritis patients seen in daily clinical practice in Japan: results from a retrospective study (REACTION study). *Mod Rheumatol*, Vol. 21, No. 2, pp. 122-133, ISSN 1439-7609

Part 3

Potential Treatments

6

The Development of Targeted Drug Delivery Systems for Rheumatoid Arthritis Treatment

Rebecca A. Bader
Syracuse Biomaterials Institute, Syracuse University
USA

1. Introduction

Despite the advent of biologics, rheumatoid arthritis continues to be closely linked with pain, functional impairment, and depression, and a significant number of those with moderate to severe rheumatoid arthritis are too disabled to work several years after onset (Sokka et al., 1999). Furthermore, biologics have increased medical costs to nearly $20,000/patient/year and side effects have hindered use by those with more advanced symptoms (Lundkvist et al., 2008). "Old" disease modifying anti-rheumatic drugs (DMARDs) are also linked to negative consequences as a result of non-specific organ toxicity. The exact cause of rheumatoid arthritis has not yet been identified and, consequently, treatment methods have not been optimally effective. Drug delivery systems may serve to reduce the necessary dosage and increase therapeutic efficacy of old and new rheumatoid arthritis treatments.

Numerous materials have been proposed as drug delivery systems for cancer, and, in recent years, the use of such materials has been increasingly extended to the treatment of rheumatoid arthritis. Liposomes, nanoparticles, micelles, and macromolecule-drug conjugates can be used to increase a drug's circulatory stability and thereby raise the probability for passive accumulation within the pannus, where permeability is enhanced. Both the specificity and therapeutic efficacy of these drug delivery systems can be further improved by combination with an active targeting moiety, such as an antibody, peptide, or polysaccharide that is specific for receptors concentrated on the surface of cells located within tissue affected by rheumatoid arthritis. The combination of passive and active targeting strategies can be used to optimize delivery of therapeutic agents to reduce toxicity and unwanted side effects and improve patient outcome. This chapter is intended to provide an overview of emerging techniques aimed at improving the efficacy of DMARDs, whilst simultaneously reducing the adverse consequences associated with non-specific targeting. Due to the nature of the disease, this review will focus only on drug delivery systems intended for systemic, rather than local/intra-articular, administration.

2. History and challenges of rheumatoid arthritis treatment

Historically, rheumatoid arthritis has been treated with a combination of anti-inflammatory drugs and immunosuppressants. Although treatment has evolved from non-steroidal anti-inflammatory drugs (NSAIDs) to disease modifying anti-rheumatic drugs (DMARDs), including modern biologics, all of the drugs in use have severe, potentially life threatening, consequences due to non-specific targeting, often in combination with impaired immune function.

Rheumatoid arthritis treatment originated wtih NSAIDs, such as aspirin and other salicylates, which act as anti-inflammatory agents by interfering with the activity of cyclooxygenase (COX) enzymes and, consequently, the production of prostaglandins (PGs), which are key mediators of the inflammatory response. Despite a lack of efficacy relative to conventional DMARDs or biologics, NSAID use in combination therapy has continued (Mottram, 2003). The long term side effects of NSAIDs include gastrointestinal and cardiovascular complications, as well as impaired renal function (Dijkmans et al., 1995).

Similar to NSAIDs, glucocorticoids (GCs), including cortisone, dexamethasone, prednisolone, and prednisone, primarily act through inhibition of PG production and are still used in current rheumatoid arthritis treatment strategies. Additionally, GCs reduce the expression of several proinflammatory proteins, including interleukin-1, -2, and -6, granulocyte macrophage-colony stimulating factor (GM-CSF), and tumor necrosis factor-α (TNF-α) (Moreland & O'Dell, 2002). Although high doses can be immunosuppressive, as well as anti-inflammatory, doses are typically kept low in rheumatoid arthritis treatment to minimize the adverse consequences that include gastrointestinal complications, an increased risk of osteoporosis, visual problems, and negative skin effects (Strand & Simon, 2003).

In the 1920s, gold salts were used to treat rheumatoid arthritis based upon the belief that the disease was triggered by an infection (Mottram, 2003). Although the link to a bacterial origin has been dispelled, gold has been classified as the earliest form of DMARD. The side effects of gold include reduced liver and renal function, as well as pulmonary complications. Consequently, the use of gold as a treatment is now limited to only severe rheumatoid arthritis patients who do not respond to other DMARDs.,

Several cytotoxic, anti-cancer agents have been adapted as DMARDs. For example, methotrexate has been in use as an oncology drug since 1950 and as a DMARD since 1970. Although the mechanism of action in rheumatoid arthritis remains largely unclear, methotrexate is speculated to either reduce proliferation of infiltrating inflammatory cells or suppress the release of pro-inflammatory cytokines (Mottram, 2003). Despite periodic liver function tests and biopsies for patients undergoing methotrexate treatment, cirrhosis and fibrosis are known side effects, and fatalities have been reported (Goodman & Polisson, 1994; Wolverton & Remlinger, 2007).

Other common DMARDs include immunosuppressants originally developed to prevent organ transplant rejection, such as cyclosporine, tacrolimus, and sirolium. The immunosuppressive properties of the latter drugs appear to be primarily due to inhibition of T-cell activation (Mottram, 2003). All of these therapeutics are nephrotoxic; consequently, creatinine levels must be monitored during treatment to assess renal dysfunction and kidney damage (Schiffelers et al., 2006; Zachariae, 1999).

A better understanding of disease progression, particularly as pertains the imbalance in pro- and anti-inflammatory cytokines, has led to the recent development of a number of biologic therapies as DMARDs, for example anti-TNF−α monoclonal antibodies such as infliximab and adalimumab. Although the latter agents are intended to be more specific, systemic inhibition of key inflammatory molecules can also have negative consequences. In particular, patients receiving treatment with biologics have an increased incidence of serious infections. Furthermore, the efficacy in individual patients is often unpredictable (Strand et al., 2007).

The pharmacokinetic profiles of most DMARDs are unfavorable (Tarner & Muller-Ladner, 2008). For example, the bioavailability, peak serum concentration, and half life of orally administered methotrexate varies considerably between patients. The large variability in pharmacokinetic parameters likely contributes to the toxicity observed in some patients (Weinblatt & Kremer, 1988). Given the high incidence of adverse side effects, in addition to variability in drug effectiveness, the application of drug delivery srategies would be a significant advancement in rheumatoid arthritis treatment.

3. Principles of drug delivery

3.1 Passive targeting

In cancer treatment, drug carrier systems with a large hydrodynamic radius to prevent renal filtration and increase circulation time can passively target diseased tissue as a result of leaky vasculature and inadequate lymphatic drainage, an effect known as "enhanced permeation and retention" (EPR) (Gillies & Frechet, 2005; Lee et al., 2006; Padilla De Jesus et al., 2002). Although inflammatory tissue, as found with rheumatoid arthritis, does not display abnormal lymphatic drainage (Xu et al., 2003), long-circulating delivery systems have been shown to selectively accumulate within the inflamed synovial tissue, i.e. the pannus (Fiehn et al., 2004; Metselaar et al., 2002; Schiffelers et al., 2006; Vanniasinghe et al., 2008; Wunder et al., 2003). The pannus possesses an increased vascular permeability similar to that of solid tumors and, consequently, the vasculature can be exploited for passive targeting in an analogous manner (Walsh, 1999). Fig. 1 illustrates the principles behind passive and active targeting of inflamed joint tissue.

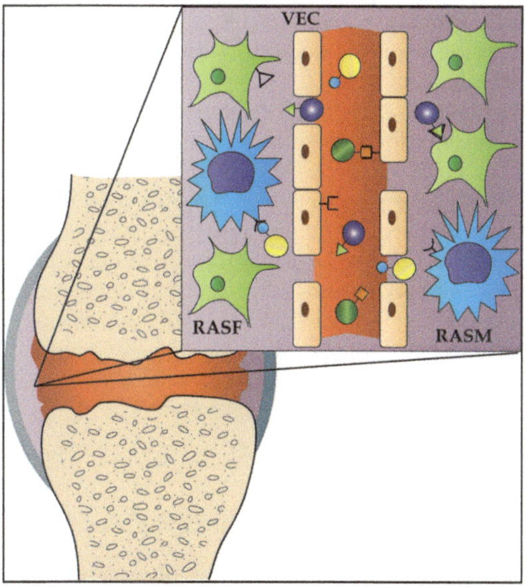

Fig. 1. Drug delivery strategies in the treatment of rheumatoid arthritis. Passive targeting of the pannus can be achieved by creating carriers that can only pass through leaky vasculature, while active targeting can be facilitated by a ligand that is specific for receptors of rheumatoid arthritis synovial fibroblasts (RASFs), rheumatoid arthritis synovial macrophages (RASMs), or activated vascular endothelial cells (VECs).

3.2 Active targeting

In addition to the potential for passive targeting, the two primary cell types found within the pannus tissue, rheumatoid arthritis synovial fibroblasts (RASFs) and rheumatoid arthritis synovial macrophages (RASMs) selectively express surface receptors, such as CD44 (Haynes et al., 1991; Johnson et al., 1993), folate receptor β (Nagayoshi et al., 2005; van der Heijden et al., 2009), and integrin $\alpha_V\beta_3$ (Wilder, 2002) that are candidates for active targeting. Angiogenic vascular endothelial cells (VECs) are also present as a result of neovascularization, and the E-selectin adhesion molecule has been identified as another viable target for drug delivery (Jamar et al., 2002).

3.3 Carrier systems

In general, drug delivery systems can be divided into two categories: polymer-drug conjugates and nanoparticulate carrier systems. "Nanoparticles" in this sense include liposomes and micelles, as well as traditional metallic and polymeric nanoparticles. As drug delivery systems have become increasing advanced, the distinction between these two categories has become less clear.

3.3.1 Polymer-drug conjugates

In 1975, Ringsdorf proposed a model for polymer-based drug delivery wherein discrete sections of a polymer backbone are used for attachment of therapeutics, solubilizers, and targeting moieties (Fig. 2) (Ringsdorf, 1975). Since this seminal manuscript, numerous macromolecular therapeutics have been synthesized and evaluated. Although initial research focused on the use of N-(2-hydroxypropyl) methacrylamide (HPMA) based upon similarity to Ringsdorf's Model, polymers with a variety of architectures and structural elements are currently being explored, including linear mono- and di-functional polymers, star polymers, and dendrimers (Fig. 3) (Kopecek et al., 2000; Peterson et al., 2003). Dendrimers can alternatively be classified as nanoparticulate carriers when drug molecules are entrapped within the interior rather than covalently linked to the surface functional groups (Gillies & Frechet, 2005; M. Liu & Frechet, 1999). Mono- and di-hydroxyl terminated poly(ethylene glycol) (PEG) have proven to be the most versatile polymers for increasing the stability, solubility, and pharmacokinetic properties of associated therapeutics, with several PEG-drug conjugates on the market for a number of indications (Joralemon et al., 2010). Only recently has this research translated to the development of macromolecular therapeutics for the treatment of rheumatoid arthritis, as discussed further in Section 4. Despite demonstrated success, polymer-drug conjugates suffer from the necessity to chemically modify the drug molecule and the potential to reduce therapeutic activity and efficacy by such modification (Haag & Kratz, 2006; Kim et al., 2009).

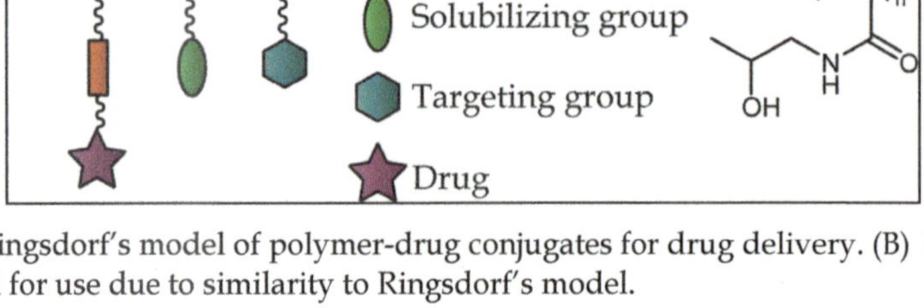

Fig. 2. (A) Ringsdorf's model of polymer-drug conjugates for drug delivery. (B) HPMA was investigated for use due to similarity to Ringsdorf's model.

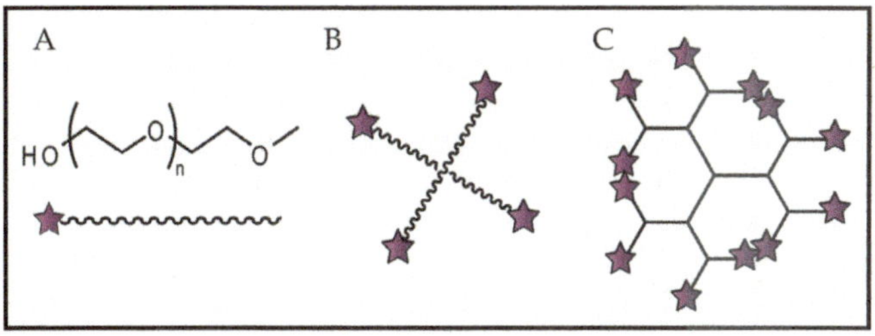

Fig. 3. Various polymer architectures investigated for use in drug delivery via polymer-drug conjugates. (A) Linear polymers, with PEG as an example, (B) star, polymers and (C) dendrimers.

3.3.2 Nanoparticulate carrier systems

Nanoparticulate carrier systems permit entrapment/encapsulation of therapeutics without modification, as is requisite for polymer-drug conjugates. The colloidal particles can range in size from 10 nm to 1 μm; however, sizes are more typically between 20 and 300 nm, thereby minimizing uptake by macrophages of the reticuloendothelial system, while permitting passive targeting of tissue with leaky vasculature. Liposomes, micelles, metallic nanoparticles, and polymeric nanoparticles constitute the most commonly used nanoparticulate carrier systems for drug delivery (Fig. 4) (Jain, 2008).

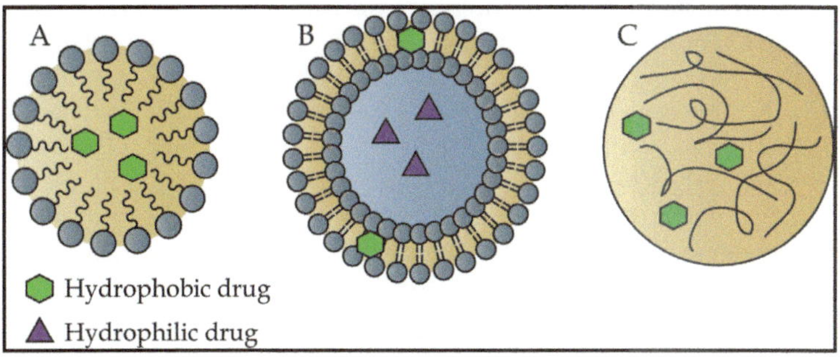

Fig. 4. Various nanoparticulate carrier systems. (A) Micelles, (B) liposomes, and (C) polymeric nanoparticles.

Liposomes are vesicles formed from phospholipid bilayers with aqueous centers. Consequently, liposomes are used to encapsulate both hydrophobic and hydrophilic drugs within the bilayer and the aqueous core, respectively. Liposomal properties are largely controlled through the choice of phospholipids, as well as the addition of sterols, particularly cholesterol, and glycolipids (Jain, 2008). Although conventional liposomes suffer from rapid uptake by the reticuloendothelial system, incorporation of PEG into the bilayer yields so called "stealth" liposomes with enhanced circulation times. Starting with the anticancer compound Doxil (Gabizon, 2001), several PEG-modified liposomes with encapsulated therapeutics have reached commercialization (Joralemon, et al., 2010). As a consequence, liposomal use has been widely studied as a potential carrier system for drug delivery for rheumatoid arthritis (Foong & Green, 1993; Konigsberg et al., 1999; Monkkonen et al., 1993; Monkkonen & Heath, 1993; Monkkonen et al., 1994; Shaw et al., 1979) .

Above a certain concentration, referred to as the critical micelle concentration (CMC), molecules that possess both hydrophobic and hydrophilic segments, such as amphipathic block-co-polymers, will self assemble to form colloidal particles with hydrophobic interiors and hydrophilic exteriors. Micelles are typically smaller than liposomes (20-50 nm) and the hydrophobic cores are used to entrap drugs that possess low aqueous solubility (Haag & Kratz, 2006). The CMC provides an indicator of stability, where systems with low CMCs are not easily disrupted or disintegrated (Oerlemans et al., 2010). Only a handful of investigators have used micelle-based drug delivery systems to improve the efficacy of DMARDs that have historically suffered from unpredictable pharmacokinetics resultant from poor solubility (Bader et al., 2011; Koo et al., 2011; Zhang et al., 2007).

Both metallic and polymeric nanoparticles are used to encapsulate drugs within the solid core. Although nanoparticles are defined as any system with a submicron (≤ 1 μm) size (van Vlerken & Amiji, 2006), most typically have sizes below 200 nm (Jain, 2008). Metallic nanoparticles include iron-oxide nanoparticles, silica-gold nanoshells, gold nanoparticles, and Quantum dots (cadmium, selenium, and zinc) (Riehemann et al., 2009; van Vlerken & Amiji, 2006). Although originally developed for cancer treatment, these technologies are currently being translated to rheumatoid arthritis treatment applications (Corthey et al., 2010). The use of metals can yield multifunctional nanoparticles whereby both therapeutic delivery and imaging are facilitated (Riehemann et al., 2009). Polymer-based nanoparticles, are advantageous in that modification permits the ready addition of the following elements: targeting ligands, environment-sensitive drug release, and biologically functional polymers.

The carrier systems discussed above can be further modified to optimize disease treatment. For example, co-administration of multiple therapeutics from one convenient platform is feasible. Additional modification with ligands specific for receptors found on diseased cells can facilitate active targeting. Furthermore, surface coating with PEG can be used to tailor circulation time (Riehemann et al., 2009; van Vlerken & Amiji, 2006). As detailed in Section 4, these technologies have only recently been applied in the realm of drug delivery for rheumatoid arthritis treatment.

3.3.3 Therapeutic release from carrier systems

Most drugs are inactive when bound to/encapsulated within the carrier system; therefore, a method that permits drug release at the diseased site is often requisite. Cellular uptake of therapeutic-loaded carrier systems typically proceeds by fluid-phase endocytosis, adsorptive endocytosis, or receptor-mediated endocytosis (Fig. 5). During each of these endocytotic processes, the pH drops from that within the extracellular space (pH $\approx$ 7.4 for healthy tissue and pH < 7.4 for diseased tissue) to pHs of ~6.0 and ~4.0 in the endosomes and lysosomes, respectively (Haag & Kratz, 2006; Petrak, 2005). Thus, the conjugate and particulate carriers can be formulated such that release is only permitted at a specified pH. Alternatively, drugs may be released after enzymes cause non-specific hydrolysis (Haag & Kratz, 2006; Kim et al., 2009). An ideal carrier system will only respond to environmental features unique to the diseased tissue, such as elevated levels of a specific enzyme. Stimuli-responsive drug delivery systems that are currently in development for the treatment of rheumatoid arthritis will be discussed in Section 5.

4. Current drug delivery systems and strategies for rheumatoid arthritis

A number of carrier systems have been designed to to improve rheumatoid arthritis treatment based upon the principles described in Section 3. These carrier systems provide an opportunity to increase the efficacy of existing rheumatoid arthritis therapeutics while reducing adverse effects. A summary of current drug delivery strategies that encompasses Sections 4 and 5 is given in Table 1.

4.1 Polymer-drug conjugates for rheumatoid arthritis treatment

Several polymer-drug conjugates have been developed to improve the therapeutic efficacy of both conventional DMARDs and biologics. A number of these compounds were only recently applied to rheumatoid arthritis after originally being developed for cancer. For example, methotrexate conjugated to human serum albumin (MTX-HSA) was shown to passively accumulate within the inflamed paws of arthritic mice. Further study revealed a reduction in cellular invasion, a downregulation of proinflammatory cytokine levels, and a decrease in cartilage damage for arthritic mice treated with MTX-HSA relative to untreated, arthritic mice. The conjugates were also useful in preventing the onset of arthritis in mice when administered prior to induction (Fiehn et al., 2004; Wunder et al., 2003). Due to the limitations of exogenous albumin, a methotrexate pro-drug has recently been developed that will react with endogenous albumin upon administration (Fiehn et al., 2008).

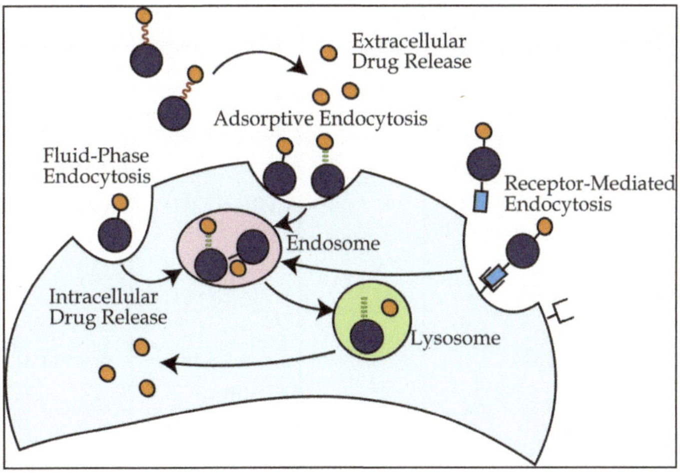

Fig. 5. Cellular uptake of carrier systems occurs by an endocytotic process. Systems can be designed to release their therapeutic payload within the extracellular space, the endosome, or the lysosome.

As mentioned in Section 3, PEG has been used extensively in all areas of drug delivery. PEG-dexamethasone conjugates were recently synthesized that reduced joint inflammation when administered intravenously to arthritis rats (Liu et al., 2010). PEGylation has been applied to biologics, in addition to conventional, small molecule therapeutics. To the authors' knowledge, the only polymer-drug conjugate to reach clinical trials for rheumatoid arthritis treatment thus far is certolizumab pegol (CDP870), a PEG conjugated TNF-α antibody fragment originally developed for treatment of Chron's disease (Barnes & Moots, 2007). Administration to a number of patients who did not respond well to conventional DMARDs, particularly methotrexate, led to a reduction in disease activity and joint damage. Unfortunately, an increase in adverse side effects was also observed (Ruiz Garcia et al.,

Type of Carrier	Material(s)	Targeting Group	Therapeutic	Reference(s)
Polymer-Drug Conjugate	Albumin	–	Methotrexate	(Wunder et al., 2003)
	PEG	–	Cathepsin-K Inhibitor	(Wang et al., 2004)
	HPMA	–	Cathepsin-K Inhibitor	(Wang et al., 2004)
	PEG	–	TNF-α Antibody Fragment	(Barnes & Moots, 2007)
	PEG	–	Dexamethasone	(Liu, et al., 2010)
	HPMA	–	Dexamethasone	(Quan et al., 2010)
	PAMAM Dendrimer	Folate	Methotrexate	(Thomas et al., 2011)
Liposome	Phospholipids Cholesterol	–	Clondronate	(Camilleri et al., 1995; Love et al., 1992)
	Phospholipids (with and without covalently linked methotrexate) Cholesterol	–	Methotrexate	(A. S. Williams, Camilleri, & Williams, 1994)
	Phospholipids Cholesterol PEG	–	Superoxide Dismutase	Corvo et al., 1999)
	Phospholipids Cholesterol PEG	–	Prendisolone	(Metselaar et al., 2002; Metselaar et al., 2003)
	Phospholipids Cholesterol	Sialyl Lewis X		(Hirai et al., 2007)
	Phosphogliv	–	Methotrexate	(Zykova et al., 2007)
	PEG-Phospholipids	Vasoactive Intenstinal Peptide	Camptothecin	(Koo et al., 2011)
	Cationic Phospholipids	–	anti-TNF-α/IL-1β/ IL-6/ IL-18 siRNA	(Khoury et al., 2008; Khoury et al., 2006)

Micelle	PEG-Poly(caprolactone)	–	Cyclosporine A	(Aliabadi et al., 2005)
	Dextran-Polyoxyethylene Cetyl Ether (POE-C_{16})	–	Cyclosporine A	(Francis et al., 2005)
	Hydroxypropyl-cellulose-(POE-C_{16})	–	Cyclosporine A	(Francis et al., 2005)
	Polysialic Acid-Decylamine	–	Cyclosporine A	(Bader et al., 2011)
Nanoparticle	PLGA	–	Betamethasone	(Higaki et al., 2005)
	PLGA-PEG	–	Betamethasone	(Ishihara et al., 2009)
	PAMAM Dendrimer	Folate	Indomethacin	(Chandrasekar et al., 2007b)
	Polyester	Ligand for E-Selectin	–	(Banquy et al., 2008).
	Cyclodextrin	–	α–Methyl-prendisolone	(Hwang et al., 2008)
	PLGA-PEG	cLABL Peptide	–	(Zhang et al., 2008)
	PEG-TRAIL Hyaluronic Acid	Hyaluronic Acid	TRAIL	(Kim et al., 2010),
	Gold Core-Gold(I)-Thiomalate	–	Gold	(Corthey, et al., 2010)
	Chitosan	Folate	IL-1R Agonist	(Fernandes et al., 2008)
	Lipid PEG	Folate	NF-κB Decoy	(Hattori et al., 2006),

Table 1. Current drug delivery strategies for rheumatoid arthritis

2011), suggesting that PEGylation may not be the ideal method to improve the efficacy of rheumatoid arthritis therapeutics.

Other polymer-drug conjugates have shown some promise *in vitro*, such as PEG and HPMA conjugated cathepsin-K inhibitor (Wang et al., 2004). Furthermore, as will be desribed in more detail in Section 5, systems such as PEG and HPMA dexamethasone conjugates are now being developed that, not only target the pannus tissue, but also selectively release the therapeutic in the targeted region (Liu, et al., 2010; Quan et al., 2010).

4.2 Liposomal carrier systems for rheumatoid arthritis treatment

Several liposome systems have been tried for improved efficacy of rheumatoid arthritis treatments. This work was pioneered by Williams, et. al., who demonstrated that technecium labelled liposomes accumulated within the synovial tissue of rheumatoid arthritis patients upon intravenous administration (Williams et al., 1986, 1987). A similar phenomenon was observed for phosphatidylcholine and cholesterol based liposomes given to arthritic rats (Love et al., 1989), and encapsulation of clondronate, an anti-inflammatory therapeutic that reduces bone resorption, resulted in a halt in disease progression and a reversal in inflammation (Camilleri et al., 1995; Love et al., 1992). The efficacy of the liposomal clondronate was attributed to depletion of the synovial macrophages (Love et al., 1992; Richards et al., 1999). Comparable results were obtained with liposomal methotrexate that was prepared by conjugation of the the γ-carboxylic acid residue to the phospholipid. The resultant liposomes yielded a significant reduction of established joint inflammation, in combination with a decrease in toxicity, relative to comparable doses of free drug (Williams et al., 1994b. Furthermore, peritoneal macrophages isolated from the liposomal methotrexate treated arthritic rats were shown to express less TNF-α and prostaglandin (PGE2) (Williams et al., 1994a)· Conventional (i.e. not PEGylated) liposomes have also been used by other investigators to improve the efficacy of aurothiomalate (Konigsberg et al., 1999).

Stealth liposomes have been used to improve the therapeutic efficacy of glucocorticoids, the use of which is often hindered by the necessity for frequent intravenous administration and by non-specific organ toxicity. Following on studies that showed an accumulation of PEG liposomes within the inflamed tissue of arthritic rats (Gabizon et al., 1994; Hong & Tseng, 2003), Metselaar et al. (2002; 2003; 2004) investigated the efficacy of prednisolone loaded liposomes. Upon administration to arthritic rats and mice, the prednisolone liposomes reversed the inflammatory response, while free prednisolone had little effect on the course of the disease. The results were attributed purely to the passive targeting capacity of the stealth liposomes (Metselaar et al., 2004; Metselaar et al., 2002; Metselaar et al., 2003). Current research is focused upon extending the use of the stealth liposomes to other glucocorticoids, including dexamethasone and budesonide, and optimizing the therapeutic index (van den Hoven et al., 2011). PEG modified liposomes have also been used to improve the efficacy of superoxide dismutase (SOD), a free radical scavenger which suffers from a short half life. When encapsulated in small, stealth liposomes, the circulation of SOD was significantly extended, and the drug passively accumulated within the joint tissue (Corvo et al., 1999).

4.3 Micelle carrier systems for rheumatoid arthritis treatment

Despite the low aqueous solubility of a number of DMARDs and glucocorticoids, micelles are a relatively unexplored drug delivery system for rheumatoid arthritis treatment. Camptothecin, originally developed as an anti-cancer drug, has recently been proposed as a new method of controlling pannus formation and reducing cartilage degradation. To circumvent problems with solubility and stability, micelles prepared from PEG-phospholipids (Ashok et al., 2004) were used for drug encapsulation. The camptothecin micelles proved to be more effective than free camptothecin at abrogating inflammation when administered to arthritic mice. The efficacy of the micelles was further increased by modification with vasoactive intenstinal peptide (VIP) due to the over expression of VIP receptor by activated synovial macrophages (Koo et al., 2011). Similarly, micelles generated from a phospholipid preparation (Phosphogliv) and loaded with methotrexate were better able to reduce inflammation when administered to arthritic rats than the drug alone (Zykova et al., 2007).

Cyclosporine A is indicated for several different conditions; therefore, micelle-based methods for improving the solubility of of this DMARD have been more thoroughly researched. Cyclosporine has been successfully encapsulated by block copolymers of PEG and poly(caprolactone) (Aliabadi et al., 2005), PEG phospholipids (Lee et al., 1999), and hydrophobically modified polysaccharides, specifically dextran and hydroxypropylcellulose (Francis et al., 2005). Recently, polysialic acid, a relatively uninvestigated polysaccharide with propertiers similar to those of PEG in regards to minimizing uptake by the reticuloendotheial system, was used to encapsulate cyclopsorine for future use in rheumatoid arthritis treatment (Bader et al., 2011). The utility of the above cyclosporine micelles *in vivo* has not yet been demonstrated.

4.4 Nanoparticle carrier systems for rheumatoid arthritis treatment

Nanoparticle systems for delivery of rheumatoid arthritis therapeutics have primarily been based upon polymers. Numerous researchers have explored the use of poly(D,L-lactic/glycolic acid) (PLGA) nanoparticles based upon their capacity to extend the circulation time and control the release of encapsulated drugs. In the realm of rheumatoid arthritis drug delivery, a glutocorticoid, betamethasone, was incorporated into PLGA nanoparticles with a size of 100-200 nm. Intravenous administration to arthritic rats and mice showed that the PLGA-betamethasone system was more effective at reducing the inflammatory response than the free glutocorticoid (Higaki et al., 2005). Targeting ability and, consequently, efficacy of the betamethasone was further improved by modifying the PLGA nanoparticles with PEG, forming so-called "stealth nanosteroids" (Ishihara et al., 2009).

Other polymeric nanoparticle systems involve covalently linking the drug molecule to one of the components so as to slow down therapeutic release, as occurs for polymer-drug conjugates, while still protecting the drug via encapsulation. For example, α-methylprednisolone was conjugated to cyclodextrin, and the resultant compound self-assembled to yield nanoparticles with a size of approximately 27 nm. When administered intravenously at a frequency of one dose per week to arthritic mice, a significantly greater reduction in synovitis and pannus formation was acheieved than that obtained for free methylprednisolone administered daily at an equivalent cumulative dose (Hwang et al., 2008). Another example is the ionic complexation of tumor necrosis factor (TNF)-related apoptosis inducing ligand (TRAIL) conjugated to PEG (PEG-TRAIL), which bears a positive charge, with negatively charged hyaluronic acid (HA) with sizes that range from 100 to 270 nm, dependent upon the relative concentration of the two components. One formulation of the HA-PEG-TRAIL complex was capable of signficantly reducing the secretion of proinflammatory mediators relative to PEG-TRAIL alone when administered subcutaneously to arthritic mice (Kim et al., 2010), thereby emphasizing the importance of nanoparticulate carrier systems. The HA may also serve as an active targeting (Section 5).

Despite the demonstrated efficacy of gold as a DMARD (Section 2), and the approval of gold nanoparticles for the treatment of rheumatoid arthritis by the FDA, little research has been conducted specifically directed towards the use of metallic nanoparticles for passive targeting in rheumatoid arthritis. The decline in the use of gold as a rheumatoid arthritis therapeutic was largely based on adverse side effects caused by non-specific toxicity. However, the synthesis of gold core-gold(I)-thiomalate nanoparticles (Au@AU(I)-TM) was recently completed. Au@Au(I)-TM bears surface carboxylate groups which may be further modified for specific drug delivery applications (Corthey et al., 2010); therefore, these nanoparticles may pave the way to a renewed interest in the use of gold in the treatment of rheumatoid arthritis.

5. Future of drug delivery for rheumatoid arthritis

The exploration of drug delivery systems for improved treatment of rheumatoid arthritis is still in the early stages. More advanced concepts that have been applied to other diseases, particularly cancer, are only beginning to be explored by rheumatoid arthritis researchers.

5.1 Active targeting strategies

Current drug delivery systems for rheumatoid arthritis have almost exclusively been developed based upon the principles of passive targeting. Specificity and, consequently, efficacy can be further improved by employing an active targeting moiety. As indicated previously, RASFs and RASMs possess receptors that can potentially be used to increase the ability of the drug carrier systems to discern pannus tissue from healthy tissue. Those receptors that have the highest potential for success are discussed in this section.

Folate receptor β (FRβ) has been identified as a viable candidate for active targeting of RASMs. Several transport mechanisms exist whereby folate and folate antagonists, including methotrexate, can enter a cell. Numerous cell types throughout the body constitutively express the reduced folate carrier (RFC), a transmembrane protein. In contrast, membrane associated folate receptors (MFRs) are restricted in expression and facilitate uptake by endocytosis. The beta isoform of MFR (FRβ) is expressed selectively by activated macrophages within the pannus tissue (Nagayoshi et al., 2005; van der Heijden et al., 2009). Thus, folate may serve as an effective means of actively targeting the pannus tissue. In support of this, folate-tagged cationic and anionic poly(amidoamine) (PAMAM) dendrimers loaded with indomethacin were more effective at treating arthritic rats than indomethacin-loaded dendrimers that were folate-free (Chandrasekar et al., 2007a; Chandrasekar et al., 2007b; Chauhan et al., 2004). Furthermore, a recent study demonstrated that PAMAM dendrimers covalently linked to both folate and methotrexate could be used to selectively deliver methotrexate to synovial macrophages (Thomas et al., 2011). Although the antifolate MTX does not have a high affinity for any MFRs, several other folate analogs have been identified that possess high affinity for FRβ with low affinities for other MFRs and the RFC (van der Heijden et al., 2009). These analogs, therefore, have strong potential to be used as active targeting moieties in the future and may possess inherent anti-rheumatic properties.

RASFs also possess an active targeting receptor in the cell surface adhesion molecule CD44, the hyaluronic acid receptor. Several studies have indicated that CD44 is upregulated in the pannus tissue relative to healthy, normal tissue (Haynes et al., 1991; Johnson et al., 1993). Furthermore, RASFs express numerous CD44 alternatively spliced variants, including long isoforms CD44v3 and CD44v6 that are associated with an enhanced invasive capacity (Croft et al., 1997). CD44 is critical to rheumatoid arthritis pathogenesis, facilitating inflammatory cell migration and signaling activation of lymphocytes (Naor & Nedvetzki, 2003). Despite evidence of upregulation and/or selective expression, the CD44 receptor has not yet been used as an active target for drug delivery in the treatment of rheumatoid arthritis. Some cancer cells also upregulate CD44, and the potential for success using this active targeting strategy has previously been illustrated by anti-cancer drug carrier systems modified with hyaluronic acid oligomers (Ossipov, 2010).

As indicated by the feasibility of passive targeting, neovascularization is a critical component of rheumatoid arthritis pathogenesis (Szekanecz & Koch, 2008). Adhesion molecules, including intercellular cell-adhesion molecule-1 (ICAM-1) and E-selectin, are upregulated within the newly formed vasculature and; therefore, the endothelium serves as another possibility for active targeting (Banquy et al., 2008; Zhang et al., 2008). Preliminary studies demonstrated that a large number of PLGA-PEG nanoparticles surface modified with a peptide specific for ICAM-1 were endocytosed by vascular endothelial cells as compared to unmodified particles (Zhang et al., 2008). A similar phenomenon was observed for polyester-based polymeric nanoparticles labeled with ligand specific for E-selectin (Banquy et al., 2008). Likewise, liposomes surface modified with the polysaccharide Sialyl Lewis X, which is known to bind selectively to E-selectin, were shown to accumulate within inflamed regions when administered intravenously to arthritic mice (Hirai et al., 2007). The vitronectin receptor, overexpressed by both angiogenic endothelial cells and RASMs (Tandon et al., 2005; Wilder, 2002), is an attractive target based upon the extensive use of Arg-Glyc-Asp (RGD) tripeptide labeled carrier systems for drug delivery to invasive tumor tissue (Hsu et al., 2007). An antibody to $\alpha_V\beta_3$, Vitaxin (ME-522), is currently being clinically developed for rheumatoid arthritis (Wilder, 2002); however, the RGD peptide sequence has not yeen been applied towards increasing the targeting ability and efficacy of existing DMARDs.

5.2 Multifunctional carrier systems

A recent push in the realm of drug delivery for cancer treatment has been the development of multifunctional carrier systems whereby a single platform can be used for the release of multiple therapeutics in a controlled fashion or for both therapeutic release and diagnostic imaging (Jabr-Milane et al., 2008; van Vlerken & Amiji, 2006). Some of the success achieved in this "theranostic" approach to cancer treatment has spilled over into the study of improved treatment methods for rheumatoid arthritis. For example, folate-conjugated radiopharmaceuticals designed to target malignant tissue showed significant accumulation in the joints of patients who also had rheumatoid arthritis (Paulos et al., 2004). Radiolabelled biologics have provided an additional example of the potential for theranostics to improve rheumatoid arthritis treatment. 99m-technetium labelled infliximab (^{99m}Tc-infliximab) was used to show a strong correlation between the amount of infliximab taken up by inflamed tissue and a reduction in symptoms and swelling (Malviya et al., 2010).

5.3 Stimuli-responsive carrier systems

As discussed in brief above, in order to be optimally effective, the drug delivery systems must release their payloads at the desired site of action, i.e. the pannus tissue. In the realm of cancer drug delivery, numerous pH- and temperature-responsive carrier systems, in the form of conjugates, dendrimers, liposomes, and micelles, have been developed (Ganta et al., 2008). Although the same potential also exists for rheumatoid arthritis drug delivery, particularly in light of the lower pH of the pannus tissue relative to native tissue, to the authors' knowledge, only two pH-responsive systems, dexamethasone-HPMA conjugates (P-Dex) and dexamethasone-PEG conjugates (PEG-DEX), have been reported. Drug release was shown to increase as the pH decreased. *In vitro* and *in vivo* tests were used to demonstrate that P-Dex and PEG-DEX are more effective than free dexamethasone in regards to reducing the production of proinflammatory mediators, preventing joint damage, and targeting inflamed tissue (Liu et al., 2010; Quan et al., 2010). In addition to temperature and pH, other environmental triggers may be used. For example, elevated elastace levels have been closely linked with inflammation and the increased enzymatic activity maybe be used for cleavage. The upregulation in enzymes may additionally serve as a means of active targeting (Meers, 2001).

5.4 Gene therapy

Given the nature of rheumatoid arthritis, gene therapy, whereby nucleic acids are introduced to a cell to either "turn off" select genes or upregulate therapeutic genes, is an attractive alternative treatment strategy (Jorgensen & Apparailly, 2010). This approach is limited, however, by the necessity for local administration and low transfection efficiency; therefore, for practical use, drug delivery systems for gene therapy will be required. Small interfering RNA (siRNA), in particular, may be used to knockdown the expression of proinflammatory proteins at the mRNA level. Cationic liposomes, referred to as lipoplexes, have been designed to facilitate systemic delivery of siRNA for rheumatoid arthritis treatment (Khoury et al., 2006, 2008). When administered intravenously to arthritic mice, anti-TNF-α, anti-IL-1β, anti IL-6, and anti IL-18 siRNA successfully reduced inflammation, bone and cartilage degradation, and secretion of a number of proinflammatory cytokines, including TNF-α and IL-1β (Khoury et al., 2006, 2008). Similarly, intraperitoneal administration of anti-TNF-α siRNA complexed with chitosan nanoparticles to arthritic mice resulted in a significant reduction in joint swelling, cartilage degradation, and inflammatory cell infiltration (Fernandes et al., 2008). Chitosan nanoparticles were also used to deliver the IL-1 receptor antagonist (IL-1Ra) gene to arthritic rats (Fernandes et al., 2008). Rats treated with the chitosan-gene delivery system showed reduced bone turnover, as well as decreased expression of IL-1β and PGE2, relative to control rats. The efficacy of the chitosan-IL-1Ra nanoparticles was further improved by modification with folate for active targeting (Fernandes et al., 2008). An innovative strategy towards gene therapy was designed by encapsulating a nuclear factor kappa B (NF-κB) decoy into stealth lipid-based nanoparticles that were surface modified with folate (Hattori et al., 2006). NF-κB regulates proinflammatory gene expression and is, therefore, a critical component of rheumatoid arthritis pathogenesis (Brown et al., 2008; Simmonds & Foxwell, 2008). *In vitro,* the nanoparticles were shown to release the NF-κB into the cytoplasm, as indicated by a reduction in NF-κB translocation into the nucleus (Hattori et al., 2006), which presumably will result in a decreased expression of proinflammatory cytokines and growth factors.

6. Conclusion

Although the advent of biologics markedly increased the number of available treatment options, numerous rheumatoid arthritis patients still use, either alone or in combination, NSAIDs, GCs, and conventional DMARDs. All of these compounds are associated with severe negative side effects resultant from non-specific organ toxicity. In some cases, the side effects necessitate the cessation of a treatment option that may be effectively altering the course of the disease. The application of drug delivery strategies, as outlined herein, promises to improve patient outcome by reducing the likelihood of an adverse reaction to NSAIDs, GCs, and biologic and conventional DMARDs. These same strategies may be extended in the future to facilitate diagnostic imaging and gene therapy, thereby further increasing the possibility of successfully controlling the progression of the disease in all people that suffer from rheumatoid arthritis.

7. References

Aliabadi, H. M., Brocks, D. R., & Lavasanifar, A. (2005). Polymeric micelles for the solubilization and delivery of cyclosporine A: pharmacokinetics and biodistribution. *Biomaterials,* 26, 35, pp. 7251-7259.

Ashok, B., Arleth, L., Hjelm, R. P., Rubinstein, I., & Onyuksel, H. (2004). In vitro characterization of PEGylated phospholipid micelles for improved drug solubilization: effects of PEG chain length and PC incorporation. *J Pharm Sci,* 93, 10, pp. 2476-2487.

Bader, R. A., Silvers, A. L., & Zhang, N. (2011). Polysialic Acid-based micelles for encapsulation of hydrophobic drugs. *Biomacromolecules,* 12, 2, pp. 314-320.

Banquy, X., Leclair, G., Rabanel, J. M., Argaw, A., Bouchard, J. F., Hildgen, P., et al. (2008). Selectins ligand decorated drug carriers for activated endothelial cell targeting. *Bioconjug Chem,* 19, 10, pp. 2030-2039.

Barnes, T., & Moots, R. (2007). Targeting nanomedicines in the treatment of rheumatoid arthritis: focus on certolizumab pegol. *Int J Nanomedicine,* 2, 1, pp. 3-7.

Brown, K. D., Claudio, E., & Siebenlist, U. (2008). The roles of the classical and alternative nuclear factor-kappaB pathways: potential implications for autoimmunity and rheumatoid arthritis. *Arthritis Res Ther,* 10, 4, pp. 212.

Camilleri, J. P., Williams, A. S., Amos, N., Douglas-Jones, A. G., Love, W. G., & Williams, B. D. (1995). The effect of free and liposome-encapsulated clodronate on the hepatic mononuclear phagocyte system in the rat. *Clin Exp Immunol,* 99, 2, pp. 269-275.

Chandrasekar, D., Sistla, R., Ahmad, F. J., Khar, R. K., & Diwan, P. V. (2007a). The development of folate-PAMAM dendrimer conjugates for targeted delivery of anti-arthritic drugs and their pharmacokinetics and biodistribution in arthritic rats. *Biomaterials,* 28, 3, pp. 504-512.

Chandrasekar, D., Sistla, R., Ahmad, F. J., Khar, R. K., & Diwan, P. V. (2007b). Folate coupled poly(ethyleneglycol) conjugates of anionic poly(amidoamine) dendrimer for inflammatory tissue specific drug delivery. *J Biomed Mater Res A,* 82, 1, pp. 92-103.

Chauhan, A. S., Jain, N. K., Diwan, P. V., & Khopade, A. J. (2004). Solubility enhancement of indomethacin with poly(amidoamine) dendrimers and targeting to inflammatory regions of arthritic rats. *J Drug Target,* 12, 9-10, pp. 575-583.

Corthey, G., Giovanetti, L. J., Ramallo-Lopez, J. M., Zelaya, E., Rubert, A. A., Benitez, G. A., et al. (2010). Synthesis and characterization of gold at gold(i)-thiomalate core at shell nanoparticles. *ACS Nano,* 4, 6, pp. 3413-3421.

Corvo, M. L., Boerman, O. C., Oyen, W. J., Van Bloois, L., Cruz, M. E., Crommelin, D. J., et al. (1999). Intravenous administration of superoxide dismutase entrapped in long circulating liposomes. II. In vivo fate in a rat model of adjuvant arthritis. *Biochim Biophys Acta,* 1419, 2, pp. 325-334.

Croft, D. R., Dall, P., Davies, D., Jackson, D. G., McIntyre, P., & Kramer, I. M. (1997). Complex CD44 splicing combinations in synovial fibroblasts from arthritic joints. *Eur J Immunol,* 27, 7, pp. 1680-1684.

Dijkmans, B. A., Janssen, M., Vandenbroucke, J. P., & Lamers, C. B. (1995). NSAID-associated upper gastrointestinal damage in patients with rheumatoid arthritis. *Scand J Gastroenterol Suppl,* 212, pp. 105-108.

Fernandes, J. C., Wang, H., Jreyssaty, C., Benderdour, M., Lavigne, P., Qiu, X., et al. (2008). Bone-protective effects of nonviral gene therapy with folate-chitosan DNA nanoparticle containing interleukin-1 receptor antagonist gene in rats with adjuvant-induced arthritis. *Mol Ther,* 16, 7, pp. 1243-1251.

Fiehn, C., Kratz, F., Sass, G., Muller-Ladner, U., & Neumann, E. (2008). Targeted drug delivery by in vivo coupling to endogenous albumin: an albumin-binding prodrug of methotrexate (MTX) is better than MTX in the treatment of murine collagen-induced arthritis. *Ann Rheum Dis,* 67, 8, pp. 1188-1191.

Fiehn, C., Muller-Ladner, U., Gay, S., Krienke, S., Freudenberg-Konrad, S., Funk, J., et al. (2004). Albumin-coupled methotrexate (MTX-HSA) is a new anti-arthritic drug which acts synergistically to MTX. *Rheumatology (Oxford),* 43, 9, pp. 1097-1105.

Foong, W. C., & Green, K. L. (1993). Treatment of antigen-induced arthritis in rabbits with liposome-entrapped methotrexate injected intra-articularly. *J Pharm Pharmacol,* 45, 3, pp. 204-209.

Francis, M. F., Cristea, M., Yang, Y., & Winnik, F. M. (2005). Engineering polysaccharide-based polymeric micelles to enhance permeability of cyclosporin A across Caco-2 cells. *Pharm Res,* 22, 2, pp. 209-219.

Gabizon, A., Catane, R., Uziely, B., Kaufman, B., Safra, T., Cohen, R., et al. (1994). Prolonged circulation time and enhanced accumulation in malignant exudates of doxorubicin encapsulated in polyethylene-glycol coated liposomes. *Cancer Res,* 54, 4, pp. 987-992.

Gabizon, A. A. (2001). Pegylated liposomal doxorubicin: metamorphosis of an old drug into a new form of chemotherapy. *Cancer Invest,* 19, 4, pp. 424-436.

Ganta, S., Devalapally, H., Shahiwala, A., & Amiji, M. (2008). A review of stimuli-responsive nanocarriers for drug and gene delivery. *J Control Release,* 126, 3, pp. 187-204.

Gillies, E. R., & Frechet, J. M. (2005). Dendrimers and dendritic polymers in drug delivery. *Drug Discov Today,* 10, 1, pp. 35-43.

Goodman, T. A., & Polisson, R. P. (1994). Methotrexate: adverse reactions and major toxicities. *Rheum Dis Clin North Am,* 20, 2, pp. 513-528.

Haag, R., & Kratz, F. (2006). Polymer therapeutics: concepts and applications. *Angew Chem Int Ed Engl,* 45, 8, pp. 1198-1215.

Hattori, Y., Sakaguchi, M., & Maitani, Y. (2006). Folate-linked lipid-based nanoparticles deliver a NFkappaB decoy into activated murine macrophage-like RAW264.7 cells. *Biol Pharm Bull,* 29, 7, pp. 1516-1520.

Haynes, B. F., Hale, L. P., Patton, K. L., Martin, M. E., & McCallum, R. M. (1991). Measurement of an adhesion molecule as an indicator of inflammatory disease activity. Up-regulation of the receptor for hyaluronate (CD44) in rheumatoid arthritis. *Arthritis Rheum,* 34, 11, pp. 1434-1443.

Higaki, M., Ishihara, T., Izumo, N., Takatsu, M., & Mizushima, Y. (2005). Treatment of experimental arthritis with poly(D, L-lactic/glycolic acid) nanoparticles encapsulating betamethasone sodium phosphate. *Ann Rheum Dis,* 64, 8, pp. 1132-1136.

Hirai, M., Minematsu, H., Kondo, N., Oie, K., Igarashi, K., & Yamazaki, N. (2007). Accumulation of liposome with Sialyl Lewis X to inflammation and tumor region:

application to in vivo bio-imaging. *Biochem Biophys Res Commun,* 353, 3, pp. 553-558.

Hong, R. L., & Tseng, Y. L. (2003). A phase II and pharmacokinetic study of pegylated liposomal doxorubicin in patients with advanced hepatocellular carcinoma. *Cancer Chemother Pharmacol,* 51, 5, pp. 433-438.

Hsu, A. R., Veeravagu, A., Cai, W., Hou, L. C., Tse, V., & Chen, X. (2007). Integrin alpha v beta 3 antagonists for anti-angiogenic cancer treatment. *Recent Pat Anticancer Drug Discov,* 2, 2, pp. 143-158.

Hwang, J., Rodgers, K., Oliver, J. C., & Schluep, T. (2008). Alpha-methylprednisolone conjugated cyclodextrin polymer-based nanoparticles for rheumatoid arthritis therapy. *Int J Nanomedicine,* 3, 3, pp. 359-371.

Ishihara, T., Kubota, T., Choi, T., & Higaki, M. (2009). Treatment of experimental arthritis with stealth-type polymeric nanoparticles encapsulating betamethasone phosphate. *Journal of Pharmacology and Experimental Therapeutics,* 329, 2, pp. 412-417.

Jabr-Milane, L., van Vlerken, L., Devalapally, H., Shenoy, D., Komareddy, S., Bhavsar, M., et al. (2008). Multi-functional nanocarriers for targeted delivery of drugs and genes. *J Control Release,* 130, 2, pp. 121-128.

Jain, K. K. (2008). Drug delivery systems - an overview. *Methods Mol Biol,* 437, pp. 1-50.

Jamar, F., Houssiau, F. A., Devogelaer, J. P., Chapman, P. T., Haskard, D. O., Beaujean, V., et al. (2002). Scintigraphy using a technetium 99m-labelled anti-E-selectin Fab fragment in rheumatoid arthritis. *Rheumatology (Oxford),* 41, 1, pp. 53-61.

Johnson, B. A., Haines, G. K., Harlow, L. A., & Koch, A. E. (1993). Adhesion molecule expression in human synovial tissue. *Arthritis Rheum,* 36, 2, pp. 137-146.

Joralemon, M. J., McRae, S., & Emrick, T. (2010). PEGylated polymers for medicine: from conjugation to self-assembled systems. *Chem Commun (Camb),* 46, 9, pp. 1377-1393.

Jorgensen, C., & Apparailly, F. (2010). Prospects for gene therapy in inflammatory arthritis. *Best Pract Res Clin Rheumatol,* 24, 4, pp. 541-552.

Khoury, M., Escriou, V., Courties, G., Galy, A., Yao, R., Largeau, C., et al. (2008). Efficient suppression of murine arthritis by combined anticytokine small interfering RNA lipoplexes. *Arthritis Rheum,* 58, 8, pp. 2356-2367.

Khoury, M., Louis-Plence, P., Escriou, V., Noel, D., Largeau, C., Cantos, C., et al. (2006). Efficient new cationic liposome formulation for systemic delivery of small interfering RNA silencing tumor necrosis factor alpha in experimental arthritis. *Arthritis Rheum,* 54, 6, pp. 1867-1877.

Kim, S., Kim, J. H., Jeon, O., Kwon, I. C., & Park, K. (2009). Engineered polymers for advanced drug delivery. *Eur J Pharm Biopharm,* 71, 3, pp. 420-430.

Kim, Y. J., Chae, S. Y., Jin, C. H., Sivasubramanian, M., Son, S., Choi, K. Y., et al. (2010). Ionic complex systems based on hyaluronic acid and PEGylated TNF-related apoptosis-inducing ligand for treatment of rheumatoid arthritis. *Biomaterials,* 31, 34, pp. 9057-9064.

Konigsberg, P. J., Debrick, J. E., Pawlowski, T. J., & Staerz, U. D. (1999). Liposome encapsulated aurothiomalate reduces collagen-induced arthritis in DBA/1J mice. *Biochim Biophys Acta,* 1421, 1, pp. 149-162.

Koo, O. M., Rubinstein, I., & Onyuksel, H. (2011). Actively targeted low-dose camptothecin as a safe, long-acting, disease-modifying nanomedicine for rheumatoid arthritis. *Pharm Res,* 28, 4, pp. 776-787.

Kopecek, J., Kopeckova, P., Minko, T., & Lu, Z. (2000). HPMA copolymer-anticancer drug conjugates: design, activity, and mechanism of action. *Eur J Pharm Biopharm,* 50, 1, pp. 61-81.

Lee, C. C., Gillies, E. R., Fox, M. E., Guillaudeu, S. J., Frechet, J. M., Dy, E. E., et al. (2006). A single dose of doxorubicin-functionalized bow-tie dendrimer cures mice bearing C-26 colon carcinomas. *Proc Natl Acad Sci U S A,* 103, 45, pp. 16649-16654.

Lee, M. K., Choi, L., Kim, M. H., & Kim, C. K. (1999). Pharmacokinetics and organ distribution of cyclosporin A incorporated in liposomes and mixed micelles. *Int J Pharm,* 191, 2, pp. 87-93.

Liu, M., & Frechet, J. M. (1999). Designing dendrimers for drug delivery. *Pharm Sci Technolo Today,* 2, 10, pp. 393-401.

Liu, X. M., Quan, L. D., Tian, J., Laquer, F. C., Ciborowski, P., & Wang, D. (2010). Syntheses of click PEG-dexamethasone conjugates for the treatment of rheumatoid arthritis. *Biomacromolecules,* 11, 10, pp. 2621-2628.

Love, W. G., Amos, N., Kellaway, I. W., & Williams, B. D. (1989). Specific accumulation of technetium-99m radiolabelled, negative liposomes in the inflamed paws of rats with adjuvant induced arthritis: effect of liposome size. *Ann Rheum Dis,* 48, 2, pp. 143-148.

Love, W. G., Camilleri, J. P., & Williams, B. D. (1992). Efficient clodronate entrapment within multilamellar and unilamellar liposomes. *J Pharmacol Toxicol Methods,* 27, 3, pp. 185-189.

Lundkvist, J., Kastang, F., & Kobelt, G. (2008). The burden of rheumatoid arthritis and access to treatment: health burden and costs. *Eur J Health Econ,* 8 Suppl 2, pp. S49-60.

Malviya, G., Conti, F., Chianelli, M., Scopinaro, F., Dierckx, R. A., & Signore, A. (2010). Molecular imaging of rheumatoid arthritis by radiolabelled monoclonal antibodies: new imaging strategies to guide molecular therapies. *Eur J Nucl Med Mol Imaging,* 37, 2, pp. 386-398.

Meers, P. (2001). Enzyme-activated targeting of liposomes. *Adv Drug Deliv Rev,* 53, 3, pp. 265-272.

Messori, L., & Marcon, G. (2004). Gold complexes in the treatment of rheumatoid arthritis. *Met Ions Biol Syst,* 41, pp. 279-304.

Metselaar, J. M., van den Berg, W. B., Holthuysen, A. E., Wauben, M. H., Storm, G., & van Lent, P. L. (2004). Liposomal targeting of glucocorticoids to synovial lining cells strongly increases therapeutic benefit in collagen type II arthritis. *Ann Rheum Dis,* 63, 4, pp. 348-353.

Metselaar, J. M., Wauben, M. H., Boerman, O. C., Van Lent, P. L., & Storm, G. (2002). Long-circulating liposomes for i.v. targeted delivery of glucocorticoids in arthritis. *Cell Mol Biol Lett,* 7, 2, pp. 291-292.

Metselaar, J. M., Wauben, M. H., Wagenaar-Hilbers, J. P., Boerman, O. C., & Storm, G. (2003). Complete remission of experimental arthritis by joint targeting of glucocorticoids with long-circulating liposomes. *Arthritis Rheum,* 48, 7, pp. 2059-2066.

Monkkonen, J., Brown, C. S., Thompson, T. T., & Heath, T. D. (1993). Liposome-mediated delivery of gallium to macrophage-like cells in vitro: demonstration of a transferrin-independent route for intracellular delivery of metal ions. *Pharm Res,* 10, 8, pp. 1130-1135.

Monkkonen, J., & Heath, T. D. (1993). The effects of liposome-encapsulated and free clodronate on the growth of macrophage-like cells in vitro: the role of calcium and iron. *Calcif Tissue Int,* 53, 2, pp. 139-146.

Monkkonen, J., Taskinen, M., Auriola, S. O., & Urtti, A. (1994). Growth inhibition of macrophage-like and other cell types by liposome-encapsulated, calcium-bound, and free bisphosphonates in vitro. *J Drug Target,* 2, 4, pp. 299-308.

Moreland, L. W., & O'Dell, J. R. (2002). Glucocorticoids and rheumatoid arthritis: back to the future? *Arthritis Rheum,* 46, 10, pp. 2553-2563.

Mottram, P. L. (2003). Past, present and future drug treatment for rheumatoid arthritis and systemic lupus erythematosus. *Immunol Cell Biol,* 81, 5, pp. 350-353.

Nagayoshi, R., Nagai, T., Matsushita, K., Sato, K., Sunahara, N., Matsuda, T., et al. (2005). Effectiveness of anti-folate receptor beta antibody conjugated with truncated Pseudomonas exotoxin in the targeting of rheumatoid arthritis synovial macrophages. *Arthritis Rheum,* 52, 9, pp. 2666-2675.

Naor, D., & Nedvetzki, S. (2003). CD44 in rheumatoid arthritis. *Arthritis Res Ther,* 5, 3, pp. 105-115.

Oerlemans, C., Bult, W., Bos, M., Storm, G., Nijsen, J. F., & Hennink, W. E. (2010). Polymeric micelles in anticancer therapy: targeting, imaging and triggered release. *Pharm Res,* 27, 12, pp. 2569-2589.

Ossipov, D. A. (2010). Nanostructured hyaluronic acid-based materials for active delivery to cancer. *Expert Opin Drug Deliv,* 7, 6, pp. 681-703.

Padilla De Jesus, O. L., Ihre, H. R., Gagne, L., Frechet, J. M., & Szoka, F. C., Jr. (2002). Polyester dendritic systems for drug delivery applications: in vitro and in vivo evaluation. *Bioconjug Chem,* 13, 3, pp. 453-461.

Paulos, C. M., Turk, M. J., Breur, G. J., & Low, P. S. (2004). Folate receptor-mediated targeting of therapeutic and imaging agents to activated macrophages in rheumatoid arthritis. *Adv Drug Deliv Rev,* 56, 8, pp. 1205-1217.

Peterson, C. M., Shiah, J. G., Sun, Y., Kopeckova, P., Minko, T., Straight, R. C., et al. (2003). HPMA copolymer delivery of chemotherapy and photodynamic therapy in ovarian cancer. *Adv Exp Med Biol,* 519, pp. 101-123.

Petrak, K. (2005). Essential properties of drug-targeting delivery systems. *Drug Discov Today,* 10, 23-24, pp. 1667-1673.

Quan, L. D., Purdue, P. E., Liu, X. M., Boska, M. D., Lele, S. M., Thiele, G. M., et al. (2010). Development of a macromolecular prodrug for the treatment of inflammatory arthritis: mechanisms involved in arthrotropism and sustained therapeutic efficacy. *Arthritis Res Ther,* 12, 5, pp. R170.

Richards, P. J., Williams, A. S., Goodfellow, R. M., & Williams, B. D. (1999). Liposomal clodronate eliminates synovial macrophages, reduces inflammation and ameliorates joint destruction in antigen-induced arthritis. *Rheumatology (Oxford)*, 38, 9, pp. 818-825.

Riehemann, K., Schneider, S. W., Luger, T. A., Godin, B., Ferrari, M., & Fuchs, H. (2009). Nanomedicine--challenge and perspectives. *Angew Chem Int Ed Engl*, 48, 5, pp. 872-897.

Ringsdorf, H. (1975). Structure and properties of pharmacologically active polymers. *J Polymer Sci*, 51, pp. 135-153.

Ruiz Garcia, V., Jobanputra, P., Burls, A., Cabello, J. B., Galvez Munoz, J. G., Saiz Cuenca, E. S., et al. (2011). Certolizumab pegol (CDP870) for rheumatoid arthritis in adults. *Cochrane Database Syst Rev*, 2, pp. CD007649.

Schiff, M. H., & Whelton, A. (2000). Renal toxicity associated with disease-modifying antirheumatic drugs used for the treatment of rheumatoid arthritis. *Semin Arthritis Rheum*, 30, 3, pp. 196-208.

Schiffelers, R. M., Banciu, M., Metselaar, J. M., & Storm, G. (2006). Therapeutic application of long-circulating liposomal glucocorticoids in auto-immune diseases and cancer. *J Liposome Res*, 16, 3, pp. 185-194.

Shaw, I. H., Knight, C. G., Thomas, D. P., Phillips, N. C., & Dingle, J. T. (1979). Liposome-incorporated corticosteroids: I. The interaction of liposomal cortisol palmitate with inflammatory synovial membrane. *Br J Exp Pathol*, 60, 2, pp. 142-150.

Simmonds, R. E., & Foxwell, B. M. (2008). Signalling, inflammation and arthritis: NF-kappaB and its relevance to arthritis and inflammation. *Rheumatology (Oxford)*, 47, 5, pp. 584-590.

Sokka, T., Kautiainen, H., Mottonen, T., & Hannonen, P. (1999). Work disability in rheumatoid arthritis 10 years after the diagnosis. *J Rheumatol*, 26, 8, pp. 1681-1685.

Strand, V., Kimberly, R., & Isaacs, J. D. (2007). Biologic therapies in rheumatology: lessons learned, future directions. *Nat Rev Drug Discov*, 6, 1, pp. 75-92.

Strand, V., & Simon, L. S. (2003). Low dose glucocorticoids in early rheumatoid arthritis. *Clin Exp Rheumatol*, 21, 5 Suppl 31, pp. S186-190.

Szekanecz, Z., & Koch, A. E. (2008). Targeting Angiogenesis in Rheumatoid Arthritis. *Curr Rheumatol Rev*, 4, 4, pp. 298-303.

Tandon, V. R., Mahajan, A., Singh, J. B., & Verma, S. (2005). Alpha V beta 3 integrin: a novel therapeutic target In rheumatoid arthritis. *JK Science*, 7, 2, pp. 61-62.

Tarner, I. H., & Muller-Ladner, U. (2008). Drug delivery systems for the treatment of rheumatoid arthritis. *Expert Opin Drug Deliv*, 5, 9, pp. 1027-1037.

Thomas, T. P., Goonewardena, S. N., Majoros, I., Kotlyar, A., Cao, Z., Leroueil, P. R., et al. (2011). Folate-targeted nanoparticles show efficacy in the treatment of inflammatory arthritis. *Arthritis Rheum*.

van den Hoven, J. M., Hofkens, W., Wauben, M. H., Wagenaar-Hilbers, J. P., Beijnen, J. H., Nuijen, B., et al. (2011). Optimizing the therapeutic index of liposomal glucocorticoids in experimental arthritis. *Int J Pharm*.

van der Heijden, J. W., Oerlemans, R., Dijkmans, B. A., Qi, H., van der Laken, C. J., Lems, W. F., et al. (2009). Folate receptor beta as a potential delivery route for novel folate antagonists to macrophages in the synovial tissue of rheumatoid arthritis patients. *Arthritis Rheum*, 60, 1, pp. 12-21.

van Vlerken, L. E., & Amiji, M. M. (2006). Multi-functional polymeric nanoparticles for tumour-targeted drug delivery. *Expert Opin Drug Deliv*, 3, 2, pp. 205-216.

Vanniasinghe, A. S., Bender, V., & Manolios, N. (2008). The Potential of Liposomal Drug Delivery for the Treatment of Inflammatory Arthritis. *Semin Arthritis Rheum*.

Walsh, D. A. (1999). Angiogenesis and arthritis. *Rheumatology (Oxford)*, 38, 2, pp. 103-112.

Wang, D., Li, W., Pechar, M., Kopeckova, P., Bromme, D., & Kopecek, J. (2004). Cathepsin K inhibitor-polymer conjugates: potential drugs for the treatment of osteoporosis and rheumatoid arthritis. *Int J Pharm*, 277, 1-2, pp. 73-79.

Weinblatt, M. E., & Kremer, J. M. (1988). Methotrexate in rheumatoid arthritis. *J Am Acad Dermatol*, 19, 1 Pt 1, pp. 126-128.

Wilder, R. L. (2002). Integrin alpha V beta 3 as a target for treatment of rheumatoid arthritis and related rheumatic diseases. *Ann Rheum Dis*, 61 Suppl 2, pp. ii96-99.

Williams, A. S., Camilleri, J. P., Topley, N., & Williams, B. D. (1994a). Prostaglandin and tumor necrosis factor secretion by peritoneal macrophages isolated from normal and arthritic rats treated with liposomal methotrexate. *J Pharmacol Toxicol Methods*, 32, 1, pp. 53-58.

Williams, A. S., Camilleri, J. P., & Williams, B. D. (1994b). Suppression of adjuvant-induced arthritis by liposomally conjugated methotrexate in the rat. *Br J Rheumatol*, 33, 6, pp. 530-533.

Williams, B. D., O'Sullivan, M. M., Saggu, G. S., Williams, K. E., Williams, L. A., & Morgan, J. R. (1986). Imaging in rheumatoid arthritis using liposomes labelled with technetium. *Br Med J (Clin Res Ed)*, 293, 6555, pp. 1143-1144.

Williams, B. D., O'Sullivan, M. M., Saggu, G. S., Williams, K. E., Williams, L. A., & Morgan, J. R. (1987). Synovial accumulation of technetium labelled liposomes in rheumatoid arthritis. *Ann Rheum Dis*, 46, 4, pp. 314-318.

Wolverton, S. E., & Remlinger, K. (2007). Suggested guidelines for patient monitoring: hepatic and hematologic toxicity attributable to systemic dermatologic drugs. *Dermatol Clin*, 25, 2, pp. 195-205, vi-ii.

Wunder, A., Muller-Ladner, U., Stelzer, E. H., Funk, J., Neumann, E., Stehle, G., et al. (2003). Albumin-based drug delivery as novel therapeutic approach for rheumatoid arthritis. *J Immunol*, 170, 9, pp. 4793-4801.

Xu, H., Edwards, J., Banerji, S., Prevo, R., Jackson, D. G., & Athanasou, N. A. (2003). Distribution of lymphatic vessels in normal and arthritic human synovial tissues. *Ann Rheum Dis*, 62, 12, pp. 1227-1229.

Zachariae, H. (1999). Renal toxicity of long-term cyclosporin. *Scand J Rheumatol*, 28, 2, pp. 65-68.

Zhang, J. X., Yan, M. Q., Li, X. H., Qiu, L. Y., Li, X. D., Li, X. J., et al. (2007). Local delivery of indomethacin to arthritis-bearing rats through polymeric micelles based on amphiphilic polyphosphazenes. *Pharm Res*, 24, 10, pp. 1944-1953.

Zhang, N., Chittasupho, C., Duangrat, C., Siahaan, T. J., & Berkland, C. (2008). PLGA nanoparticle--peptide conjugate effectively targets intercellular cell-adhesion molecule-1. *Bioconjug Chem*, 19, 1, pp. 145-152.

Zykova, M. G., Prozorovskii, V. N., Ipatova, O. M., Torkhovskaia, T. I., & Glazatov, V. V. (2007). [Antirheumatoid activity of methotrexate in phospholipid nanoparticles (Phosphogliv)]. *Biomed Khim*, 53, 4, pp. 435-441.

7

Enkorten – A Potential Drug for the Treatment of Rheumatoid Arthritis

Nedžad Mulabegović et al.*
Medical Faculty University of Sarajevo Institute of Pharmacology, Clinical Pharmacology and Toxicology Bosnia and Herzegovina

1. Introduction

Enkorten is a new potential drug for the treatment of rheumatoid arthritis, with an immunomodulatory and anti-inflammatory effect. It is a combination of two peptide components of endogenous origin: methionine-enkephalin of 5 mg and tridecactide of 1 mg (Picture 1 and 2). According to the chemical structures, these components correspond to amino acid sequences of the neuropeptide precursor proopiomelanocortin.

Generic name:	tridecactide
Chemical name:	(des-acetyl)-α-MSH-(de-amid) - α-MSH
Gross formula:	$C_{75}H_{106}N_{20}O_{19}S$
Molecular weight:	1623.85
Amino acid sequence:	H-Ser-Tyr-Ser-Met-Glu-His-Phe-Arg-Trp-Gly-Lys-Pro-Val-OH

Picture 1. Chemical characteristics of tridecactide

Generic name:	met-enkephalin 1-5 adrenorphin
Gross formula:	$C_{27}H_{35}N_5O_7S$
Molecular weight:	573.67
Amino acid sequence:	H-Tyr-Gly-Gly-Phe-Met-OH

Picture 2. Chemical characteristics of met-enkephalin

The holder of effects of the tested combination is alpha 1-13 corticotrophin–tridecactide (ACTH 1-13), composed of 13 amino acids, identical to the amino acid sequence of the alpha-melanostimulating hormone (α-MSH), but without the acetyl and amide ending. Some studies suggest that α-MSH is synthesized in the pituitary, other parts of the CNS, the placenta, and some endocrine organs - especially the adrenal, the skin and the gastrointestinal tract (Star et al, 1995; Catania et al, 2000). The presence of this neuropeptide in the mucous membrane of the gastrointestinal tract and keratinocytes of the skin suggests

* Jasna Kusturica, Maida Todić-Rakanović, Mirjana Mijanović, Fahir Bečić, Asija Začiragić, Selma Škrbo, Lejla Burnazović-Ristić, Aida Kulo and Svjetlana Loga-Zec
Medical Faculty University of Sarajevo Institute of Pharmacology, Clinical Pharmacology and Toxicology, Bosnia and Herzegovina

that it is a component of natural immunity (Catania et al, 2000a). The supposed connection between alpha-MSH and immune processes is confirmed by the clinical data on changes of its plasma level under certain pathological conditions (Lipton and Catania, 1997; Lipton et al, 2000). An increased concentration of α-MSH has been recorded in patients with an acute myocardial infarction who received thrombolytic therapy, probably as an endogenous anti-inflammatory response. This peptide has been identified in the synovial fluid of patients with rheumatoid arthritis (Star et al, 1995) and it is believed that the inflammation and joint destruction in this disease occur due to imbalances of production of proinflammatory and anti-inflammatory cytokines such as α-MSH. A higher concentration of α-MSH has been found in patients suffering from arthropathy accompanied by heavy inflammation (Lipton et al, 2000). Since α-MSH is a natural modulator peptide, its concentration is subject to intensive control to avoid excessive inhibition of the immune response. It is assumed that the increased concentration of peptides leads to downregulation of receptors in cells, which could explain the biphasic curve of the anti-inflammatory effects α-MSH (Catania et al, 2000).

The other component contained in the drug is met-enkephalin, which belongs to a group of endogenous opioid peptides, widely distributed in the CNS. All opioid peptides contain one or more copies of the simplest opioid peptides: methionine-enkefalin (tyrosine-glycine-glycine-phenylalanine-methionine) and leucine-enkephalin (tyrosine-glycine-glycine-phenylalanine-leucine) (Janković, 1991). They participate in, and modulate neurotransmission. Opioid peptides also act as growth factors that control proliferation and differentiation of cells and may participate in the process of wound healing, tissue regeneration and immune response. Enkephalins show antidepressant, antianxiety and anticonvulsive effects. They are produced in the adrenal and the hypothalamus. Met-enkephalin belongs to a group of enkephalins that are involved in transmitting signals in the nervous system, intestines, endocrine glands, bronchial tree, lymphatic and other tissues (Štambuk et al, 1996). The highest concentrations are present in the core of adrenal, hypothalamus, autonomic ganglia and the gastrointestinal tract (Janković, 1991).

Met-enkephalin as an inhibitory peptide modulates the proliferation and migration of cells, as well as the organization of tissues during development, homeostatic cell renewal, wound healing, angiogenesis, and in malignant neoplasms (Zagon et al, 2000). Physiologically, enkephalins have a signalling function in the nervous system, intestine, endocrine glands, bronchial tree, cardiovascular system, lymphatic and other tissues, and participate in the regulation of haematopoiesis (Štambuk et al, 1996). It is assumed that they participate in maintaining homeostasis of the organism exposed to stress (Mulabegović et Rakanović-Todić, 2008).

2. The place and importance of α-MSH and met-enkephalin in immunomodulation

Immunomodulatory effects of a combination of α-MSH and met-enkephalin involve several mechanisms that support the modern trend in the development of new anti-inflammatory drugs. The method of selective immunomodulation using peptides has only recently been used in immune-mediated diseases and malignant neoplasm. Immunomodulation with antigens and peptides is directed towards achieving a satisfactory long-term remission without the occurrence of toxic side effects typical for immunosuppressive drugs. It is based on two approaches: the first approach is to block the initial activation of antigen recognition of autoreactive T cells, while the second is based on downregulation of specific antigenic inflammatory response of T cells through the activation of regulatory physiological mechanisms (Štambuk et al, 1997).

Until recently it was thought that the immune/inflammatory reaction develops exclusively in the periphery. Today it is known that the nervous, endocrine and immune systems are interconnected, and that they communicate by signals that are transmitted through neuropeptides. In this way, central neurogenic influences can either enhance or modulate the peripheral response, so by analogy the treatment of inflammatory reactions could be improved by the influence of the proinflammatory signals in the central nervous system. Thus, Catania et al. (1999) suggest that one of these strategies could be based on the action of α-MSH.

In the past several years, particular attention has been given to the anti-inflammatory effects of this peptide, as a result of the introduction of α-MSH and related peptides in clinical practice for the treatment of inflammatory diseases (Getting, 2006). Undoubtedly, α-MSH, administered systemically or locally, expresses strong anti-inflammatory effects. Anti-inflammatory effects of this peptide are mediated by direct effects on cells of the immune system, as well as by indirect effects that are achieved by changing the function of non-resident immune cells of peripheral tissues (Luger and Brzoska, 2007).

Three basic mechanisms of α-MSH anti-inflammatory action can be distinguished: direct effects through melanocortin receptors on cells in the periphery (monocytes/macrophages and neutrophils); effects on glial cells; and descendent anti-inflammatory effects through melanocortin receptors on neurons (Lipton et al, 2000). These mechanisms of action correspond to the concept of neuroimmunomodulation in which nerves, endocrine and immune systems are independent networks that mutually communicate through soluble mediators such as cytokines and neuropeptides.

Multiple anti-inflammatory effects that α-MSH has have been identified in various *in vitro* systems of cell cultures. Studies of anti-inflammatory effects of α-MSH on cellular level were primarily concentrated on the issue whether and to what degree α-MSH suppresses the production of pro-inflammatory cytokines. In this respect, several studies have shown that treatment with α-MSH results in significant downregulation of pro-inflammatory cytokines such as IL-1β, IL-2, IL-4, IL-6, IL-13 and TNF-α, as well as chemokines such as IL8, Groα and interferon γ (IFNγ) (Brzoska et al, 2008). Furthermore, chemotaxis induced by IL8 in the cells of human neutrophils and monocytes has been suppressed under the influence of α-MSH (Manna et al, 2006), which indicates that the function of these types of phagocytic cells during the inflammatory response is blocked by the peptide via multiple effector pathways.

Contrary to the inhibitory effects of α-MSH on the production and activity of pro-inflammatory mediators, it has been found that α-MSH induces IL-10, a cytokine with a potent anti-inflammatory activity. Specifically, in monocytes of human peripheral blood and cultivated human monocytes, α-MSH increases the production and expression of IL-10 (Bhardway et al, 1996). Since IL-10 reduces the production of pro-inflammatory cytokines in macrophages, its upregulation could result in anti-inflammatory influences.

Studies on different cell types of human skin, including pigment cells, fibroblastic cells and dermal microvascular endothelial cells, as well as rat mast cells, showed that α-MSH is able to suppress the expression of several intracellular adhesion molecules (interstitial adhesion molecule-1 - ICAM-1 and P-selectin) induced by proinflammatory stimuli such as IFN-γ, LPS and TNF-α (Böhm et al, 2005; Hill et al, 2006; Sarkar et al, 2003). Finally, the inhibition of adhesion and transmigration of inflammatory cells may contribute to the anti-inflammatory potential of α-MSH (Böhm et al, 2005; Scholzen et al, 2003). Moreover, it was found that α-MSH inhibits the maturation of dendritic cells and downregulates the expression of co-stimulatory molecules on antigen-presenting dendritic cells, such as CD86, CD40 and CD54 (Luger, 2003; Capsoni et al, 2007).

One of the mechanisms that could explain the anti-inflammatory action of α-MSH is the suppression of pro-inflammatory non-cytokine mediators under the influence of this peptide. The inhibitory effect of α-MSH on the synthesis of prostaglandin has long been known. This peptide suppressed the synthesis of PGE in the fibroblast of foetal human lung stimulated with IL-1 (Cannon et al, 1986). The effect of α-MSH on the synthesis of PGE is cell specific. Confirmation of this is the fact that under the influence of α-MSH, TNFα–induced production of PGE2 in FM55 melanoma cells was blocked, but not in HaCaT keratinocytes (Nicolaou et al, 2004).

The induction of the inducible form of the enzyme nitric oxide synthase (iNOS) and the release of gaseous vasodilator nitric oxide (NO) after the stimulation of cells with various pro-inflammatory stressors, i.e. LPS, γ-IFN and β-amiloid, can also be suppressed under the influence of α-MSH (Tsatmali et al, 2000; Gupta et al, 2000; Caruso et al, 2007; Jung et al, 2007). The increased expression of NOS, and nitration of cellular proteins in the blood and synovial fluid of a patient with rheumatoid arthritis has been registered. Immunomodulatory effects of α-MSH realized through NO may be more important in rodent than in human cells, since human monocytes are known to contain only marginal amounts of this gaseous mediator.

Recent studies have shown that α-MSH inhibits the production of superoxide radicals in neutrophils of rats treated with LPS or forbolester (Oktar et al, 2004). Similarly, α-MSH reduced the amount of oxidative burst in HL-60 cells, a cell line of human monocytes (Manna et al, 2006). Although there is no evidence to suggest that α-MSH itself is a real radical quencher, these findings are in accordance with other reports that indicate an effect of this peptide on cellular redox balance and the process of apoptosis as well.

Regarding the release of histamine by mast cells, various effects of α-MSH have been described which are likely related to species-specific differences, the type of mast cells and experimental conditions. In mast cells obtained from rat bone marrow, α-MSH inhibited the antigen-induced histamine release together with the suppression of other pro-inflammatory cytokines (Adachi et al, 1999).

There are only a few studies that have researched the effect of α-MSH on the function of lymphocytes, probably due to the fact that the total expression of melanocortin receptors in several lymphocyte lines is low or undetectable (Andersen et al, 2005). It is known that α-MSH induces subpopulation of regulatory T lymphocytes. Regulatory T cells induced with α-MSH are characterized by the expression of CD25, CD4 and CTLA4 and production of increased levels of TGF-β2 (Namba et al, 2002). In the human system, α-MSH also expresses modulator effects on T cells. Cooper and associates (2005) found that α-MSH suppresses the proliferation of human T lymphocytes stimulated by streptokinase/streptodornase. This inhibitory effect of α-MSH was independent of the genotype MC-1R, which is highly polymorphous with more than 35 genetic variations.

Numerous effects of α-MSH on the production of inflammation mediators were a mystery to researchers until it was found that this peptide inhibits the activation of the nuclear factor kappa B (NF-κB) (Mandrika et al, 2001; Hassoun et al, 2002). This essential nuclear factor induces the transcription of many molecules involved in the inflammatory process, and therefore its inhibition results in the alteration of mediators' production and cell functions. NF-κB participates in the regulation of hundreds of genes, including those for cytokines, chemokines, factors for haematopoietic system growth, antiapoptotic factors and the inducible synthesis of nitric oxide (iNOS). Therefore, the discovery that α-MSH inhibits activation of NF-κB provides an explanation for numerous effects of this peptide on the production of mediators.

Anti-inflammatory effects of α-MSH *in vitro* have also been identified *in vivo* in various animal models. These have confirmed a number of effects of melanocortin on the production of mediators of inflammation. The anti-inflammatory activity of α-MSH in animal models of arthritis is of special interest. Repeated intraperitoneal application of the peptide twice daily resulted in a significant reduction of clinical and histological signs of adjuvant-induced experimental arthritis as compared to control animals. The efficiency of α-MSH was similar to that of prednisolone, but α-MSH did not cause significant weight loss (Ceriani et al, 1994). Some data indicate that the melanocortin receptor MC-3R may be a relevant target for the treatment of arthritis.

During the early phase of inflammation (associated with tissue destruction and activation of nociceptors) mediators of inflammation, including cytokines, chemokines, bradykinin, prostaglandins act as mediators of hyperalgesia. At the same time, the expression of peripheral opioid receptors on sensory nerve endings increases during inflammation (Rittner et al, 2003), which leads to the release of pain mediators, such as opioid peptides, somatostatin, endocannabinoids and certain cytokines. Endogenous opioid peptides, leucine and met-enkephalin act presynaptically when they inhibit the release of neurotransmitters, and postsynpatically when they suppress the activity of the postsynaptic neurone, and block the transmission of ascending pain signals (Rang, 2005).

In addition to the central nervous system, met-enkephalin influences the function of the immune system (Vujić-Redžić, 2000). It is released from polymorph nuclear cells during inflammation and periods of stress (Rittner et al, 2006). In inflammation, there is a migration of leukocytes that contain opioid peptides, and also the upregulation of opioid receptors of afferent fibres. This is supported by the fact that IL-1β is a specific inductor of expression of kappa opioid receptors (Puehler et al, 2006). Interleukin-1, together with TNF-α, is the main proinflammatory cytokine released from macrophages and many other cells, which initiates the release of other cytokines (Rajora et al, 1997).

In *in vitro* studies, it was found that T lymphocytes have opioid receptors on their surface (Wybran et al, 1985), and according to Plotnikoff and associates (1991), the effects of enkephalin are precisely related to the immune response mediated by T cells. In addition, the corticotropin-releasing hormone, similarly to the pituitary gland, appears dose-dependent locally, through delta opioid receptors, and leads to the release of opioid peptides from leukocytes and the induction of endogenous analgesia (Menzebach et al, 2003; Cabot et al, 2001).

Met-enkephalin manifests central, bimodal and dose dependent immunomodulatory effects. A bi-phasic effect was registered in *in vivo* studies on rats. High doses have suppressed, while low doses potentiated a humoral immune response (Janković and Marić, 1994). The studies *in vivo* of the immunomodulatory effect of met-enkephaline on rats showed a suppressive action of high doses of met-enkaphalin on inflammatory reactions, such as the systemic anaphylactic shock (Janković and Marić, 1987), Arthus phenomenon and postponed skin reactions to protein antigens (Marić and Janković, 1987), the rejection of allograph (Janković, 1991), arthritis (Janković, 1991) and the experimentally induced allergic encephalomyelitis (Veljić et al, 1991).

In studies conducted at the Charité University in Berlin on the effect of intraarticular application of opioids in comparison to the intraarticular application of glucocorticoids in patients with the chronic inflammatory arthritis accompanied by pain and functional impairment, according to the established hypothesis, local application of opioids led to a significant reduction of pain and inflammation, which can be explained by the activation of peripheral opioid receptors (that have been identified on peripheral sensory nerve endings), and subsequent decreases in neural excitability, transmission of nociceptive impulses, and reduced release of proinflammatory neurotransmitters (Stein et al, 2001; Mousa et al, 2001).

In summary, preclinical studies indicate that the activation of melanocortin receptors could be a new strategy to control inflammation (Catania et al, 2004). Similarly to any new therapeutic approaches, this strategy may have both advantages and disadvantages in comparison to the currently available medications. The main advantage of melanocortin in the treatment of inflammation is that its anti-inflammatory activity is not restricted to a specific mediator or a chemical process. In fact, as a consequence of reduced activation of the nuclear factor NF-κB, the collective reduction of all important molecules involved in the inflammatory process is evident.

Another positive aspect is the fact that the treatment with melanocortin peptides never reverses the inflammatory response, but modulates it. It is well known that the inflammatory response is a crucial reaction of the host that contributes to the elimination of pathogens and harmful molecules. Cytokines, which are a major component of the inflammatory process, also have a significant function in regulating the recovery of tissues, haematopoiesis and immune responses. Any agent that completely inhibits their production or action would have a detrimental impact on the host defence mechanism. Melanocortin peptides modulate the increased production of cytokines during infection or inflammation, but do not prevent their release. Besides, they do not affect the production of mediators of inflammation when being on complete rest. So, for example, alpha-1-13 corticotrophin modulates the febrile response caused by pyrogens, while on the other side, it does not cause any changes to the non-febrile temperature of the body.

The main advantage of the melanocortin in relation to the currently used anti-inflammatory drugs, particularly corticosteroids, is that neuropeptides do not reduce the microbicidal activity of neutrophils, but instead increase it. This feature could be very important in the treatment of inflammation in immunecompromised persons.

The lack of selectivity could be a potential problem when it comes to the use of natural melanocortin peptides. Today, it is clear that the melanocortins affect many body functions, including the regulation of food consumption, sexual behaviour and pigmentation. Systemic injection of non-selective peptide could, therefore, cause adverse effects by stimulating all subtypes of receptors. However, the design and synthesis of new melanocortin analogues with a selective affinity for specific receptors could greatly facilitate the achievement of target effects. Knowledge of amino acid substitution that reduces binding to all receptors can also help prevent unwanted receptor activation. (Catania et al, 2004). Another potential problem lies in the rapid splitting, or degradation of peptide molecules in the circulation and other body fluids, and natural melanocortins are no exception.

The relatively short half-life could be a problem if it is necessary to maintain the concentration in the blood. On the other hand, the fact that the peptides are not accumulated in the body reduces the likelihood of toxicity and tolerance, and allows for better control of the pharmacological effects (Catania et al, 2004).

3. Preclinical toxicological studies

Enkorten toxicity testing was conducted according to the Instructions and Rules of Good Laboratory Practice (GLP) and Harmonized Tripartite Guideline issued in 1998.

Objectives of preclinical toxicological studies were to determine the degree of toxicity of the investigated substance; to identify the target organs of toxicity and to determine the reversibility of the toxic effects; to detect the toxic effects that may help in the identification of the parameters for subsequent clinical trials and to determine the maximum tolerated dose.

Preclinical toxicological studies were carried out in rats and rabbits. The experimental animals were Wistar albino rats bred in the breeding quarters in Harlan, Italy, and the rabbit strain was HY plus giant PS 19 gene, from France. Environmental conditions for animals in the vivarium were maintained constant with daily temperature and humidity monitoring. Semisynthetic food for laboratory animals *ad libitum* and the tap water that meets the Sarajevo city water-supply criteria for drinking water were used during study. Animals were randomly divided in groups according to dose levels. Three dose levels were determined using the method of multiplication of the anticipated maximum human therapeutic dose of 10 mg of met-enkephalin (substance a) and 2 mg of alpha-MSH (substance b): the dose equivalent to the anticipated human therapeutic dose (0.071 mg /kg **a** + 0.014 mg/kg **b**); 5 times higher dose (0.355 mg/kg **a** + 0.07 mg/kg **b**); 10 times higher dose (0.71 mg/kg **a** + 0.14 mg/kg **b**). Enkorten was applied as a constant volume dose of 0.0005 ml/g according to the following dosage regime: during the first month - three times a week; during the second month - twice a week, and during the third month - once a week. The control group was treated by 0.9% of physiological NaCl solution.

Treatment was followed by a 10-day observation period. The appearance of toxic signs was monitored on a daily basis. Weighing of individual animals was performed before dosing, once a week, and before the animals were sacrificed. Daily food and water consumption per cage, as well as the stool mass were recorded on a weekly basis.

In subchronic and chronic studies, haematological and biochemical analyses were performed of the fasting blood samples taken from 12 animals from each of the experimental groups and from 24 animals from the control group, before the animals were sacrificed. The following haematological analyses were performed: hematocrit, haemoglobin concentration, red blood cell count, red blood cell morphology, total and differential white blood cell count, platelets. The following biochemical analyses were performed: Calcium (Ca^{+2}), Potassium (K^+), Sodium (Na^+), Chloride (Cl^-), Phosphorus (PO_2^{4-}), glucose, Aspartal aspartate aminotransferase (AST) , Alanine aminotransferase (ALT), alkaline phosphatase (AP), Gamma-glutamyl transpeptidase (GGT), blood urea nitrogen (BUN), total proteins, albumin, globulin, total bilirubin, creatinine, lipids, and cholinesterase.

Necropsy was performed only on the sacrificed animals (no lethality observed). Upon completion of the experiment, animals were sacrificed and both external and internal examinations of the sacrificed animals were performed. The following organs: brain, heart, lungs, liver, spleen, thymus, kidneys and adrenal glands, as well as samples of other macroscopically changed tissues were subjected to histopathological analysis.

Collected data were statistically analyzed using the Microsoft® Excel 2002 and SigmaStat programs for statistical analysis.

3.1 Acute toxicity study

The acute toxicity study was performed as the initial step of the prospective drug toxicological evaluation. Acute toxicity provides the important safety parameters for the prospective human overdose scenario and its expected clinical presentation. Traditionally, international authorities and governmental agencies had adopted the mean lethal dose as the sole measurement of acute toxicity. Testing of the rationally high doses, without detected lethality, is also acceptable and complies with the Limit Test concept (ICH, 2009; EMA, 2010).

Acute toxicity was assessed on Wistar albino rats. The study was performed as the single dose testing following intravenous (i.v.), subcutaneous (s.c.) and intraperitoneal (i.p.) application, in accordance with the Limit Test methodology. The administered multiplications were: via i.v. route 50, 100 and 200 times; via s.c. route 100, 250 and 500 times; and via i.p. route 100, 250, 500 times plus 1000 times in and additional group of males. Neither lethality, nor significant macroscopic and microscopic changes were observed at the necropsy following planned sacrificing. The necropsy and histopathological evaluation revealed no significant changes. No statistically significant differences in post-mortem organ weights were noted.

The most prominent clinical signs were noted on day 1 of the observation period. Following all three application routes, slightly reduced motor activity and the horizontal positioning of the tail was observed in all animals treated with the highest i.v. dose. There was a slight ptosis (eyelids down ¼) in a few animals in all i.v. treatment groups. Slight cyanosis and general vasoconstriction was noted in one male treated with the highest i.v. dose, and one male treated with the medium i.v. dose. Slightly slower motor activity of all treated and control animals was observed following the s.c. application. Also, slight muscular hypotonia was noted on day 3 in three males treated with the highest dose and one male treated with the lowest dose. Irregular breathing, decrease in motor activity, somnolence, ataxia, catalepsy and muscular hypotonia were observed in all males from the additional group administered i.p. with 1000 dose multiplication. A proportion of the effects noted could be attributed to the application of the large amount of fluid, since the constant volume was not respected for this group. Afterwards, the frequency and character of breathing were observed once a week and were found to remain within the physiological limits.

Intensive phonation during the manipulation with animals was registered for i.v. dosed groups. The frequency of intensive phonation intensified between days 9 and 14 of the observation period, which was not noted in control animals. Statistically significant difference was detected for increased phonation in all treatment groups of males, IVF3 and IVF2, compared to controls ($p \leq 0.000001$). Following the s.c. application, each phonation was registered, and there was no prominent difference in phonation in males, while a statistically significant difference in phonation was noted for group SCF3 ($p = 0.000001$), compared to the control.

The tested combination induced no lethality and demonstrated a low level of toxicity in high doses. The fact that neither organ or tissue damage, nor organ mass ratio differences in control and experimental groups were detected indicates that the application of the tested combination to the rats did not result in a permanent adverse toxicological effect on the examined organs. Reversible signs of toxicity disappeared with substance elimination and usually were not followed by a permanent tissue damage.

High doses of met-enkephalins produce effects on OP_3 (μ) receptors in the range of sedation, mood changes, miosis, respiratory depression and gastrointestinal disturbances (Plotnikoff et al., 1997; Brunton and Parker, 2008). The evidence of ptosis, motor activity changes, horizontal positioning of the tail or increased phonation could suggest opioid pathway engagèment. Increased intensity of phonation was clearly noted for all i.v. dosed treatment groups, but not at all in control animals (Rakanović-Todić et al, 2011).

3.2 Subacute toxicity study

The subacute toxicity study with the subcutaneous (s.c.) administration of Enkorten was conducted with three experimental groups, each of 10 Wistar albino rats (both males and females) and the control group of 20 Wistar albino rats (both males and females) during four weeks. Neither lethal outcomes nor toxic signs were observed during the study. The absence of pronounced toxicity of the substances was confirmed by the body weight gain in both experimental and control groups of animals during the study period. The ability of gaining or maintaining the body weight is considered to be a non-specific indicator of the health status of the animal (Gad and Chengelis, 1998), especially in toxicity studies with multiple applications. Furthermore, the average food and water consumption as well as the percentage ratio of stool mass were balanced between male and female groups. Neither external nor internal examination of animals sacrificed at the end of the study revealed any macroscopic pathological changes. Histopathological analysis revealed no microscopic pathological changes in tissue samples of liver, kidneys, lungs, heart, brain, spleen and thymus. All examined tissues showed a normal structure. No statistically significant differences in post-mortem organ weights were noted between male and female groups. The results of subacute toxicity study indicated that the tested combination of substances was not toxic when administered s.c. and repeatedly during four weeks (Todić et al, 2007).

3.3 Subchronic toxicity study

The subchronic toxicity study with intramuscular administration of Enkorten was conducted with three experimental groups, each of 10 Wistar albino rats (both males and females) and the control group of 15 Wistar albino rats (both males and females) during three month.

As a part of this study, the electrocardiogram (ECG) was recorded in 6 animals from each of the experimental groups (3 males + 3 females) and from the control group (3 males + 3 females), which in total amounts to 24 animals. The ECG was recorded on the day before the study commenced, as well as during the third, fifth, seventh, ninth and the eleventh week of the study and on the day before the planned sacrificing of animals. The electrocardiograph Schiller Resting ECG, connected to a personal computer was used for ECG registration. The computer program SEMA - 200 Vet (a program for ECG analysis in veterinary medicine) was used for the analysis of the registered curves. This program calculated the average values of the heart rate (FSR bits/min) and the duration of the RR interval (ms), P wave (ms), PQ interval (ms), QRS complex (ms) and QT interval (ms).

In the subchronic toxicity study, not a single lethal outcome was registered. No statistically significant differences between experimental and control groups in body weight of animals, in food and water consumption were documented. No statistically significant differences between experimental and control groups in the sensitivity to pain, frequency of breathing, were detected, nor differences in post-mortem organ weights during macroscopic examination and histopathological analysis of the tissue samples. No statistically significant differences were found between experimental and control groups in the average duration of ECG parameters and biochemical parameters in males. The results of the investigation of the Enkorten influence on the biochemical parameters in females showed the following statistically significant differences: in the values of calcium ($p = 0.046$) between the third and the first group (FG3 *vs.* FG1); in the values of sodium ($p = 0.044$) although no statistically significant differences were documented in the sodium values between the individual experimental groups and the control group; in the values of urea ($p = 0.049$) although no statistically significant differences in the urea values between the individual experimental groups and the control group were documented; in the values of ASAT ($p = 0.020$) between the first and the control group; in the values of cholinesterase ($p = 0.036$) between the first and the control group (FG1 *vs.* FGK). It may be concluded that Enkorten probably affected the values of ASAT and cholinesterase in females, whereas the differences in the values of calcium, sodium and urea were probably due to chance. The results of the haematological parameters showed no statistically significant differences. It can be concluded that the tested substance had no impact on haematological parameters. Test results of the toxic effect investigation suggested that the maximum tolerated dose for male and female rats approximately corresponds to the dose 10 times higher than the anticipated human therapeutic dose. Based on the estimates obtained, we can conclude that in the study conducted in male and female Wistar albino rats, the investigated product showed no subchronic toxicity when the multiple i.m. application of animal doses equivalent to the either anticipated human therapeutic dose, or 5 or 10 times higher dose was performed.
During the implementation of the subchronic Enkorten toxicity study in rabbits, individual cases of mortality, that cannot be linked with the activity of the test substance, have been documented in all experimental groups.

3.4 Chronic toxicity study

Based upon results of the chronic toxicity study performed on rats after the subcutaneous administration of Enkorten (three experimental groups, each of 40 Wistar albino rats and a control group) during six months, it was concluded that test substance did not show any toxic effects. In the course of the chronic toxicity study, not one lethal outcome was registered. In the course of pain sensitivity testing, the tested substance did not demonstrate a significant analgesic effect. Moreover, it was found that the tested substance increases the irritability of animals in the sense that it increases the frequency of phonation. The histopathology laboratory reports recorded no changes with respect to the mass of single organs or with respect to the macroscopic and microscopic structure of organs and tissues of experimental animals. The difference is noted in the mass of the left adrenal in the control and the first group in relation to administering the combination to male rats. Impact of tested substances on biochemical parameters in males showed statistically significant difference between the first and the control groups, as well as between the second and the control group in the values of phosphorous, alkaline phosphates, and urea. The difference in triglycerides between the first and the control group, the AST values between the second and third group and the first and the third group, the ALT values between the second and the control group were also noticed. The sifnificant difference in the values of these parameters for males may be coincidental, because the difference between the groups treated by the highest dose level and the control group was not registered. In females a statistically significant difference in calcium and potassium was registered between the treated and the control groups. The values of phosphorus and alkaline phosphatase significantly differed between the first and the control group, and urea value between the first and the control group. Triglyceride statisticaly levels of all three treated groups significantly differed from the control group values. Also, there was a significantly difference in the values of ALT between the second and the control group. These data suggest that tested substance affects the value of calcium, potassium and triglycerides in females. The value difference of other parameters can be random, because the difference between the groups treated with the highest dose level and the control group was not registered. The data on the volume and biochemical parameters of urine showed statistically non significant difference between control and other groups of animals. Statistically significant difference between the control and first group of animals was found only in glucose during the second measurement. Registered difference is probably a consequence of stress.

Statistical analyses of the results obtained after biochemical analyses were not statistically significant (including both male and female groups) for the following parameters: Ca^{+2}, K^{+}, Na^{+}, Cl^{-}, glucose, total proteins, albumins, globulins, total bilirubin, creatinine, cholesterol, cholinesterase, AST, GGT.

The tested substance has no effect on the parameters of erythrocytes, leukocytes, granulocytes, thrombocytes and lymphocytes. However, the tested substance has effects on the value of monocytes when compared to the control group, and, as far as males are concerned, also in the values of lymphocytes. The tested substance did not have effects on the volume and biochemical parameters of urea, except for the glucose report. The noted difference is, probably, the result of stress (Bečić et al, 2007).

3.5 A pilot study of the reproductive toxicity in rats

Testing was conducted at the Institute following the NTP, 2002 (NTP - National Toxicology Program - Good Science and Good Decisions - NIEHS, USA, 2002), in five months old, adult male and female laboratory Wistar albino rats (the Institute's own breeding colony).

In the first phase, Enkorten in a doubled human therapeutic dose (2HD; α-MSH 0.028 mg/kg + met-enkephalin 0.143 mg/kg) was administered once intraperitoneally (i.p.). Afterwards, animals were administered a bilateral intranasal (i.n.) dose of Enkorten eight times higher than the human therapeutic dose (8HD) per day, within two consecutive days. Administration of the substance in the above doses was carried out using the methods of crossing and gender matching. In the second phase, the same dosing protocol but with the i.n. dose increased to twenty times human therapeutic dose (20HD) was administered to the F_1 generation of male and female rats, after they reached sexual maturity. By applying the same protocol, the control group received a physiological solution. During the first and the second phase, the typical parameters of the reproductive capacity of the animals from the F_0

and F_1 generations (gestation, litter and lactation) as well as the litter of the F_1 and F_2 generations (number of offspring per litter, size, weight, growth, development and advancement until the age of 8 weeks) were followed. At the end of the study, *post mortem* analysis was performed on the tissue and reproductive organs of young male and female rats from the F_2 generation.
Comparing to controls, Enkorten did not cause any changes in the first phase of testing. In the second phase of the study, no gestation appeared in the experimental group from the F_1 generation, whereas in the remaining four groups the reproduction process was completely in accordance with the control. The number of offspring per litter ranged from 8 to 12. The size and weight of youth as well as gender contribution were fully in compliance with the control group. The development, growth, advancement of youth and lactation were progressing normally. Development was monitored until the age of 8 weeks of life, after which histopathological analysis of tissues and reproductive organs was performed. *Post mortem* analyses did not reveal significant changes in any of the young animals. No signs of teratogenicity were documented in the two generations of young rats.
Based on the observed results, it can be concluded that Enkorten did not significantly affect the process of reproduction in rats. Enkorten did not cause any teratogenic changes. Histopathological reports were completely normal.

3.6 Investigation of the effect on skin

The investigation of the effect of Enkorten on skin was conducted using the mouse ear model (according to: Hypersensitivity Test Methods: NTP-National Toxicology Program - Good Science and Good Decisions - NIEHS, USA, 2002).
Adult BALB/c male and female mice, divided into groups of 6 animals (the Institute's own breeding colony) were receiving Enkorten in 2HD (α-MSH 0.028 mg/kg + met-enkephalin 0.143 mg/kg) per day, by i.p. route, during 4 days. As an irritant, croton oil (3%, in acetone) was applied topically, in a volume of 25 µL, once, at the fifth day of the first Enkorten application. By applying the dose of Enkorten in such conditions, the irritation/inflammation process on the mouse skin caused by croton oil was inhibited by 35% compared to the control group that received the physiological solution. Enkorten action was slightly more pronounced in males during the first 24 hours.
The doubled human therapeutic dose of Enkorten, applied topically to skin in a volume of 25 µL, 6 hours prior to the irritant application (3% croton oil in acetone, in the volume of 25 µL, topically), led to the inhibition of the irritation/inflammation processes by 57% to 60%, compared to both male and female control mice.
It can be concluded that Enkorten administered preventively, in a dose equivalent to the doubled human therapeutic dose, by i.p. route, during 4 days, reduced the irritation/inflammation processes for about 35%. Compared to the control, this drug, applied once, topically, reduced irritation/inflammation processes caused on the mouse skin by 60%.

4. Pharmacokinetic study

The aim of this study was to assign the range of values of α-MSH and met-enkephalin plasma concentrations before and after the Enkorten application and to determine pharmacokinetic parameters of the test preparation (C_{max}, T_{max}, AUC, $T_{1/2}$). C_{max} (Maximum

Plasma Concentration) is the highest concentration of drug in the blood that is measured after a dose; T_{max} (Time to Reach C_{max}) is the time at which the highest plasma drug concentration occurs C_{max}; AUC (Area Under the Curve) is the measure of total plasma exposure of drug over a given time period; $T_{½}$ (Half-life) is the time required for a given drug concentration to decrease by 50%.

The study was carried out on a group of 14 healthy volunteers, ages from 18 to 30, males, of body weight and height within the standard values.

All volunteers received subcutaneously one dose of Enkorten preparation in the presumed therapeutic dose for human application. No serious side-effects were observed during the study. The available kit is not specific for the determination of α-MSH of the test preparation; thus, the cross-reactivity of physiologically present α-MSH and α-MSH component of the preparation was determined. Significant interindividual differences of α-MSH plasma concentration were found. Mean values were 21.31 - 47.56 pg/ml. Mean plasma concentration of endogenous met-enkephalin was 50.40 pg/ml. Maximum plasma concentration after Enkorten application, measured 5 minutes after the application, was 1551.86 pg/ml. The plasma half-life was 15 minutes. The concentration/time curve of met-enkephalin implies first-order kinetics (Kusturica et al, 2009).

5. Conclusion

Enkorten is an immunomodulatory preparation containing two components, α-melanocyte stimulating hormone (α-MSH) and methionine-enkefalin (met-enkephalin). α-MSH and met-enkephalin are endogenous substances of the neuropeptide group. They participate in the homeostatic processes, maintaining the biochemical link between the brain, neuroendocrine system and the immune system. The mechanism of action of both peptides directly reclines on both mechanisms of immune response development. The effect also includes analgesia, antipyretic and anti-inflammatory activities.

Pharmacodynamics of the combination shown in the studies imply great therapeutic possibilities. The presumed indication range of Enkorten encompasses diseases with inflammatory processes as the primary pathophysiological aspect (asthma, inflammatory bowel disease, rheumatoid arthritis, multiple sclerosis).

Preclinical findings indicate that the tested combination was nontoxic and well tolerated in doses applied by i.v., s.c., i.m., and i.p. routes, and therefore have the potential for safe future use as a medicine.

6. References

Adachi, S., Nakano, T., Vliagoftis, H., Metcalfe, D.D. (1999). Receptor-mediated modulation of murine mast cell function by α-melanocyte stimulating hormone. *J Immunol* 163: 3363–3368.

Andersen, G.N., Hagglund, M., Nagaeva, O., Frangsmyr, L., Petrovska, R., Mincheva-Nilsson, L., Wikberg, J.E. (2005). Quantitative measurement of the levels of melanocortin receptor subtype 1, 2, 3 and 5 and pro-opiomelanocortin peptide gene expression in subsets of human peripheral blood leucocytes. *Scand J Immunol* 61: 279–284.

Bečić, F., Mulabegović, N., Kapić, E., Rakanović-Todić, M., Kusturica, J., Ašćerić, M., Loga-Zec S. (2007). Evaluation of toxicity of combination met-encephaline and alpha-melanocyte-stimulating hormone with the aim to calculate clinical studies. 8th Congress of the European Association for Clinical Pharmacology and Therapeutics. Amsterdam, *Medimond S.r.l:* 221-226.

Bhardwaj, R.S., Becher, E., Mahnke, K., Hartmeyer, M., Schwarz, T., Scholzen, T. et al. (1997). Evidence for the differential expression of the functional alpha melanocyte stimulating hormone receptor MC-1 on human monocytes. *J Immunol* 158: 3378-3384.

Böhm, M., Eickelmann, M., Li, Z., Schneider, S.W., Oji, V., Diederichs, S., Barsh, G.S., Vogt, A., Stieler, K., Blume-Peytavi, U., Luger, T.A. (2005). Detection of functionally active melanocortin receptors and evidence for an immunoregulatory activity of α-melanocyte-stimulating hormone in human dermal papilla cells. *Endocrinology* 146: 4635–4646.

Brunton, L.L., Parker, L.K. (eds.) Goodman and Gilman's Manual of Pharmacology and Therapeutics, 1st edition. McGraw-Hill Companies, 2008; p 349-382, 1023-1036.

Brzoska, T., Luger, T.A., Maaser, C., Abels, C., Böhm, M. (2008). α-Melanocyte-Stimulating Hormone and Related Tripeptides: Biochemistry, Anti-inflammatory and Protective Effects *in Vitro* and *in Vivo*, and Future Perspectives for the Treatment of Immune-Mediated Inflammatory Diseases. *Endocrine Reviews* 29 (5): 581-602.

Cabot, P.J., Carter, L., Schäfer, M., Stein, C. (2001). Methionine-enkephalin-and Dynorphin A-release from immune cells and control of inflammatory pain. *Pain* 93(3): 207-212.

Cannon, J.G., Tatro, J.B., Reichlin, S., Dinarello, C.A. (1986). α-Melanocyte stimulating hormone inhibits immunostimulatory and inflammatory actions of interleukin 1. *J Immunol* 137: 2232–2236

Capsoni, F., Ongari, A., Colombo, G., Turcatti, F., Catania, A. (2007). The synthetic melanocortin (CKPV)(2) exerts broad anti-inflammatory effects in human neutrophils. *Peptides* 28(10): 2016-2022.

Caruso, C., Durand, D., Schiöth, H.B., Rey, R., Seilicovich, A., Lasaga, M. Activation of melanocortin 4 receptors reduces the inflammatory response and prevents apoptosis induced by lipopolysaccharide and interferon-γ in astrocytes. *Endocrinology* 148: 4918–4926.

Catania, A., Airaghi, L., Colombo, G. and Lipton, M.J. (2000). α- Melanocyte-stimulating hormone in Normal Human Physioligy and Disease States. *TEM* 11 (8): 304-308.

Catania, A., Cutuli, M., Garofalo, L., Carlin, A., Airaghi, L., Barcellini, W. and Lipton, J.M. (2000a). The neuropeptide alpha- MSH in host defence. *Amm NY Acad Sci* 917: 227-231.

Catania, A., Delgado, R., Airaghi, L., Cutuli, M., Garofalo, L., Carlin, A., Demitri, M.T., Lipton, J.M. (1999). Alfa-MSH in Systemic Inflammation: Central and Peripheral Actions. *Annals of the New York Academy of Sciences* 885:183-187.

Catania, A., Gatti, S., Colombo, G., Lipton, J.M. (2004). Targeting melanocortin receptors as a novel strategy to control inflammation. *Pharmacol Rev* 56: 1–29.

Ceriani, G., Diaz, J., Murphree, S., Catania, A., Lipton, J.M. (1994). The neuropeptide alpha-melanocyte-stimulating hormone inhibits experimental arthritis in rats. *Neuroimmunomodulation* 1: 28-32

Cooper, A., Robinson, S.J., Pickard, C., Jackson, C.L., Friedmann, P.S., Healy, E. (2005). α-Melanocyte-stimulating hormone suppresses antigen-induced lymphocyte proliferation in humans independently of melanocortin 1 receptor gene status. *J Immunol* 175: 4806–4813.

EMA: European Medicines Agency Questions and Answers on the withdrawal of the Note for guidance on single dose toxicity. Committee for Medicinal Products for Human Use. 2010: http://www.ema.europa.eu (accessed November 2, 2010).

Gad, C.S. and Chengelis P.C. Acute Toxicology Testing. Second edition. Academic Press, USA, 1998.

Getting, S.J. (2006). Targeting melanocortin receptors as potential novel therapeutics. *Pharmacol Ther* 111 (1): 1-15.

Gupta, A.K., Diaz, R.A., Higham, S., Kone, B.C. (2000). α-MSH inhibits induction of C/EBPβ-DNA binding activity and NOS2 gene transcription in macrophages. *Kidney Int* 57: 2239–2248.

Hassoun, H.T., Zou, L., Moore, F.A., Kozar, R.A., Weisbrodt, N.W., Kone, B.C. (2002). Alpha-melanocyte-stimulating hormone protects against mesenteric ischemia-reperfusion injury. *Am J Physiol Gastrointest Liver Physiol* 282: G1059–G1068.

Hill, R.P., MacNeil, S., Haycock, J.W. (2006). Melanocyte stimulating hormone peptides inhibit TNF-a signaling in human dermal fibroblast cells. *Peptides* 27: 421–430.

ICH: International Conference on Harmonisation. Guidance on Nonclinical Safety Studies for the Conduct of the Human Clinical Trials and Marketing Authorization for Pharmaceuticals M3(R2), 2009.

Jankovic, B., Maric, D. Enkephalins as regulators of inflammatory immune reactions. In: Neuropeptides and Immunoregulation. Scharrer et al. Eds. pp: 76-100, Springer-Verlag Berlin Heidelberg, 1994

Jankovic, B.D. (1991). Enkephalins and immune inflammatory reactions. *Estrallo da Acta Neurologica* 13 (XLVI) N0 5

Jankovic, B.D., Maric, D. (1987). Enkephalins and anaphylactic shock: Modulation and prevention of shock in the rat. *Immmunol Lett* 15: 153.

Jung, E.J., Han, D.J., Chang, S.H., Lim, D.G., Wee, Y.M., Kim, J.H., Koo, S.K., Choi, M., Kim, S.C. (2007). Protective effect of α-melanocyte-stimulating hormone on pancreas islet cell against peripheral blood mononuclear cell-mediated cytotoxicity in vitro. *Transplant Proc* 39: 1604–1606.

Konjevoda, P., Štambuk, N., Aralica, G., Pokrič, B. (2001). Cytoprotective effects of met-encephalin and α-MSH on ethanol induced gastric lesions in rats. *Journal of Physiology* 95: 277-281.

Konjevoda, P., Štambuk, N., Vikić-Topić, D., Boban-Blagajić, A., Vikić-Topić, S., Mrljak, V., Pavan, J., Ramadan, P., Bididn, Z. (2000). Protective effects of Met-encephalin on alcohol induced gastric lesions. *Croatica Chemica Acta* 73 (4): 1111-1121.

Kusturica, J., Mulabegović, N., Kapic, E., Krehić, J., Mandal, S. et Bečić, F. (2009). Pharmacokinetics of Encorten. *HealthMed* 3 (2):159-165.

Lipton, J.M., Catania, A., Ichiyama, T. (2000). Marshaling the anti-inflammatory influence of the neuroimmunomodulator α-MSH. *News Physiol Sci* 15: 192–195.

Lipton, M.J. and Catania, A. (1997). Anti-inflamatory actions of the neuroimunomodulator α- MSH. *Immunology today* 18 (3): 140-145.

Luger, T.A. et al. (2003). New insights into the functions of alpha-MSH and related peptides in the immune system. *Annals of the New York Academy of Sciences* 994: 133-140.

Luger, T.A., Brzoska, T. (2007). α-MSH related peptides: a new class of anti-inflammatory and immunomodulating drugs. *Annals of the Rheumatic Diseases* 66 (Suppl 3): iii52-iii55.

Mandrika, I., Muceniece, R., Wikberg, J.E. (2001). Effects of melanocortin peptides on lipopolysaccharide/interferon-γ-induced NF-κB DNA binding and nitric oxide production in macrophage-like RAW 264.7 cells: evidence for dual mechanisms of action. *Biochem Pharmacol* 61: 613–621.

Manna, S.K., Sarkar, A., Sreenivasan, Y. (2006). α-Melanocyte-stimulating hormone down-regulates CXC receptors through activation of neutrophil elastase. *Eur J Immunol* 36: 754–769.

Menzebach, A., Hirsch, J., Hempelmann, G., Welters, D. (2003). Effects of endogenous and synthetic opioid peptides on neutrophil function *in vitro. British Journal of Anaesthesia* 91(4): 546-550.

Mousa, S.A., Zhang, Q., Sitte, N., Ji, R., Stein, C. (2001). Beta-Endorphin-containing memory-cells and mu-opioid receptors undergo transport to peripheral inflamed tissue. *J Neuroimmunol* 115: 71-78.

Mulabegović, N., Rakanović-Todić, M. (2008). Pharmacodynamic Properties of Combination of Met-enkephalin and Alpha 1-13 Corticotropine. *Medicinski Arhiv* 62(1):41-4.

Namba, K., Kitaichi, N., Nishida, T., Taylor, A.W. (2002). Induction of regulatory T cells by the immunomodulating cytokines alpha-melanocyte-stimulating hormone and transforming growth factor-beta2. *J leukoc Biol* 72; 946-952.

Nicolaou, A., Estdale, S.E., Tsatmali, M., Herrero, D.P., Thody, A.J. (2004). Prostaglandin production by melanocytic cells and the effect of α-melanocyte stimulating hormone. *FEBS Lett* 570: 223–226.

Oktar, B.K., Yuksel, M., Alican, I. (2004). The role of cyclooxygenase inhibition in the effect of α-melanocyte-stimulating hormone on reactive oxygen species production by rat peritoneal neutrophils. *Prostaglandins Leukot Essent Fatty Acids* 71: 1–5.

Plotnikoff, N., Faith, R.E., Murgo, A.J., Herberman, R.B., Good, R.A. (1997). Short analytical review: Methionine enkefalin: A new cytokine-human studies. *Clinical Immunology and Immunopathology* 82(2): 99-101.

Plotnikoff, N.P., Wybran, J. (1991). Methionine enkephalin: activation of NK-K-LAK cells in AIDS patients. *Int Conf AIDS.* Jun 16-21; 7: 216 (abstract no. W.B.2139).

Puehler, W., Rittner, H.L., Mousa, S.A., Brack, A., Krause, H., Stein, C. (2006). Interleukin-1 beta contributes to the upregulation kappa opioid receptor mrna in dorsal root ganglia in response to peripheral inflammation. *Neuroscience* 16.

Rajora, N., Boccoli, G., Burns, D., Sharma, S., Catania, A.P., Lipton, J.M. (1997). α-MSH modulates local and circulating tumor necrosis factor-α in experimental brain inflammation. *The Journal of Neuroscience* 17 (6): 2181-2186.

Rakanović-Todić, M., Mulabegović, N., Becic, F., Mijanovic, M., Loga-Zec, S., Kusturica, J., Burnazović-Ristić, L., Kulo, A., Kapić, E. (2011). Acute Toxicity Study of Combination of Tridecactide and Met-Enkephalin. *Folia Medica* 46(1):13-22.

Rang, H.P., Dale, M.M., Ritter, J.M., Moore, P.K. (2005). Pharmacology. First edition in the Serb language. Edited by Z. Todorović. Belgrade. Data status, 747-752.

Rang, H.P., Dale, M.M., Ritter, J.M., Moore, P.K. (2005). Pharmacology. First edition in the Serb language. Edited by Z. Todorović. Belgrade. Data status, 217-242.

Rittner, H.L., Brack, A., Stein, C. (2003). Pro-algesic versus analgesic actions of immune cells. *Curr Opin Anaesthesiol* 16: 527-533.

Rittner, H.L., Labuz, D., Schaefer, M., Mousa, S.A., Schulz, S., Schafer, M., Stein, C., Brack, A. (2006). Pain control by CXCE2 ligands through Ca2+ regulated release of opioid peptides from polyprpho nuclear cells. *FASEB J*

Sarkar, A., Sreenivasan, Y., Manna, S.K. (2003). α-Melanocyte-stimulating hormone induces cell death in mast cells: involvement of NF-kB. *FEBS Lett* 549: 87–93.

Scholzen, T.E., Sunderkötter, C., Kalden, D.H., Brzoska, T., Fastrich, M., Fisbeck, T., Armstrong, C.A., Ansel, J.C., Luger, T.A. (2003). α-Melanocyte stimulating hormone prevents lipopolysaccharide-induced vasculitis by down-regulating endothelial cell adhesion molecule expression. *Endocrinology* 144: 360–370.

Štambuk, N., Breljak, D., Križanac-Begenez, Lj. and Boranić, M. (1996). A model of met-enkephalin induced alterations of the bone marrow cell proliferation. *Periodicum Biologorum* 96 (1): 115-118.

Štambuk, N., Brnar, V., Štambuk, V., Svoboda-Beusan, I., Rabatić, S., Mazuran, R. et al. (1997). Peptide M (Lupex(R)) immunotherapy in multiple sclerosis, optic neuritis and uveitis. *Journal of Etymology* 5(8-9): 448-464.

Star, A.R., Rajora, N., Huang, J., Stock, C.R., Catania, A., Lipton, M.J. (1995). Evidence of autocrine modulation of macrophage nitric oxide synthase by melanocyte-stimulating hormone. *Proc Natl Acad Sci USA* 92: 8016-8020.

Stein, C., Machelska, H., Schäfer, M. (2001). Peripheral analgesic and anti-inflammatory effects of opioids. *J Rheumatol* 60: 416-424.

Todić, M., Mulabegović, N., Becić, F., Kusturica, J. (2007). Subacute toxicity study of combination of adrenocorticotropine 1-13 and met-enkephalin. *Med Arh.* 61(4):199-202.

Tsatmali, M., Graham, A., Szatkowski, D., Ancans, J., Manning, P., McNeil, C.J., Graham A.M., Thody, A.J. (2000). α-Melanocyte-stimulating hormone modulates nitric oxide production in melanocytes. *J Invest Dermatol* 114: 520–526.

Veljić, J., Marić, D., Janković, B.D. (1991). Changes of experimental allergic encephalomyelitis by methionine-enkephalin injected into lateral ventricles of the rat brain. *Int J Neurosci* 59(1-3): 81-89.

Vujić-Redžić, V., Dimitrijević, M., Stanojević, S., Kovačević-Jovanović, V., Miletić, T., Radulović, J. (2000). Peripheral Effects of Methionine-Enkephalin on Inflammatory Reactions and Behavior in the Rat. *NeuroImmunoModulation* 8: 70-77.

Wybran, J., Appelboom, T., Famaey, J.P., Govaerts, A. (1985). Suggestive evidence for receptors for morphine and methionine- enkephalin on normal human blood T lymphocytes. *The Journal of Head and Face Pain* 25: 259.

Zagon, I.S., Wu, Y., McLaughlin, P.J. (1997). Opioid growth factor is present in human and mouse gastrointestinal tract and inhibits DNA synthesis. *Am J Physiol* 272 (4Pt 2): 1094-1104

8

Proteasome Targeted Therapies in Rheumatoid Arthritis

Aisha Siddiqah Ahmed
Karolinska Institutet
Sweden

1. Introduction

Rheumatoid arthritis (RA) is a chronic, systemic, autoimmune disease that primarily affects the joints. Approximately 0.5% of the adult population worldwide suffer from RA. The functional disability that results from progressive joint destruction is associated with substantial cost, significant morbidity and premature mortality [Carmona et al, 2010]. Pain and inflammation are initial symptoms followed by various degree of bone and cartilage destruction. During the last few decades' tremendous improvements have been made in search of therapies against RA. Disease modifying anti-rheumatic drugs (DMARDs) and biological therapies such as antagonists against TNF-α or IL-1 have provided efficient treatments and changed the shape of this disorder. However, the side effects, availability, and their focused approach to reduce inflammation have limited their scope. Thus there is a need of therapies targeting inflammation as well as reducing inflammatory pain and joint destruction in RA.

Cytokines are key players in pathogenesis of RA [Brennan & McInnes, 2008]. Synovial fluid from RA joints contains large quantities of cytokines secreted by macrophages, dendritic cells, neutrophils and synovial fibroblasts [Raza et al, 2005]. Cytokines such as tumor necrosis factor-α (TNF-α), interleukin-1 (IL-1) and interleukin-17 (IL-17) stimulate the production of destructive proteases. Synthesis of these pro-inflammatory mediators is regulated by the transcription factor NF-κB, controlled by the ubiquitin proteasome system (UPS) [Baldwin, 1996]. UPS is a multicatalytic system of protein degradation and present in all cell types including neurons and glia cells and regulates numerous cellular functions by selectively degrading cellular proteins.

2. Ubiquitin proteasome system

The degradation and processing of cellular proteins is critical for cell survival, growth, and cell division. Proteolysis via the proteasome pathway plays an important role in a variety of basic cellular processes. These processes are regulation of cell cycle and division, modulation of the immune and inflammatory responses, intracellular signaling, and development and differentiation [Goldberg, 2003].

Cellular proteins are mainly degraded in two ways: lysosomal degradation and ubiquitin-mediated degradation. Proteolysis in lysosomes is a non-specific process. In higher eukaryotes, membrane-associated and extracellular proteins captured during endocytosis (e.g. viral, bacterial) are destroyed in lysosomes. Degradation of the vast majority (80-90%) of intracellular proteins is proteasome mediated [Ciechanover, 2005]. The ubiquitin proteasome system (UPS) controls the degradion of proteins in the cytosol, nucleus as well as in the luminal endoplasmic reticulum in eukaryotic cells (Goldberg, 2003).

Ubiquitin-mediated degradation of a protein involves two discrete and successive steps: first, the conjugation of multiple moieties of ubiquitin (Ub) to the protein substrate; multiple copies of ubiquitin covalently bind to available lysine residues on target proteins in a three-step process. Second, recognition of polyubiquitinated proteins by the 19S proteasome complex; Ub chain is cleaved by deubiquitinated enzymes (DUB), the substrate protein is unfolded and enters the 20S core for degradation. Then the substrate protein is cleaved into smaller peptide chains (5-20 amino acids), which are further degraded into constituent amino acids and are recycled by the cell [Goldberg, 2003]. The polyubiquitin chain is also broken down by the hydrolase enzymes and free Ub molecules are recycled by the cell [Kisselev et al., 1999] (Fig. 1).

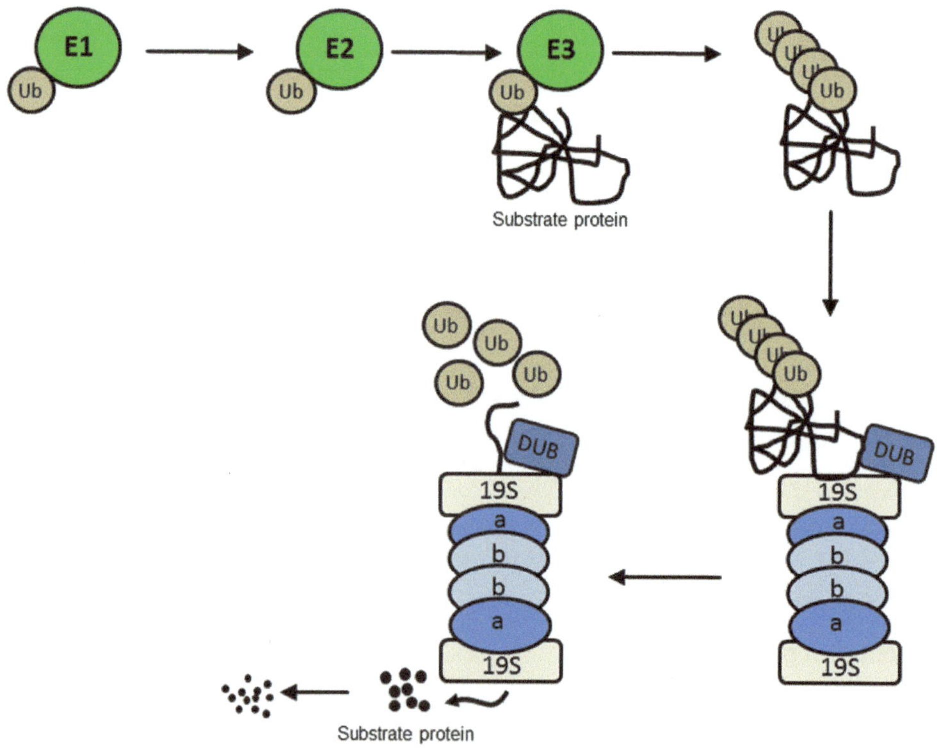

Fig. 1. The ubiquitin-dependent degradation of protein

This process has been named the "ubiquitin-dependent degradation of protein" and was first discovered by A. Ciechanover, A. Hershko, and I. Rose who were later awarded the Nobel Prize in 2004 [Sorokin et al., 2009].

2.1 Enzymatic cascade

Ubiquitin is a 76 amino acid protein conserved across eukaryotic cells. The covalent attachment of ubiquitin to a substrate protein is a highly regulated process and can be controlled at multiple points. Ubiquitin is first activated by an activating enzyme, E1. This step requires ATP to generate a high-energy thioester intermediate, E1-S~ubiquitin. The thioester attachment induces a conformational change in the E1 that promotes association with an ubiquitin carrier protein, E2. Next, activated ubiquitin is transferred to the E2 via formation of an additional high-energy thiol intermediate, E2-S~ubiquitin, leading to dissociation from the E1 [Huang et al, 2007]. In the third step, a substrate-specific ubiquitin E3 ligase interacts with the target protein-E2 ubiquitin complex to transfer ubiquitin to the target protein (Fig 2). Additional ubiquitin proteins are attached to the initial ubiquitin via a lysine linkage forming polyubiquitin chains that may be linear or branched [Kim et al, 2007; Pickart et al, 2004]. The protein must be polyubiquitinated for Ub-dependent protein degradation by the proteasome.

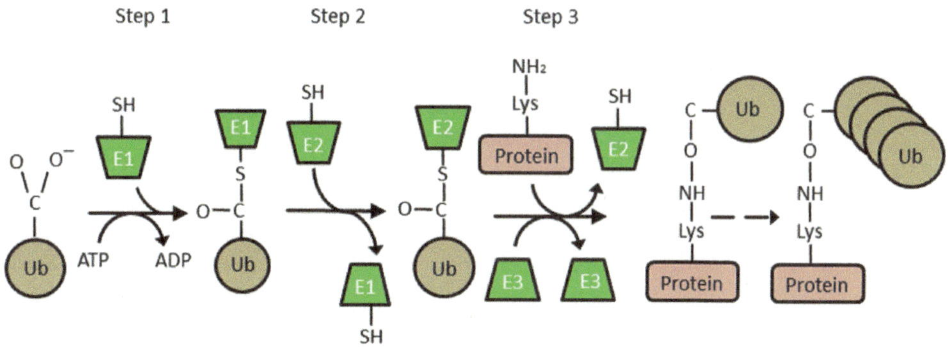

Fig. 2. Polyubiquitination of substrate protein. Ubiquitin (Ub) is activated by enzyme E1 and translocated to enzyme E2. In the last stage, E3 ligase conjugates Ub to the substrate protein.

In mammals, there are only two E1 ligases [Jin et al, 2007], but dozens of E2 ligases, and hundreds of E3 ligases. Ubiquitination specificity is determined principally by this large variety of E3 ligases, which generate the vast number of E2/E3 combinations that each target specific groups of protein substrates.

2.2 Proteasome structure

The proteasome is a cylindrical shaped structure with a molecular weight of 1,500 to 2,000 kD, located both in the cytoplasm and in nucleus in eukaryotes. It consists of two 19S regulatory complex and a core 20S catalytic complex (Fig. 3). It is also denoted the 26S proteasome [Orlowski, 1990; Ciechanover, 1998].

2.2.1 The 19S regulatory complex

Ubiquitin-tagged proteins are recognized by the 19S regulatory complex, where the ubiquitin tags are removed. ATPases with chaperone-like activity at the base of the 19S regulatory complex then unfold the protein substrates and feed them into the inner catalytic compartments of the 20S proteasome cylinder [Ciechanover, 2005]. The opening into the 20S catalytic chamber is small (approximately 1.3 nm), and significant unfolding of the substrate

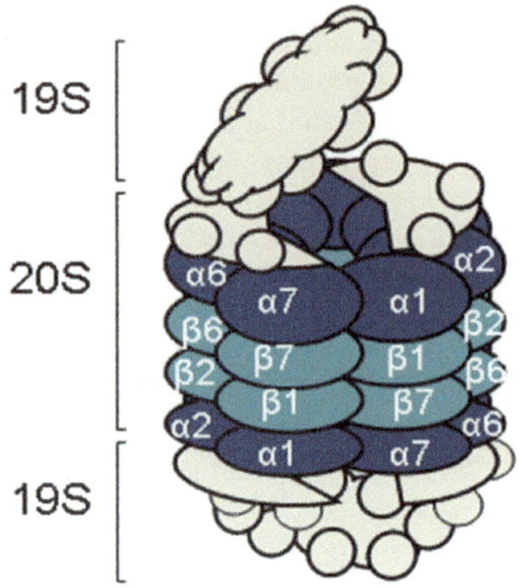

Fig. 3. The 26S proteasome, composed of two regulatory 19S and one catalytic 20S subunits.

is required for successful entering into the 20S subunit [Pickart, 2000]. A molecular gate (N-terminal tail of the α3-subunit) also guards the opening, but it is constitutively open when the 19S regulatory units are bound to the 20S proteasome [Groll, et al., 2000]. There are also multiple different 11S regulatory complexes that can replace the 19S regulator [Hill et al, 2002]. These alternate regulators do not have ATPase function and do not bind polyubiquitin chains. Proteasomes with 11S substitutions for 19S regulators have higher levels of proteolytic activity [Cascio et al, 2002; Fruh et al, 1994].

2.2.2 The 20S proteasome subunit

The 20S proteasome subunit consists of two outer and two inner rings that are stacked to form a cylindrical structure with three compartments [Lowe et al., 1995]. Each outer ring has seven alpha-subunits (α1 to α7), whereas each inner ring contains seven beta-subunits (β1 to β7) (Fig 4).

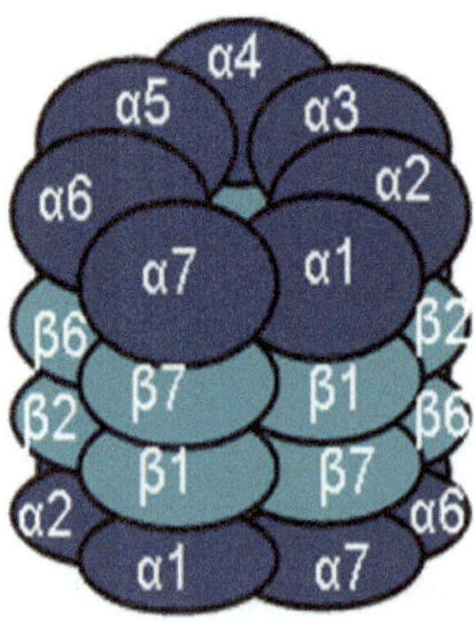

Fig. 4. The 20S proteasome.

The 20S proteasome complex has chymotryptic, tryptic, and peptidylglutamyl-like activities [Ciechanover, 2005; Orlowski, 1990]. It is conformationally flexible with active catalytic sites located on the inner surface of the cylinder where protein substrates bind. Proteins unfolded and without Ub tag, enter the inner chamber, where they are hydrolyzed by six active proteolytic sites on the - β subunits (two sites each on the β1-, β2-, and β5-subunits) into small polypeptides ranging from three to 22 amino acids in length. Proteins cannot enter the inner cylinder through the outer walls of the 20S proteasome because the gaps between the rings are tight [Lowe et al., 1995; Stein et al., 1996]. In eukaryotic cells, 26S proteasome are localized both in the cytoplasm and in the nucleus. This distribution is tissue-specific [Lowe et al., 1995].

3. UPS in immune and inflammatory response

A role for UPS in the pathogenesis of human diseases was first suggested some two decades ago. With the broad spectrum of protein substrates and the complex enzymatic machinery involved in targeting them and practically all intracellular processes being controlled by the UPS, it is not surprising that the proteasome pathway is involved in the pathogenesis of malignant, autoimmune, and neurodegenerative diseases.

The UPS plays significant role in immune and inflammatory processes. It has been shown that UPS takes part in the antigen processing in antigen presenting cells, regulates the transmission of signals from T-cell antigen receptors and the co-stimulatory CD28 molecule and is involved in activation of transcription factor-κB (NF-κB). NF-κB is the key regulator of the activity of genes of many inflammatory cytokines, chemokines and cell adhesion molecules [Sorokin, 2009]. The function of UPS in the activation of NF-kB is the most important and will be discussed here in details.

NF-kB is a family of dimeric transcription factors. The NF-kB family consists of five members: p50, p52, p65/RelA, c-rel, and RelB [Neumann & M. Neumann, 2007]. p50 and p52 are formed as a result of processing from precursors p105 and p100, respectively. The processing of p105 can be performed both by the Ub-dependent pathway by the 26S proteasome [Coux & Goldberg, 1998] and by the ATP-/Ub-independent pathway by the 20S proteasome [Moorthy, 2006]. NF-κB activation promotes the expression of variety of target genes involved in the immune response, reparation reactions, and apoptosis. These include the pro-inflammatory cytokines IL-1β and TNF-α, extracellular matrix metalloproteinase (MMPs), prostaglandins and nitric oxide. IL-1β and TNF-α, in particular, have been shown to play pivotal roles in the pathogenesis of RA both in preclinical [Han et al., 1998] and clinical studies using biological agents such as etanercept and infliximab [Carteron, 2000; Cunnane, 2001].

The UPS activate NF-κB in two stages. At first, the proteasome performs ubiquitin dependent processing of phosphorylated precursors p105 and p100 with the formation of active subunits of transcription factors p50 (NF-κB1) and p52 (NF-κB2). NF-κB is composed of p50 and p65 subunits, and in non-stimulated cells it is retained in the cytoplasm in a latent form associated with inhibitory protein IκB. Following exposure of the cell to a variety of extracellular stimuli such as cytokines, viral and bacterial products and stress, IκB is phosphorylated, poly-ubiquitinated (which is recognized by the 19S regulatory subunit of Proteasome) and is finally rapidly degraded by the 26S proteasome. The released active heterodimer is translocated into the nucleus where it activates the transcription of corresponding genes [Van Waes et al., 2007] (Fig 5).

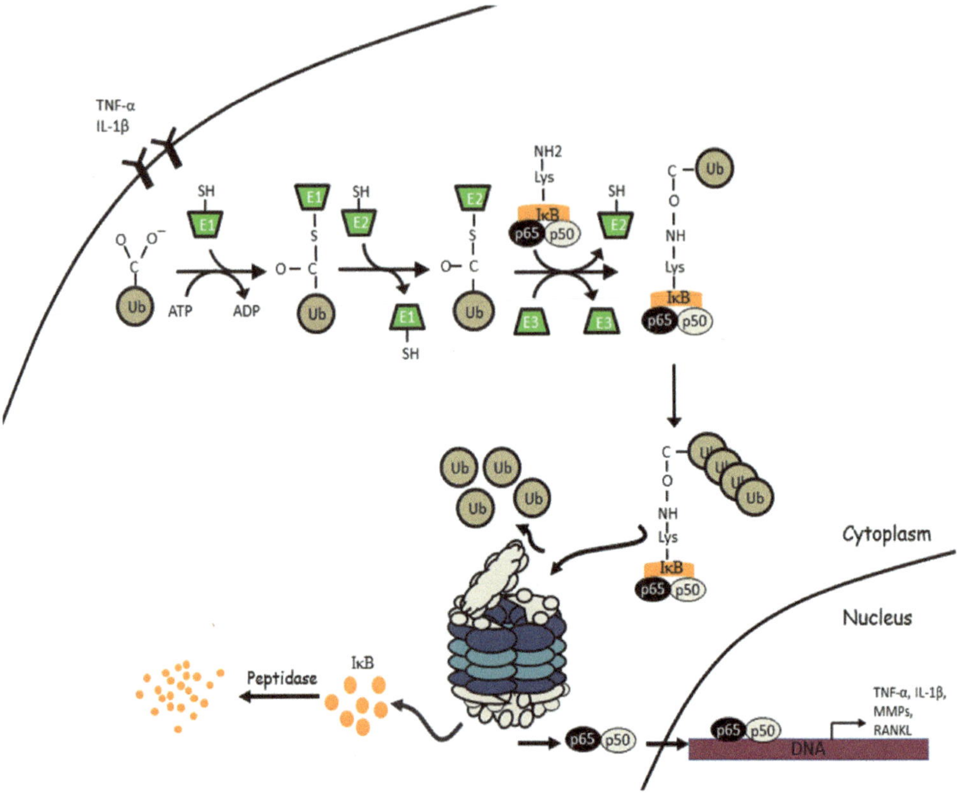

Fig. 5. Activation of Nuclear factor-κB by the proteasome system

NF-κB promotes transcription of genes which encode cytokines (TNF-α, IL-6, IL-1), stress response factors (Cyclooxygenase-2, NO), cell cycle regulators, and anti-apoptotic proteins (IAP-1, Bcl-2 family) [Delhalle et al., 2004]. The pathological activation of NF-κB is a cause of many inflammatory diseases including RA and has been an important target for therapeutic drug research in recent years [Elliott et al., 2003].

3.1 Activation of NF-κB in RA

NF-κB is one of the best-characterized transcription factors and regulates the expression of many genes, most of which encode proteins that play crucial roles in the processes of immunity and inflammation. The activation of NF-κB has been associated with the up-regulation of pro-inflammatory genes involved in several inflammatory conditions [Baldwin, 1996], and has been implicated in pathogenesis of RA [Firestein, 2004]. NF-κB activation has been studied in animal models of arthritis [Han et al., 1998; Palombella et al., 1998] and in the synovium of RA patients [Handel et al., 1995; Firestein, 2004]. NF-κB is essential for TNF-induced synovial cell activation and proliferation as several studies indicated that treatment of synovial cells with an antioxidant agent inhibited TNF-α induced NF-κB activation and transcription [Fujisawa et al., 1996]. Moreover, nuclear extracts from IL-1β stimulated human synovial fibroblasts contained p65 DNA-binding

NF-κB complexes and both the NF-κB classical oligonucleotide decoy and antisense oligonucleotide specific to p65, and they produced a concentration dependent decrease in IL-1-stimulated PGE2 production [Handel, 1995]. Additionally, NF-κB activator, IL-18 can indirectly stimulate osteoclast formation through up-regulation of RANKL production from T cells in RA synovitis [Dai et al., 2004]. Blocking of IKKβ *in vitro* with a dominant negative adenoviral construct was shown to inhibit the induction of IL-6, IL-8, and intercellular adhesion molecule-1 (ICAM-1) after stimulation with IL-1 or TNF-α [Aupperle et al., 2001].

The significance of NF-κB in inflammatory joint disease has been validated by numbers of arthritis models such as carrageenan-induced paw edema, collagen-induced arthritis and adjuvant-induced arthritis [Min et al, 2009, Campo et al, 2011, Ahmed et al., 2010]. In animal models of arthritis the activation of NF-κB appears to precede the onset of disease, and the blockade of NF-κB decreases arthritis severity [Tsao et al., 1997; Ahmed et al., 2010]. Intra-articular gene transfer of IKKβ-wild type into the joints of normal rats resulted in significant paw swelling and accompanied synovial inflammation. Increased IKK activity was detectable in the IKKβ-wt-injected ankle joints which was coincident with enhanced NF-κB-DNA-binding activity. Intra-articular gene transfer of IKKβ-dominant negative significantly ameliorated the severity of adjuvant arthritis, accompanied by a significant decrease in NF-κB DNA expression in the joints of adenoviral IKKb-dominant negative-treated animals [Tak et al., 2001].

3.1.1 NF-κB in RA joint destruction

Progressive destruction of bone and articular cartilage plays a pivotal role in the pathogenesis of RA. During joint inflammation, the inflamed synovium forms a pannus tissue, which grows into the bone and causes destruction, initially as marginal erosions at the site of synovial proliferation where bone is unprotected by hyaline cartilage. Subsequent bone destruction leads to sublaxation and deformity. Cytokines such as TNF-α, IL-1β and IL-17 stimulate the activation of bone destroying osteoaclasts, and the production of destructive proteases - matrix metalloproteinases (MMPs). MMPs have been suggested to be involved in the pathogenesis of RA and OA through their ability to degrade proteoglycans [Flannery et al., 1992; Humbry et al., 1995].

NF-κB is essential for osteoclast formation and survival through the receptor activator of the nuclear factor kappa-B ligand (RANKL) pathway [Soysa et al., 2009]. Abnormal activation of NF-κB signalling in osteoclasts has been observed in osteolytic conditions, including arthritis, Paget's disease of bone, and periodontitis [Xu et al., 2009]. Inhibition or deletion of RANKL prevents bone destruction [Zwerina et al., 2004]. Further, it is demonstrated that inhibition of IκB-kinase complex can suppress RANKL stimulated NF-κB activation and osteoclastogenesis both *in vitro* and *in vivo*. Additionally, this peptide significantly reduced the severity of collagen-induced arthritis in mice by reducing levels of TNF-α and IL-1β, and thereby abrogating joint swelling and reducing destruction of bone and cartilage [Jim et al., 2004]. Elevated levels of MMP-1 (collagenase-1) in the synovial fluid and serum of RA patients [Green et al., 2003; Yamanaka et al., 2000] and MMP-3 (stromelysin) in the synovial fluid from RA patients has been determined [Hembry et al., 1995]. Interestingly, it has been reported that NF-κB regulates synthesis of MMPs including MMP-I and MMP-3 [Thurberg et al., 1998].

4. UPS in neuronal signalling

In the nervous system, UPS is present in neurons, glia and synapses and regulates numerous functions including neuronal signalling, synapse assembly, maintenance, and function [Mengual et al., 1996]. Recent work utilizing the powerful genetic tools in *C. elegans* and *Drosophila* as well as synaptic assays in mammalian neuronal culture systems has unravelled the critical role of UPS in neuronal signaling. Active E3 ligases are identified at the synapse which participates in synaptic plasticity [Myat et al., 2002]. Moreover, localization of many E3 ligases in nucleus and synapse suggests the interplay between UPS regulation of transcriptional programs that function in synaptic modulation and local synaptic regulation of protein degradation.

UPS regulates synaptic functions by controlling levels of pre-synaptic proteins [Speese et al., 2003]. At the post-synaptic levels, the UPS regulates the surface expression and internalization of NMDA- and AMPA-glutamate receptors [Moriyoshi et al., 2004]. It has been implicated that mechanical allodynia and hyperalgesia can be prevented with NMDA-receptor antagonists [Laughlin et al., 1997]. During pathological pain UPS regulates neuronal signalling by controlling levels of synaptic proteins [Ossipov et al, 2007]. Much future work is needed to identify exact role of UPS in acute and chronic pain conditions.

5. Proteasome inhibition

Proteasome inhibitors are considered as a potential remedy for cancer, inflammation-related disorders and neurodegenerative diseases. Proteasome inhibitors can cause cellular apoptosis in proliferating cancer cells by affecting various short-lived proteins, resulting in inhibition of NF-κB activity, increased activity of p53 and Bax proteins, and accumulation of cyclin- dependent kinase inhibitors p27 and p21 [Moriyoshi et al., 2004; Van Waes et al., 2007]. Preclinical studies show that malignant, transformed, and proliferating cells are more susceptible to proteasome inhibition than cells in a resting state [Adams, 2002; Sherr, 1996].

Bortezomib is the first inhibitor of the ubiquitin-proteasome pathway to enter clinical studies [Adams et al., 1999; Richardson et al., 2003]. On the basis of a large, multicenter phase II clinical trial in which approximately one third of patients with advanced multiple myeloma (MM) had a significant response to therapy with bortezomib, on May 13th 2003, the US Food and Drug Administration granted approval for use of this drug in the treatment of patients with MM [Richardson et al., 2003]. The promising preclinical and clinical activity exhibited by bortezomib in MM and non-Hodgkin lymphomas (NHL) has confirmed the proteasome as a relevant and important target in the treatment of cancer. Several proteasome inhibitors are being tested and are in the pre-clinical and clinical phase of testing.

In the case of RA, up-regulation of the most important pro-inflammatory mediators such as TNF-α, IL-1β, IL-6, iNOS and endothelial cell adhesion molecules (e.g. vascular cell adhesion molecule 1 (VCAM-1)) are regulated by NF-κB [Van Waes et al., 2007; Han et al 1998]. Therefore RA qualifies as a potential target for proteasome inhibitors. *In vitro* and *in vivo* studies have presented encouraging results by the use of different proteasome inhibitors to reduce the NF-κB activation.

5.1 Proteasome inhibitors

Proteasome inhibitors include a variety of natural and chemically synthesized molecules which exclusively inhibit proteasome activity. The structure and function of some important classes of proteasome inhibitors are described here.

5.1.1 Peptide aldehydes

Peptide aldehydes were the first proteasome inhibitors to be developed [Palombella et al., 1994; Rock et al., 1994]. These include MG132 (Z-Leu-Leu- Leucinal-) (Fig 5), MG115 (Z-Leu-Leu-norvalinal-) and calpain inhibitor I (*N*-acetyl-Leu-Leu-norleucinal). These compounds are potent, reversible and cell permeable. MG132 is a reversible inhibitor of the chymotrypsin like activity of the proteasome.

5.1.2 Boronic acid peptides

Boronate inhibitors are much more potent than their structurally analogous peptide aldehydes [Adams et al., 1998]. These includes MG262 (Z-Leu-Leu-Leu-boronate; analogous to MG132) and PS-341 (pyrazylcarbonyl-Phe-Leu-boronate; analogous to the aldehyde PS-402). MG262 is a cell permeable and reversible inhibitors of the chymotrypsin like activity of the proteasome. PS-341 is clinically the most advanced proteasome inhibitor and inhibits the chymotrypsin like active site of the proteasome β-subunit. Its boronic acid group binds the active site threonine in the proteasome with high affinity and specificity (Fig 5).

5.1.3 Lactacystin

Lactacystin is a naturally occurring compound produced by *Streptomyces lactacystinaeus.* It selectively targets the β5 subunit of the proteasome [Fenteany et al., 1995] by covalent acylation of the amino-terminal threonine residues and is considered as an irreversible inhibitor of the proteasome. The active component of lactacystin is the highly reactive *clasto*-lactacystin β-lactone and PS-519 (Fig 5).

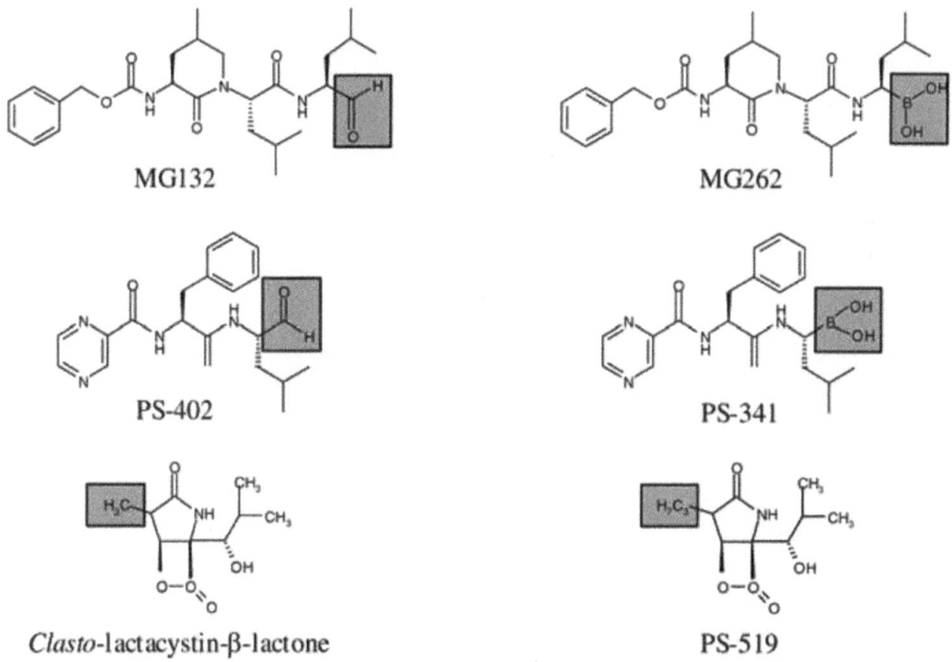

Fig. 6. Structures of selected proteasome inhibitors [Elliott et al., 2003].

5.1.4 Epoxyketones

These are naturally product proteasome inhibitors isolated from actinomycete fermentation broths by screening for antitumor activity in mice. Examples of this class include Epoxomicin and eponemycin. These compounds inhibit the chymotrypsin like site only or the chymotrypsinlike and caspaselike, respectively. In contrast to previously mentioned inhibitors, epoxomicin initially forms a covalent bond between the proteasome' s amino-terminal threonine hydroxyl at its C-terminal ketone carbonyl. This primary adduct formation is followed by formation of a stable six-membered ring adduct by a second attack by the terminal free amino group [Groll et al., 2000].

5.2 Proteasome inhibition in animal model of arthritis

Proteasome inhibitors exhibit anti-inflammatory and anti-proliferative effects. Their use in diseases characterized by these processes is thought to be promising but the effects of proteasome inhibitors on the pathogenesis of inflammatory join disorder such as RA remain quite limited. To date the effects of proteasome inhibition have been studied only in animal models of arthritis; streptococcal cell wall induced polyarthritis in rats, collagen induced arthritis and adjuvant induced arthritis (Table 1). These animal models have several clinical and pathological similarities with human rheumatoid arthritis regarding inflammation, pain, swelling, synovial hyperplasia and destruction of cartilage and bone [Kannan et al., 2005].

Animal models	Proteasome inhibitor	References
streptococcal cell wall induced polyarthritis in rat	PS-341	Palombella et al., 1998
collagen induced arthritis in mice	PS-341	Lee et al., 2009
Adjuvant induced arthritis in rat	MG132	Ahmed et al, 2010
Adjuvant induced arthritis in rat	PS-341	Yannaki et al., 2010

Table 1. List of proteasome inhibitors used in animal models of RA.

5.2.1 Proteasome inhibition and joint inflammation

Proteasome inhibitors PS-341 and MG132 have been tested in different animal models of arthritis (Table 1) with pronounced anti-inflammatory effects. Here effects of proteasome inhibitor MG132 in adjuvant induced arthritis (AIA) rat model will be discussed in details. MG132 was administered subcutaneously daily at the onset of arthritis. Two weeks of administration significantly reduced signs of inflammation including swelling, redness and warmth in ankle joints compared to vehicle treated arthritis animals. Similar effects were observed in studies where proteasome inhibitor PS-341 was administered in different arthritis models. PS-341 significantly attenuated the arthritis severity and the clinical progression of the T cell dependent chronic phase of the disease. The chronic phase of arthritis was also associated with increased serum levels of NF-κB dependent pro-inflammatory factors such as IL-1, IL-6, and nitric oxide metabolites [Palombella et al., 1998]. The expression of TNF-α, IL-1β, IL-6, MMP-3, COX-2 and iNOS were decreased in PS-341-treated animals compared to untreated [Lee et al., 2009].

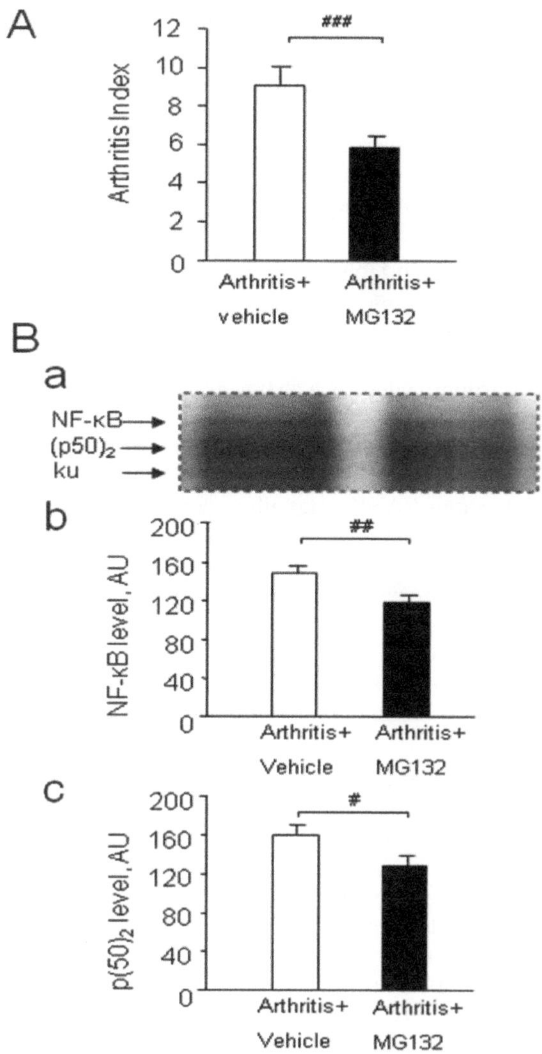

Fig. 7. Effects of proteasome inhibitor MG132 on (A) arthritis index; severity of arthritis was scored using a macroscopic scoring system according to changes in erythema and oedema in each paw (B) NF-κB and p50 activation in arthritic ankle joint of AIA rat. (a) autoradiograph of electrophoretic mobility shift assay. The upper two bands represent NF-κB and p50 homodimer complexes (indicated by arrows), (b) and (c) semi-quantification of the NF-κB and $(p50)_2$ levels.

MG132 treatment significantly down-regulated the expression of NF-κB1 (p50) in inflamed ankle joints as well as the DNA binding activity of both NF-κB and p50 homodimer in arthritic ankle joints (Fig 7 A and B). These results indicate that MG132 hinders the nuclear localization of NF-κB by retaining them in the cytosol in an inactive form bound to the inhibitory protein IκB, and also blocks UPS-mediated processing of the p105 precursor to mature p50 [Magnani et al., 2000], which is a subunit of mature NF-κB. Significantly lower levels of NF-κB dependent proinflammatory factors such as IL-1, IL-6, and nitric oxide metabolites were found in PS-341-treated animals than in control rats. Thus supporting the concept that the profound anti-inflammatory effects of PS-341 result, in part, from inhibition of NF-κB activity [Palombella et al., 1998]. Proteasome inhibitor MG132 and PS-341 treated animals gained significantly more body weight than the vehicle treated controls indicating that proteasome inhibitors given at therapeutically relevant doses were well tolerated.

5.2.2 Proteasome inhibition and joint destruction

Progressive destruction of bone and cartilage plays a pivotal role in the pathogenesis of RA. Effect of proteasome inhibitor MG132 on joint destruction was studied in AIA model [Ahmed et al., 2010]. The radiographic and histological analysis revealed that augmented cartilage and bone resorption, which is a characteristic feature of arthritis, was mitigated by the MG132 (Fig 8).

Bone resorption is a collective result of osteoclast stimulation and suppression of osteoblast precursors within the bone marrow. Previous studies have shown that NF-κB controls osteoclast activation through RANKL signalling [Soysa & Alles, 2009], while inhibition or deletion of RANKL prevents bone destruction [Zwerina et al., 2004; Pettit et al., 2001]. The protective effect of MG132 may be a consequence of with interfering osteoclast activation through the RANKL signalling pathway that is under control of NF-κB, or by enhancing the osteoblast activity. This assumption is supported by *in vitro* and *in vivo* studies indicating that the proteasome inhibitor bortezomib directly suppressed human osteoclast formation and promoted maturation of osteoblasts [Zangari et al., 2006; Mukharjee et al., 2008] and reduced joint destruction and preserved bone density in CIA mice [Lee et al., 2009].

5.2.3 Proteasome inhibition and inflammatory pain

Chronic pain is a major feature of RA and is maintained in part by long-lasting neuroplastic changes in the central and peripheral nervous system. Recent, pre-clinical studies demonstrated that the UPS is one of the systems involved in the maintenance of chronic pain by regulating proteins at pre- and post-synaptic levels [Speese, 2003; Mengual et al., 1996]. Effects of proteasome inhibitor MG132 on inflammatory pain was studied in the AIA animal model. Inflammation in joints significantly reduced the pain bearing capacity in arthritic animals as measured by the paw withdrawal threshold (PWT). Administration of MG132 significant increased PWT in arthritic animals compared to vehicle treated group (Fig 9).

Central and peripheral neuronal mechanisms are thought to play a critical role in inflammatory joint disorders, particularly with regard to inflammation and pain [Benrath, et al., 1995; Levine et al., 1985]. Sensory neuropeptides, substance P (SP) and calcitonin gene-related peptide (CGRP), are shown to participate not only in pain modulation but also in inflammatory processes. An up-regulation in the SP and CGRP expression in ankle joints and their corresponding dorsal root ganglia was demonstrated in adjuvant arthritis [Ahmed et al., 1995]. The development and progress of joint inflammation in adjuvant arthritis was significantly attenuated by using the neurotoxin capsaicin, which specifically down regulates sensory innervation [Ahmed et al., 1995]. The beneficial effects of capsaicin on joint inflammation were correlated with reduced levels of SP and CGRP in the ankle joints and corresponding DRG. Methotrexate treatment has been shown to reduce the severity of joint inflammation and destruction, partly due to its inhibitory effect on sensory

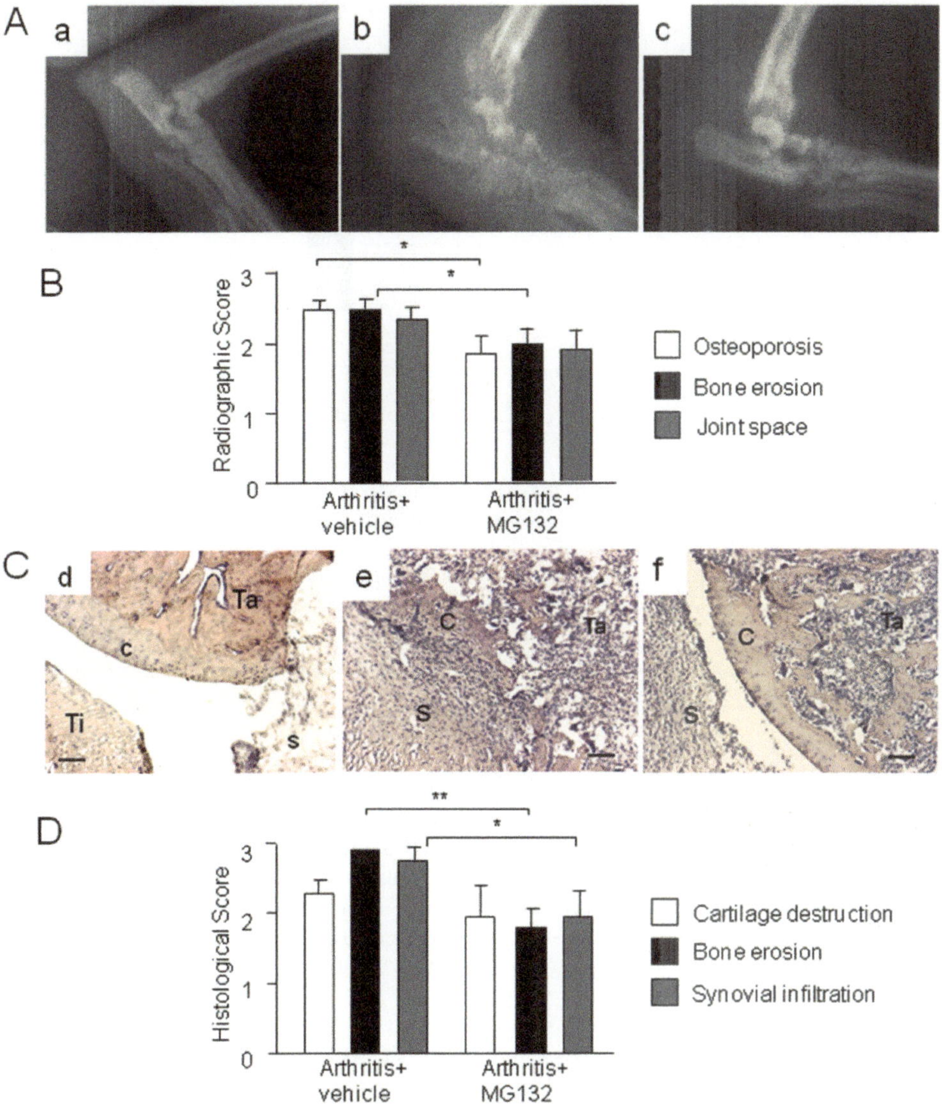

Fig. 8. Radiologic and histologic analysis of bone and cartilage destruction. A, Representative lateral view radiographs of ankle joint of (a) normal, and (b) vehicle- or (c) MG132-treated arthritic animals. B, Changes in the radiographic parameters of osteoporosis, bone erosion and joint space in ankle joints of arthritic animals treated with vehicle or MG132. C, Photomicrographs of haematoxylin and eosin stained ankle joints from (d) control rat; (e) vehicle-treated arthritic rat; and (f) MG132-treated arthritic rat. D, Changes in histologic parameters of cartilage and bone resorption and synovial infiltration in arthritic rats treated with vehicle or MG132. (c; articular cartilage, s; synovial membrane, Ti; tibia and Ta; talus). Modified results from Ahmed et al, 2010.

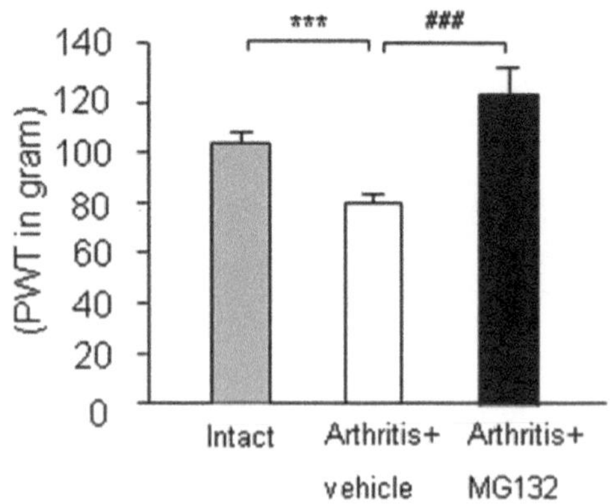

Fig. 9. Hind paw withdrawal threshold (PWT) in control and arthritic groups treated with MG132 and vehicle.

neuropeptides [Ahmed et al., 1995]. In the AIA model, strong up-regulation of SP and CGRP in the periosteum and synovium structures, which are pain sensitive and prone to inflammation, was observed. This increased SP and CGRP expression coincided with decreased pain thresholds. Administration of MG132 resulted in the normalization of pain responses as well as significantly down-regulating the expression of SP and CGRP in arthritic ankle joints (Fig 10). Results also indicate that UPS regulates inflammation induced pain behaviour and that UPS-mediated protein degradation is involved in the peripheral sensitization.

Previously it has been shown that proteasome inhibitors MG132 and epoxomicin can prevent the development of behavioural signs of neuropathic pain and abolish abnormal pain induced by sustained morphine exposure [Ossipov et al., 2009; Moss et al., 2008]. These compounds inhibited the release of DYNA and CGRP and normalized molecular changes in the spinal cord contributing to central sensitization [Ossipov et al., 2009; Moss et al., 2008]. Although the cause and neurobiological mechanisms underlying neuropathic and inflammatory pain are different, the common mechanism for the effects of proteasome inhibitors in these pathological conditions is the similar central neuronal mechanism and the activation of neurotransmission mediated by the sensory neuropeptides including SP, CGRP and dynorphins.

The dorsal root ganglia (DRG) and the spinal cord actively participate in the peripheral and central sensitization. DRG neurons have very long t-shaped axons with one end forming a sensory terminal at the skin or joints and other end synapsing in the dorsal horn of the spinal cord. In the spinal cord these neurons project to the outermost region of the spinal dorsal horn (lamina I and outer lamina II) and terminate largely on spinal neurons that project to higher-order pain centers such as the cortex and the hypothalamus in the brain.

In AIA rats, a significant increase in the SP and CGRP expression has been reported in the DRG [Ahmed et al, 1995a]. In the spinal cord an enhanced release of SP and CGRP has been recorded in the lumber dorsal horn during inflammation [Garry & Hargreaves, 1992]. Up-regulated SP expression in the DRG correlated with arthritis severity and nociceptive behavior of arthritic rats [Ahmed et al, 1995a]. This agrees with other observations that the altered expression of SP and CGRP is critical for the modulation of pain and inflammation (Ambalavanar et al., 2006; Hutchins et al., 2000). Moreover, it has been reported that

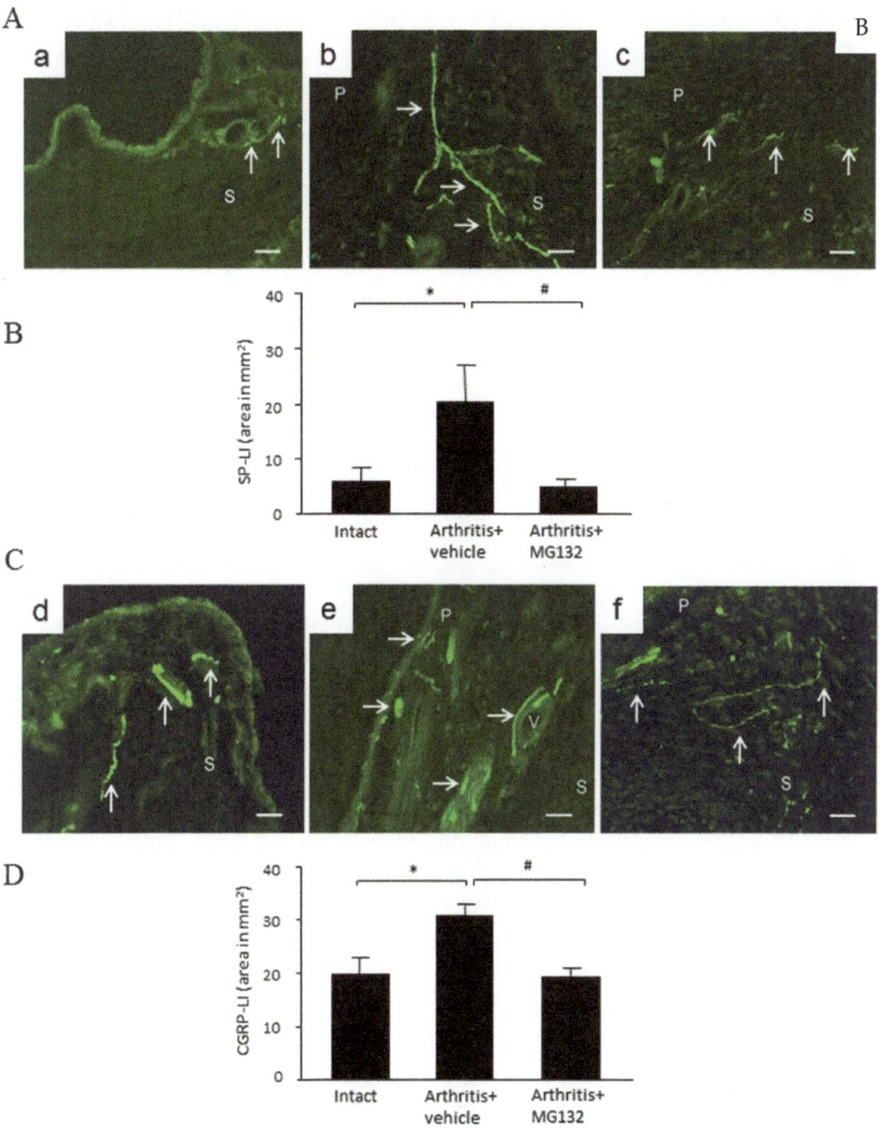

Fig. 10. Immunofluorescence micrographs and semi-quantitative analysis of SP and CGRP in rat ankles. A, Nerve fibres positive to SP in the vehicle-treated control rats (a), and in the vehicle- (b) or MG132- (c) treated arthritis rats. B, Semi-quantitative analysis of SP immunoreactive nerve fibres (immunofluorescent area) in ankle joints of the control and arthritic rats treated with vehicle or MG132. C, Nerve fibres positive to CGRP in the vehicle-treated control rats (d), and in the vehicle- (e) or MG132- (f) treated arthritis rats. D, Semi-quantitative analysis of CGRP immunoreactive nerve fibres (immunofluorescent area) in ankle joints of the control and arthritic rats treated with vehicle or MG132. (s; synovial membrane, p; periosteum and v; blood vessel). Modified results from Ahmed et al, 2010.

peripheral inflammation induces a dramatic up-regulation of PDYN biosynthesis in nociceptive neurons of the spinal dorsal horn (Przewlocki, 1987; Marvizon et al., 2009). As a future perspective it will be interesting to observe the effects of proteasome inhibition in the DRG and SC in inflammation. In the monosodium-induced model of osteoarthritis, which is a well-recognized model of osteoarthritis, MG132 treatment has normalized the up-regulated expression of SP and CGRP in the inflamed knee joints and their corresponding DRG, with reduced pain behavior [Ahmed et al, unpublished data].

6. Toxicity

The clinical application of proteasome inhibitors might be limited due to potential side effects of available compounds following chronic administration. Toxic affects might result from the accumulation of ubiquitinated proteins after inhibition of the 26S proteasome. The proteasome inhibitor bortezomib (PS-341) induced mild-to-moderate neurotoxic effects in rats [Cavaletti et al., 2007] and peripheral sensory neuropathy in cancer patients when given this compound chronically [Cata et al., 2006]. The features of bortezomib neuropathy are characteristic for a small fiber neuropathy and are characterized by a more sensory than motor neuropathy. Several observations, however, argue against these possibilities. First, in rats, the neurotoxic effects were observed when bortezomib was administered at maximum tolerated, sub-lethal doses in rats [Cavaletti et al., 2007]. Bortezomib might have induced neurotoxic effects because of the presence of a component in its activity that is blocked by the polyhydroxyl compound Tiron, this component is not involved in MG132 activity [Fernandez et al., 2006]. No effects of MG132 toxicity were apparent on motor performance during rotarod, posture, gait, exploratory and locomotor activity, or on cell death in the spinal cord, when MG132 was administered at higher doses [Ossipov et al., 2006]. Moreover, MG132 treated animals gained significantly more body weight than the vehicle treated arthritic controls [Ahmed et al., 2010]. These results indicate that proteasome inhibitor MG132 given at therapeutically relevant doses was well tolerated. This is a significant finding as the proteasome plays a central role in many intracellular functions and its inhibition might theoretically be expected to induce numerous side effects.

7. Future perspectives

Taking into account that the UPS controls important functions in eukaryotic cell, proteasome inhibitors could have been considered as toxins without any therapeutic value. Unexpectedly, proteasome inhibitors are well-tolerated drugs and do not produce adverse effects in normal cells even at high doses. Though, clinical trials indicate that use of bortezomib induces peripheral sensory neuropathy in patients, which might limit its therapeutic use. However, the reversible proteasome inhibitor such as MG132 apparently did not produce any toxic effect and was well tolerated. The use of reversible proteasome inhibitors can therefore be considered as a better alternative. It will be a future challenge to develop drugs specifically targeting the UPS, or more specifically UPS E3 ligases that select proteins for the UPS-mediated degradation, in order to treat inflammatory joint disorders. Non-toxic proteasome inhibitors alone and/or in combination with conventional RA therapies might be more effective to treat patients with this painful and debilitating arthritic disease.

8. References

Adams J, Behnke M, Chen S, Cruickshank AA, Dick LR, Grenier L, Klunder JM, Ma YT, Plamondon L, Stein RL. Potent and selective inhibitors of the proteasome: dipeptidyl boronic acids. Bioorg Med Chem Lett. 1998; 8:333–338.

Adams J, Palombella VJ, Sausville EA, Johnson J, Destree A, Lazarus DD, et al. Proteasome inhibitors: a novel class of potent and effective antitumor agents. Cancer Res. 1999;59(11):2615-22.

Adams J. Development of the proteasome inhibitor PS-341. Oncologist. 2002;7(1):9-16.

Adams J. Proteasome inhibitors as new anticancer drugs. Curr Opin Oncol. 2002;14(6):628-34.

Ahmed AS, Li J, Ahmed M, Hua L, Ossipov MH, Yakovleva T, Bakalkin G, Stark A. Attenuation of pain and inflammation in adjuvant-induced arthritis by the proteasome inhibitor MG132. Arthritis Rheum, 2010;62 (7):2160-9

Ahmed AS, Li J, Harris HE, Stark A, Bakalkin G, Ahmed M. Suppression of pain and joint destruction by inhibition of the proteasome system in experimental osteoarthritis. Pain, In Press.

Ahmed M, Bjurholm A, Schultzberg M, Theodorsson E, Kreicbergs A. Increased levels of substance P and calcitonin gene-related peptide in rat adjuvant arthritis. A combined immunohistochemical and radioimmunoassay analysis. Arthritis Rheum 1995;38:699-709.

Ahmed M, Bjurholm A, Srinivasan GR, Lundeberg T, Theodorsson E, Schultzberg M, et al. Capsaicin effects on substance P and CGRP in rat adjuvant arthritis. Regul Pept 1995;55:85-102.

Ambalavanar R, Moritani M, Moutanni A, Gangula P, Yallampalli C, Dessem D. Deep tissue inflammation upregulates neuropeptides and evokes nociceptive behaviors which are modulated by a neuropeptide antagonist. Pain. 2006;120(1-2):53-68

Aupperle K, Bennett B, Han Z, Boyle D, Manning A, Firestein G. NFkappa B regulation by I kappa B kinase-2 in rheumatoid arthritis synoviocytes. J Immunol 2001;166:2705-11.

Baldwin AS, Jr. The NF-kappa B and I kappa B proteins: new discoveries and insights. Annu Rev Immunol. 1996;14:649-83.

Benrath J, Eschenfelder C, Zimmerman M, Gillardon F. Calcitonin gene-related peptide, substance P and nitric oxide are involved in cutaneous inflammation following ultraviolet irradiation. Eur J Pharmacol 1995;293:87-96.

Brennan FM, McInnes IB. Evidence that cytokines play a role in rheumatoid arthritis. J Clin Invest 2008;118:3537–45

Campo GM, Avenoso A, Nastasi G, Micali A, Prestipino V, et al. Hyaluronan reduces inflammation in experimental arthritis by modulating TLR-2 and TLR-4 cartilage expression. Biochim Biophys Acta. 2011;1812:1170-81.

Carmona L, Cross M, Williams B, Lassere M, March L. Rheumatoid arthritis. Best Pract Res Clin Rheumatol. 2010;24:733-45.

Cascio P, Call M, Petre BM, Walz T, Goldberg AL. Properties of the hybrid form of the 26S proteasome containing both 19S and PA28 complexes. EMBO Journal. 2002;21: 2636–2645.

Cata JP, Weng HR, Lee BN, Reuben JM, Dougherty PM. Clinical and experimental findings in humans and animals with chemotherapy-induced peripheral neuropathy. Minerva Anestesiol. 2006;72(3):151-69.

Cavaletti G, Gilardini A, Canta A, Rigamonti L, Rodriguez-Menendez V, Ceresa C, et al. Bortezomib-induced peripheral neurotoxicity: a neurophysiological and pathological study in the rat. Exp Neurol. 2007;204(1):317-25.

Ciechanover A. The ubiquitin-proteasome pathway: on protein death and cell life. EMBO J 1998; 24:7151 - 7160.

Coux, O., and Goldberg, A. L. Enzymes catalyzing ubiquitination and proteolytic processing of the p105 precursor of nuclear factor kappaB1. J. Biol. Chem. 1998; 273,8820-8828.

Dai S, Hirayama T, Abbas S, Abu-Amer Y. The IkappaB kinase (IKK) inhibitor,NEMO-binding domain peptide, blocks osteoclastogenesis and bone erosion in inflammatory arthritis. J Biol Chem. 2004;279:37219–22.

Delhalle S, Blasius R, Dicato M, Diederich M. A beginner's guide to NF-kappaB signaling pathways. Ann N Y Acad Sci. 2004;1030:1-13.

Drexler HC. Activation of the cell death program by inhibition of proteasome function. Proc Natl Acad Sci U S A. 1997;94(3):855-60.

Elliott PJ and Zollner TM. Proteasome inhibition: a new anti-inflammatory strategy J Mol Med. 2003; 81:235–245.

Elliott PJ, Zollner TM, Boehncke WH. Proteasome inhibition: a new anti-inflammatory strategy. J Mol Med. 2003;81(4):235-45.

Fenteany G, Standaert RF, Lane WS, Choi S, Corey EJ, Schreiber SL. Inhibition of proteasome activities and subunit-specific amino-terminal threonine modification by lactacystin. Science. 1995;268:726-31.

Fernandez Y, Miller TP, Denoyelle C, Esteban JA, Tang WH, Bengston AL, Soengas MS. Chemical blockage of the proteasome inhibitory function of bortezomib: impact on tumor cell death. J Biol Chem 2006; 281: 1107-1118.

Firestein GS. NF-kappaB: Holy Grail for rheumatoid arthritis? Arthritis Rheum. 2004;50(8):2381-6.

Flannery CR, Lark MW, Sandy JD. Identification of a stromelysin cleavage site within the interglobular domain of human aggrecan. Evidence for proteolysis at this site in vivo in human articular cartilage. J Biol Chem 1992; 267: 1008-1014.

Fruh K, Gossen M, Wang KN, Bujard H, Peterson PA, Yang Y. Displacement of housekeeping proteasome subunits by MHC-encoded LMPs — a newly discovered mechanism for modulating the multi-catalytic proteinase complex. EMBO J. 1994;13:3236–3244.

Fujisawa K, Aono H, Hasunuma T, Yamamoto K, Mita S, Nishioka K. Activation of transcription factorNF-kappa B in human synovial cells in response to tumor necrosis factor alpha. Arthritis Rheum 1996;39:197– 203.

Garry MG, Hargreaves KM. Enhanced release of immunoreactive CGRP and substance P from spinal dorsal horn slices occurs during carrageenan inflammation. Brain Res. 1992;582:139-4

Goldberg AL. Protein degradation and protection against misfolded or damaged proteins. Nature. 2003;426:895-9.

Green MJ, Gough AK, Devlin J, Smith J, Astin P, Taylor D, et al. Serum MMP-3 and MMP-1 and progression of joint damage in early rheumatoid arthritis. Rheumatology (Oxford). 2003;42(1):83-8.

Groll M, Kim KB, Kairies N, Huber R, Crews CM. Crystal structure of epoxomicin: 20S proteasome reveals a

Grossin L, Etienne S, Gaborit N, Pinzano A, Cournil-Henrionnet C, Gerard C, et al. Induction of heat shock protein 70 (Hsp70) by proteasome inhibitor MG 132 protects articular chondrocytes from cellular death in vitro and in vivo. Biorheology. 2004;41(3-4):521-34.

Handel M, McMorrow L, Gravallese E. Nuclear factor-kappa B in rheumatoid synovium. Localization of p50 and p65. Arthritis Rheum 1995;38:1762–70.

Hembry RM, Bagga MR, Reynolds JJ, Hamblen DL. Immunolocalisation studies on six matrix metalloproteinases and their inhibitors, TIMP-1 and TIMP-2, in synovia from patients with osteo- and rheumatoid arthritis. Ann Rheum Dis. 1995;54(1):25-32.

Hill CP, Masters EI, Whitby FG. The 11S regulators of 20S proteasome activity. Curr Top Microbiol Immunol. 2002;268:73–89.

Huang DT, Hunt HW, Zhuang M, Ohi MD, Holten JM, Schulman BA. Basis for a ubiquitin-like protein thioester switch toggling E1–E2 affinity. Nature. 2007;445: 394–398.

Hutchins B, Spears R, Hinton RJ, Harper RP. Calcitonin gene-related peptide and substance P immunoreactivity in rat trigeminal ganglia and brainstem following adjuvant-induced inflammation of the temporomandibular joint. Arch Oral Biol. 2000;45(4):335-45.

Jimi E, Aoki K, Saito H, D'Acquisto F, May M, Nakamura I, et al. Selective inhibition of NF-kappa B blocks osteoclastogenesis and prevents inflammatory bone destruction in vivo. Nat Med 2004;10:617–24.

Jin J, Li X, Gygi SP, Harper JW. Dual E1 activation systems for ubiquitin differentially regulate E2 enzyme charging. Nature. 2007;447:1135–1138.

Kannan K, Ortmann RA, Kimpel D. Animal models of rheumatoid arthritis and their relevance to human disease. Pathophysiology. 2005;12(3):167-81.

Kim HT, Kim KP, Lledias F, Kisselev AF, Scaglione KM, Skowyra D, Gygi SP, Goldberg AL. Certain pairs of ubiquitin-conjugating enzymes (E2s) and ubiquitin-protein ligases (E3s) synthesize nondegradable forked ubiquitin chains containing all possible isopeptide linkages. J Biol Chem.2007;282:17375–17386.

Laughlin TM, Vanderah TW, Lashbrook J, Nichols ML, Ossipov M, Porreca F, et al. Spinally administered dynorphin A produces long-lasting allodynia: involvement of NMDA but not opioid receptors. Pain. 1997;72(1-2):253-60.

Levine JD, Collier DH, Basbaum AI, Moskowitz MA, Helms CA. Hypothesis: the nervous system may contribute to the pathophysiology of rheumatoid arthritis. J Rheumatol 1985;12:406-11.

Loughlin J. Polymorphism in signal transduction is a major route through which osteoarthritis susceptibility is acting. Curr Opin Rheumatol. 2005;17(5):629-33.

Lowe J, Stock D, Jap B, Zwickl P, Baumeister W, Huber R. Crystal structure of the 20S proteasome from the archaeon T. acidophilum at 3.4 A resolution. Science. 1995;268(5210):533-9.

Marvizon JC, Chen W, Murphy N. Enkephalins, dynorphins, and beta-endorphin in the rat dorsal horn: an immunofluorescence colocalization study. J Comp Neurol. 2009;517(1):51-68

Mengual E, Arizti P, Rodrigo J, Gimenez-Amaya JM, Castano JG. Immunohistochemical distribution and electron microscopic subcellular localization of the proteasome in the rat CNS. J Neurosci. 1996;16(20):6331-41.

Min SW, Kim NJ, Baek NI, Kim DH. Inhibitory effect of eupatilin and jaceosidin isolated from Artemisia princeps on carrageenan-induced inflammation in mice. J Ethnopharmacol. 2009;125:497-500.

Moorthy, A. K., Savinova, O. V., Ho, J. Q., Wang, V. Y., Vu, D., and Ghosh, G. (2006) EMBO J., 25, 1945-1956.

Moriyoshi K, Iijima K, Fujii H, Ito H, Cho Y, Nakanishi S. Seven in absentia homolog 1A mediates ubiquitination and degradation of group 1 metabotropic glutamate receptors. Proc Natl Acad Sci U S A. 2004;101(23):8614-9.

Moss A, Blackburn-Munro G, Garry EM, Blakemore JA, Dickinson T, Rosie R, et al. A role of the ubiquitin-proteasome system in neuropathic pain. J Neurosci 2002;22:1363-72.

Mukherjee S, Raje N, Schoonmaker JA, Liu JC, Hideshima T, Wein MN, et al. Pharmacologic targeting of a stem/progenitor population in vivo is associated with enhanced bone regeneration in mice. J Clin Invest. 2008;118(2):491-504.

Neumann, M., and Naumann, M. Beyond IkappaBs: alternative regulation of NF-kappaB activity. FASEB J., 2007; 21, 2642-2654.

Ossipov MH, Bazov I, Gardell LR, Kowal J, Yakovleva T, Usynin I, et al. Control of chronic pain by the ubiquitin proteasome system in the spinal cord. J Neurosci. 2007;27(31):8226-37.

Palombella VJ, Conner EM, Fuseler JW, Destree A, Davis JM, Laroux FS, Wolf RE, Huang J, Brand S, Elliott PJ, Lazarus D, McCormack T, Parent L, Stein R, Adams J, Grisham MB (1998) Role of the proteasome and NF-kappaB in streptococcal cell wall-induced polyarthritis. Proc Natl Acad Sci USA 95:15671-15676

Palombella VJ, Rando OJ, Goldberg AL, Maniatis T. The ubiquitin-proteasome pathway is required for processing the NF-kappa B1 precursor protein and the activation of NFkappa B. Cell. 1994; 78:773–785.

Pettit AR, Ji H, von Stechow D, Muller R, Goldring SR, Choi Y, et al. TRANCE/RANKL knockout mice are protected from bone erosion in a serum transfer model of arthritis. Am J Pathol. 2001;159(5):1689-99.

Pickart CM, Fushman D. Polyubiquitin chains: polymeric protein signals. Curr Opin Chem Biol.2004;8:610–616.

Przewlocki R. Opioid peptides in relation to antinociception. Pol J Pharmacol Pharm. 1987;39(5):609-21.

Raza K, Falciani F, Curnow SJ, Ross EJ, Lee CY, et al. Early rheumatoid arthritis is characterized by a distinct and transient synovial fluid cytokine profile of T cell and stromal cell origin. Arthritis Res Ther. 2005;7:R784-95.

Richardson PG, Barlogie B, Berenson J, Singhal S, Jagannath S, Irwin D, et al. A phase 2 study of bortezomib in relapsed, refractory myeloma. N Engl J Med. 2003;348(26):2609-17.

Rock KL, Gramm C, Rothstein L, Clark K, Stein R, Dick L, Hwang D, Goldberg AL. Inhibitors of the proteasome block the degradation of most cell proteins and the generation of peptides presented on MHC class I molecules. Cell. 1994;78:761–771

Sherr CJ. Cancer cell cycles. Science. 1996;274(5293):1672-7.

Soysa NS, Alles N, Shimokawa H, Jimi E, Aoki K, Ohya K. Inhibition of the classical NF-kappaB pathway prevents osteoclast bone-resorbing activity. J Bone Miner Metab. 2009;27(2):131-9.

Speese SD, Trotta N, Rodesch CK, Aravamudan B, Broadie K. The ubiquitin proteasome system acutely regulates presynaptic protein turnover and synaptic efficacy. Curr Biol. 2003;13(11):899-910.

Stein RL, Melandri F, Dick L. Kinetic characterization of the chymotryptic activity of the 20S proteasome. Biochemistry. 1996;35(13):3899-908.

Tak P, Gerlag D, Aupperle K, van de Geest D, Overbeek M, Bennett B, et al. Inhibitor of nuclear factor kappaB kinase beta is a key regulator of synovial inflammation. Arthritis Rheum 2001;44:1897–907.

Thurberg BL, Collins T. The nuclear factor-kappa B/inhibitor of kappa B autoregulatory system and atherosclerosis. Curr Opin Lipidol. 1998;9(5):387-96.

Tsao PW, Suzuki T, Totsuka R, Murata T, Takagi T, Ohmachi Y, et al. The effect of dexamethasone on the expression of activated NF-kappa B in adjuvant arthritis. Clin Immunol Immunopathol. 1997;83(2):173-8.

Valdes AM, Van Oene M, Hart DJ, Surdulescu GL, Loughlin J, Doherty M, et al. Reproducible genetic associations between candidate genes and clinical knee osteoarthritis in men and women. Arthritis Rheum. 2006;54(2):533-9.

Van Waes C, Yu M, Nottingham L, Karin M. Inhibitor-kappaB kinase in tumor promotion and suppression during progression of squamous cell carcinoma. Clin Cancer Res. 2007;13(17):4956-9.

Xu J, Wu HF, Ang ES, Yip K, Woloszyn M, Zheng MH, et al. NF-kappaB modulators in osteolytic bone diseases. Cytokine Growth Factor Rev. 2009;20(1):7-17.

Yamanaka H, Matsuda Y, Tanaka M, Sendo W, Nakajima H, Taniguchi A, et al. Serum matrix metalloproteinase 3 as a predictor of the degree of joint destruction during the six months after measurement, in patients with early rheumatoid arthritis. Arthritis Rheum. 2000;43(4):852-8.

Zangari M, Yaccoby S, Cavallo F, Esseltine D, Tricot G. Response to bortezomib and activation of osteoblasts in multiple myeloma. Clin Lymphoma Myeloma. 2006;7(2):109-14.

Zwerina J, Hayer S, Tohidast-Akrad M, Bergmeister H, Redlich K, Feige U, et al. Single and combined inhibition of tumor necrosis factor, interleukin-1, and RANKL pathways in tumor necrosis factor-induced arthritis: effects on synovial inflammation, bone erosion, and cartilage destruction. Arthritis Rheum. 2004;50(1):277-90.

9

Role of Adrenomedullin in Patients with Rheumatoid Arthritis

Etsuo Chosa, Hiroaki Hamada and Toshiyuki Ohkura
Division of Orthopaedic Surgery, Department of Medicine of Sensory and Mortor Organs, Faculty of Medicine, University of Miyazaki
Japan

1. Introduction

The mechanism of arthritis including rheumatoid arthritis (RA) has not been clarified enough in terms of its molecular biology. However, owing to advances in techniques to produce monoclonal antibodies and genetic engineering techniques to produce recombinant proteins, targeted therapies have progressed. Tumor necrosis factor-alpha (TNF-α), interleukin-1 (IL-1), interleukin-6 (IL-6), and T-cells (CD28) are representative targets, and therapies targeting them have produced epoch-making results in the treatment of RA. In this text, we report the role and effects of therapy with adrenomedullin as a novel, promising targeted therapy.

Adrenomedullin (ADM) is a peptide that was discovered by the assay-based monitoring of platelet cAMP activity (Kitamura et al., 1993). This protein shows not only marked vasodilatory but also *in vivo* and *in vitro* anti-inflammatory activities (Isumi et al., 1998).

To determine the efficacy of ADM in patients with RA, we researched the plasma level of ADM and its correlation with the plasma CRP level. The result showed that the plasma ADM level in patients with RA was twice that in healthy controls and strongly correlated with the blood CRP level, and the ADM level in synovial tissue in patients with RA was 3 times that in patients with osteoarthritis (Chosa et al., 2003). Then, thorough research is needed to examine whether the cultured RA synoviocytes are related to the ADM *in vitro*. The result showed that ADM was produced from RA synoviocytes and reduced the IL-6 level in cultured media (Fig. 5). These results suggest the close involvement of ADM in arthritis in RA. Therefore, to examine the therapeutic efficacy of intra-articular ADM injection, we injected ADM into the joint of a rabbit model of adjuvant arthritis, and confirmed the inhibition of arthritis at an early stage. These findings suggest the potentiality of ADM as a novel drug for the treatment of arthritis in RA (Okura et al., 2008).

2. Measured adrenomedullin (ADM) in patients with RA

2.1 Patient background

For measurement of plasma ADM, the study population consisted of 26 patients with RA aged 58–73 years (mean ± SD 62 ± 4 yrs), 10 with osteoarthritis (OA) aged 59–76 years

(68 ±8), and 10 healthy volunteer controls aged 50-66 years (57 ± 5). All subjects were female.

To clarify further the reason for the increase in plasma ADM, joint fluid, synovial tissue, and cartilage were measured by radioimmunoassay (RIA). These were acquired from surgical subjects during total knee arthroplasty in patients with RA (n = 6) and OA (n = 6). All patients with RA were classified as stage 4, functional class 2, according to the criteria of the American Rheumatism Association (ARA) (Clegg & Ward, 1987); they were medicated with only DMARDs and NSAIDs without steroid. All patients with OA were classified as stage 4 to 5, according to the Kellgren-Lawrence radiographic staging system (Kellgren & Lawrence, 1958). Since plasma ADM concentration has been reported to be elevated in patients with hypertension, renal failure, systemic infections, myocardial infarction, and heart failure (Ishimitsu et al., 1994; Nishikimi et al., 1995; Kobayashi et al., 1996), patients and controls with these conditions were excluded.

2.2 Methods of measuring ADM levels in plasma, joint fluid and joint tissues

2.2.1 Methods measuring the plasma and joint fluid ADM level

Blood and joint fluid samples were transferred into tubes containing 1 mg/ml EDTA-2Na and 500 kallikrein inhibitory units/ml of aprotinin for measurement of ADM. The plasma was kept at -30°C until assayed. Levels of plasma ADM and joint fluid ADM were measured by IRMA using specific kits (AM RIA Shionogi) developed by Shionogi Pharmaceutical Co. Ltd., Osaka, Japan. The limit of detection of human AM is 0.5 pmol/l for these kits.

2.2.2 Extraction of ADM in joint tissues

For measuring ADM levels of acquired joint fluids, samples were acidified with acetic acid to a final concentration of 1.0 M and centrifuged at 3000 rpm for 5 min, while synovium and cartilage specimens were acidified with acetic acid to a final concentration of 1.0 M and boiled for 10 min to inactivate proteases. The samples were then homogenized and centrifuged for 90 min at 12,000 rpm. The supernatant of samples was applied to a Sep-Pak C18 cartridge (Millipore-Waters, Milford, MA, USA). After the cartridge was washed with 10% CH_3CN in 0.1% trifluoroacetic acid, the absorbed materials were eluted with 50% CH_3CN in 0.1% trifluoroacetic acid. The eluted samples were dried by speed vacuum, freeze-dried and stored at -30°C until assayed.

2.2.3 Radioimmunoassay for ADM

The RIA for ADM was performed as described previously (Kitamura et al., 1994). The incubation buffer for RIA was 0.05 M sodium phosphate buffer (pH 7.4), containing 0.5% BSA, 0.5% Triton X-100, 0.08 M NaCl, 0.025 M EDTA 2Na, 0.05% NaN_3, and 500 KIU/ml trasylol. A disposable plastic tube (10 × 75 mm) was used for assaying. All assay procedures were performed at 4°C. Both standard ADM and unknown samples (100 µl) were incubated with anti-ADM antiserum diluent (200 µl) for 12 h before the tracer solution (125I-AM, 18,000-20,000 counts/min in 100 µl) was added. After incubation for 16 h, anti-rabbit IgG goat serum diluent (100 µl) was added. After standing for 24 h, the tubes were centrifuged at 3000 rpm for 30 min at 4°C and the radioactivity of the precipitate was measured using an Aloka ARC-600 gamma counter.

2.3 Result of ADM in plasma, joint fluid and joint tissues in patients with RA Discussion of joint ADM level in patients with RA

It has been reported that some collagenous disorders show increased levels of plasma ADM (Yudoh et al., 1999). We measured and compared plasma ADM concentrations in patients with RA and healthy controls, finding that patients with RA exhibited a 1.7-fold increase in plasma ADM levels (Table 1).

	Tolal ADM (fmol / ml)	Mature ADM (fmol / ml)
Healthy controls	11.64±2.8	1.34±0.9
RA patients	18.35±6.9	1.80±1.4
OA patients	12.88±1.9	1.42±0.8

Table 1. Blood adrenomedullin (ADM) levels in RA and OA patients and healthy controls

All values are expressed as means ± SD.※$p < 0.01$. Patients with RA demonstrated high plasma concentration of ADM (18.35 ± 6.9 fmol/ml) compared to healthy controls (11.64 ± 2.8 fmol/ml) and OA patients (12.88 ± 1.9 fmol/ml)

Moreover, plasma ADM levels in patients with RA were also found to be significantly correlated to CRP levels (Fig. 1). In RA, CRP correlates with disease activity and response to therapy. Our patient data did not include RA disease activity, excluding RA functional class classification. Hamada et al. (2010) stated that no autologous antibody such as rheumatoid factor or anti-CCP antibody showed significant correlation with plasma ADM level. In addition, there was no correlation with disease activity scores such as DAS-28. DAS-28 is not only dependent on the inflammatory level, so the plasma ADM level may escalate before escalation of the activity in synovitis or the amount of actual synovial inflammation (Hamada et al., 2010). Therefore, our results suggest that ADM levels are increased in patients with RA and investigated that they might be correlated with disease activity. Moreover, ADM concentration in the joint fluid of RA patients (10.8 ± 4.3 fmol/ml) was significantly higher than that of OA patients (7.2 ± 1.8 fmol/ml) (Fig. 2).

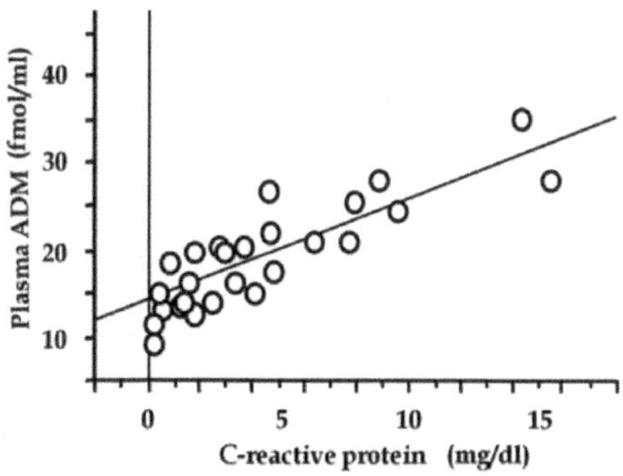

Fig. 1. Correlation between plasma AM and C-reactive protein

A significant positive correlation was observed between AM and CRP (correlation coefficient = 0.685, $p < 0.01$). Plasma ADM and plasma CRP levels were found to be well correlated. The correlation coefficient between CRP and AM was 0.685, $p < 0.01$.

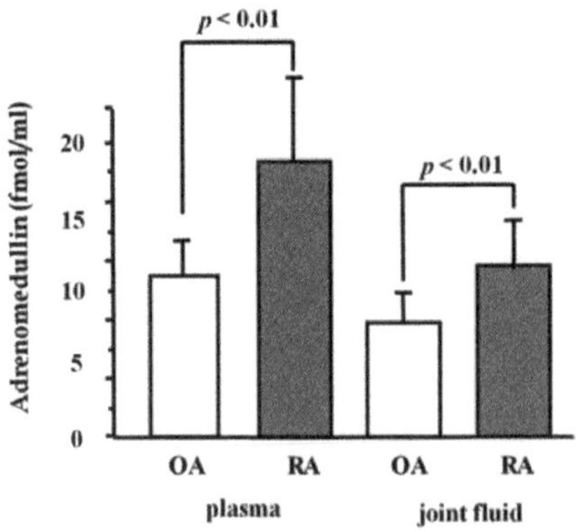

Fig. 2. Concentration of ADM between RA and OA in plasma and joint fluid

Patients with RA demonstrated high plasma concentration of ADM (18.35 ± 6.9 fmol/ml) compared to OA patients (12.88 ± 1.9 fmol/ml). ADM concentration in the joint fluid of RA patients (10.8 ± 4.3 fmol/ml) was significantly higher than that of OA patients (7.2 ± 1.8 fmol/ml)

We applied conventional radioimmunoassay (RIA) to determine ADM concentration in tissues. RA is characterized by the presence of inflammatory synovitis accompanied by destruction of joint cartilage and bone. The concentration of ADM in the synovium of RA patients was 3.2-fold higher than that of OA patients (Fig. 3). In addition, the concentration of ADM in plasma of RA patients was 1.4-fold higher than that of OA patients (Table 2). To determine the relationship between plasma ADM and arthritis in patients with RA, we compared ADM levels in joint fluid of RA and OA patients. Joint fluid is similar in composition to plasma, which explains the similarly significant increases in ADM concentration in both plasma and joint fluid in patients with RA compared with those with OA ($p < 0.01$) (Fig. 2). These observations indicate that the reason for this high concentration of ADM might be secretion from synovial stromal cells or secretion from synovial vascular wall cells. However, the mechanism by which plasma and joint fluid ADM levels increase in patients with RA remains unknown.

Several tissues including vessels secrete ADM, and elevated ADM could conceivably be caused by secretion from vascular cells in general. When we consider the results, in which ADM levels in the synovium of RA patients were higher than those of OA patients, we may assume that synovitis is one reason for the increased ADM concentration in synovium and joint fluid, and may partially contribute to the increase in ADM levels in plasma. Our results indicate the possibility that ADM participates in the pathophysiology of joint lesions in patients with RA. Together with the fact that ADM is known to inhibit the secretion of cytokines from several cell lines (Isumi et al., 1999; Kamoi et al., 1995), the findings seem to validate the assumption that production and secretion of ADM in synovium are strongly correlated with anti-inflammation in arthritis. Thus, the elevation of plasma ADM levels may be related to the anti-inflammatory response. Clementi et al. (1999) investigated the anti-inflammatory effect of ADM in rats, finding that ADM production in several cell lines was strongly induced by stimulation of a group of inflammatory cytokines including interleukin 1 and tumor necrosis factor-α (TNF-α) (Hofbauer et al., 2002). Some studies report that ADM acts as a circulating vasoactive hormone in blood, and plays an anti-inflammatory role in the prevention of local infection and inflammation, thus contributing to host defense systems (Ueda et al., 1999; Elsasser & Kahl, 2002). From these observations, we speculate that ADM may play a role in the pathophysiology of inflammation as well as in the regulation of joint disorders.

Synovitis inevitably plays a role in the destruction of joint surface, so we measured the concentration of ADM in articular cartilage. We found the ADM concentration in cartilage was lower than that of other tissues (Fig. 2). While the concentration of ADM in normal human articular cartilage has not been determined, an immunohistochemical study has reported that normal human articular chondrocytes produce ADM (Fig. 4) (Asada et al., 1999). No statistically significant difference was found in the articular cartilage concentration of ADM in RA and OA patients (Fig. 3). We therefore speculate that this may be because our samples were from cases that consisted of end-stage arthritis, with advanced degeneration and differentiation of the cartilage. A thorough investigation of the role of ADM in cartilage pathophysiology is necessary.

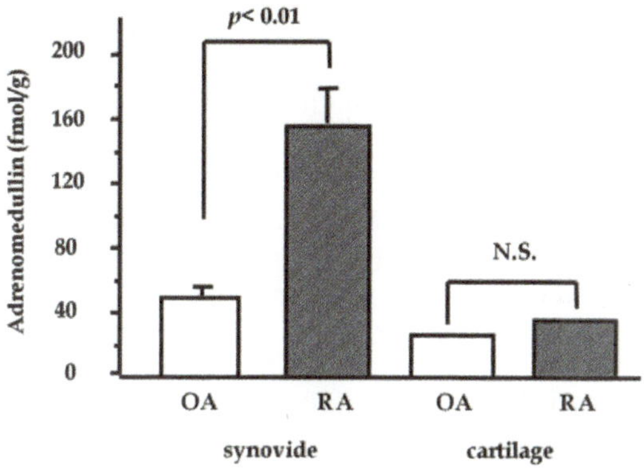

Fig. 3. Concentration of ADM for synovium and articular cartilage in patients with OA and RA

RA patients showed higher concentrations of ADM in synovium compared to OA patients. *p < 0.01; **not significant. In cartilage, there is no significantly difference between the concentration of OA and RA

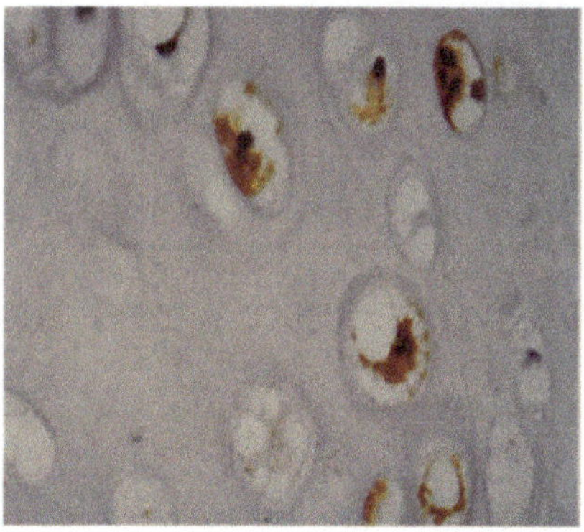

Fig. 4. Novel distribution of adrenomedullin-immunoreactive cells in human cartilage

Hyaline cartilage: Chondrocytes are positive for ADM. (donated from Prof. Asada, Miyazaki University)

We observed that plasma ADM concentration in patients with RA was higher than that of healthy controls, and plasma ADM and plasma CRP levels were found to be well correlated. Our data suggest that plasma ADM levels increase with the activity of RA. We conclude that ADM probably plays a part in the regulation of the inflammatory process of RA, and its plasma and/or joint fluid levels could be used as an index of the degree of RA. Therefore, we investigated the role of ADM in inflammation in cultured RA synoviocytes (fibroblast-like synovium) in a subsequent investigation.

3. Effiency of ADM in cultured synovia (fibroblast-like synoviocytes)

3.1 Methods of ADM study in cultured FLS

3.1.1 Fibroblast-like synoviocytes (FLS) culture

Synovial tissue specimens were collected under sterile conditions from 6 patients with RA. Specimen collection occurred during total knee arthroplasty in all patients with RA. All RA patients fulfilled 1987 American College of Rheumatology criteria for RA. All of them were treated with only NSAIDs, DMARDs and hyaluronic acid injection into the joint before samples were obtained. The methods of FLS culture was described previously (Nanki, et al., 2001).

3.1.2 Characterization of secreted ADM

To examine the molecular forms of ADM, extracts of cells cultured on a 100-mm dish and 15 ml of the conditioned medium (1%FBS) were analyzed by reverse-phase high-performance liquid chromatography (HPLC) with a column of TSK ODS 120 A (Tosoh, Tokyo, Japan). A linear gradient of 10% to 60% acetonitrile was run in 0.1% trifluoroacetic acid for 60 minutes and the ir-AM level in each fraction was measured by RIA. The recovery of ir-ADM from this HPLC system was greater than 80%.

3.2 IL-6 secretion was inhibited in cultured FLS after addition of ADM

The present study demonstrated that cultured RA synoviocytes expressed the mRNA for ADM and also actively secreted ADM (Fig. 5). The active secretion of ADM by RA synoviocytes seems to be similar to its active secretion by endothelial cells (Hojo et al., 2001; Uemura et al., 2002). ADM in the culture medium seemed to be actual AM because reverse-phase HPLC revealed that most of the ADM secreted into the medium emerged at the

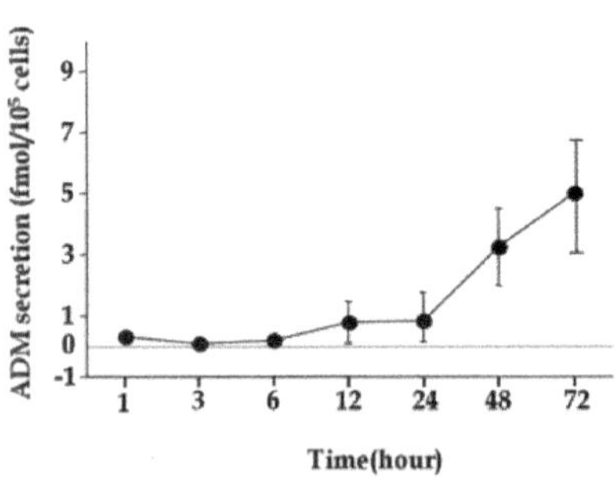

Fig. 5. Time course curve for secretion of AM and intracellular ADM

The cells were incubated for the indicated time-periods in serum free medium, and the ADM was determined by RIA. Intracellular ADM was too low to be determined.

identical elution position to that of authentic human ADM (1-52), which is the full-length human ADM peptide (Fig. 6). The minor peak that was eluted earlier was thought to be oxidized ADM containing methione sulfoxide. The intracellular ADM concentration remained extremely low in RA synoviocytes (Fig. 5), suggesting that these cells constitutively secrete ADM. Thus, RA synoviocytes seem to secrete ADM rapidly after its synthesis, with little intracellular storage.

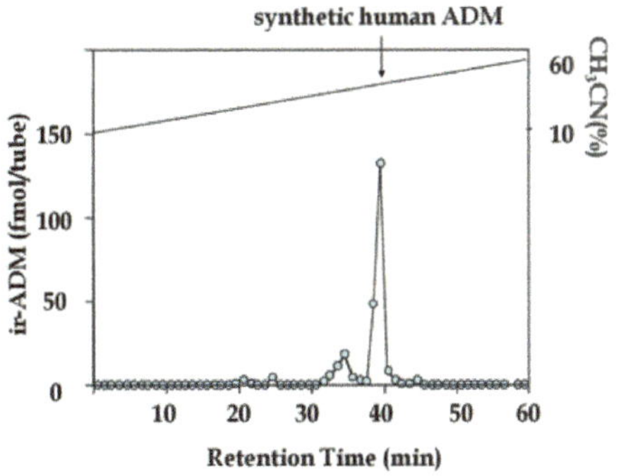

Fig. 6. Analysis by reverse-phase HPLC of immunoreactive adrenomedullin (ir-ADM) secreted into the media

A linear gradient of acetonitrile of 10% to 60% was made in 0.1% trifluoroacetic acid for 60 minutes at a flow rate of 1.0mL/min. The arrow indicates the elution position of synthetic human AM. The specificity of the RIA was clarified.

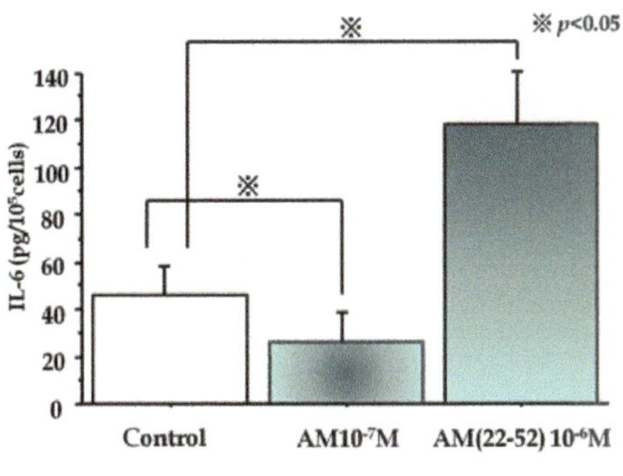

Fig. 7. Inhibitory effect of ADM about the IL-6 secretion into the media in cultured FLS

Effects of ADM 22-52 10^{-6}M (ADM blocker) on control level of IL-6 secretion in cultured fibroblast like synoviocytes (FLS) donated from RA patients. Serum-starved FLS were incubated 24 hours. Values are the means±SEM of six wells examined. Each was compared with the cells incubated with 1%FBS media (control). Each set of experiments was repeated three times and identical results were obtained.

When the synoviocytes reached confluence, ADM (10^{-8} M) was added to the culture media. After 24 hours, the level of IL-6 in culture media significantly decreased. Moreover, ADM (22-52), which is an ADM antagonist, elevated the level of IL-6 in culture media (Fig. 7).

These observations lead us to conclude that ADM inhibited the secretion of IL-6 and regulated the IL-6 production in the cultured RA synoviocytes.
Besides the findings in our study, a similar report stated that ADM reduced constitutive production of IL6 from RA synoviocytes in a dose-dependent manner. A high concentration of ADM (>10-8 mmol/l) significantly reduced constitutive production of IL6 compared with a low concentration of ADM (<10-9 mmol/l) (p=0.0029) (Nanke et al., 2003). Then, we tried to inject ADM into the knee in antigen-induced arthritis in rabbits.

4. Adrenomedullin injection to the knee in antigen-induced arthritis (AIA) in rabbits

4.1 Methods

4.1.1 Induction of antigen-induced arthritis

The AIA rabbit model was developed as described by Consden and colleagues (Consden et al., 1971). Briefly, rabbits were anesthetized by an intravenous injection of pentobarbital sodium and were immunized by 1.2 ml intradermal injections of 6 mg/ml ovalbumin (Sigma-Aldrich, St Louis, MO, USA) in saline emulsified with an equal volume of TiterMax Gold (TiterMax, Norcross, GA, USA). The rabbits were re-immunized in the same manner 30 days later. Seven days after the second immunization, the rabbits underwent skin testing following a 0.1 ml intradermal injection of a solution of 200 μg/ml ovalbumin in saline. Animals exhibiting a welt of 13 mm or greater after 24 hours were confirmed as 'immunized'. Twelve days after the second immunization, the 'immunized' rabbits were anesthetized and arthritis was induced by 0.5 ml bilateral knee intra-articular injections of a solution of 20 mg/ml ovalbumin in saline.

4.1.2 Treatment protocol

Twenty-four hours after arthritis induction, the rabbits were anesthetized and different doses of ADM (1 ng to 3 μg; Peptide Institute Inc., Osaka, Japan) dissolved in 0.3 ml saline were injected into the knee joint spaces or 0.3 ml saline was injected into the contralateral knee joint spaces as controls. For time-course experiments, ADM and saline were injected into the knee joint spaces daily for 7 days and 20 days. The rabbits were sacrificed on day 8 (n = 5 in each group) and day 21 (n = 3 in each group).

4.1.3 Joint swelling

To evaluate the grade of arthritis/inflammation, joint swelling was assessed by measuring the maximum diameter of the swollen joint using calipers. The swelling was compared with that at the same level on the contralateral knee, treated with saline.

4.1.4 Histological evaluation

For histological evaluation, rabbits were given an overdose of pentobarbital 8 days and 21 days after arthritis induction. The infrapatellar fat pads were harvested from dissected knees and were cut longitudinally, perpendicular to the patella ligament in the middle of the infrapatellar fat pad. The tissues were fixed in 10% buffered formaldehyde and embedded in paraffin wax, and sections 3 μm thick were obtained. The specimens were stained with H & E and Mallory-Azan stains. The area of the infrapatellar fat pad was measured using AxioVision software (release 4.3; ZEISS, Oberkochen, Germany).

Inflammatory cells, including lymphocytes and plasma cells, were counted in the superficial and deep portions of the infrapatellar fat pads (three fields under ×200 magnification in each portion) in H & E-stained specimens. The inflammatory cell count was performed by two independent observers.
To measure the collagen volume, the images of sections with Mallory–Azan stain were projected onto a color imaging analysis system (Mac SCOPE version 2.3.2; Mitani, Fukui, Japan). In each section, 10 separate sites were analyzed at ×40 magnification. The collagen volume fraction was obtained by calculating the mean ratio of connective tissue to the total tissue area.

4.1.5 Measurement of cytokine mRNA

Total RNA was extracted from the infrapatellar fat pad with TRIzol reagent (Invitrogen, Carlsbad, CA, USA) according to the manufacturer's protocol and was then reverse-transcribed into cDNA with the SuperScript First-Strand Synthesis System for RT-PCR kit (Invitrogen). To measure rabbit TNFα, IL-6, vascular endothelial growth factor (VEGF), transforming growth factor beta (TGFβ), and β-actin mRNA levels, we used the quantitative RT-PCR method of real-time quantitative PCR.

4.2 Result after joint injection of ADM in AIA rabbit

4.2.1 Adrenomedullin concentration in plasma

We measured the plasma ADM concentration before and 15, 30, 60 and 120 minutes after intra-articular injection of 3 µg ADM (n = 6). No significant change, however, was observed in the plasma concentration of ADM (Figure (Figure1).1). The intra-articular injection of ADM did not therefore increase the level of ADM in plasma.

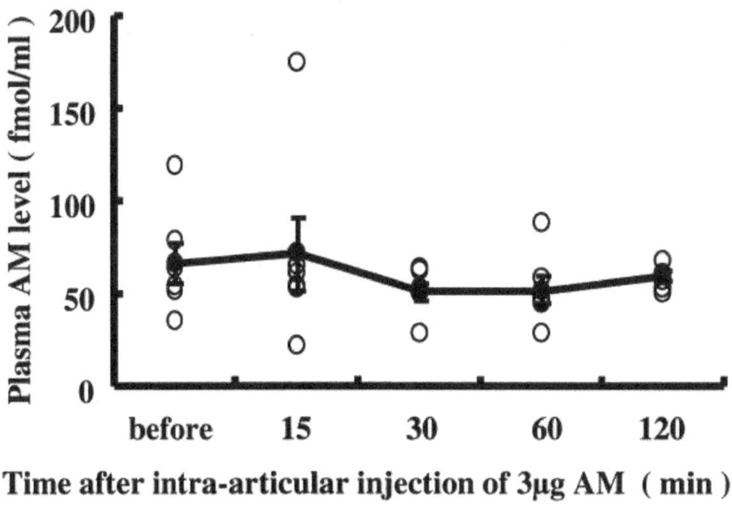

Fig. 8. Sequential concentrations of plasma ADM following intra-articular ADM injection in rabbits with antigen-induced arthritis.

Whole-blood samples (total 1 ml) were taken from a peripheral artery in the rabbit ear using a 22-gauge needle before and 15, 30, 60 and 120 minutes after intra-articular injection of 3 µg adrenomedullin (AM). The plasma AM concentration was measured using an immunoenzymometric assay kit (n = 6). White circles, plasma AM levels in rabbits; black circles, average plasma AM levels at each time point after intra-articular injection of 3 μg AM. Data expressed as the mean ± SEM. Each of plasma ADM level was not significantly.

4.2.2 Joint swelling

To evaluate the anti-inflammatory effect of ADM on arthritis, we used calipers to measure joint swelling in ADM-treated knees and compared the swelling with that at the same level on the contralateral knees, treated with saline. In rabbits with AIA treated with daily injections of ADM or saline into the knee joint spaces for 7 days, 3 μg ADM significantly reduced joint swelling compared with contralateral knees after day 5. No significant decrease in joint swelling was observed, however, in knees treated with <0.1 μg ADM (Fig. 9a and 10).

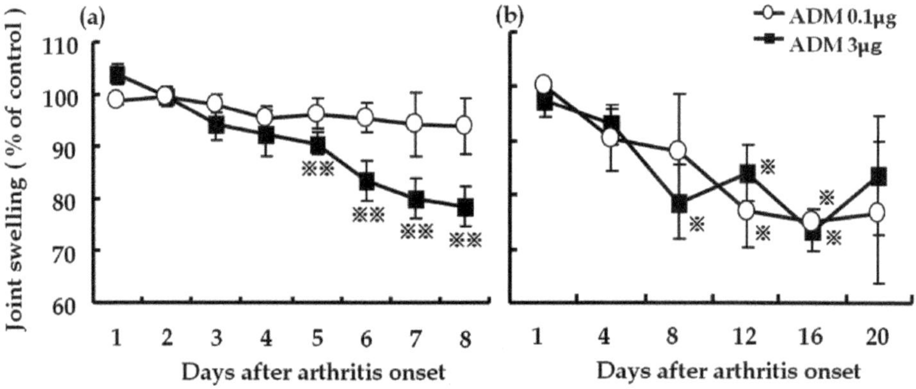

Fig. 9. Adrenomedullin reduced joint swelling in rabbits with antigen-induced arthritis.

(a) Joint swelling progress in rabbits with AIA treated with daily intra-articular injections of ADM or saline for 7 days (n = 5 in each group). Daily intra-articular injections of 3 μg ADM significantly decreased joint swelling compared with contralateral knees after day 5. No significant decrease in joint swelling was observed in knees treated with <0.1 μg ADM.
(b) Joint swelling progress in rabbits with AIA treated with daily intra-articular injections of ADM or saline for 20 days (n = 3 in each group). Daily intra-articular injections of 0.1 μg and 3 μg ADM showed a tendency to reduce joint swelling throughout the experiment, and significantly decreased joint swelling on days 12 and 16 and on days 8, 12 and 16, respectively, compared with contralateral control knees. Daily intra-articular injections of 1 ng and 0.01 μg ADM did not ameliorate joint swelling throughout the experiments (data not shown). Data expressed as the mean ± standard error of the mean. *P < 0.05 and **P < 0.01, compared with contralateral knees.

In rabbits with AIA treated for 20 days with daily injections of ADM or saline into the knee joint spaces, 0.1 μg and 3 μg ADM showed a tendency to reduce joint swelling throughout the experiment - and significantly decreased joint swelling on days 12 and 16 and on days 8, 12 and 16, respectively, compared with contralateral knees (Fig. 9b). Daily intra-articular injections of 1 ng and 0.01 μg ADM, however, did not ameliorate joint swelling (data not shown).

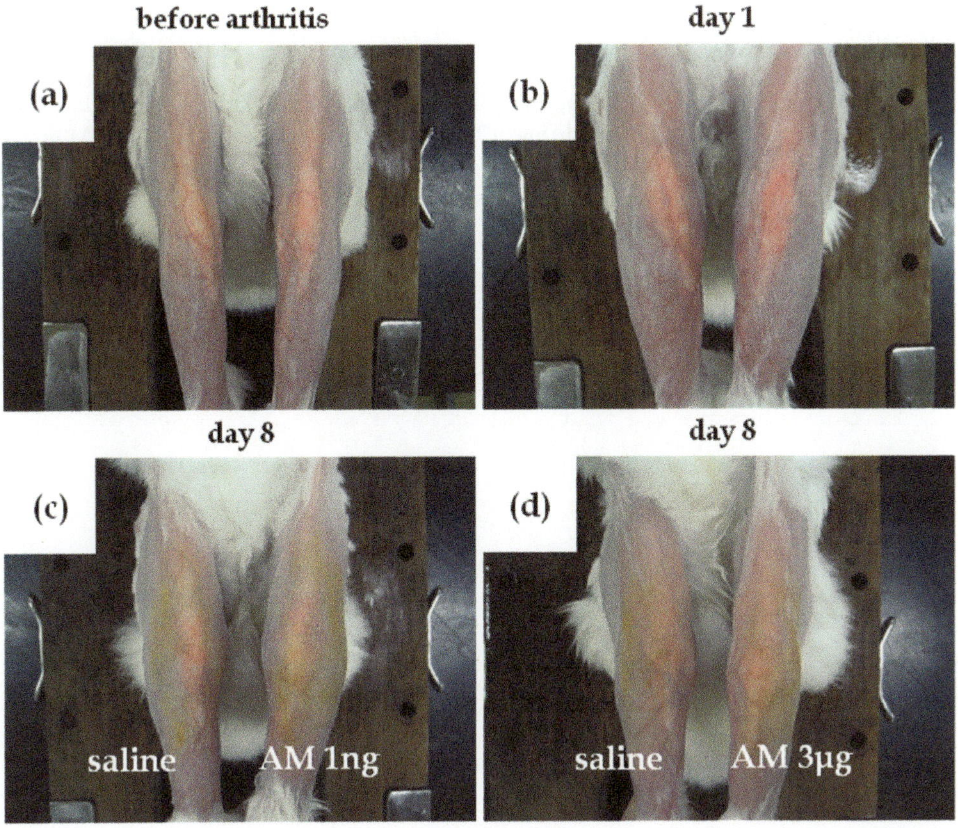

Fig. 10. Macroscopic pathology of joint swelling in rabbits with antigen-induced arthritis

(a) Photograph taken before arthritis onset. **(b)** Photograph taken 24 hours after arthritis onset. **(c)** The left knee of the rabbit with antigen-induced arthritis (AIA) was treated with daily intra-articular injections of 1 ng ADM for 7 days and the right knee was treated with daily intra-articular injections of saline for 7 days. Photograph taken 8 days after arthritis onset. **(d)** The left knee of the rabbit with AIA was treated with daily intra-articular injections of 3 μg ADM for 7 days and the right knee was treated with daily intra-articular injections of saline for 7 days. Photograph taken 8 days after arthritis onset.

4.2.3 Histological findings

The infrapatellar fat pads harvested from control knees on day 8 showed a dense inflammatory reaction, including edematous changes in the synovial interstitium, intracellular edema in the infrapatellar fat pads, hyperplasia of synovial surface cells and widespread infiltration of inflammatory cells in the infrapatellar fat pads (Fig. 11d,e,f). In contrast, these inflammatory reactions were suppressed in the knees treated with ADM for 7 days. In particular, edematous changes in the synovial interstitium, intracellular edema in the infrapatellar fat pads and infiltration of inflammatory cells in the deep portion of the infrapatellar fat pads were significantly reduced (Fig. 11a,b,c). The infrapatellar fat pads harvested from control knees on day 21 also showed a severe inflammatory reaction. Edematous changes in the synovial interstitium, hyperplasia of synovial surface cells and widespread infiltration of inflammatory cells throughout the infrapatellar fat pads were observed (Fig. 12d,e,f). In the knees treated with ADM for 20 days, these inflammatory reactions were ameliorated. ADM treatment significantly suppressed infiltration of inflammatory cells in the deep portion of the infrapatellar fat pads (Fig. 12a,b,c).

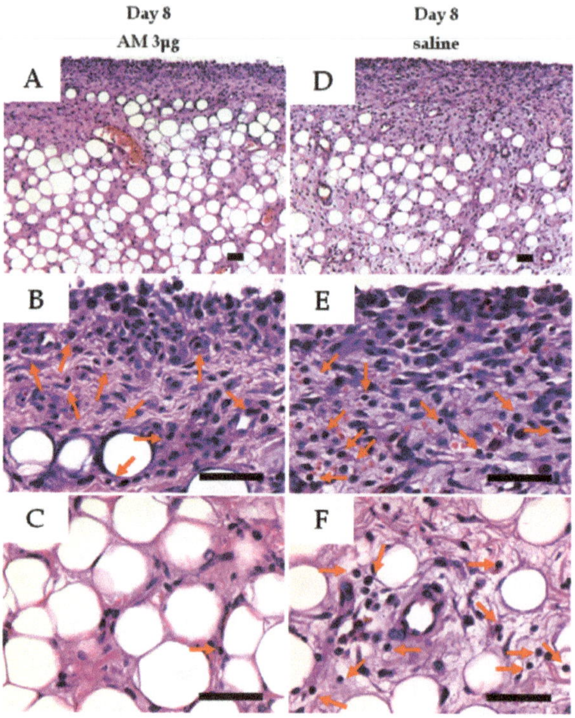

Fig. 11. Histological analysis of infrapatellar fat pad harvested from rabbit knees 8 days after arthritis onset

Rabbits with antigen-induced arthritis (AIA) were treated with daily injections of ADM or saline (control) into the knee joint spaces for 7 days. Tissues were sectioned longitudinally perpendicular to the patella ligament in the middle of the tissue, and were stained with H & E. **(a)**, **(b)**, **(c)** AIA rabbit knee was treated with daily intra-articular injections of 3 μg ADM for 7 days. (a) Low-magnification image (×100). (b), (c) High-magnification images (×400) of the superficial portion and the deep portion of (a), respectively. **(d)**, **(e)**, **and (f)** the contralateral knee of (a), (b) and (c) was treated with daily intra-articular injections of saline for 7 days. (d) Low-magnification image (×100). (e), (f) High-magnification images (×400) of the superficial portion and the deep portion of (d), respectively. Arrows indicate inflammatory cells. Bar = 50 μm.

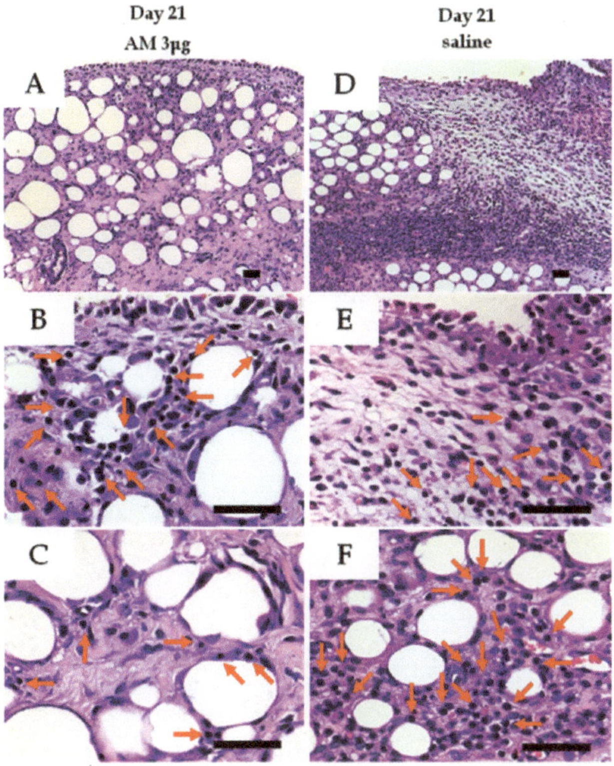

Fig. 12. Histological analysis of infrapatellar fat pad harvested from rabbit knees 21 days after arthritis onset

Rabbits with antigen-induced arthritis (AIA) were treated with daily injections of ADM or saline (control) into the knee joint spaces for 20 days. **(a)**, **(b)**, **(c)** AIA rabbit knee was treated with daily intra-articular injections of 3 μg AM for 20 days. (a) Low-magnification image (×100). (b), (c) High-magnification images (×400) of the superficial portion and the deep portion of (a), respectively. **(d)**, **(e)**, **and** **(f)** the contralateral knee of (a), (b) and (c) was treated with daily intra-articular injections of saline for 20 days. (d) Low-magnification image (×100). (e), (f) High-magnification images (×400) of the superficial portion and the deep portion of (d), respectively. Arrows indicate inflammatory cells. Bar = 50 μm.

4.2.4 Collagen volume in infrapatella fat pads treated with Adrenomedullin

To observe the effect of ADM on fibrosis of the infrapatellar fat pads harvested on day 21, we examined the collagen volume ratio of the infrapatellar fat pad histologically using Mallory-Azan staining. The collagen volume ratio was significantly increased in ADM-treated knees by 39% and 31% at 0.1 μg and 3 μg ADM, respectively, compared with control knees (Fig. 13 and 14). The effects of ADM on these pathological tissue changes, however, were not observed in knees treated with low-dose ADM.

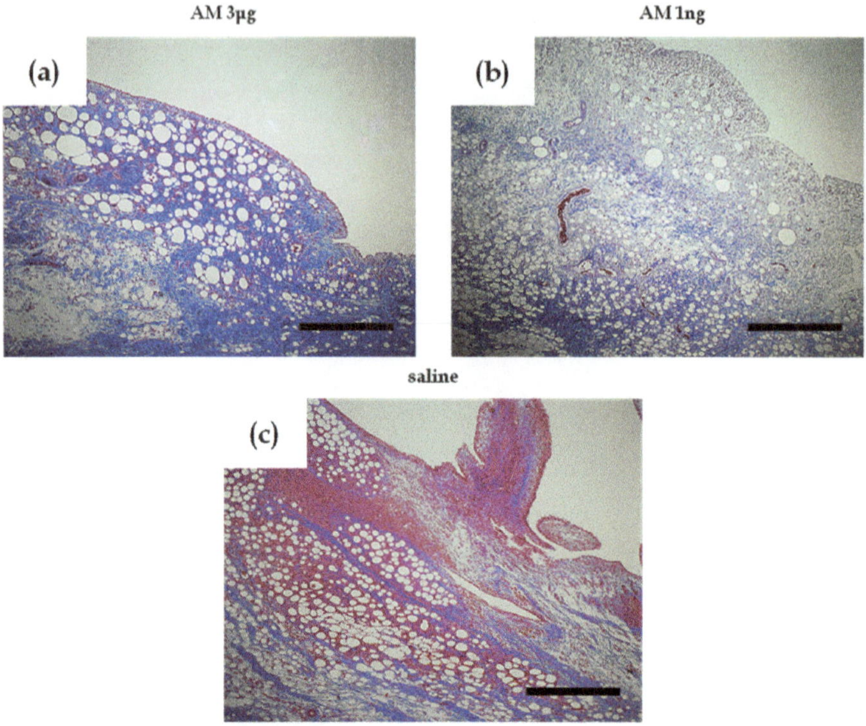

Fig. 13. Histological analysis of infrapatellar fat-pad sections stained with Mallory - Azan from rabbits with antigen-induced arthritis

The tissues were sectioned longitudinally perpendicular to the patella ligament in the middle of the tissue, and were stained with Mallory - Azan. **(a)** AIA rabbit knee was treated with daily intra-articular injections of 3 μg ADM for 20 days. **(b)** AIA rabbit knee was treated with daily intra-articular injections of 1 ng ADM for 20 days. **(c)** The contralateral knee of (a) was treated with daily intra-articular injections of saline for 20 days. Photographs taken at ×40 magnification. Bar = 500 μm.

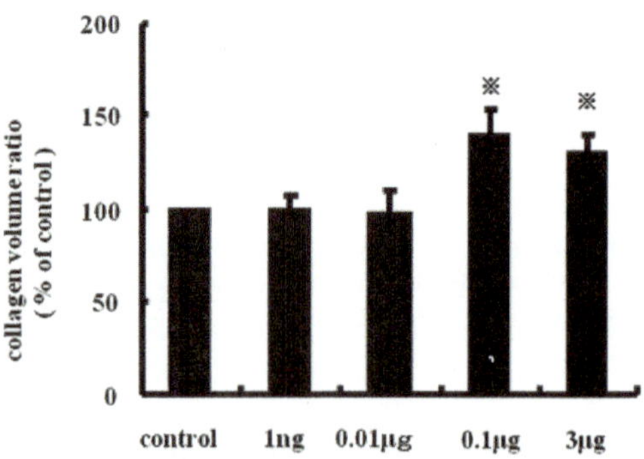

Fig. 14. Quantitative evaluation of collagen volume in the infrapatellar fat pad

The collagen volume ratio was increased in ADM-treated knees by 39% and 31% at 0.1 µg and 3 µg ADM, respectively. Data expressed as the mean ± standard error of the mean. $*P < 0.05$, compared with contralateral knees.

4.2.5 Cytokines

To elucidate the mechanism of the anti-inflammatory effects of AM in inflamed joints, we investigated the effect of AM on cytokine mRNA expression linked to AIA. Treatment with AM reduced TNFα mRNA expression in a dose-dependent manner. Daily intra-articular injections of 3 µg AM significantly suppressed the TNFα mRNA level by 21% and 49% at day 8 and day 21, respectively, compared with controls (Fig. 15a). In contrast, AM dose-dependently increased IL-6 mRNA expression. Daily intra-articular injections of 3 µg AM significantly increased the IL-6 mRNA level by 45% and 121% at day 8 and day 21, respectively, compared with controls (Fig. 15b). Although the VEGF mRNA level was suppressed by 10% at 3 µg AM on day 8, we did not observe a dose-dependent effect of AM on VEGF mRNA expression (Fig. 15d). AM treatment did not significantly alter the TGFβ mRNA level (Fig. 15c).

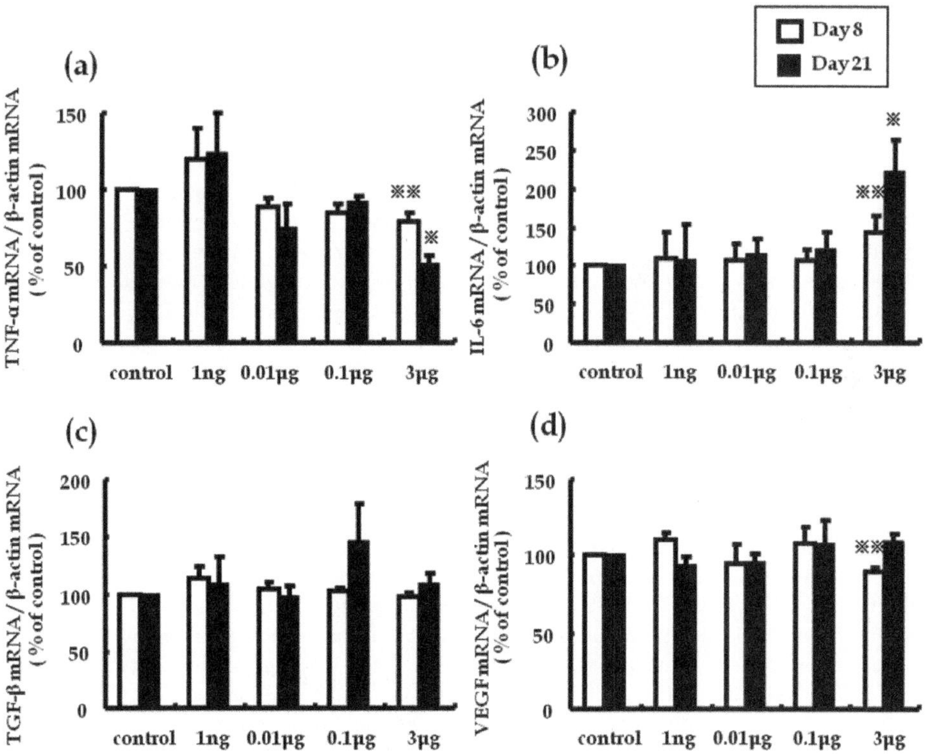

Fig. 15. Effect of adrenomedullin on cytokine mRNA expression linked to antigen-induced arthritis

Expression levels of TNFα, IL-6, transforming growth factor beta (TGFβ), and vascular endothelial growth factor (VEGF) mRNA in the infrapatellar fat pads were determined by real-time quantitative PCR. **(a)** ADM treatment reduced TNFα mRNA expression in a dose-dependent manner. Daily intra-articular injections of 3 μg ADM significantly suppressed the TNFα mRNA level by 21% and 49% at day 8 and day 21, respectively. **(b)** ADM increased IL-6 mRNA expression in a dose-dependent manner. Daily intra-articular injections of 3 μg AM significantly increased the IL-6 mRNA level by 45% and 121% at day 8 and day 21, respectively. **(c)** ADM treatment did not alter the TGFβ mRNA level. **(d)** Although the VEGF mRNA level was suppressed by 10% at 3 μg AM on day 8, a dose-dependent effect of ADM on VEGF mRNA expression was not observed. Open and closed columns represent the data at day 8 ($n = 5$ in each group) and day 21 ($n = 3$ in each group), respectively. Data expressed as the mean ± SEM. *$P < 0.05$ and **$P < 0.01$, compared with contralateral knees

4.3 Therapeutic efficacy of ADM injection to the knee in AIA in rabbits

In the present study we have shown that daily injections of ADM into the knee joint spaces of rabbits with AIA ameliorated the inflammatory response associated with the disease. Treatment with ADM reduced joint swelling, and reduced the expression of TNFα mRNA, edematous changes and the number of infiltrating inflammatory cells in the synovial tissue.

We observed that ADM suppressed joint swelling (Fig. 9 and 10). Histologically, ADM treatment reduced edematous changes and increased the ratio of connective tissue in the infrapatellar fat pad (Fig. 13 and 14). A previous study showed that TNFα induced cytoskeletal reorganization of endothelial cells and increased endothelial permeability by stimulating TNF receptors 1 and 2 (Ferrero et al., 2001). In addition, TNFα facilitates the ability of VEGF to promote excessive vascular permeability (Clauss et al., 2001). TNFα also suppresses the expression of matrix genes and the induction of connective tissue growth factor by TGFβ during the wound healing response (Leask & Abraham, 2004). TNFα therefore aggravates edematous changes and suppresses the fibrotic response of the tissue. Moreover, ADM was shown to reduce endothelial hyperpermeability induced by hydrogen peroxide, thrombin, and *Escherichia coli* hemolysin (Hippenstiel et al., 2002).

Two research groups reported recently that ADM signaling deficiency in mice resulted in midgestation death and massive edema. The cause of this edema was shown to be a result of fragility and hyperpermeability of blood vessels in one group and to be a failure of lymphatic vessel growth in the other (Ichikawa et al., 2008; Fritz et al., 2008). The evidence from these studies suggests that ADM plays an important role in preventing edema. From these observations, we speculate that ADM not only suppresses the production of TNFα, but also directly and indirectly inhibits edematous changes in the inflamed joint.

Although RA is a chronic and systemic inflammatory disorder of unknown etiology, TNFα has been shown to play a central role in the pathogenesis of RA (Moreland et al., 1997; Elliott et al., 1993; Arend et al., 1995). TNFα stimulates the proliferation of synovial cells and the production of matrix metalloproteinases by chondrocytes and synovial cells, and induces the release of other proinflammatory cytokines, leading to joint destruction (Arend et al., 1995; Nishimoto et al., 2000). We have shown that daily injections of ADM into the knee joint spaces of rabbits with AIA suppressed the expression of TNFα mRNA in the synovial tissue in a dose-dependent manner (Fig. 15a). It has been reported that ADM suppressed the secretion of TNFα from lipopolysaccharide-stimulated RAW 264.7 macrophages and NR8383 macrophages (Wong et al., 2005; Kubo et al., 1998; Wu et al., 2003). Because the major source of TNFα in inflamed synovial tissue of RA is due to macrophages (Chu et al., 1991) it is plausible that ADM suppresses the production of TNFα from activated macrophages in inflamed synovial tissue.

On the contrary, we found that ADM increased IL-6 mRNA expression in the synovial tissue (Fig.15b). Our results agree with previous findings on the effects of ADM on IL-6 production. ADM is reported to augment the production of IL-6 from NR8383 cells and Swiss 3T3 fibroblast cells stimulated with lipopolysaccharide or cytokines (Isumi et al., 1998). Several observations support the concept that IL-6 is an anti-inflammatory cytokine (Tilg et al., 1997). IL-6 has been shown to have a suppressive effect on TNFα and IL-1β production in peripheral blood mononuclear cells and exerts its anti-inflammatory effects in hepatitis by reducing the production of TNF (Schindler et al., 1990; Mizuhara et al., 1994). Our results therefore lead us to speculate that the mechanism involved in the anti-inflammatory effects of ADM is related to suppression of TNFα in inflamed synovial tissue directly or through IL-6 production.

Overproduction of IL-6 has been observed and is known to cause unfavorable clinical symptoms in immune-inflammatory diseases such as RA. Overproduction of IL-6 induces the production of rheumatoid factors and increases antibody levels, the platelet count, C-reactive protein levels, and serum amyloid A protein levels in RA (Nishimoto et al., 2000). Treatment with a humanized anti-IL-6 receptor antibody has also been shown to reduce RA disease activity (Nishimoto et al., 2004). The effect of ADM on IL-6 production might therefore be an undesirable adverse effect in RA therapy. Plasma ADM levels have been reported to increase with RA disease activity and in the acute or flare phase of myocardial infarction and sepsis (Chosa et al., 2003; Yudoh et al., 1999; Kobayashi et al., 1996; Hirata et al., 1996). Recent studies have shown that ADM administration in the acute phase reaction of several disease models produced significant protective effects in organs against inflammation and oxidative stress (Kawai et al., 2004; Nakamura et al., 2004; Yang et al., 2002). Miyashita and colleagues reported that ADM administration to prevent ischemic brain damage in mice less than 72 hours after the ischemic event showed significant therapeutic effects, whereas ADM administration more than 72 hours after stroke onset produced no significant therapeutic effects (Miyashita et al., 2006).

From these observations and our study findings, we speculate that the effects of ADM may be dependent on the tissue environment and the disease state; that is, the role and effects of ADM in inflammation may change during the inflammatory process. ADM acts as a strong anti-inflammatory agent in the acute or flare phase of inflammation, but in the chronic phase of inflammation ADM may act not only as an anti-inflammatory agent but also as a proinflammatory agent. It is therefore important to consider the time of administration, the route of administration and the dosage schedule of ADM in the treatment of RA.

5. Conclusions

In our study, plasma ADM level was found to be elevated in patients with RA and the origin of ADM was shown to be synovial tissue. ADM may exert anti-inflammatory effects because the cultured RA synoviocytes secrete ADM, have ADM receptors, and inhibit IL-6 production. Therefore, the effects of daily intra-articular injections of ADM into the knees of rabbits with AIA were examined. The results suggest that ADM suppresses the inflammatory response in inflamed joints by inhibiting the expression of TNFα mRNA and increasing IL-6 mRNA level.

Although ADM may have anti-inflammatory properties, the effect of ADM on IL-6 production in inflamed synovial tissue might be an undesirable adverse effect in RA therapy. Further research is necessary to investigate the drug effects, the time of administration, and the dosage schedules of intra-articular injection of ADM in the treatment of RA.

6. Acknowledgment

The authors would like to thank Prof. Kazuo Kitamura for his helpful discussion, Prof. Yujiro Asada for the offer of sample in the immunohistochemical study, and Ms Mariko Tokashiki for technical support in measurement of the plasma AM concentration.

7. References

Arend WP & Dayer JM. (1995) Inhibition of the production and effects of interleukin-1 and tumor necrosis factor alpha in rheumatoid arthritis. *Arthritis Rheum.* Vol. 38, pp. 151–160

Asada Y, Hara S, Marutsuka K, Kitamura K, Tsuji T, Sakata J, Sato Y, Kisanuki A, Eto T & Sumiyoshi A. (1999) Novel distribution of adrenomedullin-immunoreactive cells in human tissues. *Histochem Cell Biol*, Vol. 112, pp. 185-191.

Clementi G, Caruso A, Cutuli VM, Prato A, Mangano NG, Amico-Roxas M. (1999) Antiinflammatory activity of adrenomedullin in the acetic acid peritonitis in rats. *Life Sci* Vol.65, pp. 203-8.

Chosa E, Hamada H, Kitamura K, Eto T & Tajima N.(2003) Increased plasma and joint tissue adrenomedullin concentrations in patients with rheumatoid arthritis compared to those with osteoarthritis. *J Rheumatol.* Vol. 30, pp. 2553–2556.

Chu CQ, Field M, Feldmann M & Maini RN. (1991) Localization of tumor necrosis factor alpha in synovial tissues and at the cartilage–pannus junction in patients with rheumatoid arthritis. *Arthritis Rheum.* Vol. 34, pp. 1125–1132.

Clauss M, Sunderkötter C, Sveinbjörnsson B, Hippenstiel S, Willuweit A, Marino M, Haas E, Seljelid R, Scheurich P, Suttorp N, Grell M & Risau W. (2001)A permissive role for tumor necrosis factor in vascular endothelial growth factor-induced vascular permeability. *Blood.* Vol. 97, pp. 1321–29.

Clegg DO & Ward JR. (1987) Diagnostic criteria in rheumatoid arthritis. *Scand J Rheumatol Suppl.* Vol. 65, pp. 3-11. Review

Consden R, Doble A, Glynn LE & Nind AP. (1971) Production of a chronic arthritis with ovalbumin. Its retention in the rabbit knee joint. *Ann Rheum Dis.* Vol. 30, pp. 307–315.

Elliott MJ, Maini RN, Feldmann M, Long-Fox A, Charles P, Katsikis P, Brennan FM, Walker J, Bijl H, Ghrayeb J, et al. (1993) Treatment of rheumatoid arthritis with chimeric monoclonal antibodies to tumor necrosis factor alpha. *Arthritis Rheum.* Vol. 36, pp. 1681–1690.

Elsasser TH & Kahl S. (2002) Adrenomedullin has multiple roles in disease stress: development and remission of the inflammatory response. *Microsc Res Tech* Apr 15 Vol. 57. pp. 120-9.

Ferrero E, Zocchi MR, Magni E, Panzeri MC, Curnis F, Rugarli C, Ferrero ME & Corti A. (2001) Roles of tumor necrosis factor p55 and p75 receptors in TNF-α-induced vascular permeability. *Am J Physiol Cell Physiol.* Oct. Vol. 281, pp. c1173–c1179.

Fritz-Six KL, Dunworth WP, Li M & Caron KM. (2008) Adrenomedullin signaling is necessary for murine lymphatic vascular development. *J Clin Invest.* Vol. 118, pp. 40–50.

Hamada H, Saisyo K, Sekimoto T, Chosa E. (2010) Plasma adrenomedullin and proadrenomedullin N-terminal 20 peptide in patients diagnosed as having early rheumatoid arthritis. *Mod Rheumatol.* Aug. Vol. 20(4), pp. 89-95.

Hip.penstiel S, et al. (2002) Adrenomedullin reduces endothelial hyperpermeability. *Circ Res.*(91):618–625.

Hofbauer KH, Schoof E, Kurtz A & Sandner P. (2002) Inflammatory cytokines stimulate adrenomedullin expression through nitric oxide-dependent and -independent pathways. *Hypertension,* Vol. 39, pp. 161-7.

Hirata Y, Mitaka C, Sato K, Nagura T, Tsunoda Y, Amaha K, Marumo F. (1996) Increased circulating adrenomedullin, a novel vasodilatory peptide, in sepsis. *J Clin Endocrinol Metab.* Vol. 81, pp. 1449–1453.

Hojo Y, Ikeda U, Ohya K, Ichida M, Kario K, Takahashi M, Ikeda M, Minota S, Isumi Y, Minamino N, Ishimitsu T & Shimada K. (2001, Apr) Interaction between monocytes and vascular endothelial cells induces adrenomedullin production. *Atherosclerosis.* Vol. 155 (2), pp. 381-7.

Ichikawa-Shindo Y, Sakurai T, Kamiyoshi A, Kawate H, Iinuma N, Yoshizawa T, Koyama T, Fukuchi J, Iimuro S, Moriyama N, Kawakami H, Murata T, Kangawa K, Nagai R & Shindo T. (2008) The GPCR modulator protein RAMP2 is essential for angiogenesis and vascular integrity. *J Clin Invest.* Vol. 118, pp.29–39.

Ishimitsu T, Nishikimi T, Saito Y, Kitamura K, Eto T, Kangawa K, Matsuo H, Omae T & Matsuoka H. (1994) Plasma levels of adrenomedullin, a newly identified hypotensive peptide, in patients with hypertension and renal failure. *J Clin Invest.* Vol. 94, pp. 2158-61.

Isumi Y, Minamino N, Kubo A, Nishimoto N, Yoshizaki K, Yoshioka M, Kangawa K & Matsuo H. (1998) Adrenomedullin stimulates interleukin-6 production in Swiss 3T3 cells. *Biochem Biophys Res Commun.* Vol. 244, pp. 325–331.

Isumi Y, Kubo A, Katafuchi T, Kangawa K & Minamino N. (1999) Adrenomedullin suppresses interleukin-1 beta-induced tumor necrosis factor-alpha production in Swiss 3T3 cells. *FEBS Lett* Vol. 463, pp. 110-4.

Kamoi H, Kanazawa H, Hirata K, Kurihara N, Yano Y & Otani S. (1995) Adrenomedullin inhibits the secretion of cytokine-induced neutrophil chemoattractant, a member of the interleukin-8 family,from rat alveolar macrophages. *Biochem Biophys Res Commun* Vol. 21, pp. 1031-5.

Kawai J, Ando K, Tojo A, Shimosawa T, Takahashi K, Onozato ML, Yamasaki M, Ogita T, Nakaoka T & Fujita T. (2004) Endogenous adrenomedullin protects against vascular response to injury in mice. *Circulation,* vol. 109, pp. 1147–1153.

Nanki T, Nagasaka K, Hayashida K, Saita Y and Miyasaka N.(2001) Chemokines regulate IL-6 and IL-8 production by fibroblast-like synoviocytes from patients with rheumatoid arthritis *J Immunol.* Nov 1; Vol. 167(9):5381-5

Kellgren JH & Lawrence JL. (1958) Osteoarthritis and disc degeneration in an urban population. *Ann Rheum Dis.* Vol. 17, pp. 388-97.

Kitamura K, Kangawa K, Kawamoto M, Ichiki Y, Nakamura S,Matsuo H & Eto T (1993) Adrenomedullin: a novel hypotensive peptide isolated from human pheochromocytoma. Biochem Biophys Res Commun Vol. 192, pp. 553–560

Kitamura K, Ichiki Y, Tanaka M, Kawamoto M, Emura J, Sakakibara S, Kangawa K, Matsuo H & Eto T. (1994) Immunoreactive adrenomedullin in human plasma. FEBS Lett Vol. 341, pp. 288-90.

Kita T, Kitamura K, Hashida S, Morishita K & Eto T. (2003) Plasma adrenomedullin is closely correlated with pulse wave velocity in middle-aged and elderly patients. *Hypertens Res.* Vol. 26, pp. 887–893

Kobayashi K, Kitamura K, Hirayama N, Date H, Kashiwagi T, Ikushima I, Hanada Y, Nagatomo Y, Takenaga M, Ishikawa T, Imamura T, Koiwaya Y & Eto T. (1996) Increased plasma adrenomedullin in acute myocardial infarction. *Am Heart J.* Vol. 131, pp. 676–680.

Kubo A, Minamino N, Isumi Y, Katafuchi T, Kangawa K, Dohi K & Matsuo H. (1998) Production of adrenomedullin in macrophage cell line and peritoneal macrophage. *J Biol Chem.* Vol. 273, pp. 16730–16738.

Leask A & Abraham DJ. (2004) TGF-β signaling and the fibrotic response. *FASEB J* Vol. 18, pp. 816–827.

Miyashita K, Itoh H, Arai H, Suganami T, Sawada N, Fukunaga Y, Sone M, Yamahara K, Yurugi-Kobayashi T, Park K, Oyamada N, Sawada N, Taura D, Tsujimoto H, Chao TH, Tamura N, Mukoyama M & Nakao K. (2006) The neuroprotective and vasculo-neuro-regenerative roles of adrenomedullin in ischemic brain and its therapeutic potential. *Endocrinology.* Vol.147, pp. 1642–1653.

Mizuhara H, O'Neill E, Seki N, Ogawa T, Kusunoki C, Otsuka K, Satoh S, Niwa M, Senoh H & Fujiwara H. (1994) T cell activation-associated hepatic injury: mediation by tumor necrosis factors and protection by interleukin 6. *J Exp Med.* Vol.179, pp. 1529–1537.

Moreland LW, Baumgartner SW, Schiff MH, Tindall EA, Fleischmann RM, Weaver AL, Ettlinger RE, Cohen S, Koopman WJ, Mohler K, Widmer MB & Blosch CM. (1997) Treatment of rheumatoid arthritis with a recombinant human tumor necrosis factor receptor (p75)-Fc fusion protein. *N Engl J Med.* Vol. 337, pp. 141–147.

Nakamura R, Kato J, Kitamura K, Onitsuka H, Imamura T, Cao Y, Marutsuka K, Asada Y, Kangawa K & Eto T. (2004) Adrenomedullin administration immediately after myocardial infarction ameliorates progression of heart failure in rats. *Circulation.* Vol. 110, pp. 426–431.

Nishikimi T, Saito Y, Kitamura K, Ishimitsu T, Eto T, Kangawa K, Matsuo H, Omae T & Matsuoka H. (1995) Increased plasma levels of adrenomedullin in patients with heart failure. *J Am Coll Cardiol.* Vol. 26, pp. 1424-31.

Nishimoto N, Ito A, Ono M, Tagoh H, Matsumoto T, Tomita T, Ochi T & Yoshizaki K. (2000) IL-6 inhibits the proliferation of fibroblastic synovial cells from rheumatoid arthritis patients in the presence of soluble IL-6 receptor. *Int Immunol.* Vol. 12, pp. 187–193.

Nanke Y, Kotake S, Yonemoto K, Saito S, Tomatsu T, Kamatani N. (2003) Adrenomedullin in synovial fluids from patients with rheumatoid arthritis inhibits interleukin 6 production from synoviocytes. *Ann Rheum Dis.* Jan, Vol. 62(1), pp. 82-3.

Nishimoto N, Kishimoto T & Yoshizaki K. (2000) Anti-interleukin 6 receptor antibody treatment in rheumatic disease. *Ann Rheum Dis.* Vol. 59 (Suppl 1), pp. i21–i27.

Nishimoto N, Yoshizaki K, Miyasaka N, Yamamoto K, Kawai S, Takeuchi T, Hashimoto J, Azuma J & Kishimoto T. (2004) Treatment of rheumatoid arthritis with humanized anti-interleukin-6 receptor antibody: a multicenter, double-blind, placebo-controlled trial. *Arthritis Rheum.* Vol. 50, pp. 1761–1769.

Okura T, Marutsuka K, Hamada H, Sekimoto T, Fukushima T, Asada Y, Kitamura K, Chosa E. (2008) Therapeutic efficacy of intra-articular adrenomedullin injection in antigen-induced arthritis in rabbits. Arthritis Res Ther. Vol. 10(6), pp133. Epub

Schindler R, Mancilla J, Endres S, Ghorbani R, Clark SC, Dinarello CA. (1990) Correlations and interactions in the production of interleukin-6 (IL-6), IL-1, and tumor necrosis factor (TNF) in human blood mononuclear cells: IL-6 suppresses IL-1 and TNF. *Blood.* Vol. 75, pp. 40–47.

Tilg H, Dinarello CA & Mier JW. (1997) IL-6 and APPs: anti-inflammatory and immunosuppressive mediators. *Immunol Today.* Vol. 18, pp. 428–432.

Ueda S, Nishio K, Minamino N, Kubo A, Akai Y, Kangawa K, Matsuo H, Fujimura Y, Yoshioka A, Masui K, Doi N, Murao Y & Miyamoto S. (1999) Increased plasma levels of adrenomedullin in patients with systemic inflammatory response syndrome. *Am J Respir Crit Care Med* Vol. 160, pp. 132-6.

Uemura T, Kato J, Kuwasako K, Kitamura K, Kangawa K & Eto T. (2002) Aldosterone augments adrenomedullin production without stimulating pro-adrenomedullin N-terminal 20 peptide secretion in vascular smooth muscle cells. *J. Hypertension* Vol. 20 (6), pp. 1209-14

Wong LY, Cheung BM, Li YY & Tang F. (2005) Adrenomedullin is both proinflammatory and antiinflammatory: its effects on gene expression and secretion of cytokines and macrophage migration inhibitory factor in NR8383 macrophage cell line. *Endocrinology.* Vol. 146, pp. 1321–1327.

Wu R, Zhou M & Wang P. (2003) Adrenomedullin and adrenomedullin binding protein-1 downregulate TNF-α in macrophage cell line and rat Kupffer cells. *Regul Pept.* Vol. 112, pp. 19–26.

Yang S, Zhou M, Fowler DE & Wang P. (2002) Mechanisms of the beneficial effect of adrenomedullin and adrenomedullin-binding protein-1 in sepsis: down-regulation of proinflammatory cytokines. *Crit Care Med.* Vol. 30, pp. 2729–2735.

Yudoh K, Matsuno H & Kimura T. (1999) Plasma adrenomedullin in rheumatoid arthritis compared with other rheumatic diseases. *Arthritis Rheum*, Vol. 42, pp. 1297-8.

Zagariya A, Bhat R, Navale S, Chari G & Vidyasagar D. (2006) Inhibition of meconium-induced cytokine expression and cell apoptosis by pretreatment with captopril. *Pediatrics*. Vol. 117, pp. 1722–1727

10

Targeting DAMP Activation of Toll-Like Receptors: Novel Pathways to Treat Rheumatoid Arthritis?

Theresa H. Page and Kim S. Midwood
Kennedy Institute of Rheumatology, Imperial College of Science, Technology and Medicine, London
UK

1. Introduction

Inflammation is a necessary response to infection and injury by which the invading pathogen and/or damaged cells are cleared. Under normal circumstances this is a tightly controlled and transient process. However, in conditions such as rheumatoid arthritis (RA) these regulatory mechanisms appear inactive or ineffective such that inflammation progresses unchecked. This results in the pain, swelling and bone and cartilage destruction that define this disease.

The etiology of RA initiation is still uncertain, but increasing evidence points to a key role for the toll-like receptor (TLR) family in driving aberrant inflammation in the joint. TLRs were originally identified as receptors for exogenous pathogen associated molecular patterns (PAMPs) of bacterial, fungal or viral origin, which initiate inflammation in response to microbial infection. Perhaps of more interest in the context of RA however, is the role that these molecules play in the recognition of endogenous danger signals or DAMPs (damage associated molecular patterns).

DAMPs are generated by both infection-induced and sterile tissue damage. They include a wide range of molecules including intracellular proteins such as high mobility group protein 1 (HMGB1), cell derived nucleic acids and extracellular matrix molecules such as tenascin-C and fibrinogen. High levels of DAMPs are present in both the RA synovium and in the peripheral circulation in RA patients. Accumulating evidence from both human studies and experimental animal models now suggests that these molecules may be critical to the persistence of the inflammatory state in RA. Moreover, targeting TLRs and their downstream signalling pathways is emerging as a potentially tractable means for treating a range of inflammatory conditions, including RA and its associated pathologies.

Here we focus on the current literature that demonstrates a role for DAMPs in driving chronic inflammation in RA. We will discuss the mechanistic differences between PAMP and DAMP mediated activation of TLRs; and highlight how these data have already informed novel pathways to develop improved therapies for RA and how future therapeutic strategies may further evolve.

2. The cellular basis of RA and current therapies

RA is a systemic, chronic, progressive autoimmune inflammatory disease which affects approximately 1% of the population worldwide. The disease is polyarticular, and is characterised by synovitis, pannus formation, neovascularisation and hyperplasia caused by the infiltration of leukocytes. This in turn leads to the destruction of cartilage, tendon and bone, and the associated joint stiffness, swelling and pain that is the hallmark of this disease. Systemic symptoms also include inflammation in distil areas of the body, including the lungs, pericardium and pleura. Vasculitis, atherosclerosis, myocardial infarction and stroke are consequently commonly linked to RA.

The cells infiltrating the affected joint space are central to the pathology of RA, and include B cells, T cells, and cells of the monocyte/macrophage lineage as well as fibroblast-like synoviocytes. In their activated state within the affected joint these cells produce auto-antibodies such as those against citrullinated proteins (CCP) and immunoglobulin (Rheumatoid factor (RF)), tissue degrading enzymes such as the matrix metalloproteaes (MMPs), as well as pro-inflammatory molecules such as TNF, Interleukin (IL)-6 and IL-1 that are central to tissue destruction, disease chronicity, and the maintenance of the inflammatory state. The ability of some cell types (B cells and RA synovial fibroblasts) to migrate to other sites has also been proposed as a precipitating event in the spread of disease to other joints (Lefevre et al., 2009).

TARGET	NAME	FORM	STATUS
All rapidly dividing cells	Methotrexate Other DMARDs eg Sulphalazine, Cyclosporin, Corticosteriods	Drugs (anti-metabolites, anti-inflammatory)	Clinical use
B cells	[1]Rituximab (CD 20), [2]MDX-1342 (CD19), [3]anti-BAFF, [4]anti-CD16, [5]Eculizumab (complement C5),	[1, 2, 5]Humanised Ig, [2]human non-glycosylated Ig,	[1]Clinical use [2,3,4] Pre-clinical [5]Approved for human use - not RA
T cells	Abatacept (CTLA4)	Fusion protein	Clinical use
Cytokines [1-5]TNF, [6]IL-6R, [7]IL-1, [8]VEGF	[1]Etanercept, [2]Adalimumab, [3]Infliximab, [4]Golimumab, [5]Certolizumab, [6]Tocilizumab, [7]Anakinra, [8]Bevacizumab	[1]Fusion protein. [2,4,5,6]Human Ig, [3]chimeric mouse/human Ig, [7]IL-1R antagonist	Clinical use
Signalling molecules [1]IKK2, [2]PDE4, [3]p38, [4]Btk, [5]Syk, [6]JAK3	[1, 2,3] Multiple, [4]CG11746, [4]PC132765, [6]CP-690550, [5]R788 (anti-Syk)	Small molecule inhibitors	Pre-clinical

Table 1. Current RA therapies

Knowledge of the processes responsible for disease activity and progression has lead to significant advances in the treatment of RA in the last 30 years. Early treatment, within months of the onset of persistent symptoms, is recommended, and at the present time usually takes the form of disease modifying anti-rheumatic drugs (DMARD) such as methotrexate. In more recent years however, the choice of treatment for RA has expanded significantly, and importantly now utilises agents that are less globally immunosuppressive than methotrexate (Weinblatt et al., 1985) (Table 1). These newer therapies target either specific cell types, such as B and T cells that present within the inflamed synovium, or their products (Genovese et al., 2008; Tedder, 2009; Townsend et al., 2010; Buch et al., 2011). Indeed, anti-cytokine therapies have revolutionised the treatment of RA in recent years. In particular, the use of anti-TNF biologicals such as Adalimumab, Etanercept and Infliximab have become the treatment of choice in those who do not respond to conventional DMARDs (Taylor et al., 2009), although biologicals that target other pro-inflammatory cytokines are also approved for use. These include Tocilizumab (anti-IL-6R) (Fleischmann et al., 2006; Jones et al., 2010) and Anakinra, a recombinant IL-1 receptor antagonist, as well as Bevacizumab, an antibody that targets vascular endothelial growth factor (VEGF) and hence may reduce neovascularisation that pannus formation depends upon. A variety of small molecule inhibitors designed to target critical elements of the B cell receptor, T cell receptor or cytokine signalling pathways such as inhibitors of IKK2, PDE4 and Btk (Bruton's tyrosine kinase), have shown interesting results in some animal models of arthritis, as have clinical trials with the syk inhibitor R788 (Podolin et al., 2005; Lindstrom et al., 2010; Di Paolo et al., 2011). The p38 inhibitors however, which showed such promise in animal models have not lived up to expectations in clinical trials and have not progressed beyond phase II (Genovese, 2009).

Despite the significant advances made with this arsenal of therapies, the goal of achieving sustained remission of RA has remained elusive and even with long term DMARD and biologic therapy is relatively uncommon. The efficacy of treatments is also unpredictable. Thus, a significant proportion of patients do not respond adequately to first line DMARD treatment and are then moved on to biologics. Even here, approximately 40% of patients do not respond to anti-TNF therapy for example. Moreover, many of these treatments are accompanied by significant side-effects, ranging from injection site reactions, increased infection rates and neutropenia to the potential for an increased risk of malignancies (van Vollenhoven, 2009).

When taking a global view of all the therapies for RA, either in use in the clinic, in early trials, in animal models, or in *in vitro* studies, it becomes clear that all are designed to target the ongoing process of inflammation. Namely the cells present in the joint during the inflammatory process, or their soluble products (cytokines), rather than targeting a causative agent for RA. However, for RA sufferers a single causative agent has not, and probably will never, be defined. Rather, RA is a complex disease with a multi-factorial etiology. It's prevalence in women (3:1 female to male ratio) suggests a hormonal contribution, and there are clear links to environmental factors such as smoking as well as a predisposition to RA with certain HLA haplotypes (Bax et al., 2011). Genetic and twin studies also suggest a strong environmental influence as well as a genetic link. As a tractable causative agent or single predisposing gene is therefore unlikely to be identified, a therapy that will treat disease in the early stages, that will prevent progression to a chronic state and thereby allow the inflammatory state to resolve, thereby preventing tissue damage, bone and cartilage destruction and progression, remains the holy grail of many researchers.

Given that RA is an inflammatory condition it is likely that a precipitating event initiates a state of inflammation. In the normal individual, inflammation is invariably initiated in response to danger signals sensed by a series of cellular receptors known as pattern recognition receptors (PRRs). PRRs were originally defined by their ability to recognise and respond to invading pathogens (bacterial, viral, fungal) but are now increasingly linked to the detection of damaged 'self' molecules known as DAMPs. A large body of evidence has emerged in the last decade implicating one particular family of PRRs, the TLRs, in driving inflammation during RA.

3. The toll-like receptors

TLRs are a highly conserved family of PRRs. With the most recent addition of murine TLR13 (Shi et al., 2011), 14 mammalian TLRs have been reported to date, with 10 human subtypes. All TLRs are type I transmembrane proteins comprising an extracellular domain of multiple leucine rich repeats (LRRs), a single membrane spanning α-helix and a cytoplasmic Toll/IL-1 receptor (TIR) homology signalling domain.

TLRs can be classified according to their subcellular localization: the endosomal TLRs 3, 7, 8 and 9 reside in intracellular compartments, whilst the others are found at the plasma membrane. This distribution also reflects the ligand specificity of TLRs; the cell surface receptors predominantly recognize pathogenic and self surface elements, whereas endosomal receptors primarily sense nucleic acids. Recognition of ligand triggers receptor dimerization which in turn triggers a multitude of signalling cascades leading to the expression of pro-inflammatory mediators such as cytokines and chemokines, which are designed to combat the perceived danger. In this way the body mounts an effective immune response (reviewed in (Piccinini et al., 2010). The TLR ligands that induce such a response include both PAMPs and DAMPs, and a more detailed list of them, with particular reference to those found in RA, can be found in Table 2. Thus, TLRs are critical for both the response to invading pathogens and the response to 'sterile' tissue damage.

3.1 TLRs and RA pathology

TLRs are expressed on a variety of different cell types, many of which are found within the inflamed rheumatoid joint, including myeloid cells, fibroblasts, epithelial and endothelial cells. In humans the first evidence linking the presence of TLRs with RA pathology arose from the comparison of TLR expression between normal or non-inflamed joints and RA joints. Significant up-regulation of a number of TLRs was observed in both synovial tissue and circulating immune cells isolated from RA patients. Table 3 depicts the specific pattern of expression of these TLRs in RA.

TLR	PAMP	SOURCE	DAMP	SOURCE
TLR1	Triacyl lipoprotein	Bacteria	β-defensin 3	Released from activated/necrotic cells
TLR2	Lipoprotein	Bacteria, Viruses, Parasites	HSP60, 70, Gp96, HMGB1, HMGB1-nucleosome complexes, β-defensin 3, surfactant proteins A and	Released from activated/necrotic cells

			D, eosinophil derived neurotoxin, antiphospholipid antibodies, serum amyloid A,cardiac myosin, PAUF, CEP, monosodium urate crystals	
			Biglycan, versican	Induced upon tissue damage
			Hyaluronic acid fragments	Degradation of tissue
TLR3	dsRNA	Viruses	mRNA	Released from activated/necrotic cells
TLR4	Lipopolysaccharide (LPS)	Bacteria, Viruses	HMGB1, surfactant proteins A and D, β-defensin 2, HSP60, 70, 72, 22, Gp96, S100A8, S100A9, neutrophil elastase, antiphospholipid antibodies, lactoferrin, serum amyloid A, oxidised LDL, saturated fatty acids, resistin, PAUF, monosodium urate crystals	Released from activated/necrotic cells
			Biglycan, fibronectin EDA, fibrinogen, tenascin-C	Induced upon tissue damage
			Heparin sulphate fragments, hyaluronic acid fragments	Degradation of tissue
TLR5	Flagellin	Bacteria	Unknown	Unknown
TLR6	Diacyl lipoprotein	Bacteria, Viruses	Unknown	Unknown
TLR7/8	ssRNA	Bacteria, Viruses	Antiphospholipid antibodies, ssRNA, cardiac myosin	Released from activated/necrotic cells
TLR9	CpG-DNA	Bacteria, Viruses, Protazoa	IgG-chromatin complexes, mitochondrial DNA	Released from activated/necrotic cells
TLR10	Unknown	Unknown	Unknown	Unknown
TLR11	Profilin-like molecule	Protazoa	Unknown	Unknown

DAMPs in red have been reported in the RA joint.

Table 2. Exogenous and endogenous activators of human TLRs.

TLR	EXPRESSION	F	REFERENCE
TLR1	Protein in DCs> macrophages > fibroblasts from RA joint	nd	(Tamaki et al., 2011)
TLR2	mRNA in RA synovial tissue, protein in DCs and macrophages but not T cells or fibroblasts from RA joint	yes	(Sacre et al., 2007) (Tamaki et al., 2011).
	mRNA in RA > OA or non arthritic joints, at synovial lining, sites of attachment and invasion into cartilage or bone, around small vessels and in areas of infiltrating lymphocytes (fibroblasts not macrophages or T cells)	yes	(Seibl et al., 2003)
	Protein in RA > OA or healthy joints in synovial lining, sublining and perivascular regions	nd	(Radstake et al., 2004)
	Protein in RA blood monocytes, tissue macrophages	yes	(Iwahashi et al., 2004; Huang et al., 2007)
	Protein in fibroblasts from RA > OA joints > healthy skin	yes	(Kim et al., 2007)
TLR3	mRNA and protein in RA > OA or healthy synovium, in fibroblasts of the synovial lining and sublining, and in the perivascular areas	yes	(Brentano et al., 2005; Roelofs et al., 2005)
	Protein in fibroblasts from early RA > OA or healthy synovium	yes	(Ospelt et al., 2008)
TLR4	mRNA in RA synovial tissue, protein in DCs and macrophages but not T cells or fibroblasts from RA joint	yes	(Sacre et al., 2007) (Tamaki et al., 2011) (Huang et al., 2007)
	Protein in synovial tissue from RA > OA > healthy joints, in early and longstanding RA	yes	(Radstake et al., 2004) (Ospelt et al., 2008)
	Protein in RA synovial fibroblasts	yes	(Kim et al., 2007; Wu et al., 2010)
TLR5	Protein in DCs> macrophages > fibroblasts from RA joint	nd	(Tamaki et al., 2011)
TLR6	Protein in DCs> macrophages > fibroblasts from RA joint	nd	(Tamaki et al., 2011)
TLR7	Protein in RA synovium > OA or healthy joints	yes	(Roelofs et al., 2005; Roelofs et al., 2009)
TLR9	Protein in DCs> macrophages > fibroblasts from RA joint	nd	(Tamaki et al., 2011)

nd = not determined

F= function = the ability of the TLR to respond to its cognate ligand in each cell/ tissue type

Table 3. Distribution of TLR expression in the RA joint

Further studies using *ex vivo* human disease models have provided evidence of a functional role for TLRs in driving inflammation in RA. Adenoviral over expression of dominant negative Myd88, an adaptor molecule required for signalling by all TLRs except TLR3, inhibited cytokine synthesis in RA synovial cells (Sacre et al., 2007). The naturally occurring TIR signalling antagonist single-immunoglobulin interleukin-1 receptor-related (SIGIRR) is also efficacious in suppressing cytokine synthesis in these cells (Drexler et al., 2010). Together these data suggest that TLRs may contribute to synovial inflammation but do not rule out the possibility that IL-1-mediated signalling, which shares the TIR-myd88 derived framework, is responsible for these findings, nor do they pinpoint any specific TLR.

3.2 Which TLRs are important in RA?

Evidence of a role in RA for both cell surface TLRs and endosomal TLRs in human disease is accumulating. In particular, over expression of dominant negative Mal, an adaptor protein required exclusively by TLR2 and 4, has been shown to inhibit cytokine and protease synthesis in RA synovial cells, supporting the contribution of these two family members to the synthesis of pro-inflammatory mediators in the RA joint (Sacre et al., 2007). Blockade of the function of TLR2 and 4 using neutralizing antibodies has also been reported, and while commercially available antibodies to either TLR2 or TLR4 had no effect on cytokine production in isolated RA synovial cells at 10 μg/ml (Sacre et al., 2007), 1 μg/ml of an anti-TLR2 antibody (OPN301) inhibited spontaneous cytokine release in RA tissue explants as effectively as anti-TNF antibodies (Nic An Ultaigh et al., 2011). Inhibition of TLR4 by the naturally occurring antagonist LPS isolated from *Bartonella Quintana*, also partially inhibited cytokine release in RA synovial biopsies (Abdollahi-Roodsaz et al., 2008). Stimulation of TLRs 2, and 4 has also been shown to induce cytokine synthesis in cell cultures isolated from RA synovia (Sacre et al., 2008). While the same workers found that TLRs 7 and 9 were not responsive to their respective ligands in RA cultures, stimulation of TLRs 3 and 8 did increase cytokine production.

The contribution of endosomal TLRs to cytokine synthesis in RA is also supported by other studies; chloroquine, which prevents intracellular TLR function by inhibiting endosomal acidification, reduces cytokine release in synovial cells (Sacre et al., 2008). The selective serotonin reuptake inhibitors, antidepressant drugs fluoxetine and citalopram and the antidepressant small molecule mianserin are also efficacious in inhibiting synovial cell cytokine release (Sacre et al., 2010). These drugs also inhibit TLR3, -7, -8 and -9 activity, by mechanisms which are yet unknown. More specifically, the small molecule imiquimod, which targets TLR8, also inhibited the production of TNF from human RA synovial membranes (Sacre et al., 2008). There have also been anecdotal reports of improved symptoms in RA patients taking anti-depressants (Krishnadas et al., 2011). Taken together these studies suggest a significant role for TLR2 and 4 as well as the endosomal TLRs 3 and 8 in human disease.

3.3 The role of TLRs in animal models of RA

In addition to studies in human tissue, the contribution of TLRs to inflammation and joint destruction has been examined in rodent models of arthritis. Mice with targeted deletions in TLRs have demonstrated that specific family members are important in driving disease pathogenesis *in vivo*.

Many experimental models of joint disease utilize TLR ligands to initiate or sustain disease induction, making interpretation of the contribution of each TLR to disease induction or progression difficult (Joosten et al., 2003; Frasnelli et al., 2005; Lee et al., 2005). However, in a serum transfer model where induction of arthritis occurs independently of TLR administration, disease was not sustained in TLR4 null mice (Choe et al., 2003). Likewise, the severity of spontaneous, IL-17 driven arthritis in mice lacking IL-1RA is significantly reduced when crossed with TLR4 null mice, concomitant with blunted expression of IL-17 suggesting a key role for TLR4. In this model TLR2 null mice showed increased disease severity whereas TLR9 knockout had no effect on disease (Abdollahi-Roodsaz et al., 2008).
Whilst most data point towards a role for TLR4 in disease progression in mice *in vivo*, recent data have also suggested a role for the endosomal TLRs. Fluoxetine and citalopram reduce disease progression in murine collagen induced arthritis (Sacre et al., 2010). TLR3 was found to be the most significantly up-regulated TLR during pristine induced arthritis in rats, where it appeared in the spleen early after disease initiation. Stimulation of TLR3 with polyI:C also exacerbated disease severity and silencing TLR3 expression reduced disease severity in these animals (Meng et al., 2010).
Despite evidence from human studies highlighting the contribution of TLR8 in synovial inflammation, the lack of activation of murine TLR8 by its cognate ligand suggests this PRR is not biologically active in mice (Heil et al., 2004). Nor is TLR10 present in mice (Hasan et al., 2005). This makes investigation of the *in vivo* function of these TLRs challenging. Combined with the fact that TLR signalling and gene activation is species-specific, notably most recently highlighted by examination of the differences in human and murine TLR4-mediated nickel recognition that confers contact hypersensitivity specifically to man (Schmidt et al., 2010), extrapolation of data between species should be undertaken cautiously.

3.4 Targeting TLRs as a therapy in RA

Studies examining the blockade of TLRs in mouse models have confirmed the importance of TLRs in disease and have provided evidence that TLR antagonism may be a viable means to reduce inflammation in RA. Treatment with LPS from *Bartonella quintana* and ST2 protein expressed by mast cells and T helper cell type 2 (Th2) inhibits TLR4-mediated signalling in experimental models of arthritis, resulting in disease amelioration (Leung et al., 2004; Abdollahi-Roodsaz et al., 2007). Further evidence for a role for the endosomal TLRs in CIA has also come from studies with short DNA oligonucleotides (ODNs). These act as Immunoregulatory Sequences (IRS) and inhibit endosomal TLR activity (Barrat et al., 2005; Ranjith-Kumar et al., 2008; Lenert, 2010). Prophylactic administration of ODNs in CIA and CpG-induced arthritis has been shown to abrogate disease progression (Zeuner et al., 2002; Dong et al., 2004).
In the light of the wealth of evidence implicating TLRs in both animal models of RA and in human disease considerable commercial, pharmaceutical activity has also been focused on designing TLR inhibitors for use in treating RA. TLR antagonists in preclinical development for RA include NI-0101, a TLR4 specific antibody developed by NovImmune, OPN305, a TLR2 specific antibody developed by Opsona, VTX-763, a small molecule inhibitor targeting TLR8 developed by VentiRx Pharmaceuticals and DV-1179, a DNA based TLR7/9 antagonist, developed by Dynavax. There are also several compounds currently in trial. For example, Heat shock protein 10 (HSP10) (chaperonin 10) which can inhibit LPS mediated

TLR4 activation, has improved symptoms in all RA patients tested, causing disease remission in 3 out of 23 in a small clinical trial (Vanags et al., 2006). Cbio et al are also examining the recombinant analogue of HSP10, XToll®, in a phase II clinical trial for RA. The DNA-based TLR7/9 antagonist, IMO-3100, developed by Idera, has also shown promising results *in vivo* for several autoimmune disease models. Phase I clinical trials of IMO-3100 in healthy subjects are underway and it appears to be well tolerated with no major adverse effects; in addition to reducing the release of cytokines such as TNF and IL-1 in these subjects.

Taken together, data from human, animal and pharmaceutical studies suggests a significant role for TLRs 2 and 4, in addition to the endosomal TLRs in synovial inflammation, in RA. Intriguingly however, the identity of the factor or factors that mediate this activation is not clear.

4. Which TLR activators drive chronic inflammation in RA?

Infection has long been purported to be a key underlying factor in RA pathogenesis. However, whilst pathogenic stimuli may trigger inflammation in RA, a causative infectious agent for RA has not been found and there is little evidence to suggest that PAMPs generate sustained joint inflammation (Schumacher et al., 1999; Chen et al., 2003). In contrast, data implicating DAMPs in RA pathogenesis have emerged from a number of independent studies in which factors derived from the serum, synovial fluid or synovial cells of RA patients can activate TLR mediated signalling pathways (Brentano et al., 2005; Roelofs et al., 2005; Sacre et al., 2007).

DAMPs are endogenous molecules that are immunologically silent in healthy tissues but become active upon tissue injury. They include intracellular molecules released from necrotic cells or secreted from activated cells, extracellular matrix molecule fragments created by tissue damage or proteolysis and extracellular matrix molecules that are specifically expressed upon tissue injury. In normal circumstances they act as danger signals that alert the organism to tissue damage and initiate the process of tissue repair. In addition to this physiological role however, there is evidence which indicates that DAMPS also contribute to the pathogenesis of many inflammatory and autoimmune diseases characterized by aberrant TLR activation including RA.

High levels of some DAMPs are detected in the destructive milieu of the RA joint (Table 2) (reviewed in (Piccinini et al., 2010), where they are hypothesized to drive chronic inflammation by invoking a perpetual destructive cycle where inflammation leads to the creation of new stimulators of inflammation (Roelofs et al., 2008). A number of approaches have been taken to examine the effect of DAMP administration, deletion or blockade in animal models of arthritis and data supporting the role of specific molecules in such models are summarized in Table 4.

In particular, the administration of the fibronectin EDA domain (FNEDA), fibrinogen, HMGB-1 and tenascin-C intra-articularly to mice provokes pathological inflammation *in vivo*, (Pullerits et al., 2003; Gondokaryono et al., 2007; Midwood et al., 2009). Moreover, targeted deletion of tenascin-C protects mice from experimental disease; synovial inflammation is induced but is transient and little tissue destruction occurs in contrast to wild type mice (Midwood et al., 2009) suggesting that tenascin-C plays a crucial role in disease chronicity.

DAMP	Effect of intra-articular administration in mice	Reference
Fibrinogen	Induced joint inflammation that is inhibited by CTLA4-Ig	(Ho et al., 2010; Yue et al., 2010)
FNEDA	Induced TLR4 dependent transient ankle swelling, cytokine synthesis, synovial inflammation	(Gondokaryono et al., 2007)
HMGB1	Induced synovial inflammation, some pannus formation	(Pullerits et al., 2003)
Tenascin-C	Induced TLR4 dependent joint inflammation and tissue erosion	(Midwood et al., 2009)
	Effect of targeted deletion in mice	
Tenascin-C	Protected from persistent synovial inflammation, joint erosion and tissue destruction in antigen induced arthritis	(Midwood et al., 2009)
	Effect of blockade in murine disease model	
HMBG1	Polyclonal antibodies or the DNA binding box A domain reduced severity of established joint disease in collagen induced arthritis	(Andersson et al., 2004)
HSP90	SNX-7081 (inhibitor) ameliorated disease, joints returned to normal in collagen induced arthritis	(Rice et al., 2008)
Neutrophil elastase	ONO-5046 (inhibitor) reduced incidence and severity of disease, ablated cartilage destruction in collagen induced arthritis	(Kakimoto et al., 1995)

Table 4. Evidence supporting the role of specific DAMPs in driving inflammation in RA

5. The role of citrullination

The mechanism underlying the switch from DAMPs that initiate controlled tissue repair, to those that mediate chronic, uncontrolled inflammation is still unclear, but recent evidence suggests that the process of citrullination may play a key role in this event. Citrullination is a post-translational event whereby peptidyl arginine deaminase enzymes convert arginine residues on susceptible molecules to citrulline.

Fibrinogen, a DAMP and TLR4 agonist, has been shown to be citrullinated in the RA joint (Sebbag et al., 2006; van Beers et al., 2010), which potentiates its activation of TLR4 and enhances its activity within immune complexes (Sokolove et al., 2011). Moreover, immunization with citrullinated, but not native, fibrinogen induces a T cell dependent murine arthritis (Ho et al., 2010; Yue et al., 2010). In addition, citrullination modifies the antigenicty of fibrinogen by creating new epitopes preferentially recognized by HLA DR (James et al., 2010). Whilst the accumulation of citrullinated proteins is a hallmark of many autoimmune diseases, unique to RA is the loss of tolerance to these epitopes. Anti-citrullinated protein antibodies (ACPAs) are present in ~65% of RA patients but are found in only <1% of individuals who do not have RA. Appearing before any evident symptoms, they correlate with poor prognosis; progressive joint destruction and low remission (Scott et al., 2010). Largely used diagnostically, emerging evidence suggests that ACPAs actively contribute to disease pathogenesis as their adoptive transfer enhances experimental murine arthritis (Kuhn et al., 2006; Uysal et al., 2009). Investigation of which DAMPs are pathologically post translationally modified in this and other ways may reveal the antigens that drive autoimmunity; thereby shedding light on RA disease pathogenesis.

In summary therefore, the presence of DAMPs within the RA synovia or their elevated levels within the peripheral circulation of patients, implicates their involvement in disease pathology. This hypothesis is now underscored by evidence in animal models of RA that includes the effects on disease after targeted deletion of DAMPs, the induction of disease by administration of DAMPS as well as the manipulation of DAMP function / expression. However, whilst targeted deletion of a particular DAMP is possible in the mouse it is clearly not a viable therapeutic option in the clinic. A more achievable goal is to target the receptors or signalling pathways involved in DAMP activity, an approach that requires a detailed understanding of both.

6. Distinct mechanisms of DAMP versus PAMP-mediated TLR activation

Whilst there is now clear evidence for a role for endosomal TLRs -3 and -8, their ligands are still to be defined; all DAMPS that have been implicated in RA to date mediate their effects via either TLR2 or 4 (Tables 2 and 4). However, despite considerable evidence implicating TLRs -2 and -4 in RA, there is also conflicting evidence. In particular, the inability of some function blocking antibodies to prevent spontaneous cytokine production in isolated RA synovial cells (Sacre et al., 2007), and the protective effect of TLR2 deletion in murine arthritis (Abdollahi-Roodsaz et al., 2008) might suggest that these TLRs are not important in RA. Moreover, SNPs of TLR2 and TLR4 or polymorphisms in human TLR4 that prevent LPS responsiveness do not correlate with RA disease susceptibility. For example, the Asp299Gly mutation in TLR4 (Kilding et al., 2003; Radstake et al., 2004) or Arg677Trp and Arg753Gln polymorphisms in TLR2 (Sanchez et al., 2004) that prevent PAMP induced activation of cells show no significant association with RA.

However, the apparent discordance with SNP data and some antibody studies may be accounted for by the idea that the mechanism of TLR activation by DAMPs is unlikely to be the same as that used by the pathogenic activation of TLRs. LPS-relevant SNPs and antibodies that prevent LPS-TLR4 association may therefore not be applicable to TLR4:DAMP association. Indeed, studies with HMGB1, HSPs and tenascin-C, all DAMPS that have been implicated in RA, have revealed differences in the gene expression profiles and cytokines produced by these DAMPs when compared to LPS. This disparity was despite the uniform use of the TLR4 receptor. Thus, whilst HMGB1 and LPS induce many of the same genes in neutrophils from septic patients, there are also distinct differences, in particular in the expression of IL-8 (Silva et al., 2007). HSP60 is able to induce IFN alpha production in peritoneal macrophages and bone marrow derived DCs where LPS cannot (Osterloh et al., 2007), and tenascin-C exhibits a different profile of cytokine induction in RA synovial fibroblasts to LPS, being unable to induce IL-8 in these cells (Midwood et al., 2009). The induction of different gene patterns implies that the DAMPS are using TLR4 in a different way from the PAMPs. This is perhaps not surprising when we consider that TLR4 recognises a wide variety of ligands, ranging from HSPs to lipids to breakdown products of the extracellular matrix (Piccinini et al., 2010) and it is unlikely that the TLR4 molecule would be able to recognise such a diverse repertoire of molecules in the same way. This is borne out by findings from crystallography studies which have revealed three basic mechanisms for TLR:PAMP association. Thus, the crystal structure of the extracellular domain of TLR3 complexed with ds RNA reveals that this molecule interacts directly with residues on the external surface of the TLR3 homodimer (Liu et al., 2008). More recent modelling of TLRs 7 and 9 also suggests direct ligand binding to the TLR molecule (Kubarenko et al., 2010). In contrast, TLR1:TLR2 hetero-dimerisation results in the formation of a hydrophobic pocket into which the lipopeptide PAM3Cys fits (Jin et al., 2007). Lastly, the structure of the TLR4:MD2:LPS complex reveals that LPS does not initially make direct contact with TLR4, but rather first binds to MD2, altering its conformation and allowing it to bind to and cause homodimerisation of TLR4 (Park et al., 2009). In this case, TLR4 residues important for LPS activity include those required for MD2 binding and those required for receptor homodimerisation. TLR4 responses to LPS also require the presence of CD14 which facilitates the transfer of LPS to MD2.

Our knowledge of the receptor complexes used by DAMPs is far from complete, but it is already clear that these molecules have a further level of complexity in their receptor organisation. Thus, of those that require TLR4, some, such as HSP70, biglycan and s100 also require both CD14 and MD2 for activity. Others, such as Gp96, HMGB1 and fibronectin EDA require only MD2, whilst another group that includes surfactant protein A and lactoferrin require only CD14 (Piccinini et al., 2010). The last, and probably the most diverse group of DAMPs use co-receptors or accessory molecules that are distinct from CD14 and MD2. Immune complexes of citrullinated fibrinogen for example have recently been shown to use a combination of Fcgamma receptors and TLR4 (Sokolove et al., 2011), and may also use CD11b/ CD18 (Barrera et al., 2011). A-SAA, which has been associated with RA and uses the TLR2 receptor has been shown to also use both CD36 and FPRL-1 as co-receptors, while low molecular weight hyaluronan forms complexes with TLR2 and CD44, and biglycan, which may use both TLR2 and TLR4, uses a variety of molecules including CD14, MD2, P2x4 and NLRP3 (Babelova et al., 2009). Other DAMPs such as tenascin-C do not use CD14 or MD2 (Midwood et al., 2009). Whether they bind directly to TLR4 or use an as yet undefined co-receptor molecule(s) is unclear at present.

Because of their alternative use of co-receptor molecules, DAMPs are therefore likely to use different residues on the TLR4 molecule than those used by LPS, so it may not be surprising that SNPs that affect LPS binding and antibodies designed to prevent LPS activation of TLR4 are inactive in RA where DAMP mediated activation of TLR4 may be critical to disease pathology. This hypothesis is confirmed by studies of the D299G and T399I mutations in TLR4. These have been shown to prevent LPS activation, but to enhance the ability of TLR4 to respond to fibrinogen. (Hodgkinson et al, 2008)

The signalling mechanisms used by DAMPs are also not well defined, and there is very little data available at present to suggest therapeutic targets for DAMPs. However, the use of TLR molecules suggests that many of the same pathways activated by PAMPs may be relevant. This has been confirmed by recent studies of oxidised LDL signalling (a TLR4 DAMP), which shows activation of many familiar pathways such as those involving IKK and the MAP kinases. Studies with tenascin-C also show that MyD88 signalling is important in response to this molecule (Midwood et al., 2009). Any differences between DAMP and LPS mediated signalling pathways are likely to come from the DAMP use of alternative co-receptors. Molecules such as CD36, CD44 and integrins already have defined signalling pathways. Whether DAMP signalling will prove to be simply a combination of TLR:MyD88 driven pathways and those emanating from any co-receptor molecules remains to be defined. It is more likely however, that the signal transduction mechanism of DAMPs will be a result of a combination of both pathways, where each is able to modulate / modify the other.

Examples of other molecules able to modify TLR signalling pathways, and consequently TLR-induced cytokine production are already established in the literature, and in particular a number of molecules that contain ITAM motifs have been shown to modulate TLR signalling pathways (Ivashkiv, 2008). Some such as TREM1 appear to cooperate with TLR molecules, amplifying the production of pro-inflammatory cytokines (Bleharski et al., 2003) whilst others such as the FcγR and the CD300F molecule inhibit TLR signalling (Wang et al., 2010). Other cell surface molecules able to modulate TLR activity include the TAM (Tyro3, Axl, Mer) receptors and SIGIRR (Rothlin et al., 2007; Drexler et al., 2010). The mechanisms responsible for these activities are varied and include ITAM mediated changes in IL-10 production and the induction of inhibitory signalling molecules. Conversely, recent data has emerged detailing a requirement for TLR4 in CD16 signalling revealing that TLRs in their turn can modulate other signalling pathways (Rittirsch et al., 2009).

7. Conclusion

In conclusion, it is clear that whilst the advent of specific biological therapies for the treatment of RA has significantly improved treatment of this disease in the last 10 years, there is still a significant un-met clinical need for therapies that target the cause of disease chronicity rather than its consequences.

Increasing evidence from *in vitro* studies, murine models of disease, and human studies, suggests that the TLRs play a significant role in RA. In particular, TLRs 2 and 4 and the intracellular TLRs 3 and 8 are increasingly regarded as key to the pathogenesis of this disease. However, PAMPs derived from infectious agents are not found in RA joints and are unlikely to be the causative TLR ligands in RA. Rather, there is now increasing evidence that endogenously derived DAMPs, either in their native form or in a citrullinated state, are able to drive the chronicity of RA. DAMPs comprise an enormously diverse subset of molecules and targeting them as a form of RA therapy could be achieved in a number of different ways. Many of these approaches have already found some success in other fields, but have yet to be tested in RA.

For example, for DAMPs whose expression is specifically up-regulated during inflammation it may be possible to manipulate this induction of expression at the genetic level. This approach has been taken in a murine lung carcinoma model where knockdown of versican expression in Lewis lung carcinoma cell lines (LLC) ablated their tumorigenic capability, promoting mouse survival and reduced metastasis. Conversely, over expression of versican in LLC lines with low innate metastatic potential increased lung metastasis (Kim et al., 2009).

The use of micro RNAs (miRNAs) to manipulate gene expression is also attracting considerable attention. MicroRNAs are endogenous RNAs that post-transcriptionally modulate gene expression (reviewed in (Guo et al., 2010). Not surprisingly, regulation of gene expression by microRNAs has also been extended to the TLR signalling paradigm (reviewed in (O'Neill et al., 2011)) where they impose several levels of regulation on the TLR signalling axis. For example, miR-155, miR-21 and miR-147 regulate the expression of TLRs 2-4, downstream signalling mediators such as MyD88 and TRIF, as well as transcription factors NF-κB and IRF3 (reviewed in (O'Neill et al., 2011)). Recent studies have reported that miR-155, miR-146a and miR-203 are upregulated in RA synovial fibroblasts, resulting in altered cytokine and MMP synthesis (Stanczyk et al., 2008; Li et al., 2010; Stanczyk et al., 2011). These insights may create a novel approach to limiting excessive TLR activation during inflammation.

A second method of modulating DAMP activity in RA may be to block their production or level of expression. Indeed, ethyl pyruvate, stearoyl lysophosphatidylcholine and nicotine have already been shown to be efficacious in ameliorating experimental sepsis by preventing HMGB1 release (Ulloa et al., 2003; Wang et al., 2004; Chen et al., 2005). However, the mechanism by which they do so is unclear and these compounds are likely also to affect numerous other cell processes. HMGB1 is released from cells by two distinct mechanisms: it is either liberated from cells undergoing necrosis (Scaffidi et al., 2002), or it is hyperacetylated and then actively secreted from stimulated cells. Other DAMPs including the S100 proteins are also secreted in the same way (Foell et al., 2007) and targeting this pathway therefore may potentially offer a means to modulate the release of intracellular DAMPs. Other DAMPs are generated by the degradation of extracellular matrix and inhibition of this process may also be therapeutically beneficial. This has already been tested in the case of immune stimulatory heparin sulphate (HS) fragments which are released from the ECM as a result of elastase activity (Brunn et al., 2005). Injection of elastase into the peritoneal cavity of mice caused the release of HS and induced sepsis, nearly as effectively as direct injection of HS or LPS (Johnson et al., 2004). Thus therapeutic measures aimed at

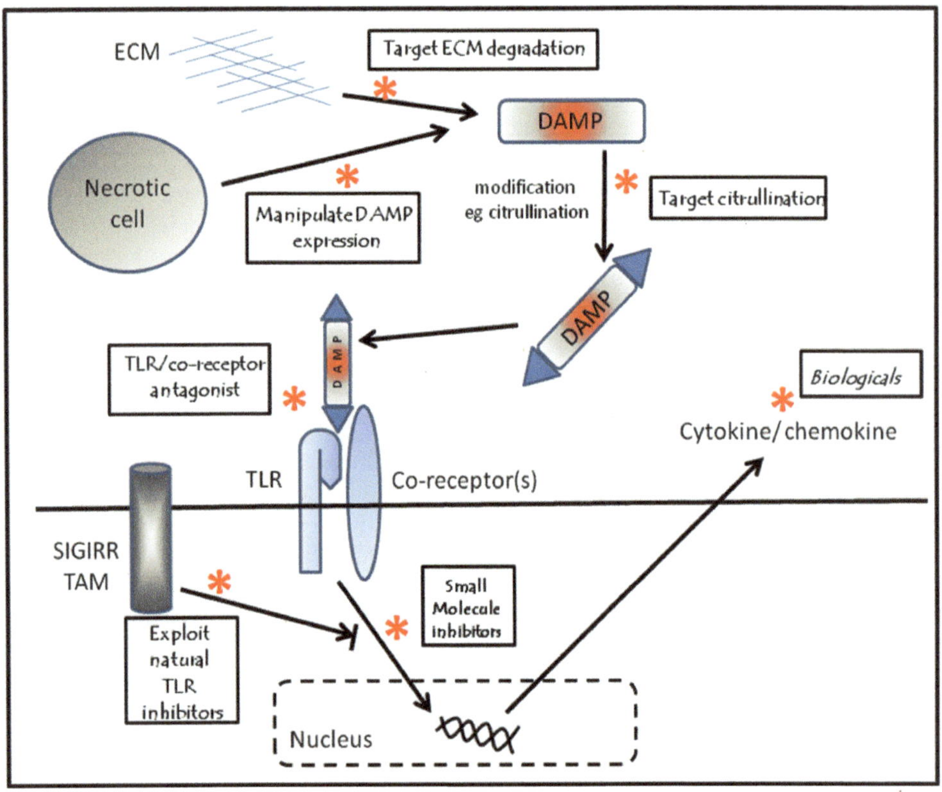

Red star = Potential site of DAMP manipulation.

Fig. 1. Potential sites at which DAMP activity could be modulated for therapeutic advantage.

blocking elastase could reduce the production of endogenous TLR4 activators. Indeed, pre-treatment with neutrophil elastase inhibitor before induction of hepatic ischemia-reperfusion injury has already been shown to ameliorate liver damage (Uchida et al., 2009).
Thirdly, as we have discussed here, targeting the TLRs that are critical for DAMP recognition is increasingly considered as a viable therapeutic option in RA. This can take the form of agents that antagonise DAMP:TLR association as has been tested with the antagonistic TLR2 and TLR4 antibody studies and the DNA based TLR7/9 antagonist IMO-3100 and with the studies on *Bartonella Quintana* LPS and the ST2 protein. Other approaches tested so far include the use of antagonistic bent oligonucleotides that have a high affinity for HMGB1 and suppress HMGB1-induced proliferation and migration of smooth muscle cells *in vitro* (Musumeci et al., 2007). An engineered mutant fragment of HMGB1 (HMGB1 Mut (102-105)) that carries two glycine substitutions has also been shown to decrease TNF release induced by the full-length HMGB1 protein in human monocyte cultures (Yuan et al., 2008). In addition, the N-terminal domain of thrombomodulin, an endothelial anticoagulant cofactor, has been shown to exert anti-inflammatory effects in a model of lethal endotoxemia partly by binding to and sequestering HMGB1 (Abeyama et al., 2005). Targeting the DAMP co-receptor molecules may also prove to be a viable therapeutic approach.
TLR signalling pathways, activated during DAMP recognition, would also represent tractable targets in RA and the success in *in vitro* studies and animal models of RA of small molecule inhibitors directed against signalling molecules such as p38, IKK2, PDE4, Syk and Btk may in large part be due to their effect on DAMP mediated signalling pathways. In addition, it will be interesting to see if DAMP-mediated signalling pathways are subject to the same control mechanisms as PAMP-mediated TLR signals. The role of naturally occurring molecules such as SIGIRR and SARM which are reported to modulate TLR signalling, as are the TAM receptors Tyro3, Axl and Mer. Many of these have not been examined in the context of DAMP:TLR activity and may yield further areas of study.
In summary, it is now clear that the TLR:DAMP axis represents a key point in RA pathology that will be susceptible to therapeutic attack. However, in order to mount such an attack we need to understand a number of key points: which DAMPs are relevant to RA pathology?; how are these DAMPs produced and / or modulated to become pathogenic?; how do the TLRs recognise DAMPs, including the role of co-receptor molecules?; and which signals are generated? The field of DAMP research in RA should prove to be an exciting one for many years.

8. Acknowledgements

The authors are supported by funding from Arthritis Research UK.

9. References

"www.opsona.com."

Abdollahi-Roodsaz, S., L. A. Joosten, et al. (2008). "Shift from toll-like receptor 2 (TLR-2) toward TLR-4 dependency in the erosive stage of chronic streptococcal cell wall arthritis coincident with TLR-4-mediated interleukin-17 production." *Arthritis Rheum* 58(12): 3753-3764.

Abdollahi-Roodsaz, S., L. A. Joosten, et al. (2008). "Stimulation of TLR2 and TLR4 differentially skews the balance of T cells in a mouse model of arthritis." *J Clin Invest* 118(1): 205-216.

Abdollahi-Roodsaz, S., L. A. Joosten, et al. (2007). "Inhibition of Toll-like receptor 4 breaks the inflammatory loop in autoimmune destructive arthritis." *Arthritis Rheum* 56(9): 2957-2967.

Abeyama, K., D. M. Stern, et al. (2005). "The N-terminal domain of thrombomodulin sequesters high-mobility group-B1 protein, a novel antiinflammatory mechanism." *J Clin Invest* 115(5): 1267-1274.

Andersson, U. and H. Erlandsson-Harris (2004). "HMGB1 is a potent trigger of arthritis." *J Intern Med* 255(3): 344-350.

Babelova, A., K. Moreth, et al. (2009). "Biglycan, a danger signal that activates the NLRP3 inflammasome via toll-like and P2X receptors." *J Biol Chem* 284(36): 24035-24048.

Barrat, F. J., T. Meeker, et al. (2005). "Nucleic acids of mammalian origin can act as endogenous ligands for Toll-like receptors and may promote systemic lupus erythematosus." *J Exp Med* 202(8): 1131-1139.

Barrera, V., O. A. Skorokhod, et al. (2011). "Host fibrinogen stably bound to hemozoin rapidly activates monocytes via TLR-4 and CD11b/CD18-integrin: a new paradigm of hemozoin action." *Blood* 117(21): 5674-5682.

Bax, M., J. van Heemst, et al. (2011). "Genetics of rheumatoid arthritis: what have we learned?" *Immunogenetics*.

Bleharski, J. R., V. Kiessler, et al. (2003). "A role for triggering receptor expressed on myeloid cells-1 in host defense during the early-induced and adaptive phases of the immune response." *J Immunol* 170(7): 3812-3818.

Brentano, F., O. Schorr, et al. (2005). "RNA released from necrotic synovial fluid cells activates rheumatoid arthritis synovial fibroblasts via Toll-like receptor 3." *Arthritis Rheum* 52(9): 2656-2665.

Brunn, G. J., M. K. Bungum, et al. (2005). "Conditional signaling by Toll-like receptor 4." *FASEB J* 19(7): 872-874.

Buch, M. H., J. S. Smolen, et al. (2011). "Updated consensus statement on the use of rituximab in patients with rheumatoid arthritis." *Ann Rheum Dis* 70(6): 909-920.

Chen, G., J. Li, et al. (2005). "Suppression of HMGB1 release by stearoyl lysophosphatidylcholine:an additional mechanism for its therapeutic effects in experimental sepsis." *J Lipid Res* 46(4): 623-627.

Chen, T., M. Rimpilainen, et al. (2003). "Bacterial components in the synovial tissue of patients with advanced rheumatoid arthritis or osteoarthritis: analysis with gas chromatography-mass spectrometry and pan-bacterial polymerase chain reaction." *Arthritis Rheum* 49(3): 328-334.

Choe, J. Y., B. Crain, et al. (2003). "Interleukin 1 receptor dependence of serum transferred arthritis can be circumvented by toll-like receptor 4 signaling." *J Exp Med* 197(4): 537-542.

Di Paolo, J. A., T. Huang, et al. (2011). "Specific Btk inhibition suppresses B cell- and myeloid cell-mediated arthritis." *Nat Chem Biol* 7(1): 41-50.

Dong, L., S. Ito, et al. (2004). "Suppressive oligonucleotides protect against collagen-induced arthritis in mice." *Arthritis Rheum* 50(5): 1686-1689.

Drexler, S. K., P. Kong, et al. (2010). "SIGIRR/TIR-8 is an inhibitor of Toll-like receptor signaling in primary human cells and regulates inflammation in models of rheumatoid arthritis." *Arthritis Rheum* 62(8): 2249-2261.

Fleischmann, R. M., J. Tesser, et al. (2006). "Safety of extended treatment with anakinra in patients with rheumatoid arthritis." *Ann Rheum Dis* 65(8): 1006-1012.

Foell, D., H. Wittkowski, et al. (2007). "Mechanisms of disease: a 'DAMP' view of inflammatory arthritis." *Nat Clin Pract Rheumatol* 3(7): 382-390.

Frasnelli, M. E., D. Tarussio, et al. (2005). "TLR2 modulates inflammation in zymosan-induced arthritis in mice." *Arthritis Res Ther* 7(2): R370-379.

Genovese, M. C. (2009). "Inhibition of p38: has the fat lady sung?" *Arthritis Rheum* 60(2): 317-320.

Genovese, M. C., M. Schiff, et al. (2008). "Efficacy and safety of the selective co-stimulation modulator abatacept following 2 years of treatment in patients with rheumatoid arthritis and an inadequate response to anti-tumour necrosis factor therapy." *Ann Rheum Dis* 67(4): 547-554.

Gondokaryono, S. P., H. Ushio, et al. (2007). "The extra domain A of fibronectin stimulates murine mast cells via toll-like receptor 4." *J Leukoc Biol* 82(3): 657-665.

Guo, H., N. T. Ingolia, et al. (2010). "Mammalian microRNAs predominantly act to decrease target mRNA levels." *Nature* 466(7308): 835-840.

Hasan, U., C. Chaffois, et al. (2005). "Human TLR10 is a functional receptor, expressed by B cells and plasmacytoid dendritic cells, which activates gene transcription through MyD88." *J Immunol* 174(5): 2942-2950.

Heil, F., H. Hemmi, et al. (2004). "Species-specific recognition of single-stranded RNA via toll-like receptor 7 and 8." *Science* 303(5663): 1526-1529.

Ho, P. P., L. Y. Lee, et al. (2010). "Autoimmunity against fibrinogen mediates inflammatory arthritis in mice." *J Immunol* 184(1): 379-390.

Hodgkinson, C.P. and Patel. K. et al. (2008). "Functional Toll-like receptor 4 mutations modulate the response to fibrinogen." *Thromb Haemost.* 100(2): 301-307.

Huang, Q., Y. Ma, et al. (2007). "Increased macrophage activation mediated through toll-like receptors in rheumatoid arthritis." *Arthritis Rheum* 56(7): 2192-2201.

Ivashkiv, L. B. (2008). "A signal-switch hypothesis for cross-regulation of cytokine and TLR signalling pathways." *Nat Rev Immunol* 8(10): 816-822.

Iwahashi, M., M. Yamamura, et al. (2004). "Expression of Toll-like receptor 2 on CD16+ blood monocytes and synovial tissue macrophages in rheumatoid arthritis." *Arthritis Rheum* 50(5): 1457-1467.

James, E. A., A. K. Moustakas, et al. (2010). "HLA-DR1001 presents "altered-self" peptides derived from joint-associated proteins by accepting citrulline in three of its binding pockets." *Arthritis Rheum* 62(10): 2909-2918.

Jin, M. S., S. E. Kim, et al. (2007). "Crystal structure of the TLR1-TLR2 heterodimer induced by binding of a tri-acylated lipopeptide." *Cell* 130(6): 1071-1082.

Johnson, G. B., G. J. Brunn, et al. (2004). "Cutting edge: an endogenous pathway to systemic inflammatory response syndrome (SIRS)-like reactions through Toll-like receptor 4." *J Immunol* 172(1): 20-24.

Jones, G. and C. Ding (2010). "Tocilizumab: a review of its safety and efficacy in rheumatoid arthritis." *Clin Med Insights Arthritis Musculoskelet Disord* 3: 81-89.

Joosten, L. A., M. I. Koenders, et al. (2003). "Toll-like receptor 2 pathway drives streptococcal cell wall-induced joint inflammation: critical role of myeloid differentiation factor 88." *J Immunol* 171(11): 6145-6153.

Kakimoto, K., A. Matsukawa, et al. (1995). "Suppressive effect of a neutrophil elastase inhibitor on the development of collagen-induced arthritis." *Cell Immunol* 165(1): 26-32.

Kilding, R., M. Akil, et al. (2003). "A biologically important single nucleotide polymorphism within the toll-like receptor-4 gene is not associated with rheumatoid arthritis." *Clin Exp Rheumatol* 21(3): 340-342.

Kim, K. W., M. L. Cho, et al. (2007). "Human rheumatoid synovial fibroblasts promote osteoclastogenic activity by activating RANKL via TLR-2 and TLR-4 activation." *Immunol Lett* 110(1): 54-64.

Kim, S., H. Takahashi, et al. (2009). "Carcinoma-produced factors activate myeloid cells through TLR2 to stimulate metastasis." *Nature* 457(7225): 102-106.

Krishnadas, R. and J. Cavanagh (2011). "Sustained remission of rheumatoid arthritis with a specific serotonin reuptake inhibitor antidepressant: a case report and review of the literature." *J Med Case Reports* 5: 112.

Kubarenko, A. V., S. Ranjan, et al. (2010). "Comprehensive modeling and functional analysis of Toll-like receptor ligand-recognition domains." *Protein Sci* 19(3): 558-569.

Kuhn, K. A., L. Kulik, et al. (2006). "Antibodies against citrullinated proteins enhance tissue injury in experimental autoimmune arthritis." *J Clin Invest* 116(4): 961-973.

Lang, K. S., M. Recher, et al. (2005). "Toll-like receptor engagement converts T-cell autoreactivity into overt autoimmune disease." *Nat Med* 11(2): 138-145.

Lartigue, A., P. Courville, et al. (2006). "Role of TLR9 in anti-nucleosome and anti-DNA antibody production in lpr mutation-induced murine lupus." *J Immunol* 177(2): 1349-1354.

Leadbetter, E. A., I. R. Rifkin, et al. (2002). "Chromatin-IgG complexes activate B cells by dual engagement of IgM and Toll-like receptors." *Nature* 416(6881): 603-607.

Lee, E. K., S. M. Kang, et al. (2005). "Essential roles of Toll-like receptor-4 signaling in arthritis induced by type II collagen antibody and LPS." *Int Immunol* 17(3): 325-333.

Lefevre, S., A. Knedla, et al. (2009). "Synovial fibroblasts spread rheumatoid arthritis to unaffected joints." *Nat Med* 15(12): 1414-1420.

Lenert, P. S. (2010). "Classification, mechanisms of action, and therapeutic applications of inhibitory oligonucleotides for Toll-like receptors (TLR) 7 and 9." *Mediators Inflamm* 2010: 986596.

Leung, B. P., D. Xu, et al. (2004). "A novel therapy of murine collagen-induced arthritis with soluble T1/ST2." *J Immunol* 173(1): 145-150.

Li, J., Y. Wan, et al. (2010). "Altered microRNA expression profile with miR-146a upregulation in CD4+ T cells from patients with rheumatoid arthritis." *Arthritis Res Ther* 12(3): R81.

Lindstrom, T. M. and W. H. Robinson (2010). "A multitude of kinases--which are the best targets in treating rheumatoid arthritis?" *Rheum Dis Clin North Am* 36(2): 367-383.

Liu, L., I. Botos, et al. (2008). "Structural basis of toll-like receptor 3 signaling with double-stranded RNA." *Science* 320(5874): 379-381.

Meng, L., W. Zhu, et al. (2010). "Toll-like receptor 3 upregulation in macrophages participates in the initiation and maintenance of pristane-induced arthritis in rats." *Arthritis Res Ther* 12(3): R103.

Midwood, K., S. Sacre, et al. (2009). "Tenascin-C is an endogenous activator of Toll-like receptor 4 that is essential for maintaining inflammation in arthritic joint disease." *Nat Med* 15(7): 774-780.

Musumeci, D., G. N. Roviello, et al. (2007). "Bent oligonucleotide duplexes as HMGB1 inhibitors: a comparative study." *Nucleosides Nucleotides Nucleic Acids* 26(10-12): 1447-1450.

Nic An Ultaigh, S., T. P. Saber, et al. (2011). "Blockade of Toll-like receptor 2 prevents spontaneous cytokine release from rheumatoid arthritis ex vivo synovial explant cultures." *Arthritis Res Ther* 13(1): R33.

O'Neill, L. A., F. J. Sheedy, et al. (2011). "MicroRNAs: the fine-tuners of Toll-like receptor signalling." *Nat Rev Immunol* 11(3): 163-175.

Ospelt, C., F. Brentano, et al. (2008). "Overexpression of toll-like receptors 3 and 4 in synovial tissue from patients with early rheumatoid arthritis: toll-like receptor expression in early and longstanding arthritis." *Arthritis Rheum* 58(12): 3684-3692.

Osterloh, A., U. Kalinke, et al. (2007). "Synergistic and differential modulation of immune responses by Hsp60 and lipopolysaccharide." *J Biol Chem* 282(7): 4669-4680.

Park, B. S., D. H. Song, et al. (2009). "The structural basis of lipopolysaccharide recognition by the TLR4-MD-2 complex." *Nature* 458(7242): 1191-1195.

Piccinini, A. M. and K. S. Midwood (2010). "DAMPening inflammation by modulating TLR signalling." *Mediators Inflamm* 2010.

Podolin, P. L., J. F. Callahan, et al. (2005). "Attenuation of murine collagen-induced arthritis by a novel, potent, selective small molecule inhibitor of IkappaB Kinase 2, TPCA-1 (2-[(aminocarbonyl)amino]-5-(4-fluorophenyl)-3-thiophenecarboxamide), occurs via reduction of proinflammatory cytokines and antigen-induced T cell Proliferation." *J Pharmacol Exp Ther* 312(1): 373-381.

Pullerits, R., I. M. Jonsson, et al. (2003). "High mobility group box chromosomal protein 1, a DNA binding cytokine, induces arthritis." *Arthritis Rheum* 48(6): 1693-1700.

Radstake, T. R., B. Franke, et al. (2004). "The Toll-like receptor 4 Asp299Gly functional variant is associated with decreased rheumatoid arthritis disease susceptibility but does not influence disease severity and/or outcome." *Arthritis Rheum* 50(3): 999-1001.

Radstake, T. R., M. F. Roelofs, et al. (2004). "Expression of toll-like receptors 2 and 4 in rheumatoid synovial tissue and regulation by proinflammatory cytokines interleukin-12 and interleukin-18 via interferon-gamma." *Arthritis Rheum* 50(12): 3856-3865.

Ranjith-Kumar, C. T., K. E. Duffy, et al. (2008). "Single-stranded oligonucleotides can inhibit cytokine production induced by human toll-like receptor 3." *Mol Cell Biol* 28(14): 4507-4519.

Rice, J. W., J. M. Veal, et al. (2008). "Small molecule inhibitors of Hsp90 potently affect inflammatory disease pathways and exhibit activity in models of rheumatoid arthritis." *Arthritis Rheum* 58(12): 3765-3775.

Rittirsch, D., M. A. Flierl, et al. (2009). "Cross-talk between TLR4 and FcgammaReceptorIII (CD16) pathways." *PLoS Pathog* 5(6): e1000464.

Roelofs, M. F., S. Abdollahi-Roodsaz, et al. (2008). "The orchestra of Toll-like receptors and their potential role in frequently occurring rheumatic conditions." *Arthritis Rheum* 58(2): 338-348.

Roelofs, M. F., L. A. Joosten, et al. (2005). "The expression of toll-like receptors 3 and 7 in rheumatoid arthritis synovium is increased and costimulation of toll-like receptors 3, 4, and 7/8 results in synergistic cytokine production by dendritic cells." *Arthritis Rheum* 52(8): 2313-2322.

Roelofs, M. F., M. H. Wenink, et al. (2009). "Type I interferons might form the link between Toll-like receptor (TLR) 3/7 and TLR4-mediated synovial inflammation in rheumatoid arthritis (RA)." *Ann Rheum Dis* 68(9): 1486-1493.

Rothlin, C. V., S. Ghosh, et al. (2007). "TAM receptors are pleiotropic inhibitors of the innate immune response." *Cell* 131(6): 1124-1136.

Sacre, S., M. Medghalchi, et al. (2010). "Fluoxetine and citalopram exhibit potent antiinflammatory activity in human and murine models of rheumatoid arthritis and inhibit toll-like receptors." *Arthritis Rheum* 62(3): 683-693.

Sacre, S. M., E. Andreakos, et al. (2007). "The Toll-like receptor adaptor proteins MyD88 and Mal/TIRAP contribute to the inflammatory and destructive processes in a human model of rheumatoid arthritis." *Am J Pathol* 170(2): 518-525.

Sacre, S. M., S. K. Drexler, et al. (2007). "Could toll-like receptors provide a missing link in chronic inflammation in rheumatoid arthritis? Lessons from a study on human rheumatoid tissue." *Ann Rheum Dis* 66 Suppl 3: iii81-86.

Sacre, S. M., A. Lo, et al. (2008). "Inhibitors of TLR8 reduce TNF production from human rheumatoid synovial membrane cultures." *J Immunol* 181(11): 8002-8009.

Sanchez, E., G. Orozco, et al. (2004). "Polymorphisms of toll-like receptor 2 and 4 genes in rheumatoid arthritis and systemic lupus erythematosus." *Tissue Antigens* 63(1): 54-57.

Scaffidi, P., T. Misteli, et al. (2002). "Release of chromatin protein HMGB1 by necrotic cells triggers inflammation." *Nature* 418(6894): 191-195.

Schmidt, M., B. Raghavan, et al. (2010). "Crucial role for human Toll-like receptor 4 in the development of contact allergy to nickel." *Nat Immunol* 11(9): 814-819.

Schumacher, H. R., Jr., T. Arayssi, et al. (1999). "Chlamydia trachomatis nucleic acids can be found in the synovium of some asymptomatic subjects." *Arthritis Rheum* 42(6): 1281-1284.

Scott, D. L., F. Wolfe, et al. (2010). "Rheumatoid arthritis." *Lancet* 376(9746): 1094-1108.

Sebbag, M., N. Moinard, et al. (2006). "Epitopes of human fibrin recognized by the rheumatoid arthritis-specific autoantibodies to citrullinated proteins." *Eur J Immunol* 36(8): 2250-2263.

Seibl, R., T. Birchler, et al. (2003). "Expression and regulation of Toll-like receptor 2 in rheumatoid arthritis synovium." *Am J Pathol* 162(4): 1221-1227.

Shi, Z., Z. Cai, et al. (2011). "A novel Toll-like receptor that recognizes vesicular stomatitis virus." *J Biol Chem* 286(6): 4517-4524.

Silva, E., J. Arcaroli, et al. (2007). "HMGB1 and LPS induce distinct patterns of gene expression and activation in neutrophils from patients with sepsis-induced acute lung injury." *Intensive Care Med* 33(10): 1829-1839.

Sokolove, J., X. Zhao, et al. (2011). "Immune complexes containing citrullinated fibrinogen costimulate macrophages via Toll-like receptor 4 and Fcgamma receptor." *Arthritis Rheum* 63(1): 53-62.

Stanczyk, J., C. Ospelt, et al. (2011). "Altered expression of microRNA-203 in rheumatoid arthritis synovial fibroblasts and its role in fibroblast activation." *Arthritis Rheum* 63(2): 373-381.

Stanczyk, J., D. M. Pedrioli, et al. (2008). "Altered expression of MicroRNA in synovial fibroblasts and synovial tissue in rheumatoid arthritis." *Arthritis Rheum* 58(4): 1001-1009.

Tamaki, Y., Y. Takakubo, et al. (2011). "Expression of Toll-like Receptors and Their Signaling Pathways in Rheumatoid Synovitis." *J Rheumatol* 38(5): 810-820.

Taylor, P. C. and M. Feldmann (2009). "Anti-TNF biologic agents: still the therapy of choice for rheumatoid arthritis." *Nat Rev Rheumatol* 5(10): 578-582.

Tedder, T. F. (2009). "CD19: a promising B cell target for rheumatoid arthritis." *Nat Rev Rheumatol* 5(10): 572-577.

Townsend, M. J., J. G. Monroe, et al. (2010). "B-cell targeted therapies in human autoimmune diseases: an updated perspective." *Immunol Rev* 237(1): 264-283.

Uchida, Y., M. C. Freitas, et al. (2009). "The inhibition of neutrophil elastase ameliorates mouse liver damage due to ischemia and reperfusion." *Liver Transpl* 15(8): 939-947.

Ulloa, L., F. M. Batliwalla, et al. (2003). "High mobility group box chromosomal protein 1 as a nuclear protein, cytokine, and potential therapeutic target in arthritis." *Arthritis Rheum* 48(4): 876-881.

Uysal, H., R. Bockermann, et al. (2009). "Structure and pathogenicity of antibodies specific for citrullinated collagen type II in experimental arthritis." *J Exp Med* 206(2): 449-462.

van Beers, J. J., R. Raijmakers, et al. (2010). "Mapping of citrullinated fibrinogen B-cell epitopes in rheumatoid arthritis by imaging surface plasmon resonance." *Arthritis Res Ther* 12(6): R219.

van Vollenhoven, R. F. (2009). "Treatment of rheumatoid arthritis: state of the art 2009." *Nat Rev Rheumatol* 5(10): 531-541.

Vanags, D., B. Williams, et al. (2006). "Therapeutic efficacy and safety of chaperonin 10 in patients with rheumatoid arthritis: a double-blind randomised trial." *Lancet* 368(9538): 855-863.

Wang, H., H. Liao, et al. (2004). "Cholinergic agonists inhibit HMGB1 release and improve survival in experimental sepsis." *Nat Med* 10(11): 1216-1221.

Wang, L., R. A. Gordon, et al. (2010). "Indirect inhibition of Toll-like receptor and type I interferon responses by ITAM-coupled receptors and integrins." *Immunity* 32(4): 518-530.

Weinblatt, M. E., J. S. Coblyn, et al. (1985). "Efficacy of low-dose methotrexate in rheumatoid arthritis." *N Engl J Med* 312(13): 818-822.

Wu, C. Y., P. L. Chi, et al. (2010). "TLR4-dependent induction of vascular adhesion molecule-1 in rheumatoid arthritis synovial fibroblasts: Roles of cytosolic phospholipase A(2)alpha/cyclooxygenase-2." *J Cell Physiol* 223(2): 480-491.

Yuan, Z., J. Chen, et al. (2008). "Construction and characterization of the HMGB1 mutant as a competitive antagonist to HMGB1 induced cytokines release." *Biochem Biophys Res Commun* 372(4): 703-707.

Yue, D., W. Brintnell, et al. (2010). "CTLA-4Ig blocks the development and progression of citrullinated fibrinogen-induced arthritis in DR4-transgenic mice." *Arthritis Rheum* 62(10): 2941-2952.

Zeuner, R. A., K. J. Ishii, et al. (2002). "Reduction of CpG-induced arthritis by suppressive oligodeoxynucleotides." *Arthritis Rheum* 46(8): 2219-2224.

11

Targeting the Metabolism and Receptors of Sphingosine-1-Phosphate for the Treatment of Rheumatoid Arthritis

Sylvain G. Bourgoin, Chenqi Zhao
and Maria J. Fernandes
Laval University
Canada

1. Introduction

Sphingolipids belong to a major class of lipids that are ubiquitously synthesized by eukaryotic cells and are characterized by their sphingoid backbone and primary structural roles in membrane formation. Over the past two decades, sphingolipids have emerged as a source of important signalling molecules in addition to their structural functions (Merrill et al., 1997). In particular, sphingosine-1-phosphate (S1P), is a unique signalling molecule that has the ability to act as an intracellular second messenger, as well as an extracellular stimulus through specific G protein-coupled receptor (GPCRs) (Pyne and Pyne, 2000; Spiegel and Milstien, 2003; Van Brocklyn et al., 1998). S1P has been shown to mediate a variety of fundamental biological processes including cell proliferation, migration, invasion, angiogenesis, vascular maturation and lymphocyte trafficking. The intracellular level of S1P is tightly regulated by the equilibrium between its synthesis by sphingosine kinases (SphKs) and its degradation by S1P phosphatases (SPPs) and S1P lyase (SPL) (Saba and Hla, 2004). Activation of SphKs by a variety of agonists, including growth factors, cytokines and hormones, increases intracellular S1P. Once generated, S1P can either act intracellularly as a second messenger or be secreted out of the cell and act extracellularly by binding to and signalling through S1P receptors expressed on the surface of the same cell or nearby cells in autocrine and/or paracrine manners (Alvarez et al., 2007). Many of the biological effects of S1P are mediated by its binding to and activation of its specific receptors S1P1–S1P5 (Ishii et al., 2004). Alterations in S1P signalling, as well as in the enzymes involved in its synthesis and metabolism, have been observed in many types of pathological situations such as angiogenesis, metastasis, and autoimmunity.

The role played by S1P in the autoimmune disease rheumatoid arthritis (RA) has recently emerged. Activated SphK and elevated levels of S1P have been detected in the synovium and synovial fluids of patients with RA, respectively (Kamada et al., 2009; Kitano et al., 2006; Lai et al., 2008). In addition, exogenously applied S1P in cultured synovial fibroblasts from RA patients causes cell migration, production of cytokines/chemokines, expression of cyclooxygenase-2 and prostaglandins, as well as cell proliferation and survival (Kitano et al., 2006; Zhao et al., 2008). These results suggest a biological function for the SphK/S1P/S1P receptor (S1PR) axes in RA disease progression. In this review we summarize the current understanding of how S1P metabolism and signalling impact the biology of inflammation in

RA. We also discuss the potential therapeutic benefit of modulators of S1P metabolism and S1P receptors, including SphK/SPL inhibitors, FTY-720, S1P receptor antagonists, and anti-S1P monoclonal antibodies, in the treatment of RA.

2. S1P biosynthesis, metabolism and secretion

All cells are able to generate S1P during the normal physiologic metabolism of sphingolipids (Hla, 2004). Generally, systemic and local concentrations of S1P are tightly regulated by the balance between its synthesis and degradation via three enzyme families, including SphKs (SphK1 and SphK2), SPPs (SPP1 and SPP2), and SPL (Fig. 1). SphKs generate S1P through phosphorylation of its precursor, sphingosine, while SPPs reversibly convert S1P back to sphingosine by removing the phosphate (Xia et al., 2000). Irreversible degradation of S1P is carried out by a single enzyme SPL, which cleaves S1P into ethanolamine phosphate and hexadecenal, representing the last step in the sphingolipid degradation pathway (Xia et al., 2000).

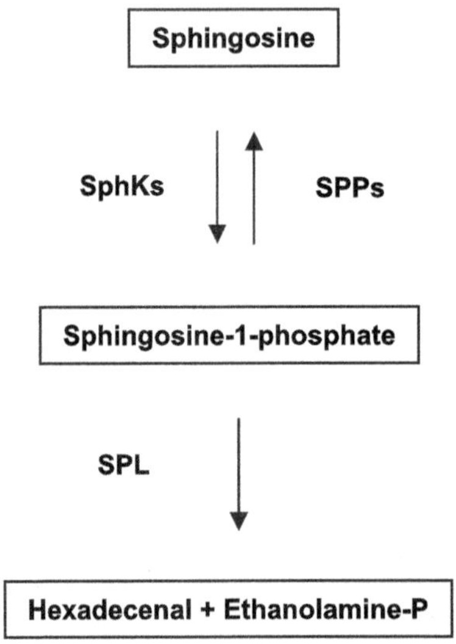

Fig. 1. S1P metabolism pathway. S1P homeostasis is tightly regulated by the balance between its synthesis and degradation via three enzyme families: (1) sphingosine kinases (SphK1 and SphK2), which generate S1P through phosphorylation of its precursor, sphingosine, (2) S1P phosphatases (SPP1 and SPP2), which reversibly convert S1P back to sphingosine, and (3) S1P lyase (SPL), which irreversibly degrades S1P to generate ethanolamine phosphate and hexadecenal.

SphK is represented by two different isoforms (SphK1 and SphK2). Although both SphK1 and SphK2 can phosphorylate sphingosine, SphK1 produces the majority of S1P in cells (Kohama et al., 1998). SphKs can be activated by a large variety of agonists, including growth factors (such as platelet-derived growth factor, vascular endothelial growth factor, epidermal growth factor and hepatocyte growth factor), cytokines (such as TNF-α), steroid hormones (such as estradiol), and GPCR ligands (such as lysophosphatidic acid (LPA) and S1P) (reviewed in (Alvarez et al., 2007; Spiegel and Milstien, 2003; Taha et al., 2006)). Following cellular activation by these agonists, SphK1 can be activated through: 1)

phosphorylation and translocation to the plasma membrane, 2) interaction with acidic phospholipids such as phosphatidic acid produced by phospholipase D (Delon et al., 2004), and 3) possible association with other proteins. All or parts of these mechanisms may be required for full activation of SphK1 (Takabe et al., 2008). Phosphorylation of SphK1 leads to its translocation to the plasma membrane where its substrate sphingosine is located, resulting in the production of S1P (Johnson et al., 2002; Pitson et al., 2005). S1P, in turn, activates specific S1P receptors present on the surface of the same cell or on nearby cells in autocrine and/or paracrine manners (Alvarez et al., 2007). The "inside-out" export of intracellularly generated S1P is crucial for many S1P functions (Takabe et al., 2008).
The mechanism by which S1P is exported from the inside to the outside of cells after synthesis is not fully understood. Several lines of evidence suggest the involvement of the ATP-binding cassette (ABC) family of transporters in S1P secretion (Kobayashi et al., 2006; Mitra et al., 2006; Sato et al., 2007). Mitra et al. (2006) revealed that the release of S1P from mast cells is regulated by ABCC1. Similarly, the ABCA1 transporter is critical for the release of S1P from astrocytes (Sato et al., 2007). In breast cancer the export of S1P mediated by ABCC1 and ABCG2 transporters is stimulated by estrogen receptor-α (Takabe et al., 2010). Altogether, these studies suggest that members of the family of ABC transporters may be important for export of S1P out of cells.

3. S1P receptors and downstream signalling pathways

S1P evokes diverse biological functions by binding to its ubiquitously-expressed and specific cell surface receptors. So far, five S1P receptors, designated as S1P1/Edg1, S1P2/Edg5, S1P3/Edg3, S1P4/Edg6, and S1P5/Edg8, have been identified (An et al., 1997; Im et al., 2000; Lee et al., 1998; Van Brocklyn et al., 2000; Yamazaki et al., 2000). These receptors were initially named "Edg" receptors as they belong to the so-called endothelial differentiation gene (Edg) family; however "S1P receptors" is now preferred (Chun et al., 2002). S1P receptors are GPCRs that share high similarity with each other and with LPA receptors. S1P receptors exhibit variable tissue distribution, for example, S1P1, S1P2, and S1P3 are widely expressed in various tissues, whereas the expression of S1P4 and S1P5 is more restricted to cells of the immune system and nervous system, respectively (reviewed in (Sanchez and Hla, 2004)). Upon binding to S1P receptors, S1P activates downstream signalling pathways, leading to a variety of cellular responses such as proliferation, cell migration, actin cytoskeletal rearrangement, and adherens junction assembly (Kluk and Hla, 2002; Taha et al., 2004). Each S1P receptor is coupled to a specific heterotrimeric G protein ($G_{i/o}$, G_q and $G_{12/13}$), which, when activated, dissociates into its α and $\beta\gamma$ subunits and transduces signals toward the downstream pathways. Particularly, S1P1 is coupled predominantly to $G_{i/o}$, through which it activates: 1) Rho kinase and tyrosine kinases, leading to cytoskeletal rearrangement (Garcia et al., 2001); 2) MAPK, leading to angiogenesis (Lee et al., 1999); and 3) Akt, leading to cell chemotaxis (Lee et al., 2001). On the other hand, S1P2 and S1P3 are linked predominantly to G_q and $G_{12/13}$, through which they activate phospholipase C leading to Ca^{2+} mobilization (Ancellin and Hla, 1999) and positive or negative modulation of Rho and thus of cell migration (Sugimoto et al., 2003). More detailed information on the various signalling pathways turned on by S1P receptor activation is discussed in previous reviews (Choi et al., 2008; Rosen et al., 2009).
It is known that S1P can also act intracellularly to enhance cell proliferation and suppress apoptosis independently of S1P receptors (Rosenfeldt et al., 2001; Van Brocklyn et al., 1998). In plants and yeast, which do not express S1P receptors, for instance, intracellular S1P

regulates stomatal aperture (Coursol et al., 2005) or stress responses and survival (Jenkins and Hannun, 2001), respectively. Similarly, in mammalian cells intracellular S1P regulates calcium release independently of inositol trisphosphate formation and of S1P receptor activation (Blom et al., 2005). S1P also signals within the nucleus by binding to and inhibiting histone deacetylases HDAC1 and HDAC2, leading to the epigenetic regulation of gene expression (Hait et al., 2009). Further studies are needed, however, to reveal the intracellular second messenger functions of S1P.

4. Role of SphK/S1P/S1PR signalling in rheumatoid arthritis

4.1 Rheumatoid arthritis

Rheumatoid arthritis (RA) is an autoimmune disease characterized by chronic inflammation of the joint synovium, synovial hyperplasia and a massive infiltration of inflammatory cells into the affected joints, leading to the progressive destruction of cartilage and bone (Feldmann et al., 1996a). The inciting agent that triggers the development of RA is unknown; however, the disease is clearly an inflammatory process since the critical events in RA are largely coordinated by complex interplays of proinflammatory cytokines, chemokines, and matrix metalloproteinases produced by both synovial resident cells and infiltrating cells (Feldmann et al., 1996b; McInnes and Schett, 2007). These inflammatory mediators are involved in many pathological processes in RA. Increasing evidence demonstrates,

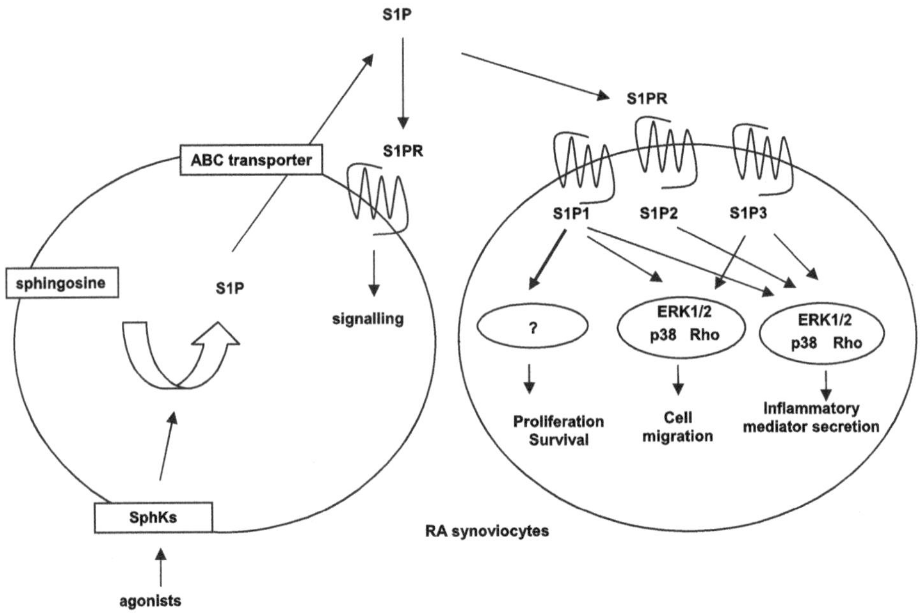

Fig. 2. S1P metabolism and signalling in RA synoviocytes. A range of agonists including growth factors, hormones, angiogenic factors and other stimuli activate SphKs through phosphorylation. S1P is then generated and exported out of the cells by ABC transporters to act on the same cell (autocrine) or on nearby cells (paracrine). S1P engages with its receptors (S1P1-3) to mediate a diverse array of signalling pathways, impacting fundamental biological processes that are integral to the pathogenesis of RA, such as cell proliferation and survival, cell migration, and inflammatory mediator secretion.

however, that the activation of RA synoviocytes can be maintained in the absence of inflammatory cytokines (Muller-Ladner et al., 1996), indicating the involvement of biologically active mediators other than inflammatory cytokines in RA disease progression. Emerging evidence suggests a role for S1P metabolism and signalling in various aspects of the pathogenesis of RA. Recent *in vitro* and *in vivo* studies evaluated the potential role of S1P synthesis, catabolism enzymes and S1P signalling in RA (Fig. 2).

4.2 S1P expression and SphK activity in RA synovium and synovial fluids

Several studies reveal high levels of S1P in RA synovial tissues and fluids (Kitano et al., 2006; Lai et al., 2008). Kitano et al. (2006) reported elevated levels of S1P in synovial fluids of RA patients (1078 pM/ml) in comparison to those of osteoarthritis (OA) patients (765 pM/ml). The S1P content in RA synovial fluids was significantly higher than those in serum (400 pM/ml) or plasma (100 pM/ml) from normal people. Lai et al. (2008) also measured the amount of S1P by a competitive ELISA and detected up to 17 μM S1P in RA synovial fluids, which was more than five fold higher than that found in OA synovial fluids (3 μM). The increased level of S1P could be responsible for the recruitment and the infiltration of immune cells into the synovium (see section 4.2.2). Pi et al. (2006) also showed that peripheral blood B lymphoblastoid cell lines derived from patients with RA exhibit a high level of S1P synthesis.

SphK expression and activity were also demonstrated in RA. Increased SphK1 expression and activity were found in RA B lymphoblastoid cell lines, which were implicated as the underlying mechanism of impaired Fas-mediated death signalling in RA (Pi et al., 2006). More recently, SphK2 was shown to be expressed in rheumatoid synovial fibroblasts *in vivo* and *in vitro* and associated with the up-regulation of S1P production (Kamada et al., 2009). Surprisingly, FTY-720 (2-amino-2-[2-(4-octylphenyl) ethyl] propane-1, 3-diol hydrochloride), a sphingosine analog that is phosphorylated to the active metabolite FTY-720-phosphate (FTY-720-P) by SphK2 (Brinkmann et al., 2002; Mandala et al., 2002), induces apoptosis of synovial fibroblasts. This effect could be due, at least in part, to FTY-720-P-mediated degradation of specific S1P receptors (Matloubian et al., 2004). Corroborating this observation, we reported that S1P protects synovial fibroblasts from ongoing apoptosis (Zhao et al., 2008). Using the mouse model of collagen-induced arthritis (CIA), Lai et al. (2009) highlighted distinct roles for SphK1 and SphK2 in regulating cell growth and survival. The *in vivo* administration of SphK1 siRNA reduced inflammation whereas mice treated with SphK2 siRNA resulted in a more aggressive disease and greater secretion of proinflammatory cytokines (IL-6, TNF-α and IFN-α) by immune cells. How and why SphK1 and SphK2 exert distinct opposing roles in the regulation of inflammatory arthritis remains unclear and may be related to the location of S1P production (Maceyka et al., 2005). The role of SphK2 in chronic inflammatory diseases remains ambiguous since the selective inhibitor of SphK2 ABC249640 has been reported to reduce bone and cartilage degradation in the mouse models of adjuvant-induced arthritis (AIA) and of CIA (Fitzpatrick et al., 2011). The SphK1 signalling pathway is activated in RA (Limaye et al., 2009). In the mouse model of CIA, administration of a non-specific pharmacological inhibitor of SphKs, *N,N*-dimethylsphingosine (DMS), and a siRNA approach to knockdown the SphK1 isoform, markedly suppressed joint pathologies such as adjacent cartilage and bone erosion, synovial hyperplasia, and infiltration of inflammatory cells into the joint compartment (Lai et al., 2008). Moreover, SphK1 deficiency in hTNF-α transgenic mice that develop arthritis at an early age was related to less synovial inflammation and bone erosion (Baker et al., 2010). To

our knowledge the effect of specific inhibitors of SphK1, such as BML-258 (Paugh et al., 2008), has not been tested in animal models of arthritis.
At present, evidence for roles of SPPs and SPL in RA is limited. However, up-regulation of SPP2 was detected in samples of skin lesions from patients with psoriasis, a chronic inflammatory skin disease (Mechtcheriakova et al., 2007). Interestingly, elevated mRNA expression of SPP1 and SPL was observed in RA synoviocytes compared to non-arthritic synoviocytes (Zhao et al., unpublished data).

4.3 S1P receptor expression in RA synovial fibroblasts

In RA, the abnormal growth and erosive activity of synovial fibroblasts suggest that these cells are important contributors to chronic inflammation. During RA disease progression, synovial fibroblasts become hyperplasic and closely interact with infiltrated immune cells to form the aggressive pannus tissue that eventually promotes joint destruction (reviewed in (Feldmann et al., 1996a)). Synovial fibroblasts have been reported to express three of five known S1P receptors, S1P1-3 (Kitano et al., 2006; Nochi et al., 2008; Zhao et al., 2008). Expression of S1P1 in RA synovial tissues was significantly higher compared to that of OA synovial tissues (Kitano et al., 2006). Moreover, pretreatment of synovial fibroblasts with TNF-α, the well-recognized critical cytokine in RA, resulted in up-regulation of S1P3 receptor expression in synovial fibroblasts, which likely contributes to the synergistic production of inflammatory cytokines/chemokines upon subsequent exposure to S1P (Zhao et al., 2008).

4.4 S1P signalling in RA pathophysiology

4.4.1 S1P signalling in migration of synovial fibroblasts and osteoclasts

As constituents of the synovial pannus in RA, synovial fibroblasts have long been considered as key players in the aggressive destruction of cartilage and bone (Shiozawa et al., 1983). Using an *in vitro* wound-closing assay, we previously reported that S1P could induce synoviocyte migration (Zhao et al., 2008). S1P-induced cell migration is mediated through the activation of extracellular signal-regulated kinase-1 and -2 (ERK1/2), as well as p38 mitogen-activated protein kinase (MAPK) and of Rho kinase. S1P-driven motility of synoviocytes was mainly via S1P1 and S1P3 receptor activation since the effect of S1P was mimicked by the S1P1 receptor agonist (SEW2871) but abolished by S1P1/3 (VPC23019) and S1P3 (CAY10444) receptor antagonists.
S1P has also been shown to induce chemotaxis and regulate migration of osteoclasts and their precursors *in vitro* and *in vivo* (Ishii et al., 2009). Cells bearing the properties of osteoclast precursors express S1P1 receptors and migrate along an S1P gradient *in vitro*. The S1P1 agonist, SEW2871, stimulated motility of osteoclast precursors-containing monocytoid populations *in vivo*. In addition, osteoclast/monocyte lineage-specific conditional S1P1 knockout mice show osteoporotic changes due to increased osteoclast attachment to the bone surface, suggesting a crucial role of the S1P-S1P1 receptor axis in regulating the migratory behaviour of osteoclast precursors and bone mineral homeostasis.

4.4.2 S1P signalling in the secretion of cytokines/chemokines and lipid mediators

In the inflamed RA synovium, large amounts of pro-inflammatory cytokines and chemokines may contribute directly to cartilage and bone erosion by promoting matrix metalloproteinase (MMP) production and suppressing chondrocyte/osteoclast functions (Feldmann et al., 1996b). Previous studies from our group and others demonstrated that exogenously applied S1P could stimulate synovial fibroblasts to release various inflammatory mediators, including cytokines, chemokines, and prostaglandin E_2 (PGE_2) (Kitano et al., 2006; Zhao et al., 2008). S1P administration strongly stimulated the secretion of IL-8 (interleukin-8), IL-6, MCP-1 (monocyte chemotactic protein-1), and RANTES (regulated on activation normal T cells expressed and secreted) via S1P2 and S1P3 receptors. The signalling pathways involved in S1P-mediated cytokine/chemokine secretion were dependent on ERK1/2, p38 MAPK, and Rho kinase activation. These cytokines/chemokines may subsequently increase the recruitment of inflammatory cells such as neutrophils into the synovium, as chemokines such as IL-8 exhibit selective chemotactic activity for neutrophils, whereas MCP-1, MIP-1α (macrophage inflammatory protein-1α), MIP-1β (macrophage inflammatory protein-1β), and RANTES primarily attract monocytes (Koch, 2005). S1P may therefore contribute to the regulation and maintenance of the inflammatory response in RA, in part through stimulation of multiple cytokine/chemokine secretion by synovial fibroblasts. SphK/S1P signalling was also implicated in cell-contact-mediated proinflammatory cytokine/chemokine secretion in RA synovium without additional exogenous stimulation. Lai et al. (2008) used peripheral blood mononuclear cells from RA patients in cell-cell contact experiments. They discovered that activated peripheral T lymphocytes from RA patients induced substantial production of TNF-α, IL-1β, IL-6, MCP-1 and MMP-9 by autologous peripheral monocytes. Importantly, treatment with a potent SphK inhibitor, DMS, significantly suppressed production of these cytokines. The results suggest the importance of SphK/S1P signalling in cell-contact-mediated inflammatory mediators, which is relevant to RA pathology.

Regarding PGE_2, S1P was reported to stimulate COX-2 expression and super-production of PGE_2 by RA synovial fibroblasts (Kitano et al., 2006; Nochi et al., 2008). PGE_2 is an autocrine lipid mediator derived from arachidonic acid metabolism by cyclooxygenases (COX-1 or COX-2) (Ghosh et al., 2004). High levels of PGE_2 were detected in synovial fluids of RA patients (Hidaka et al., 2001; Lettesjo et al., 1998). PGE_2 has pro-inflammatory properties and contributes to the pathogenesis of arthritis, since PGE_2 stimulates angiogenesis in the rheumatoid synovium (Ben-Av et al., 1995) and triggers bone resorption by osteoclasts (Mino et al., 1998). Thus, S1P may aggravate synovial hyperplasia, inflammation and angiogenesis through the induction of COX-2 and PGE_2 in RA synovial tissues. Indeed, the COX-2-PGE_2 axis has been suggested to play an important role in arthritic diseases by stimulating inflammation, angiogenesis, and osteoclastic bone destruction (Martel-Pelletier et al., 2003).

4.4.3 S1P signalling in the proliferation and survival of RA synovial fibroblasts, B lymphoblastoid cells and chondrocytes

Abnormal proliferation and resistance to apoptosis of synovial fibroblasts have been suggested to contribute directly to the hyperplasia of the rheumatoid synovium (Ospelt et al., 2004). Indeed, S1P appears capable of increasing cell survival and inhibiting apoptosis of various cell types, including B lymphoblastoid cells derived from RA patients (Pi et al., 2006). We previously demonstrated that S1P, through S1P1, protected synovial fibroblasts from apoptosis (Zhao et al., 2008). In our study we were not able to demonstrate a significant effect of S1P on RA synoviocyte proliferation, although Kitano et al. (2006) reported a small stimulatory effect of S1P on cell proliferation. Nonetheless these studies suggest that S1P can induce the proliferation of synovial fibroblasts, which may contribute to synovial hyperplasia (Knedla et al., 2007). S1P was also reported to aggravate arthritis by inducing chondrocyte proliferation through the stimulation of COX-2 and PGE_2 production and via the activation of ERK (Kim et al., 2006; Masuko et al., 2007).

4.4.4 Synergistic action of S1P and TNF-α on synovial fibroblast functions

TNF-α is central to RA pathogenesis as the pro-inflammatory cytokine not only stimulates the production of other inflammatory mediators but also directly triggers the activation of synovial cells and osteoclasts leading to the irreversible damage of soft tissues and bone (Olsen and Stein, 2004). Several studies have suggested that S1P and TNF-α might synergize in their regulation of synovial fibroblast functions. On the one hand, the expression of S1P3 receptor was enhanced by TNF-α, leading to amplified secretion of cytokines/chemokines, including IL-6, IL-8, MCP-1, and RANTES (Zhao et al., 2008). On the other hand, S1P enhanced TNF-α-mediated COX-2 expression and production of PGE_2 by RA synoviocytes (Kitano et al., 2006). Thus, the elevated levels of TNF-α seen in RA synovium may increase S1P synthesis via activation of SphKs and make synovial fibroblasts more responsive to S1P possibly through up-regulation of S1P receptor expression. The synergy between TNF-α and S1P may eventually exacerbate the clinical manifestations of RA, including enhanced synovial tissue invasion by aggressive fibroblasts (due to enhanced cell mobility), synovial hyperplasia (due to proliferation and survival of synoviocytes), and exacerbated inflammation (due to over production of inflammatory mediators).

5. Potential S1P-targeted therapy for RA

Despite great efforts devoted to the development of new therapeutic targets for RA, currently used drugs have limitations in their use for the treatment of RA. As discussed in the above sections, S1P appears to be an important modulator of many aspects of the pathogenesis of RA. Manipulation of endogenous local and systemic amounts of bioactive S1P by inhibiting metabolic enzymes such as SphKs and SPL, by applying S1P-blocking agents such as FTY-720, VPC23019 and JTE-013 or anti-S1P antibodies is thus a promising approach for the treatment of RA. Studies targeting S1P metabolism and signalling for the treatment of RA are summarized in Table 1.

5.1 Targeting S1P metabolism

5.1.1 Reducing S1P formation with sphingosine kinase inhibitors

Blockade of SphK1 activity in the mouse model of CIA significantly suppressed articular inflammation and joint destruction, reduced disease severity, and down-regulated proinflammatory cytokine production and inflammatory cell recruitment into the synovium (Lai et al., 2009). Decreasing S1P production by inhibiting SphK activity is, therefore, a promising therapeutic option in chronic inflammatory arthritis. Indeed, the inhibition of S1P synthesis by blocking SphKs activity has proven useful as an anti-inflammation strategy in cancer therapy *in vitro* and in animal models (Billich et al., 2005; Bonhoure et al., 2006; French et al., 2006; Gamble et al., 2006; Leroux et al., 2007).

5.1.2 Downregulation of S1P receptor activity with S1P lyase inhibitors

SPL catalyzes the irreversible degradation of intracellular S1P to hexadecenal and phosphoethanolamine. It is the major and constitutively active S1P-degrading enzyme in cells and tissues (Fig. 1). As a result, S1P concentrations in tissues are maintained at very low levels. Inhibition of SPL leads to the accumulation of S1P in various tissues (Schwab et al., 2005). Treatment with SPL inhibitor results in accumulation of S1P in lymphoid tissues

Approach and reagent	Mechanism of action	Target	Experimental system	Reference
Inhibition of SphK activity				
N,N-dimethylsphingosine (DMS, SphK inhibitor)	Reduces S1P formation	SphK1 and SphK2	*In vivo*	Lai et al., 2008
ABC249640 (SphK2 inhibitor)	Reduces S1P formation	SphK2	*In vivo*	Fitzpatrick et al., 2011
siSphK1	Reduces S1P formation	SphK1	*In vivo*	Lai et al., 2008
Inhibition of SPL activity				
SPL inhibitor	Downregulates S1PR activity	SPL	Clinical trial	Bagdanoff et al., 2010
Sequestration of S1P				
S1P specific antibody	Depletes extracellular S1P	S1P	*In vivo*	Visentin et al., 2006
Blocking S1PR				
FTY-720 (sphingosine analogue)	Down-regulates S1PRs and renders cells unresponsive to S1P	S1P1, S1P3, S1P4 and S1P5	*In vivo*	Matsuura et al., 2000; Tsunemi et al.; Wang et al., 2007
VPC23019 (S1P1/3 antagonist), CAY10444 (S1P3 antagonist) and JTE-013 (S1P2 antagonist)	Block S1P binding to S1PR	S1P1-3	*In vitro*	Kitano et al., 2006; Zhao et al., 2008

Table 1. Targeting the SphK/S1P/S1PR signalling pathway in RA.

and induces premature internalization of the exit-signal-sensing S1P1 receptor on lymphocytes (Schwab et al., 2005). S1P1 receptor internalization renders lymphocytes unresponsive to S1P, preventing their egress from the thymus and lymph nodes (Lo et al., 2005). One physiological outcome of this systemic redistribution of lymphocytes is potent immunosuppression, which offers new opportunities for developing immunoregulatory agents to treat autoimmune and inflammatory diseases (Gardell et al., 2006; Huwiler and Pfeilschifter, 2008; Mandala et al., 2002; Rosen et al., 2003; Zhang and Schluesener, 2007). Indeed, SPL-deficient mice showed resistance to various inflammatory and autoimmune challenges (Bagdanoff et al., 2009; Bandhuvula et al., 2007; Vogel et al., 2009). The evaluation of a synthetic SPL inhibitor, LX2931, is currently underway in phase II clinical trials in RA patients (Bagdanoff et al., 2010).

5.1.3 Depletion of extracellular S1P with S1P antibody

Specific antibodies against S1P have been developed and are currently being tested in clinical studies for the treatment of cancer, fibrosis, inflammation, macular degeneration, diabetic retinopathy, glaucoma, and other diseases (Graler and Goetzl, 2004). The antibodies are thought to bind S1P and reduce the extracellular pool of bioactive S1P (Sabbadini, 2006). Indeed, a preclinical study using blocking S1P antibodies to prevent tumor progression was recently reported (Visentin et al., 2006). In this hallmark study, a specific monoclonal antibody recognizing S1P was administered to mice harboring human cancer xenografts. The intervention reduced, and in some cases completely eliminated, tumour formation and accompanying tumour angiogenesis. The results suggest that antibody-mediated inhibition of S1P signalling may be developed as a strategy for inhibiting pannus formation and angiogenesis in RA.

5.2 Targeting S1P receptors

S1P and its receptors are powerful regulators of various critical functions of RA synoviocytes. Targeting these cells with specific S1P receptor agonists or antagonists can modulate specific inflammatory responses locally and systemically by altering cell migration, cytokine and chemokine secretion, and proliferation/survival. RP-001, a potent S1P1 receptor agonist with properties similar to those reported for FTY-720 on S1P1 receptor degradation and lymphocyte sequestration from the blood, was recently characterized (Cahalan et al., 2011). The short half-life of RP-001 *in vivo*, however, disqualifies this compound for clinical use.

5.2.1 S1P receptor agonists, FTY-720

The immunosuppressant drug FTY-720 (fingolimod) was originally described as a sphingosine analogue that is phosphorylated *in vivo* by SphK2 to a S1P agonist for all S1P receptors except S1P2 (Brinkmann et al., 2002; Mandala et al., 2002). Further studies revealed that FTY-720-P not only activates S1P receptors, it also down-regulates them and consequently renders cells unresponsive to S1P (Matloubian et al., 2004). FTY-720 has been suggested to play a major role in autoimmune disease, such as multiple sclerosis [reviewed in (Nicholas et al., 2011)]. Multiple sclerosis is a common neurological disability, in which autoreactive T-cells migrate across the blood–brain barrier and attack myelin sheaths, leading to demyelination and axonal damage. FTY-720 deprives thymocytes and lymphocytes by downregulating S1P receptors and interfering with S1P signalling necessary for their egress from secondary lymphoid tissues (Cyster, 2005; Graler and Goetzl, 2004; Kappos et al., 2006; Matloubian et al., 2004). The results of a Phase II clinical trial evaluating the efficacy and safety of FTY-720 for treating relapsing multiple sclerosis showed that the annualized relapse rate of the FTY-720 group was significantly decreased (Kappos et al., 2006). FTY-720 was recently FDA-approved for the treatment of multiple sclerosis (Strader et al., 2011).

The effects of FTY-720 have been examined in several animal models of arthritis (Matsuura et al., 2000; Tsunemi et al., 2010; Wang et al., 2007). In the study of Wang et al. (2007), CIA rats were treated daily with FTY-720 for 28 days and the arthritis index was measured. Radiological analysis revealed that FTY-720-treated CIA rats had less joint damage in comparison to untreated CIA rats. Moreover, while histological assessment showed that CIA rats suffered from inflammatory cell infiltration and synovial hyperplasia in their joints,

FTY-720 treatment clearly reduced these pathological parameters. Similarly, Matsuura et al. (2000) compared FTY-720 with two other anti-rheumatic compounds, mizoribine and prednisolone, in the rat models of CIA and AIA. FTY-720 completely suppressed the increase in hind paw volume and bone destruction to normal control levels by inhibiting leukocyte accumulation in the arthritic joint. Moreover, FTY-720 was shown to possess anti-arthritic activity with a wider margin of safety in AIA and CIA models as compared to mizoribine and prednisolone. A recent study by Tsunmi et al. (2010) revealed that FTY-720 administration suppressed the progression of laminarin-induced arthritis in SKG mice. FTY-720 treatment decreased IL-6 and TNF-α expression by synovial fibroblasts, diminished the number of inflammatory cells migrating into the joints, and suppressed bone destruction.

5.2.2 S1P receptor antagonists

Blocking S1P receptor activity by using S1P receptor antagonists may lead to promising therapeutic strategies for patients suffering from RA. Despite the lack of more comprehensive *in vivo* data, considerable progress has been made in the identification of the S1P receptors regulating synovial fibroblast migration, production of cytokines/chemokines and PGE_2, proliferation, and survival. Several compounds targeting S1P receptors have also been used to decipher the biological roles of S1P receptors. The S1P1/3 antagonist VPC23019 and S1P3 antagonist CAY10444 blocked S1P-mediated synoviocyte migration and cytokine secretion, whereas the S1P2 antagonist JTE-013 attenuated S1P-mediated cytokine secretion (Kitano et al., 2006; Zhao et al., 2008). The pharmacokinetics, bioavailability and metabolic characteristics of these S1P antagonists are essential to advance *in vivo* studies and for therapeutic intervention. Indeed, pharmacological approaches have been developed to block the action of S1P in the context of cancer progression (reviewed in Peyruchaud, 2009).

6. Conclusion

In summary, SphKs and S1P/S1PR signalling appear to play essential roles in modulating RA pathogenesis. The SphK1 pathway is activated and likely plays a pro-inflammatory role in mouse models of inflammatory arthritis. It is fascinating that the blockade of SphK1 activity results in the simultaneous reduction of several inflammatory responses such as pro-inflammatory cytokines and inflammatory cell infiltration into the synovium. Excessive S1P and enhanced S1P receptor expression are detected in the synovium of RA patients. S1P and signalling through S1P receptors induce expression of inflammatory cytokines and suppress apoptosis of B lymphoblastoid cells and fibroblast-like synoviocytes. Although the possible mechanism by which S1P exerts its activity in RA remains to be fully characterized, further understanding of S1P metabolism and S1P receptor expression by synovial tissues represents an exploitable objective for the development of novel chemotherapeutic agents in the treatment of RA.

7. Acknowledgment

The authors would like to thank Ms. Lynn Davis for her editorial assistance. The works cited in the review from the authors' laboratory were supported by research grants from the Canadian Arthritis Network and the Arthritis Society of Canada.

8. References

Alvarez, S. E., et al., 2007. Autocrine and paracrine roles of sphingosine-1-phosphate. Trends Endocrinol Metab. 18, 300-7.

An, S., et al., 1997. Identification of cDNAs encoding two G protein-coupled receptors for lysosphingolipids. FEBS Lett. 417, 279-82.

Ancellin, N., Hla, T., 1999. Differential pharmacological properties and signal transduction of the sphingosine 1-phosphate receptors EDG-1, EDG-3, and EDG-5. J Biol Chem. 274, 18997-9002.

Bagdanoff, J. T., et al., 2010. Inhibition of sphingosine 1-phosphate lyase for the treatment of rheumatoid arthritis: discovery of (E)-1-(4-((1R,2S,3R)-1,2,3,4-tetrahydroxybutyl)-1H-imidazol-2-yl)ethanone oxime (LX2931) and (1R,2S,3R)-1-(2-(isoxazol-3-yl)-1H-imidazol-4-yl)butane-1,2,3,4-tetraol (LX2932). J Med Chem. 53, 8650-62.

Bagdanoff, J. T., et al., 2009. Inhibition of sphingosine-1-phosphate lyase for the treatment of autoimmune disorders. J Med Chem. 52, 3941-53.

Baker, D. A., et al., 2010. Genetic sphingosine kinase 1 deficiency significantly decreases synovial inflammation and joint erosions in murine TNF-alpha-induced arthritis. J Immunol. 185, 2570-9.

Bandhuvula, P., et al., 2007. A rapid fluorescence assay for sphingosine-1-phosphate lyase enzyme activity. J Lipid Res. 48, 2769-78.

Ben-Av, P., et al., 1995. Induction of vascular endothelial growth factor expression in synovial fibroblasts by prostaglandin E and interleukin-1: a potential mechanism for inflammatory angiogenesis. FEBS Lett. 372, 83-7.

Billich, A., et al., 2005. Basal and induced sphingosine kinase 1 activity in A549 carcinoma cells: function in cell survival and IL-1beta and TNF-alpha induced production of inflammatory mediators. Cell Signal. 17, 1203-17.

Blom, T., et al., 2005. Enhancement of intracellular sphingosine-1-phosphate production by inositol 1,4,5-trisphosphate-evoked calcium mobilisation in HEK-293 cells: endogenous sphingosine-1-phosphate as a modulator of the calcium response. Cell Signal. 17, 827-36.

Bonhoure, E., et al., 2006. Overcoming MDR-associated chemoresistance in HL-60 acute myeloid leukemia cells by targeting sphingosine kinase-1. Leukemia. 20, 95-102.

Brinkmann, V., et al., 2002. The immune modulator FTY720 targets sphingosine 1-phosphate receptors. J Biol Chem. 277, 21453-7.

Cahalan, S. M., et al., 2011. Actions of a picomolar short-acting S1P agonist in S1P-eGFP knock-in mice. Nat Chem Biol. 7, 254-6.

Choi, J. W., et al., 2008. Biological roles of lysophospholipid receptors revealed by genetic null mice: an update. Biochim Biophys Acta. 1781, 531-9.

Chun, J., et al., 2002. International Union of Pharmacology. XXXIV. Lysophospholipid receptor nomenclature. Pharmacol Rev. 54, 265-9.

Coursol, S., et al., 2005. Arabidopsis sphingosine kinase and the effects of phytosphingosine-1-phosphate on stomatal aperture. Plant Physiol. 137, 724-37.

Cyster, J. G., 2005. Chemokines, sphingosine-1-phosphate, and cell migration in secondary lymphoid organs. Annu Rev Immunol. 23, 127-59.

Delon, C., et al., 2004. Sphingosine kinase 1 is an intracellular effector of phosphatidic acid. J Biol Chem. 279, 44763-74.

Feldmann, M., et al., 1996a. Rheumatoid arthritis. Cell. 85, 307-10.

Feldmann, M., et al., 1996b. Role of cytokines in rheumatoid arthritis. Annu Rev Immunol. 14, 397-440.

Fitzpatrick, L. R., et al., 2011. Attenuation of arthritis in rodents by a novel orally-available inhibitor of sphingosine kinase. Inflammopharmacology. 19, 75-87.

French, K. J., et al., 2006. Antitumor activity of sphingosine kinase inhibitors. J Pharmacol Exp Ther. 318, 596-603.

Gamble, J. R., et al., 2006. Phenoxodiol, an experimental anticancer drug, shows potent antiangiogenic properties in addition to its antitumour effects. Int J Cancer. 118, 2412-20.

Garcia, J. G., et al., 2001. Sphingosine 1-phosphate promotes endothelial cell barrier integrity by Edg-dependent cytoskeletal rearrangement. J Clin Invest. 108, 689-701.

Gardell, S. E., et al., 2006. Emerging medicinal roles for lysophospholipid signaling. Trends Mol Med. 12, 65-75.

Ghosh, M., et al., 2004. Role of cytosolic phospholipase A(2) in prostaglandin E(2) production by lung fibroblasts. Am J Respir Cell Mol Biol. 30, 91-100.

Graler, M. H., Goetzl, E. J., 2004. The immunosuppressant FTY720 down-regulates sphingosine 1-phosphate G-protein-coupled receptors. FASEB J. 18, 551-3.

Hait, N. C., et al., 2009. Regulation of histone acetylation in the nucleus by sphingosine-1-phosphate. Science. 325, 1254-7.

Hidaka, T., et al., 2001. Dynamic changes in cytokine levels in serum and synovial fluid following filtration leukocytapheresis therapy in patients with rheumatoid arthritis. J Clin Apher. 16, 74-81.

Hla, T., 2004. Physiological and pathological actions of sphingosine 1-phosphate. Semin Cell Dev Biol. 15, 513-20.

Huwiler, A., Pfeilschifter, J., 2008. New players on the center stage: sphingosine 1-phosphate and its receptors as drug targets. Biochem Pharmacol. 75, 1893-900.

Im, D. S., et al., 2000. Characterization of a novel sphingosine 1-phosphate receptor, Edg-8. J Biol Chem. 275, 14281-6.

Ishii, I., et al., 2004. Lysophospholipid receptors: signaling and biology. Annu Rev Biochem. 73, 321-54.

Ishii, M., et al., 2009. Sphingosine-1-phosphate mobilizes osteoclast precursors and regulates bone homeostasis. Nature. 458, 524-8.

Jenkins, G. M., Hannun, Y. A., 2001. Role for de novo sphingoid base biosynthesis in the heat-induced transient cell cycle arrest of Saccharomyces cerevisiae. J Biol Chem. 276, 8574-81.

Johnson, K. R., et al., 2002. PKC-dependent activation of sphingosine kinase 1 and translocation to the plasma membrane. Extracellular release of sphingosine-1-phosphate induced by phorbol 12-myristate 13-acetate (PMA). J Biol Chem. 277, 35257-62.

Kamada, K., et al., 2009. Expression of sphingosine kinase 2 in synovial fibroblasts of rheumatoid arthritis contributing to apoptosis by a sphingosine analogue, FTY720. Pathol Int. 59, 382-9.

Kappos, L., et al., 2006. Oral fingolimod (FTY720) for relapsing multiple sclerosis. N Engl J Med. 355, 1124-40.

Kim, M. K., et al., 2006. Sphingosine-1-phosphate stimulates rat primary chondrocyte proliferation. Biochem Biophys Res Commun. 345, 67-73.

Kitano, M., et al., 2006. Sphingosine 1-phosphate/sphingosine 1-phosphate receptor 1 signaling in rheumatoid synovium: regulation of synovial proliferation and inflammatory gene expression. Arthritis Rheum. 54, 742-53.

Kluk, M. J., Hla, T., 2002. Signaling of sphingosine-1-phosphate via the S1P/EDG-family of G-protein-coupled receptors. Biochim Biophys Acta. 1582, 72-80.

Knedla, A., et al., 2007. Developments in the synovial biology field 2006. Arthritis Res Ther. 9, 209.

Kobayashi, N., et al., 2006. Sphingosine 1-phosphate is released from the cytosol of rat platelets in a carrier-mediated manner. J Lipid Res. 47, 614-21.

Koch, A. E., 2005. Chemokines and their receptors in rheumatoid arthritis: future targets? Arthritis Rheum. 52, 710-21.

Kohama, T., et al., 1998. Molecular cloning and functional characterization of murine sphingosine kinase. J Biol Chem. 273, 23722-8.

Lai, W. Q., et al., 2008. Anti-inflammatory effects of sphingosine kinase modulation in inflammatory arthritis. J Immunol. 181, 8010-7.

Lai, W. Q., et al., 2009. Distinct roles of sphingosine kinase 1 and 2 in murine collagen-induced arthritis. J Immunol. 183, 2097-103.

Lee, M. J., et al., 1999. Vascular endothelial cell adherens junction assembly and morphogenesis induced by sphingosine-1-phosphate. Cell. 99, 301-12.

Lee, M. J., et al., 2001. Akt-mediated phosphorylation of the G protein-coupled receptor EDG-1 is required for endothelial cell chemotaxis. Mol Cell. 8, 693-704.

Lee, M. J., et al., 1998. Sphingosine-1-phosphate as a ligand for the G protein-coupled receptor EDG-1. Science. 279, 1552-5.

Leroux, M. E., et al., 2007. Sphingolipids and the sphingosine kinase inhibitor, SKI II, induce BCL-2-independent apoptosis in human prostatic adenocarcinoma cells. Prostate. 67, 1699-717.

Lettesjo, H., et al., 1998. Synovial fluid cytokines in patients with rheumatoid arthritis or other arthritic lesions. Scand J Immunol. 48, 286-92.

Limaye, V., et al., 2009. Chronic increases in sphingosine kinase-1 activity induce a pro-inflammatory, pro-angiogenic phenotype in endothelial cells. Cell Mol Biol Lett. 14, 424-41.

Lo, C. G., et al., 2005. Cyclical modulation of sphingosine-1-phosphate receptor 1 surface expression during lymphocyte recirculation and relationship to lymphoid organ transit. J Exp Med. 201, 291-301.

Maceyka, M., et al., 2005. SphK1 and SphK2, sphingosine kinase isoenzymes with opposing functions in sphingolipid metabolism. J Biol Chem. 280, 37118-29.

Mandala, S., et al., 2002. Alteration of lymphocyte trafficking by sphingosine-1-phosphate receptor agonists. Science. 296, 346-9.

Martel-Pelletier, J., et al., 2003. Cyclooxygenase-2 and prostaglandins in articular tissues. Semin Arthritis Rheum. 33, 155-67.

Masuko, K., et al., 2007. Sphingosine-1-phosphate attenuates proteoglycan aggrecan expression via production of prostaglandin E2 from human articular chondrocytes. BMC Musculoskelet Disord. 8, 29.

Matloubian, M., et al., 2004. Lymphocyte egress from thymus and peripheral lymphoid organs is dependent on S1P receptor 1. Nature. 427, 355-60.

Matsuura, M., et al., 2000. Effect of FTY720, a novel immunosuppressant, on adjuvant- and collagen-induced arthritis in rats. Int J Immunopharmacol. 22, 323-31.

McInnes, I. B., Schett, G., 2007. Cytokines in the pathogenesis of rheumatoid arthritis. Nat Rev Immunol. 7, 429-42.

Mechtcheriakova, D., et al., 2007. Sphingosine 1-phosphate phosphatase 2 is induced during inflammatory responses. Cell Signal. 19, 748-60.

Merrill, A. H., Jr., et al., 1997. Sphingolipids--the enigmatic lipid class: biochemistry, physiology, and pathophysiology. Toxicol Appl Pharmacol. 142, 208-25.

Mino, T., et al., 1998. Interleukin-1alpha and tumor necrosis factor alpha synergistically stimulate prostaglandin E2-dependent production of interleukin-11 in rheumatoid synovial fibroblasts. Arthritis Rheum. 41, 2004-13.

Mitra, P., et al., 2006. Role of ABCC1 in export of sphingosine-1-phosphate from mast cells. Proc Natl Acad Sci U S A. 103, 16394-9.

Muller-Ladner, U., et al., 1996. Synovial fibroblasts of patients with rheumatoid arthritis attach to and invade normal human cartilage when engrafted into SCID mice. Am J Pathol. 149, 1607-15.

Nicholas, R., et al., 2011. Development of oral immunomodulatory agents in the management of multiple sclerosis. Drug Des Devel Ther. 5, 255-74.

Nochi, H., et al., 2008. Stimulatory role of lysophosphatidic acid in cyclooxygenase-2 induction by synovial fluid of patients with rheumatoid arthritis in fibroblast-like synovial cells. J Immunol. 181, 5111-9.

Olsen, N. J., Stein, C. M., 2004. New drugs for rheumatoid arthritis. N Engl J Med. 350, 2167-79.

Ospelt, C., et al., 2004. Synovial activation in rheumatoid arthritis. Front Biosci. 9, 2323-34.

Paugh, S. W., et al., 2008. A selective sphingosine kinase 1 inhibitor integrates multiple molecular therapeutic targets in human leukemia. Blood. 112, 1382-91.

Peyruchaud, O., 2009. Novel implications for lysophospholipids, lysophosphatidic acid and sphingosine 1-phosphate, as drug targets in cancer. Anticancer Agents Med Chem. 9, 381-91.

Pi, X., et al., 2006. Sphingosine kinase 1-mediated inhibition of Fas death signaling in rheumatoid arthritis B lymphoblastoid cells. Arthritis Rheum. 54, 754-64.

Pitson, S. M., et al., 2005. Phosphorylation-dependent translocation of sphingosine kinase to the plasma membrane drives its oncogenic signalling. J Exp Med. 201, 49-54.

Pyne, S., Pyne, N. J., 2000. Sphingosine 1-phosphate signalling in mammalian cells. Biochem J. 349, 385-402.

Rosen, H., et al., 2003. Rapid induction of medullary thymocyte phenotypic maturation and egress inhibition by nanomolar sphingosine 1-phosphate receptor agonist. Proc Natl Acad Sci U S A. 100, 10907-12.

Rosen, H., et al., 2009. Sphingosine 1-Phosphate Receptor Signaling. Annu Rev Biochem.

Rosenfeldt, H. M., et al., 2001. EDG-1 links the PDGF receptor to Src and focal adhesion kinase activation leading to lamellipodia formation and cell migration. FASEB J. 15, 2649-59.

Saba, J. D., Hla, T., 2004. Point-counterpoint of sphingosine 1-phosphate metabolism. Circ Res. 94, 724-34.

Sabbadini, R. A., 2006. Targeting sphingosine-1-phosphate for cancer therapy. Br J Cancer. 95, 1131-5.

Sanchez, T., Hla, T., 2004. Structural and functional characteristics of S1P receptors. J Cell Biochem. 92, 913-22.

Sato, K., et al., 2007. Critical role of ABCA1 transporter in sphingosine 1-phosphate release from astrocytes. J Neurochem. 103, 2610-9.

Schwab, S. R., et al., 2005. Lymphocyte sequestration through S1P lyase inhibition and disruption of S1P gradients. Science. 309, 1735-9.

Shiozawa, S., et al., 1983. Morphologic observations in the early phase of the cartilage-pannus junction. Light and electron microscopic studies of active cellular pannus. Arthritis Rheum. 26, 472-8.

Spiegel, S., Milstien, S., 2003. Sphingosine-1-phosphate: an enigmatic signalling lipid. Nat Rev Mol Cell Biol. 4, 397-407.

Strader, C. R., et al., 2011. Fingolimod (FTY720): A Recently Approved Multiple Sclerosis Drug Based on a Fungal Secondary Metabolite. J Nat Prod. 74, 900-7.

Sugimoto, N., et al., 2003. Inhibitory and stimulatory regulation of Rac and cell motility by the G12/13-Rho and Gi pathways integrated downstream of a single G protein-coupled sphingosine-1-phosphate receptor isoform. Mol Cell Biol. 23, 1534-45.

Taha, T. A., et al., 2004. Sphingosine-1-phosphate receptors: receptor specificity versus functional redundancy. Biochim Biophys Acta. 1682, 48-55.

Taha, T. A., et al., 2006. Sphingosine kinase: biochemical and cellular regulation and role in disease. J Biochem Mol Biol. 39, 113-31.

Takabe, K., et al., 2010. Estradiol induces export of sphingosine 1-phosphate from breast cancer cells via ABCC1 and ABCG2. J Biol Chem. 285, 10477-86.

Takabe, K., et al., 2008. "Inside-out" signaling of sphingosine-1-phosphate: therapeutic targets. Pharmacol Rev. 60, 181-95.

Tsunemi, S., et al., 2010. Effects of the novel immunosuppressant FTY720 in a murine rheumatoid arthritis model. Clin Immunol. 136, 197-204.

Van Brocklyn, J. R., et al., 2000. Sphingosine-1-phosphate is a ligand for the G protein-coupled receptor EDG-6. Blood. 95, 2624-9.

Van Brocklyn, J. R., et al., 1998. Dual actions of sphingosine-1-phosphate: extracellular through the Gi-coupled receptor Edg-1 and intracellular to regulate proliferation and survival. J Cell Biol. 142, 229-40.

Visentin, B., et al., 2006. Validation of an anti-sphingosine-1-phosphate antibody as a potential therapeutic in reducing growth, invasion, and angiogenesis in multiple tumor lineages. Cancer Cell. 9, 225-38.

Vogel, P., et al., 2009. Incomplete inhibition of sphingosine 1-phosphate lyase modulates immune system function yet prevents early lethality and non-lymphoid lesions. PLoS One. 4, e4112.

Wang, F., et al., 2007. Reduction of CD4 positive T cells and improvement of pathological changes of collagen-induced arthritis by FTY720. Eur J Pharmacol. 573, 230-40.

Xia, P., et al., 2000. An oncogenic role of sphingosine kinase. Curr Biol. 10, 1527-30.

Yamazaki, Y., et al., 2000. Edg-6 as a putative sphingosine 1-phosphate receptor coupling to Ca(2+) signaling pathway. Biochem Biophys Res Commun. 268, 583-9.

Zhang, Z., Schluesener, H. J., 2007. FTY720: a most promising immunosuppressant modulating immune cell functions. Mini Rev Med Chem. 7, 845-50.

Zhao, C., et al., 2008. Specific and overlapping sphingosine-1-phosphate receptor functions in human synoviocytes: impact of TNF-alpha. J Lipid Res. 49, 2323-37.

12

Modern Pharmacological Approaches to Therapies: Substances Tested in Animal Models of Rheumatoid Arthritis

Katarina Bauerova[1], Silvester Poništ[1], Radomir Nosal'[1], Maria Stančikova[2] and Jozef Rovensky[2]
[1]*Institute of Experimental Pharmacology and Toxicology, Slovak Academy of Sciences,*
[2]*National Institute of Rheumatic Diseases*
Slovakia

1. Introduction

Preclinical research on animal models of rheumatoid arthritis (RA) is very important for alerting the healthcare and scientific community and pharmaceutical companies of the existence of new or "forgotten" molecules. Most antirheumatics have side-effects when used in higher doses and/or within long-term dosage. Combinatory therapy is expected to have a higher efficacy without increased toxicity. Methotrexate (MTX) has become the main immunosuppressive substance used in the treatment of patients with RA. However, the use of MTX has to be limited due to its toxic manifestations, e.g. abdominal disorder, alopecia, oral ulcers, and cytopenia (Alarcon et al., 1989). Ineffectiveness of treatment can be also observed. In the survey of McKendry and Dale (McKendry & Dale, 1993), due to the risk of treatment, termination was substantiated in 75% of patients with RA taking MTX for 60 months. An adverse drug effect proved to be a more common reason for treatment termination (53%) compared to loss/lack of beneficial effect (22%), other reasons (16%), or lost of follow-up (9%). On the other hand, the therapeutic efficacy of MTX can be increased by combination with other synthetic drugs or inhibitors of TNF-α (Smolen et al., 2010). Application of biological therapy (antibodies or soluble receptors of TNF-α, IL-1 and IL-6) represents a great progress in the therapy of RA. Yet biological treatment is also frequently combined with MTX (Maini et al., 1998; Weinblatt et al., 1999). There are countless possibilities for combinations with MTX. Many substances were neglected when they failed to show good efficacy in monotherapy compared to standard antirheumatics. They would not get a second chance if the expected reduction of clinical parameters (mainly edema of joints) did not materialize, despite the fact that they improved many biochemical disease markers. Our research in the last years was focused on evaluation of new therapeutics for the combinations of the classical immunosuppressive treatment with immunomodulators and compounds affecting reduction/oxidation homeostasis.

Development of drugs for the therapy of RA has been very intensive in recent years. Biological therapy targeted on neutralizing the effect of antiinflammatory cytokines, particularly TNF-α, IL-1 and IL-6, by using antibodies or soluble receptors provided a great progress in RA therapy. However, not even these expensive drugs are able to cure RA definitely, although they remarkably inhibit the development of arthritis and improve the life quality of patients. Following treatment interruption, a fast development of RA occurs. Biological therapy also has adverse effects, such as development of resistance and secondary infections. For these reasons, the search for new drugs which could avoid these infections or suppress them is still an up-to-date problem. As already mentioned, the most frequently applied conventional drug for RA has been MTX. Its application is usually additional to the biological therapy or it is used in combination with other conventional drugs. Intensive immunosuppressive treatment with MTX or biological therapy adversely affects immunological homeostasis of the organism and increases the risk of infections. For these reasons, there is a search for alternative immunomodulatory approaches, which could minimize side effects of immunosuppressive therapy on cellular and humoral immunity. One possibility is represented by the combination of immunosuppressive and immunostimulatory substances or compounds regulating redox balance of the organism. Their application can establish immunological and redox homeostasis and increase resistance of the organism to infections.

The focus of this chapter is mostly on substances of natural origin possessing antiinflammatory, antioxidative or immunomodulating properties along with minimal side effects when administered to animals. The safety of long-term therapy of RA is very important, because patients with RA are usually treated for two or more decades. We describe our results obtained in adjuvant arthritis (AA) with endogenous antioxidants as carnosine and coenzyme Q_{10}, glucomannan and Imunoglukan®, as well as selected extracts and compounds from plants. These results will be confronted with results of other authors from preclinical and clinical studies. The aim is to present an overview of the potential of new compounds for the therapy of RA with the focus on approving their ability for combination therapy with methotrexate.

2. Adjuvant arthritis: An animal model for preclinical evaluation of new antirheumatics

In AA the injection of rats with complete or incomplete adjuvant induces polyarthritis, possibly by way of a mechanism involving heat shock proteins. Arthritis induced in rats with intradermal injection of adjuvants containing mycobacteria is an animal model often used for evaluation of potential antirheumatic drugs. This model is also a good methodological tool for investigation of pathological mechanisms in RA. An intradermal injection, into the base of the tail, with heat-killed *Mycobacterium tuberculosis* in incomplete Freund´s adjuvant (IFA) results in destructive arthritis within 14 days in susceptible Dark Agouti or Lewis inbred rat strains. AA can also be induced with cell walls from other bacterial types in IFA, although the arithrogenicity varies (Joe et al., 1999). In many experiments, the induction of arthritis is achieved also with *Mycobacterium butyricum* in IFA (Akiyama et al., 2005; Bauerova et al., 2006, 2009). Basic clinical manifestations of AA are paw swelling, infiltration of mononuclear and polymorphonuclear phagocytes into joints, formation of pannus, periostitis and erosions of cartilage and bone (Williams et al., 1998). The intensity of AA development is described by so-called "basic clinical parameters", i.e. arthritic score, hind paw edema, which are usually measured once a week over the whole duration of the experiment. Increased synthesis of TNF- α, IL-1 and IL-6 is detected as early as day four after adjuvant injection. The disease progresses rapidly over several weeks in what appears clinically to be a monophasic process. Granulocytes and autoreactive CD41

cells play major roles in the disease. Humoral immune mechanisms appear not to contribute to the disease process (Joe et al., 1999).
AA has been extensively used for pharmaceutical testing, and therefore much data exists for comparison in humans. While this model does not mimic perfectly the condition of human arthritis, it is easily reproducible, well defined and has proven useful for the development of new therapies for arthritis, as exemplified also by cytokine blockade therapies (Bendele et al., 1999). AA has been used in the evaluation of nonsteroidal inflammatory drugs, such as phenylbutazone and aspirin during the early 1960s, and later COX-2 inhibitors such as celecoxib were studied. AA in rats shares many features with human arthritis, including genetic linkage, synovial $CD4^+$ cells and T cell dependence. On the contrary, one of the major differences between the AA model and human arthritis is simply that the inciting agent is known in the model, though the need for any specific antigen is controversial.

2.1 Markers applied in adjuvant arthritis

The parameters characterizing efficacy of the substances tested on the immunological, oxidative and inflammatory processes will be reported in this chapter. The spectrum of these parameters is suitable for the description of AA development and provides optimal possibilities for studying pharmacological influence of the substances tested as well as for the elucidation of the mechanisms of their action. In our laboratory, plasma and blood samples were collected regularly from animals in light anesthesia. Tissue samples were collected at the end of the experiment after sacrificing the anesthesised animals. The end of the experiment was mostly day 28 after injection of *Mycobacterium butyricum*. All characteristics monitored could be divided into three groups: clinical, biochemical and immunological parameters. For data interpretation and statistical analysis the data were expressed in terms of arithmetic mean ± S.E.M. In all cases the untreated arthritis group was compared with healthy control animals (*-symbol), the treated arthritis groups were compared with the untreated arthritis animals (+-symbol). For significance calculations the unpaired Student's t-test (two samples unequal variance) was used with the following significance designations extremely significant ($p < 0.001$), highly significant ($p < 0.01$), significant ($p < 0.05$); not significant ($p > 0.05$).

2.1.1 Clinical markers

We monitored one basic clinical parameter: the hind paw volume (HPV). The HPV increase was calculated as the percentage increase in the HPV on a given experimental day relative to the HPV at the beginning of the experiment. The hind paw volume was recorded on days 1, 14, 21, and 28 with the use of an electronic water plethysmometer (UGO BASILE, Comerio-Varese, Italy). In one of our previous experiments, we confirmed that this clinical parameter became significantly modified starting around day 14 and its significant increase in comparison with healthy controls is maintained until the end of the experiment (Bauerova et al., 2007).

2.1.2 Biochemical markers

Numerous studies have suggested an important role of oxidative stress (OS) in the pathogenesis of RA (Bauerova & Bezek, 1999; Bohanec et al., 2009). Several clinical studies as well as preclinical studies using animal models of RA have documented an imbalance in the body's redox homeostasis to a more pro-oxidative environment, suggesting that therapies

which restore the redox balance may have beneficial effects on the disease process. The role of reactive oxygen species (ROS) in the etiology of RA is supported by numerous studies documenting that not only the damaging effects of ROS but also the role that ROS play in regulating various inflammatory processes contributes to the pathogenesis of the disease (Kunsch et al., 2005). The net effect of redox signaling is highly specific changes in gene expression and in the cellular phenotype. Therefore, by serving as second messengers, ROS/reactive nitrogen species are not only toxic agents but also mediators of physiological function (Giustarini et al., 2004; Poli et al., 2004). Considering these facts, we monitored parameters of OS together with the inflammatory marker plasma C-reactive protein (CRP). For the determination of rat plasma CRP concentration, the ELISA kit from Immunology Consultant Laboratories, Inc. (ICL) was used. CRP comparable to HPV was already significantly increased in arthritic rats on day 14 (Bauerova et al., 2010).
γ-Glutamyltransferase (GGT), as a non-specific marker of inflammation and OS, has been assessed in different cells and tissues of the lymphatic system – T-lymphocytes, macrophages, spleen and thymus tissue (Koner et al., 1997). The ectoenzyme form of GGT is not present on non-active peripheral T-lymphocytes, but its expression rises after activation of native T-lymphocytes. In other tissues, GGT is essential for "scavenging" glutathione metabolites (mostly γ-glutamyl) and their transport into cells, where GSH is synthesized *de novo* (Carlisle et al., 2003). GGT is an important component of inflammatory processes since its activity is closely connected with the overall antioxidant status of the organism. In our experiments, GGT in the joint from the hind paw (cartilage and soft tissue without bone) and in spleeen tissue was determined at the end of the experiment, on day 28. The activity of GGT was measured by the method of (Orlowski & Meister, 1970), modified by (Ondrejickova et al., 1993). We found that the activity of GGT was approximately 3–6 times higher in AA animals than in healthy controls in the spleen and 1.4–2.3 times higher in the joint (Bauerova et al., 2006, 2008b, 2009; Sotnikova et al., 2009). We assume that the increased activity of GGT in AA is a result of elevated systemic OS. The finding that the GGT activity is also elevated in peripheral joint tissue is in good agreement with clinical studies of patients with RA who had increased levels of GGT not only in the serum and urine but also in synovial fluid (Rambabu et al., 1990). In one of our studies we showed a good correlation between GGT activity in joint tissue and the HPV of arthritic animals (Bauerova et al., 2006). GGT expression has been detected in active lymphocytes that accumulate at the inflammation region, as observed in RA. Ishizuka et al. (2007) found that neutralizing antibodies against GGT had a therapeutic effect on joint destruction in collagen-induced arthritis in mice. Elevated expression and activity of GGT in joint tissue is a good marker for synovial inflammation and bone resorption. Substances able to reduce the activity and/or expression of GGT could be important for RA therapy. OS, a consequence of chronic inflammatory processes occurring in AA, increased after the experimental day 14, which was also the onset of clinical manifestations of the disease. OS increased the consumption of endogenous antioxidants in plasma and thus caused a lowering of the plasma antioxidant capacity, measured as the total antioxidant status with RANDOX® TAS kit (Bauerova et al., 2009, Mihalova et al., 2007). A frequently used marker of lipid peroxidation is malondialdehyde (MDA), assessed as an adduct with thiobarbituric acid (TBA). We used the substances reacting with thiobarbituric acid measured in plasma at 535nm (Brown & Kelly, 1996). Clinical studies have shown increased plasmatic levels of MDA in patients with RA (Baskol et al., 2005, 2006; Sarban et al., 2005). The level of MDA in the plasma of arthritic animals was also elevated (Bauerova et al., 2008b, 2009; He et al., 2006; Sotnikova et al., 2009;

Strosova et al., 2008, 2009; Tastekin et al., 2007). In recent years, methods based on chemiluminescence and fluorescence measurements have been widely used for determination of ROS, RNS and lipid peroxidation metabolites. Fluorescent protein adducts are derivatives formed by reaction of secondary metabolites of lipid peroxidation (especially HNE and MDA) with free amino groups of proteins (Aldini et al., 2007; Requena et al., 1996). In murine and human serum, albumin protein fraction was identified as the most fluorescent fraction of proteins (Tsuchida et al., 1985). Several authors have suggested that protein adducts with secondary metabolites of lipid peroxidation also have immunogenic properties and may play a significant role in the pathogenesis of auto-immune diseases including RA (Kurien et al., 2006; Tuma, 2002). This highlights the importance of monitoring these adducts in auto-immune, chronic inflammatory diseases. The presence of oxidative damage in AA plasma was evaluated in our experiments also by measurement of fluorescence adducts in plasma. Two types of aldehydes were measured: HNE and MDA adducts of proteins (Biasi et al., 1995; Tsuchida et al., 1985). In rat AA, we were the first to monitor the HNE and MDA protein adducts in a time profile (Ponist et al., 2010). The level of HNE adducts was slightly increased already on day 7. The maximal level of HNE adducts was reached on day 14, and then it slowly decreased to the control level (day 28). Similar changes were recorded in the level of MDA adducts during the experiment, except that they were still significantly elevated on day 21 (Ponist et al., 2010). The time course of lipid peroxidation measured by the MDA protein adducts resembles the temporal pattern of ROS production by phorbol myristate acetate (PMA) - stimulated neutrophils measured by chemiluminescence of whole blood of arthritic animals, with maximum on day 14 and 21 (Nosal et al., 2007). Recent evidence from animal models of RA emphasizes the importance of neutrophils in the initiation and progression of AA (Cross et al., 2006). There are multiple experimental studies dedicated to neutrophil-generated chemiluminescence of whole blood (Arnhold et al., 1994; Cedergren et al., 2007; Miesel et al., 1996) and of synovial fluid (Arnhold et al., 1994; Cedergren et al., 2007), depending on the disease severity in patients with RA. An increase in whole blood chemiluminescence (2–8 fold) was shown in RA patients compared with healthy volunteers (Miesel et al., 1996). The results published by Nosal (Nosal et al., 2007) are in good agreement with this finding. Arthritic animals had significantly elevated spontaneous chemiluminescence from the seventh experimental day until the end of experiment (day 28). Neutrophils in whole blood of AA animals reacted excessively to stimulation with PMA and produced 6–9 times more ROS. The development of AA in rats was also accompanied with an increase in blood neutrophil count when compared with control animals (Nosal et al., 2007). Oxidative damage to the tissues in AA was demonstrated - ROS levels in the joint and the spleen were analysed by chemiluminiscence assessment (Drabikova et al., 2009). Measurements in the joint were completed by spectrophotometric analysis of myeloperoxidase activity in an experiment focused on evaluation of therapeutic effects of two stilbenoids in AA (Macickova et al., 2010). In this study, myeloperoxidase (MPO) activity in the hind paw joint homogenate of arthritic rats was approx. 3-times higher than in healthy controls. This finding is of importance as MPO is the most abundant enzyme in neutrophils. It is a marker of OS and ROS generated by MPO can deplete the NO level in vascular endothelium (Brennan & Hazen, 2003). MPO enhances the binding of leukocytes, including monocytes and neutrophils, to the endothelium (Johansson et al., 1997). Vascular endothelial cells are also capable of secreting various cytokines, which are potent chemoattractants for neutrophils. Both MPO and cytokines participate in the recruitment of cells into the area of inflammation. Lefkowitz et al. (1999) reported that MPO may be an important mediator in the inflammatory response.

Moreover, in the scale of systemic OS parameters, phagocytosis, oxidative burst and metabolic activity of rat granulocytes isolated from peripheral blood were monitored. Flow cytometric analysis was used for these measurements, according to the method published by Kronek et al. (2010) and modified for the model of AA (Bauerova et al., 2010a). Interestingly, increased production of ROS by neutrophils recorded by whole blood chemiluminiscence measurements emerged already in an early phase of disease, on the day 7. We therefore decided to investigate this finding more precisely using flow cytometry. Another reason was that the changes in neutrophils occur before the clinical parameter HPV starts to be increased. Due to arthritis, both phagocytosis and oxidative burst were already significantly increased on experimental day 7. Metabolic activity of neutrophils as the percentage of double positive cells (simultaneously phagocytotic and positive for oxidative burst) was decreased. This finding could be explained by an increased number of "arthritic" neutrophils, which are positive only for oxidative burst and therefore are not counted as double positive cells (Bauerova et al., 2010a). Further we analyzed in plasma the level of one of the most important endogenous antioxidants in rats - coenzyme Q_9 (CoQ_9). Significant changes in the levels of CoQ_9 and/or CoQ_{10} have been noted in a wide variety of diseases in both animal and human studies. These changes may be caused by impairment in CoQ biosynthesis or excessive utilization of CoQ by the body, or any combination of these processes (Bauerova et al., 2008a; Littarru et al., 1991). In this experiment, we focused on evaluating the CoQ_9 plasmatic levels as the dominant form of CoQ in rats. Its concentration is about 10 times higher than the concentration of CoQ_{10} (Dallner & Sindelar, 2000). In AA the arthritis process increases significantly the level of CoQ_9 in comparison with healthy controls. Evidently, the arthritic processes stimulate the synthesis of CoQ_9 and its transport to plasma. In addition to monitoring lipid peroxidation, also protein oxidation was followed up in AA. Arthritis, similarly to many other diseases, is accompanied by oxidative damage of plasma proteins induced by the action of free radicals. Protein carbonyls (aldehydes and ketones) are produced directly by oxidation or *via* reactions with other molecules generated by the oxidation process. The assay of protein carbonyls as biomarkers of OS in various diseases is with advantage used in diagnostics because of the relatively early formation and relative stability of carbonylated proteins (Dalle-Donne et al., 2003). The ability of certain compounds to reduce the amount of carbonyls is considered as one of the indirect proofs of their antioxidant activity. In our AA experiments, enzyme linked immunosorbent assay (ELISA) was used most frequently for quantitative determination of protein carbonyls in plasma (Buss et al., 1997). The first measurement of protein carbonyls in our experiments with AA was performed in a study with carboxymethyl (1/3)-b-D-glucan isolated from *Saccharomyces cerevisiae* administered to arthritic rats (Kogan et al., 2005). In this study, the content of carbonyls in the arthritic animals increased significantly in comparison with healthy controls and protein carbonyl determination in plasma was performed according to the method described by (Levine et al., 1990) and modified in agreement with the previously applied experimental conditions (Bauerova et al., 2002). Also in the following experiments with AA we found significant damage of proteins caused by oxidative stress accompanying arthritis (Bauerova et al., 2005b; Strosova et al., 2009). In addition to determination of protein carbonyls in plasma, we performed an assay of carbonyls in brain tissue and applied it as a marker of antioxidative properties of carnosine evaluated for monotherapy of AA (Ponist et al., 2011). Protein carbonyls in brain tissue homogenates were significantly elevated, comparable to protein carbonyls in plasma. This novel finding emphasizes the systemic role of OS in chronic inflammatory diseases such as AA, with oxidatively modified proteins, not only in directly affected tissues (cartilage, bone and skeletal muscle).

2.1.3 Immunological markers

RA is associated with elevated levels of IL-1 in the synovium. IL-1 is closely related to inflammation and articular damage in several arthritis models and it is therefore generally accepted that IL-1 has a pivotal role in the pathophysiology of RA. In particular, IL-1 is a potent stimulator of synoviocytes, chondrocytes and osteoblasts. Moreover, IL-1 is a key mediator of synovial inflammation and pannus formation (Dinarello & Moldawer, 2002). It has a severe impact on different cell populations and exerts biological effects, e.g. increased synthesis of acute phase reactants. IL-1α is secreted by monocytes/macrophages activated via TNF-α and/or bacterial endotoxin. Furthermore, IL-1α markedly potentiates the toxic effect of TNF-α in animal experiments (Waage, et al., 1991). In the AA model used in our experiments, IL-1α was significantly increased in plasma on day 14 and also on day 28 (Bauerova et al., 2007, 2009; Bauerova et al., 2010a). The course of plasma levels of both pro-inflammatory cytokines IL-1α and TNF-α in AA was very similar, with the maximum on day 14 and with decreasing levels on days 21 and 28 in comparison to day 14 (Bauerova et al., 2009). These results are of importance as TNF-α controls the gene expression of various cytokines and chemokines in different cell types engaged in the host immune response to infection and triggers the cascade of cytokines acting in the inflammatory response. The efficient biological activities of TNF-α include direct activation of T- and B-lymphocytes, macrophages, and natural killer cells, release of acute-phase proteins, and endothelial cell activation. The activated monocyte or macrophage represents the primary source for TNF-α, especially after IFN-γ priming. TNF-α is a key regulator of other pro-inflammatory cytokines such as IL-1α, IL-6, and IL-8. Further, we followed the course of monocyte chemoattractant protein 1 (MCP-l) (Bauerova et al., 2009). This chemokine is mainly expressed by macrophages in response to a wide range of cytokines, e.g. TNF-α and IL-1.

In this experiment, the significant maximum of MCP-1 plasma level measured on day 21 and the following decrease is in close association with kinetics of both TNF-α and IL-1α. According to the target cell specificity, MCP-1 was postulated to play a pathognomonic role in various diseases with monocyte cell infiltration. MCP-1 is a member of the CC chemokine subfamily that modulates monocyte chemotaxis both *in vitro* (Oppenheim et al., 1991) and *in vivo* (Rollins, 1996; Volejnikova et al., 1997). MCP-1 displays chemotactic activity for monocytes and basophils but not for neutrophils or eosinophils. Expression of MCP-1 has been detected in a number of pathologic conditions associated with monocyte aggregation, including atherosclerosis, arthritis, and glomerulonephritis (Rollins, 1996). The synovial fluid (SF) and serum MCP-1 concentrations are significantly higher in RA patients. This suggests that MCP-1 is mainly produced locally by activated cells, where it may exacerbate and sustain inflammation by attracting proinflammatory leukocytes, predominantly monocytes (Stankovic et al., 2009). Substances that can suppress the production of MCP-1 have shown beneficial effects in animal models of arthritis (Guglielmotti et al., 2002; Inoue et al., 2001). A completely different picture was revealed for IL-4. The level of this anti-inflammatory cytokine was increasing with time with the maximum observed on day 28 in AA animals (Bauerova et al., 2009). IL-4 is a pleiotropic cytokine produced by mature Th2 cells and mastocyte- and/or basophil-derived cells. IL-4 has marked inhibitory effects on the expression and release of monocyte-derived pro-inflammatory cytokines, e.g. IL-1, TNF-α,

IL-6, IL-8, and MIP- 1α. It was shown to suppress macrophage cytotoxic activity, parasite killing, and macrophage-derived nitric oxide production (Vannier, et al., 1992). In our experiments, detection of plasma IL-1α, IL-4, TNF-α, and MCP-1 was done by the flowcytometric (Cytomics FC 500, Beckman Coulter Inc. Fullerton, USA) fluorescent bead-based multiplex assay Rat Cytokine Flow Cytomix Multiplex (Bender Med System, GmbH., Austria). Additionally for determination of IL-1α in plasma an ELISA kit from Bender MedSystems or from R&D Systems Quantikine® was used and to as assessed MCP in plasma by Instant ELISA kit from eBioscience®.

3. Newer experimental therapies with antioxidants evaluated in AA

Oxygen metabolism has an important role in the pathogenesis of RA. ROS produced in the course of cellular oxidative phosphorylation and by activated phagocytic cells during oxidative bursts exceed the physiological buffering capacity and result in OS. The excessive production of ROS can damage proteins, lipids, nucleic acids, and matrix components. They also serve as important intracellular signaling molecules that amplify the synovial inflammatory-proliferative response. Repetitive cycles of hypoxia and reoxygenation associated with changes in synovial perfusion are postulated to activate hypoxia-inducible factor-1α and nuclear factor-κB, two key transcription factors that are regulated by changes in cellular oxygenation and cytokine stimulation, and that in turn orchestrate the expression of a spectrum of genes critical to the persistence of synovitis. Understanding of the complex interactions involved in these pathways might allow the development of novel therapeutic strategies for RA (Hitchon & El-Gabalawy, 2004). Free radicals from oxygen metabolism destroy antioxidant systems (Harris, 2003). Researchers such as Heliovaara et al. (1994) have suggested that enzymatic and/or nonenzymatic antioxidant systems are impaired in RA. RA patients are therefore exposed to oxidant stress (Harris, 2003). Consequently, a number of different activities of antioxidant enzymes, such as superoxide dismutase, glutathione peroxidase, catalase, and glutathione reductase have been reported to be effective in treating RA (Blake et al., 1981; Mazetti et al., 1996; Shah & Vohora, 2002). Some other researchers found that RA patients were more inclined to lipid peroxidation because of the reduced antioxidant defense system (Rowley et al., 1984; Gambhir et al., 1997). The synovial fluids from patients with RA were found to present high levels of antioxidant damage (Miyata et al., 1998; Chapman et al., 1999). According to Babior (2000) reactive oxidants are essential tools for the pathogenesis of RA.

There is widespread availability and interest in the use of antioxidant supplementation by patients with inflammatory arthritis, although proof of efficacy is modest. A traditional Mediterranean diet relatively high in antioxidants improved RA disease and functional status after 3 months compared with a standard 'Western' diet, although clinical improvement was not associated with any significant change in plasma levels of antioxidants (Heliovaara et al., 1994; Skoldstam et al., 2003). In a separate study of patients with RA, supplementation with the antioxidants vitamin A, E, and C increased plasma antioxidant levels with a corresponding decrease in MDA, a key marker of OS; however, a clinical response was not reported (Jaswal et al., 2003). Specific supplementation of oral vitamin E, the major lipid-soluble antioxidant in human plasma, erythrocytes, and tissue, had no effect on RA disease activity or indices of inflammation but did improve pain, suggesting a role in central analgesia mechanisms (Edmonds et al., 1997). Various forms of antioxidant therapy have demonstrated promising results in experimental arthritis models (Bandt et al., 2002; Cuzzocrea et al., 2000; Venkatraman & Chu, 1999).

As resulted also from our previous experiments (Bauerova et al., 2005a, 2005b, 2008a, 2008b, 2009, Drabikova et al., 2009; Drafi et al., 2010; Jancinova et al., 2009; Kogan et al., 2005; Macickova et al., 2010; Ponist et al., 2010; Sotnikova et al., 2009; Strosova et al., 2008, 2009), all performed in the AA model, substances with antioxidant properties have a high potency to be used in therapy of RA. They decreased the progression of AA when administered to rats with AA over the period of 28 days. For our experiments, we chose substances with antioxidative properties and low toxicity. These antioxidative substances were synthetic antioxidants, as pyridoindol derivatives, and natural substances possessing antioxidative properties. We chose compounds and extracts isolated from plants, polysaccharides isolated from yeast and mushrooms and finally also endogenous antioxidants. An overview of some selected results is given below along with new unpublished data to provide complex information about administration of antioxidants in AA.

3.1 Natural substances isolated from plants

The world of plants is an unlimited source of compounds with healing effects, including antiinflammtory, antioxidative and immunomodulating properties. We chose some of them for our experiments with AA. Figure 1 compares all these plant ingredients concerning their effect on the basic clinical parameter - change of hind paw volume (HPV), together with selected parameters of OS as plasmatic TBARS and GGT assessed in spleen and joint tissue homogenates. We compared the effect of *Boswellia serrata* extract (Bo), *Arctostaphylos uva-ursi* extract (UV), *Zingiber officinale* extract (Zg) in combination with two previous extracts (Bo-UV-Zg), sesame oil in combination with *Arctostaphylos uva-ursi* extract (Bo-So), arbutin (Ar), curcumin (CU), Pycnogenol® (PYC) and two stilbenoids - pinosylvin (PIN) and pterostilbene (PTE). The compounds and extracts were all given per os in a single dose immediately after induction of AA and were administered daily until the end of the experiment - experimental day 28. The experimental protocol was approved by the Ethics Committee of the Institute of Experimental Pharmacology and Toxicology and by the Slovak State Veterinary and Food Administration. AA was induced by a single intradermal injection of heat-inactivated *Mycobacterium butyricum* in incomplete Freund's adjuvant (Difco Laboratories, Detroit, MI, USA) to male Lewis rats. The injection was performed near the tail base. All experiments included healthy animals (HC), arthritic animals not treated (AA), arthritic animals treated with the compounds/extracts studied. The oral daily doses used were 30 mg/kg b.w for AA-PIN and AA-PTE, 10 mg /kg b.w for A-PYC, 50 mg/kg b.w for AA-UV, AA-Bo, AA-Bo-So, AA-Ar and AA-CU, 50+25+25 mg/kg b.w for the mixture AA-Bo-UV-Zg and 0.1 ml/kg b.w. for sesame oil. For statistical analysis of the obtained data the same procedure was applied in all experimental cases. The data for all parameters are expressed as arithmetic mean ± S.E.M. For significance calculations unpaired Student`s *t*-test was used with *$p<0.05$ (significant), **$p<0.01$ (very significant), ***$p<0.001$ (extremely significant). The arthritis group was compared with healthy control animals (*-symbol). The treated arthritis groups were compared with untreated arthritis (+-symbol). In each experimental group 8–10 animals were used. In Figure 1 the reduction of HPV and OS parameters is illustrated in relation to untreated arthritic rats (100% represented by dot-and-dash line). The situation for AA is complicated due to the dominant involvement of Th 1-driven autoimmune etiopathology. OS in this animal model occurs as a reaction to autoimmune processes. Under these conditions, control of OS is of secondary importance, although it could enhance immunomodulatory therapy of RA (Bauerova et al., 2011). Figure 1 clearly shows that plant-related treatment is not enough for successful improvement of

HPV (excluding pinosylvin) although some of the compounds and extracts tested (e.g. UV, Ar , CU, Bo-So or Bo-UV-Zg) achieved a biochemical improvement in the body redox state expressed as reduction of plasmatic TBARS and GGT activity assessed in joint and spleen. Moreover, CU was found to be a potent inhibitor of neutrophil functions in experimental arthritis. AA was accompanied by an increased number of neutrophils in blood and by a more pronounced spontaneous as well as PMA stimulated chemiluminescence. Whereas the arthritis-related alterations in neutrophil count and in spontaneous chemiluminescence were not modified by CU, the increased reactivity of neutrophils to PMA was less evident in CU-treated animals. The effects of CU were comparable with those of methotrexate. CU was found to be a potent inhibitor of neutrophil functions (Jancinova et al., 2009). As neutrophils are considered to be cells with the greatest capacity to inflict damage within diseased joints, the observed effects could support the beneficial use of CU in RA treatment. Further the beneficial effect of sesame oil (So) administered alone on markers of OS accompanying AA was demonstrated not only by decrease of plasma TBARS, decrease of GGT activity in the joint and spleen tissues, but also the level of protein carbonyls, TAC in plasma and activity of NAGA in serum and in the kidney were improved, yet not significantly. In HPV the maximal increase was found on day 28 of AA, and at the same time we observed a

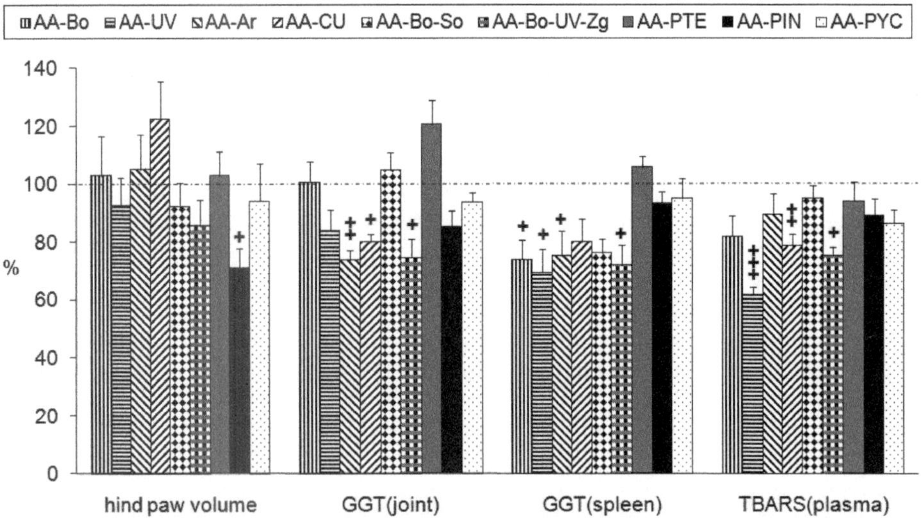

Fig. 1. Comparison of the effect of different plant treatments in adjuvant arthritis (AA) on reduction of hind paw volume (HPV) and on GGT (γ-glutamyltransferase) activity in spleen and joint and level of TBARS (thiobarbituric acid reactive substances) in plasma measured on experimental day 28. Changes in parameters are illustrated in relation to untreated arthritic rats (100% represented by dot-and-dash line). The data were expressed as arithmetic mean ± S.E.M. Statistical significance was evaluated applying Student's t-test for independent variables: +P < 0.05, ++P < 0.01, and +++P < 0.001 compared to untreated arthritic animals. *Boswellia serrata extract* (Bo), *Arctostaphylos uva-ursi extract* (UV), *Zingiber officinale extract* (Zg), combination of three previous extracts (Bo-UV-Zg), sesame oil in combination with *Arctostaphylos uva-ursi* extract (Bo-So), arbutin (Ar), curcumin (CU), Pycnogenol® (PYC), pinosylvin (PIN) and pterostilbene (PTE).

significant decrease of aortic endothelium-dependent relaxation. Administration of So resulted in mild, non-significant decrease of hind paw swelling and in significantly increased acetylcholine-evoked relaxation of aorta (Sotnikova et al., 2009).

3.1.1 Pinosylvin and methotrexate combination in AA

PIN [3′,5′-dihydroxystilbene] and PTE [3,5-dimethoxy-4′-hydroxystilbene] used in our experiments were synthesized and purified by Šmidrkal et al. (2010) and Harmatha et al. (2011). PIN and PTE are natural substances from the stilbenoid group, wide-spread in a variety of plants. They are chemically related to resveratrol. Both substances studied inhibited significantly the chemiluminescence (CL) of whole human blood and the CL of isolated human neutrophils (Perečko et al. 2008). The new information on the inhibitory effect of PIN and PTE on HPV, production of ROS and MPO activity suggests that the protective effect of PIN may be beneficial in controlling inflammation in experimental AA (Macickova et al., 2010). PIN was also the most effective in reducing HPV on day 28, when administered in the dose of 30 mg/kg b.w. per os (Fig. 1). According to these findings we chose PIN as a suitable candidate for combination therapy with methotrexate (MTX). In the combination AA-PIN+MTX, arthritic animals were treated twice a week with MTX in the oral dose of 0.4 mg/kg b.w. and daily with PIN in the oral dose of 50 mg/kg b.w. Monotherapy was performed with the same doses. In addition to the routine statistical analysis the combination treatment was compared to individual MTX treatment (#-symbol). In arthritic rats, PIN potentiated the antiarhritic effect of MTX on days 14 and 21, evaluated as decrease of HPV (Table 1). Activity of GGT in spleen homogenate (Table 2), plasma levels of MCP-1 and CRP (Table 3) were not improved by addition of PIN to MTX, due to the prominent effect of MTX alone on these parameters. Arthritic animals showed an increase in OS, evaluated as plasma levels of TBARS. PIN enhanced the antioxidant effect of MTX (Table 2) (Bauerova et al., 2010b).

HPV (%)	Day 14	Day 21	Day 28
CO	8.48 ±0.69	12.98 ±0.97	17.05 ±0.83
AA	33.68 ±5.22 ***	87.24 ±7.50 ***	81.62 ±7.20 ***
AA-PIN	26.30 ±2.61	86.02 ±4.56	84.03 ±5.51
AA-MTX	7.57 ± 0.87 +++	13.14 ± 2.22 +++	16.22 ± 2.10 +++
AA-PIN-MTX	4.34 ± 0.79 +++ / ##	7.49 ± 1.14 +++ / #	11.44 ± 1.16 +++

Table 1. Hind paw volume (HPV) changes in an experiment with methotrexate (MTX) and pinosylvine (PIN) in monotherapy and in combination therapy PIN+MTX measured in time profile. The data were expressed as arithmetic mean ± S.E.M. Statistical significance was evaluated applying Student's t-test for independent variables: *P < 0.05, **P < 0.01, and ***P < 0.001 compared to control healthy animals (CO); +P < 0.05, ++P < 0.01, and +++P < 0.001 compared to untreated arthritic animals (AA); #P < 0.05, ##P < 0.01, and ###P < 0.001 compared to methotrexate monotherapy (AA-MTX).

Parameters	CO	AA	AA-PIN	AA-MTX	AA-PIN-MTX
TBARS (nmol/ml)	10.59±0.23	19.10±0.53 ***	17.89±0.47	14.33±0.95 +++	11.78±0.47 +++/#
Activity of GGT in spleen (†)	19.977±1.843	90.45±4.52 ***	85.90±4.07	37.38±2.95 +++	35.47±1.89 +++

† - nmol 4-nitroaniline / min / g tissue

Table 2. Plasmatic level of TBARS (thiobarbituric acid reactive substances) and activity of GGT (γ-glutamyltransferase) in spleen measured on experimental day 28 in an experiment with methotrexate (MTX) and pinosylvine (PIN) in monotherapy and in combination therapy PIN+MTX. For statistical analysis of data see table 1.

Parameters	CO	AA	AA-PIN	AA-MTX	AA-PIN-MTX
MCP-1 (μg/ml)	6.896±0.438	14.089±1.159 ***	9.470±0.603 ++	8.446±0.616 ++	8.316±0.257 ++
CRP (μg/ml)	337.4±14.8	722.6±49.3 ***	662.7±19.6	385.4±27.4 +++	366.2±8.8 +++

Table 3. Plasmatic level of MCP-1 (monocyte chemotactic protein-1) and CRP (C-reactive protein) measured on experimental day 14 in an experiment with methotrexate (MTX) and pinosylvine (PIN) in monotherapy and in combination therapy PIN+MTX. For statistical analysis of data see table 1.

Effect of PIN and MTX, applied separately or in combination, was further studied on spontaneous and stimulated chemiluminescence and neutrophil count in blood of arthritic rats. In rats treated with MTX, all the arthritis-induced changes were significantly reduced and this inhibition became more pronounced when MTX was applied along with PIN. MTX alone decreased neutrophil count, spontaneous and stimulated chemiluminescence by 28%, 41% and 43%, respectively, whereas in combination with PIN, it inhibited these parameters by 59%, 69% and 63%, respectively. Monotherapy with PIN failed to induce any detectable changes either in the number of neutrophils or in oxidant concentration (Jancinova et al., 2010).

RA is a common severe joint disease affecting all age groups. It is thus of great importance to develop new strategies for its treatment. As disease modifying anti-rheumatic drugs (DMARDs) often have side effects at high doses and/or during long-term administration, increased efficacy without increased toxicity is expected for combination therapy of RA. MTX, a folic acid antagonist, has become the predominant immunosuppressive agent used in the treatment of patients with RA (Williams et al., 1985). MTX acts mainly on actively proliferating cells during the S-phase of proliferation, suppresses macrophage function, modulates interleukin-1 (IL-1) and superoxide anion production, and inhibits neutrophil chemotaxis (Moreland et al., 1997). Furthermore, MTX treatment was shown to decrease synovial collagenase gene expression in patients with RA (Genestier et al., 2000). The effects of MTX in vivo may be mediated by reducing cell proliferation, increasing the rate of apoptosis of T cells, increasing endogenous adenosine release, altering the expression of cellular adhesion molecules, influencing production of cytokines, humoral responses and bone formation (Wessels et al., 2008). The use of MTX has been limited by some of its toxic manifestations, such as abdominal discomfort, alopecia, oral ulcerations, and cytopenia (Alarcon et al., 1989). In this case a lowering of the dose could be beneficial and this could be achieved by combination therapy, for which we could recommend PIN, as indicated by the results of our studies.

3.2 Natural substances isolated from yeast and mushrooms

The control of inflammation in RA patients by natural and synthetic substances with anti-inflammatory and/or antioxidant and immunomodulatory effects, which are safe also during long-term administration, could become a relevant part of RA therapy. Modulation of OS accompanying RA can offer a new approach and crucially modify treatment of this disease. The key goal of this proposal will be the investigation of the combination of immunosuppressive therapy of MTX with immunomodulators-antioxidants with the aim to achieve enhancement of its efficacy in RA treatment, which would enable dosage reduction in clinical conditions and, consequently, decrease the frequency of occurrence of its dose-dependent side effects. Thus new ways of supplementary or combinatory RA therapy are of great importance. The aim is to find an alternative or additive to classical RA therapy with natural molecules without side effects possessing immunomodulatory, antiinflammatory, and antioxidative properties.

In recent decades, polysaccharides isolated from botanical sources (mushrooms, algae, lichens, and higher plants) have attracted a great deal of attention in the biomedical arena because of their broad spectrum of therapeutic properties and relatively low toxicity (Tzianabos, 2000). Plant and mushroom polysaccharides reveal immunomodulatory effects that depend on polysaccharide structure and molecular weight (low molecular weight - inhibition, high molecular weight - activation) (Schepetkin & Quinn, 2006). Prokopova (Prokopova et al., 1993) were the first to describe a therapeutic effect of simple carbohydrates on AA. We were first to report on the protective antioxidant and antiinflammatory activities of carboxylated (1-3)-beta-D-glucan isolated from *Saccharomyces cerevisiae* in Lewis rats with AA (Kogan et al., 2005). Glucomannans (GM) from *Candida utilis* were evaluated in the same model. The antiarthritic activity for cell-wall GM was associated with antioxidant activity *in vivo* (Bauerova et al., 2006; Mihalova et al., 2007). In the following experiment, the beneficial action of GM was revealed mainly in HPV decrease. Further a decrease of the activity of GGT in the spleen, hind paw joint and muscle tissue homogenates, decrease of the plasmatic activity of N-acetyl-beta-D-glucosaminidase (NAGA), and finally suppression of lysozyme and peroxidase activity assessed in peritoneal macrophages were observed in arthritic animals treated with GM. All these findings speak in favor of the antiinflammatory activity of GM. Moreover, a significant improvement of the arthritis induced suppression of total antioxidant status and decrease of the level of the arthritis-associated protein carbonyls in plasma were detected. In this experiment two doses of GM - 5 and 7.5 mg/kg b.w. were evaluated successfully. Peroral and intraperitoneal ways of administration were also compared (Bauerova et al., 2008b). In the following study, we tested the effect of GM in a higher dose of 15 mg/kg b.w. administered per os. On day 28 after *Mycobacterium butyricum* induced AA, GM was found to reduce HPV. Neutrophil count in whole blood was significantly increased on day 28 after induction of AA, yet GM in the dose of 15 mg/kg b.w. did not change it significantly. The spontaneous and PMA-induced CL was significantly increased in whole blood of rats with AA in comparison with healthy controls. GM 15 mg/kg b.w. decreased spontaneous as well as PMA-stimulated CL. CL of spleen and joint in rats with AA was significantly increased in comparison with controls (3.38±1.07 mV/1mg wet weight *vs.* 1.33±0.16 mV/1mg wet weight, and 6.63±1.34 mV/100mg wet weight *vs.* 1.11±0.11 mV/100mg wet weight). GM significantly decreased CL of joints, while CL of the spleen was not affected by GM. The obtained results showed that GM reduced ROS generation in arthritic rats. The predominant decrease of extracellular ROS production suggests a protective effect of GM against tissue damage, especially in the hind paw joint of arthritic rats (Drabikova et al., 2009).

Further we decided to compare the effect of GM to Imunoglukan®, a beta-(1,3/1,6)-D-glucan (IMG), which was isolated from *Pleurotus ostreatus*. Figure 2 shows a comparison of the effect of GM and IMG on HPV as well as on OS parameters. GM was tested in two doses: 7.5 (GM1) and 15 mg/kg b.w (GM2). IMG was evaluated also in two doses: 1 (IMG1) and 2 mg/kg b.w. (IMG2). The experimental and statistical design was the same as described in section 3.1. of this chapter. Both GM as IMG were effective in reducing HPV and improving the oxidative status. As no clear dose dependency was shown, we chose for the next experiment higher doses with the aim to detect the more effective immunomodulator for combinatory therapy with MTX. The experiment included healthy intact animals as reference controls (CO), arthritic animals without any drug administration (AA), and arthritic animals with the administration of GM (AA-GM) in the oral daily dose of 15 mg/kg b.w. and of IMG (AA-IMG) in the oral daily dose of 2 mg/kg b.w. Table 4 shows that as to the capability of lowering the HPV no differences between GM and IMG were found. However, as to the antioxidant potential expressed as a more prominent decrease of

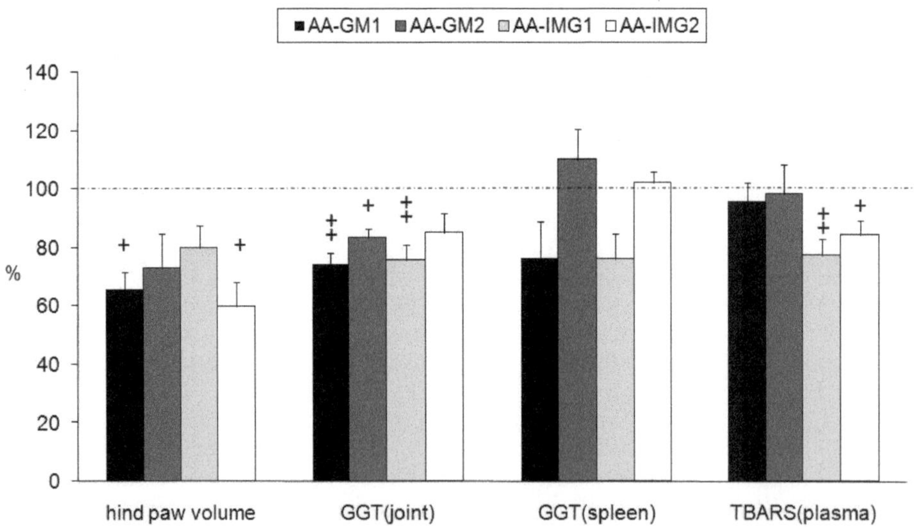

Fig. 2. Comparison of the effect of different glucomannan (GM) and Imunoglukan® (IMG) doses used as monotherapy in adjuvant arthritis (AA) on hind paw volume (HPV), GGT (γ-glutamyltransferase) activity in spleen and joint and level of TBARS (thiobarbituric acid reactive substances) in plasma measured on experimental day 28. Changes in parameters are illustrated in relation to untreated arthritic rats (100% represented by dot-and-dash line). For statistical analysis of data see Fig. 1.

TBARS accompanied with a more pronounced increase of TAS measured in plasma on day 28, IMG was more effective than GM.

Parameters	CO	AA	AA-GM	AA-IMG
HPV (%)	17.20±1.81	91.45±10.61 ***	66.57±3.84 +	54.50±7.77 +
TAS (mmol/l)	1.02±0.21	0.52±0.20 *	0.89±0.18	1.16±0.13 +
TBARS (nmol/ml)	3.50±0.20	5.90±0.20 ***	5.70±0.30	4.70±0.30 ++

Table 4. Changes in hind paw volume (HPV), plasmatic TAS (total antioxidant status) and plasmatic TBARS (thiobarbituric acid reactive substances) in an experiment with glucomannan (GM) and Imunoglukan® (IMG) measured on experimental day 28. For statistical analysis of data see table 1.

The good antioxidative and antiinflammatory effect of IMG stimulated us to study in a more complex way its effect on the course of the main cytokines/chemokines in AA. Daily administration of IMG suppressed significantly the levels of pro-inflammatory cytokines IL-1α (Table 5) and TNF-α (Table 6) on all days monitored. Moreover, the observed

IL-1α (pg/ml)	Day 14	Day 21	Day 28
CO	186.44±77.42	N.M.	N.M.
AA	732.90±128.56 ***	588.58±272.50	633.06±117.40 *
AA-IMG	339.80±117.40 +	168.88±38.98 +	184.40±18.44 +

N.M. - not measured

Table 5. Plasma level of IL-1 α (interleukin-1α) in an experiment with Imunoglukan® (IMG) analyzed in time profile. For statistical analysis of data see table 1.

TNF-α (pg/ml)	Day 14	Day 21	Day 28
CO	59.64±13.58	N.M.	N.M.
AA	202.10±26.23 ***	100.15±28.35	100.65±42.85
AA-IMG	98.58±27.43 ++	49.50±4.30 +	29.45±2.90 +

N.M. - not measured

Table 6. Plasma level of TNF-α (tumor necrosis factor-α) in an experiment with Imunoglukan® (IMG) analyzed in time profile. For statistical analysis of data see table 1.

inhibitory effect of IMG became stronger with time. After IMG treatment, the MCP-1 level was also decreasing significantly on days 14 and 21 (Table 7). The time course of the MCP-1 level was found to be comparable for treated and untreated arthritis animals. The level of cytokine IL-4 was increasing with time – the maximum was observed on day 28 in AA animals. IMG exerted probably an indirect time dependent inhibitory effect on this cytokine (Table 8).

MCP-1 (pg/ml)	Day 14	Day 21	Day 28
CO	229.44±4.87	N.M.	N.M.
AA	360.62±51.26 **	559.52±98.22 ***	363.28±89.57 *
AA-IMG	187.42±28.06 ++	363.28±89.57 +	287.42±108.02

N.M. - not measured

Table 7. Plasma level of MCP-1 (monocyte chemotactic protein-1) in an experiment with Imunoglukan® (IMG) analyzed in time profile. For statistical analysis of data see table 1.

IL-4 (pg/ml)	Day 14	Day 21	Day 28
CO	10.50±4.90	N.M.	N.M.
AA	25.00±10.75	31.78±11.26 *	40.43±4.58 ***
AA-IMG	23.05±4.50	10.15±4.15 +	7.70±3.85 +++

N.M. - not measured

Table 8. Plasma level of IL-4 (interleukin-4) in an experiment with Imunoglukan® (IMG) analyzed in time profile. For statistical analysis of data see table 1.

On the basis of all the obtained results with GM and IMG, we finally chose IMG for combinatory treatment of AA with MTX.

3.2.1 Imunoglukan® and methotrexate combination in AA

The study of Rovensky et al (Rovensky et al., 2011) was focused on the effect of IMG on inflammatory and arthritic markers in rats with AA during basal treatment with MTX. The treatment was prophylactic, which means that the animals were treated immediately after administration of the adjuvant, with the same design as used in our previous experiments. The results of our investigation confirmed the already reported effect of MTX treatment in rats with AA (Connolly et al., 1988; Welles et al., 1985). MTX at a dose of 1 mg/kg/week (0.5 mg/kg twice a week) suppressed but did not prevent arthritis development. In our study, MTX significantly suppressed the hind paw swelling and decreased arthrogram scores. IMG alone decreased both the hind paw swelling and the arthrogram on days 21 and 28. The remarkable finding was that IMG potentiated the beneficial effect of MTX; reduction of hind paw swelling and arthrogram scores on days 21 and 28 were more significant compared to the rats treated with MTX alone. Hetland et al. (1998) showed that β-glucan reduced growth of *Mycobacterium tuberculosis* in macrophage cultures and had a protective effect against *Mycobacterium bovis*, BCG infection in BALB/c mice (Hetland & Sandven, 2002). Certain microbes, fungi and viruses led to the generation and activation of autoimmune T cells resulting in the development of a particular autoimmune disease in genetically susceptible individuals. Thus IMG, an effective activator of the immune system may also be beneficial in humans in preventing or eliminating bacterial infections, which are known to induce reactive arthritis. In our studies, we tested the pure β-glucan - Imunoglukan® isolated from *Pleurotus ostreatus*. This β-glucan decreased arthritis development in rats and had an additional and beneficial effect to that of MTX treatment.

3.3 Endogenous antioxidants

Inflammation is one of the leading causes of mortality in the western world. Much evidence suggests a major role for dysregulation of the immune response to toxic stress (Itoh et al., 2003; Lynn & Golenbock, 1992). The intensive production of ROS associated with inflammation generally results in OS (Macdonald et al., 2003). Under conditions of high OS, the abilities of cells to eliminate ROS become exhausted, and dietary sources of antioxidants are requirered (Novoselova et al., 2009). We studied two important endogenous antioxidants - coenzyme Q_{10} (CoQ) and carnosine (CARN) as supplementary therapy in AA with the aim to contribute to the alternatives for dietetary complementary healing of RA. In Figure 3, two dose of CoQ - 20 (CoQ1) and 200 mg/kg b.w. (CoQ2) are compared with one dose of CARN - 150 mg/kg b.w. The experimental and statistical design was the same as described in section 3.1.

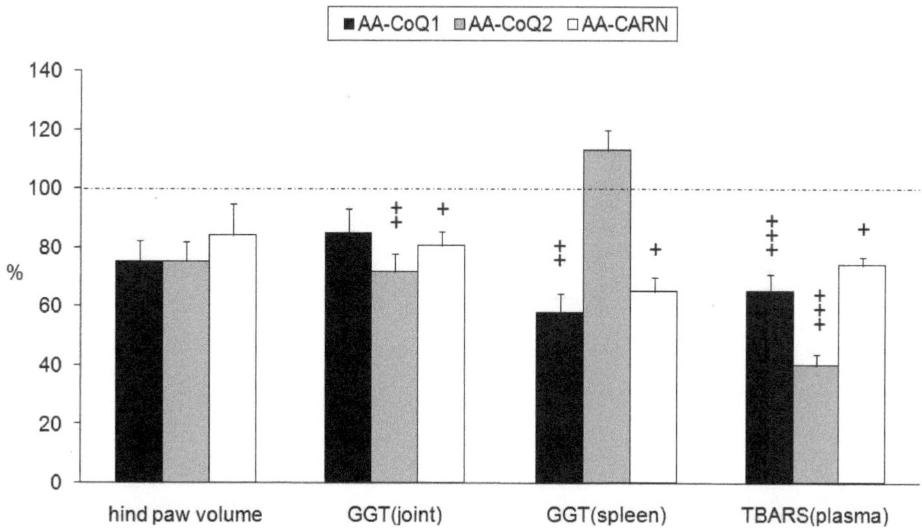

Fig. 3. Comparison of the effect of carnosine (CARN) and two different doses of coenzyme Q_{10} (CoQ) used as monotherapy in adjuvant arthritis (AA) on hind paw volume (HPV), GGT (γ-glutamyltransferase) activity in spleen and joint and level of TBARS (thiobarbituric acid reactive substances) in plasma measured on experimental day 28. Changes in parameters are illustrated in relation to untreated arthritic rats (100% represented by dot-and-dash line). For statistical analysis of data see Fig. 1.

Both antioxidants tended to improve HPV (not significantly) and significantly corrected the parameters of OS. No dose dependency was shown with exception of CoQ influence on GGT in spleen. In the next experiments we evaluated CARN in monotherapy of AA and CoQ in the lower dose for combinatory therapy with MTX in AA. The obtained results are described below.

3.3.1 Carnosine in monotherapy of AA

Carnosine (CARN) is a dipeptide consisting of β-alanine and L-histidine. It was shown to be a specific constituent of excitable tissues of all vertebrates accumulating in amounts exceeding that of ATP (Boldyrev & Severin, 1990). The antioxidant capacity of this compound is well documented, as well as its pH buffering, osmoregulating, and metal-chelating abilities (Boldyrev, 1990). A potentially useful characteristic of CARN is its ability to act as an anti-glycating agent (Boldyrev, 2002; Boldyrev, 2005; Hipkiss et al., 1998; Hipkiss & Brownson, 2000), to quench superoxide anion and hydroxide radical (Pavlov, et al. 1993; Rubtsov et al., 1991) and to neutralize 4-hydroxy-nonenal (HNE) and other toxic aldehydes (Aldini et al., 2002, 2011, Liu et al., 2003). In order to study the efficiency of carnosine as geroprotector, senescence accelerated mice (SAM), which have increased levels of ROS and deficiency of antioxidant capacity, was used (Boldyrev et al., 2001; Yuneva et al., 2002). CARN decreased the content of protein carbonyls and lipid peroxides in their blood, demonstrating normalization of oxidative metabolism in SAM tissues as a cause of increased life span. Oxygen metabolism has an important role in the pathogenesis of RA. ROS produced in excessive amounts under some pathological states, exceed the physiological ROS buffering capacity and result in OS. Excessive production of ROS can damage proteins, lipids, nucleic acids, and matrix components (Bauerova & Bezek, 1999). With respect to this fact we evaluated CARN in AA. The aim of this study was to assess whether administration of CARN in AA would ameliorate inflammation and disease progression. CARN beneficially affected the clinical parameter HPV in the model of AA measured in time profile (days 14, 21 and 28), significantly on day 14 (Table 9).

HPV (%)	Day 14	Day 21	Day 28
CO	8.81±1.91	11.67±2.54	13.09±2.61
AA	40.84±4.53 ***	91.32±6.00 ***	88.42±5.44 ***
AA-CARN	23.58±4.88 +	72.76±12.91	74.19±9.60

Table 9. Hind paw volume (HPV) changes in an experiment with carnosine (CARN) evaluated as monotherapy in time profile. For statistical analysis of data see table 1.

Activity of GGT in joint was significantly reduced by CARN administration (Table 10). Markers of redox imbalance in plasma (TBARS, and protein carbonyls) were significantly decreased (Table 10). Protein carbonyls in brain tissue homogenates were significantly elevated and were decreased by CARN to control values (Table 10). The reduction of immunological markers of inflammation (IL-1α and MCP-1) in plasma by CARN is a result supporting its anti-inflammatory activity (Table 11).

In the present experiment, the GGT activity was elevated in peripheral joint tissue. This finding is in good agreement with clinical studies of patients with RA who had increased levels of GGT not only in serum and urine but also in synovial fluid (Rambabu et al., 1990). CARN effectively reduced the activity of GGT in joint. Administration of CARN lowered the level of secondary products of lipid peroxidation in plasma measured as TBARS. Cheng (Cheng et al., 2011) showed that CARN, but not other conventional antioxidants, could protect neurons against MDA-induced injury through decomposition of protein cross-linking and may serve as a novel agent in the treatment of neurodegenerative diseases. The "anti-carbonyl" effect of CARN administration was also evidenced by other authors (Aldini et al., 2010).

Parameters	CO	AA	AA-CARN
Activity of GGT in joint (†)	11.03±1.81	26.30±2.04 ***	21.22±1.28 +
Protein carbonyls in plasma (nmol/mg protein)	0.15±0.01	0.20±0.01 **	0.14±0.02 +
Protein carbonyls in brain tissue (nmol/mg protein)	10.68±0.78	17.57±0.96 ***	12.98±0.53 +
TBARS (nmol/ml)	1.60±0.12	2.38±0.10 **	1.44±0.12 ++

† - nmol 4-nitroaniline / min / g tissue

Table 10. Activity of GGT(γ-glutamyltransferase) in joint, plasmatic TBARS (thiobarbituric acid reactive substances), and protein carbonyls in plasma and brain measured on experimental day 28 in an experiment with carnosine (CARN) evaluated as monotherapy. For statistical analysis of data see table 1.

We found that CARN was effective in decreasing protein carbonyls in plasma as well as in brain tissue homogenate of arthritic rats. These findings might provide, at least partially, an explanation for the antiinflammatory activity of CARN in chronic autoimmune disease, such as RA. The action of CARN resulted in decreased systemic inflammation in AA, monitored by plasmatic level of proinflammatory cytokine IL-1α and chemokine MCP-1. CARN was also effective in reducing the MCP-1 level in plasma in our experiment, suggesting that it may have a good potential in the treatment of chronic inflammatory diseases including RA where IL-1 and MCP-1 are involved.

Parameters	CO	AA	AA-CARN
IL-1α (pg/ml)	47.55±3.63	70.5±5.94 *	49.87±4.13 +
MCP-1 (pg/ml)	5345.70±734.30	7946.50±878.70 *	5422.00±658.50 +

Table 11. IL-1α (interleukin-1α) and MCP-1 (monocyte chemotactic protein-1) measured on experimental day 28 in an experiment with carnosine (CARN) evaluated as monotherapy. For statistical analysis of data see table 1.

3.3.2 Coenzyme Q_{10} in combination with MTX in AA

Based on our results with mitochondrial energetics modification and the observed anti-inflammatory and antioxidant effects (Bauerova et al., 2005a, 2008a; Gvozdjakova et al., 2004; Ponist et al., 2007), we chose CoQ_{10} as a candidate for combinatory therapy of RA. Patients with RA often suffer muscle weakness and atrophy. It is assumed that progressive muscle atrophy in RA patients is caused by damaged myofibrils and impaired mitochondria (De Palma et al., 2000). Disruption of mitochondrial bioenergetics caused by free radicals is involved in the development of myopathies. OS-caused alteration of mitochondrial functions can manifest in different manners (Cardoso et al., 1999). Leakage of free radicals from the respiratory chain leads to damaged mitochondrial membrane, proteins, DNA and inhibits oxidative phosphorylation (Luft, 1995; Miesel et al., 1996). Maneiro et al. (2003) found inhibition of functions of complex II and III of the respiratory chain and higher frequency of energetically "exhausted" mitochondria in chondrocytes of patients with osteoarthritis compared to healthy donors. In light of these findings, we decided to support the impaired mitochondrial functions by CoQ_{10} supplementation and thus to reduce the increased OS in AA. Some evidence from the literature showed that antirheumatic therapies which increased the level of CoQ_{10} were able to slow down RA progression (Comstock et al., 1997; Knekt et al., 2000; Kucharska et al., 2005). The hind-paw muscle of arthritic animals lies very close to the inflamed joint and could be also sensitive to joint inflammation (Ponist et al., 2007). Moreover, AA is a systemic inflammatory disease and we might also expect impairment in myocardial mitochondrial functions. We found that the reactions of skeletal muscle and myocardium muscle on CoQ supplementation in AA were different, which was not so surprising in view of their different structure and functions in the organism (Gvozdjakova et al., 2007). The results with solubilized CoQ_{10} (water-soluble form) indicated its therapeutic effect in the experimental model of AA (Bauerova et al., 2005a, 2008a; Gvozdjakova et al., 2004; Ponist et al., 2007). These findings are of potential significance in the treatment of patients with RA.

The aim of the present study was to examine the combined effect of CoQ_{10} and MTX on the progression of AA. For this purpose, we used monitoring of HPV along with evaluation of OS and inflammation markers assessed in plasma and tissues. The experiments included healthy animals (CO), arthritic animals not treated (AA), arthritic animals treated with coenzyme Q_{10} (AA-CoQ), arthritic animals treated with methotrexate (AA-MTX), and arthritic animals treated with the combination of CoQ_{10} and methotrexate (AA-MTX+CoQ). The two latter groups received a daily oral dose of 20 mg/kg b.w. of CoQ_{10} either alone or with methotrexate in the oral dose of 0.3 mg/kg b.w. twice a week. AA-MTX was performed as a reference treatment. CoQ_{10} supplementation to arthritis animals slightly decreased the HPV on all experimental days (Table 12). In the present study, the decreasing effect of MTX monotherapy on hind paw swelling was evident on all monitored days (Table 12). The significance of this effect was a confirmation of its well known antiarthritic effect, which we proved also previously on the AA model (Jurcovicova et al., 2009; Nosal et al., 2007; Rovensky et al., 2009). As shown in Table 12, the combination therapy was the most effective in decreasing the HPV of arthritic animals on all experimental days selected. Moreover, for day 14, we found a statistically significant difference between MTX monotherapy and its combination with CoQ_{10}. These promising clinical results were further completed by measurements of HNE- and MDA-protein adducts and protein carbonyls in plasma (Table 13). Changes in all groups with arthritis were calculated with respect to the control value assessed for healthy control animals on experimental day 28. The dashed line represents the value of control as 100%. We obtained a good agreement of HPV with the parameters of OS: the effect was increasing in the order CoQ_{10} alone, MTX alone, combination of CoQ_{10} and MTX. The most pronounced effect found for the combination of MTX and CoQ_{10} was significant for all OS parameters compared with non-treated arthritic animals. Moreover, the combination decreased all parameters close to the control group values, being more effective than the individual substances (Table 13).

HPV (%)	Day 14	Day 21	Day 28
CO	6.228±0.942	13.64±1.891	14.874±1.744
AA	42.411±7.411 ***	81.083±7.901 ***	68.629±8.952 ***
AA-CoQ	28.094±4.515	77.635±3.599	59.949±6.039
AA-MTX	13.307±2.673 ++	23.793±4.946 +++	26.996±8.201 ++
AA-CoQ+MTX	4.965±1.026 +++ / #	12.552±2.328 +++	19.571±2.426 ++

Table 12. Hind paw volume (HPV) changes in an experiment with coenzyme Q_{10} (CoQ) and methotrexate (MTX) evaluated as monotherapy and combination therapy (CoQ+MTX) in time profile. For statistical analysis of data see table 1.

As shown in Table 14, the arthritis process increases significantly the level of CoQ_9 in comparison with healthy controls. The effect of therapy on this phenomenon unveils a picture comparable to that found for other OS parameters (Table 13). The combination therapy was again the most effective and significant in comparison to the untreated arthritis group and the improvement was on the level of CO (Table 14). Table 14 shows also that the effects of the given treatments on the AA-increased IL-1α levels are very close to the effects illustrated in table 13. The improving effect on the increased cytokine plasmatic levels is raising in the order CoQ_{10}, MTX and CoQ_{10}+MTX. Furthermore, a statistically significant difference was found between MTX monotherapy and its combination with CoQ_{10}. For the local inflammatory parameter – the activity of GGT in joint homogenate – an approximately double increase was recorded on comparing arthritic animals with CO (Table 14). The treated groups presented similar results as already described for IL-1α. All these findings suggest that the cycles of GGT and CoQ are not directly coupled.

Oxidative stress parameters (%)	Protein carbonyls	HNE-protein adducts	MDA-protein adducts
AA	189.49±3.19 ***	125.80±8.74 ***	131.56±13.13 ***
AA-CoQ	169.74±3.19 +	114.03±9.41	112.92±4.49
AA-MTX	146.50±4.78 +++	111.31±7.85 +	101.49±7.45 ++
AA-CoQ+MTX	122.93±3.886 +++	91.66±8.571 +++ / #	85.376±5.129 +++ / # # #

Table 13. Protein carbonyls, HNE (4-hydroxynonenal) and MDA (malondialdehyde)-protein adducts levels in plasma measured on experimental day 28 in an experiment with coenzyme Q_{10} (CoQ) and methotrexate (MTX) evaluated as monotherapy and combination therapy (CoQ+MTX). Changes in all groups with arthritis were calculated compared to the control value assessed for healthy control animals on experimental day 28. For statistical analysis of data see table 1.

Parameters	CO	AA	AA-CoQ	AA-MTX	AA-CoQ +MTX
IL-1α (pg/ml)	42.95±7.88	87.11±8.52 **	67.76±13.59	38.27±4.21 ++	14.83±0.90 ++ / # #
Activity of GGT in joint (†)	9.38±0.76	16.08±0.96 ***	16.16±1.07	6.83±1.21 +++	9.60±1.05 +++
CoQ_9 in plasma (nmol/l)	154±7.70 **	241±21.28	189±16.51	209±21.75	158±12.65 +

† - nmol 4-nitroaniline / min / g tissue

Table 14. GGT (γ-glutamytransferase) activity in joint, IL-1α (interleukin-1α) and CoQ_9 (coenzyme Q_9) levels in plasma measured on experimental day 28 in an experiment with coenzyme Q_{10} (CoQ) and methotrexate (MTX) evaluated as monotherapy and combination therapy (CoQ+MTX). For statistical analysis of data see table 1.

The functionality of peripheral blood neutrophils in AA was evaluated by phagocytosis, oxidative burst and metabolic activity (Table 15).

Both phagocytosis and oxidative burst were increased due to arthritis. The immunosuppressive effect of MTX was demonstrated in lowering all characteristics of the functionality of peripheral blood neutrophils, not only in comparison with arthritis but also with CO. The addition of CoQ_{10} to MTX modulated all processes back to the level of CO. The observed immunoenhancing activity of CoQ_{10} may prove beneficial in MTX routine treatment. In this experiment, flow cytometric determination of the functionality of neutrophils was first applied for an experimental model on rats.

Parameters	CO	AA	AA-CoQ	AA-MTX	AA-CoQ +MTX
Phagocytosis (%)	41.90±3.56	51.28±3.51 *	55.48±4.07	30.07±1.44 ++	46.60±7.38 ##
Oxidative burst (%)	27.36±3.44	43.70±3.97 *	42.95±6.29	19.97±0.47 ++	31.07±8.98
Metabolic activity (%)	40.38±2.04	30.56±5.10 *	39.13±3.07	21.20±0.61 ++	34.79±7.81 ##

Table 15. Functional parameters of neutrophils measured on experimental day 7 in an experiment with coenzyme Q_{10} (CoQ) and methotrexate (MTX) evaluated as monotherapy and combination therapy (CoQ+MTX) of AA. For statistical analysis of data see table 1.

In summary, combined administration of CoQ_{10} and MTX suppressed arthritic progression in rats more effectively than did MTX alone. This finding may become a beneficial contribution to the treatment of RA. Restoration of redox homeostasis in chronic inflammatory diseases may be of significant importance in new therapeutic strategies.

4. Conclusion

In the past our research team, using the AA model, has monitored OS and inflammation in time course using different clinical and biochemical/immunological markers, and at the same time we have assessed the efficacy of the administered experimental substances with regard to their ability to reduce OS and inflammatory processes. In our experiments on AA rats we observed a beneficial effect of administration of low molecular weight antioxidants (coenzyme Q and carnosine), high molecular weight immunomodulators/antioxidants (glucomannan, Imunoglukan®) and compounds related to plants (curcumin, arbutin, pinosylvin, sesame oil, and extracts from *Boswellia serrata*, *Arctostaphylos uva-ursi* and *Zingiber officinale*).

In light of these results, we proceeded in the search for the most suitable therapeutic substance (an antioxidant/immunomodulator) with the ability to improve the therapy of RA with MTX. The aim was to find a potential enhancement of the antirheumatic effect of MTX in particular combinations compared to monotherapy. Carnosine, coenzyme Q, pinosylvin and Imunoglukan® were selected for assessment of a combinatory therapy with MTX. The already performed experiments on arthritic rats with pinosylvin, Imunoglukan® and coenzyme Q confirmed the hypothesis about the beneficial effect of adding a suitable immunomodulator/antioxidant to the therapy with MTX. Final safety and efficacy of these approaches calls for further more detailed research not only in preclinical but also in clinical conditions.

5. Acknowledgment

The authors wish to thank Dr. Magda Kouřilova, PhD. for correction of the English language. Experimental work was supported by grants VEGA 2/0045/11; VEGA 2/0090/08; VEGA 2/0003/10; APVV-51-017905; APVV-3015-07, APVV-21-055205 and

APVV-0052-10. Study with Coenzyme Q_{10} was performed in the frame of CNR/SAS bilateral project 2010-2012: "*In vitro* and *in vivo* models of arthritic processes for studying the mechanisms of inflammation and oxidative stress link-up. New perspectives for arthritis". Study with carnosine was performed in the frame of RAMS/SAS bilateral project 2010-2012: "Regulation of cytokine synthesis during inflammation development in brain and other tissues"
Imunoglukan® was donated from Pleuran s.r.o. company (Bratislava, Slovak Republic). Glucomannan was isolated by Martin Pajtinka (Institute of Chemistry, Slovak Academy of Sciences, Bratislava, Slovak Republic). Pinosylvin and pterostilbene were prepared by Prof. Jan Šmidrkal (Institute of Chemical Technology, Prague, Czech Republic) and Ing. Juraj Harmatha, PhD (Institute of Organic Chemistry and Biochemistry, Academy of Sciences of Czech Republic). Coenzyme Q_{10} in the form of Li-Q-Sorb® was purchased from Tishcon Corp., USA and carnosine was purchased from Hamary Chemicals Ltd., Japan. Pycnogenol® was obtained from VULM, s.r.o., Modra, Slovak Republic. All other used plant-related compounds and extracts were provided by assoc. Prof. Daniela Kostalova (Faculty of Pharmacy, Comenius University, Bratislava, Slovak Republic).

6. References

Akiyama, T., Mori, S., Mashiba, T., Miyamoto, K., Komatsubara, S., Cao, Y., Manabe, T., Norimatsu, H., Dobashi, H. & Tokuda, M. (2005) Incadronate disodium inhibits joint destruction and periarticular bone loss only in the early phase of rat adjuvant-induced arthritis. *Journal of Bone and Mineral Metabolism,* Vol. 23, No. 4, (December 2004) pp. 295-301, ISSN 1435-5604

Alarcon, G. S., Tracy, I. C. & Blackburn, W.D. Jr. (1989) Methotrexate in rheumatoid arthritis. Toxic effects as the major factor in limiting long-term treatment. *Arthritis & Rheumatism,* Vol. 32, No.6, (Jun 1989) pp. 671-676, ISSN 1529-0131

Aldini, G., Carini, M., Beretta, G., Bradamante, S. & Facino, R.M. (2002) Carnosine as a quencher of 4-hydroxynonenal: through what mechanism of reaction? *Biochemical and Biophysical Research Communications,*Vol. 298, No. 5, (November 2002) pp. 699–706, ISSN 0006-291X

Aldini, G., Dalle-Donne, I., Facino, R.M., Milzani, A. & Carini, M. (2007) Intervention strategies to inhibit protein carbonylation by lipoxidation derived reactive carbonyls. *Medical Care Research and Review,* Vol. 27, No. 6, (November 2007) pp. 817–868, ISSN 1552-6801

Aldini, G., Orioli, M., Rossoni, G., Savi, F., Braidotti, P., Vistoli, G., Yeum, K.J., Negrisoli, G. & Carini, M. (2010) The carbonyl scavenger carnosine ameliorates dyslipidemia and renal function in zucker obese rats. *Journal of Cellular and Molecular Medicine,*Vol. 15, No. 6, (Jun 2010) pp. 1339-54, ISSN 1582-4934

Arnhold, J., Sonntag, K., Sauer, H., Häntzschel, H. & Arnold. K. (1994) Increased native chemiluminescence in granulocytes isolated from synovial fluid and peripheral blood of patients with rheumatoid arthritis. *Journal of Bioluminescence and Chemiluminescence,* Vol. 9, No. 2, (March - April 1994) pp. 79–86, ISSN 1099-1271

Babior, B.M. (2000) Phagocytes and oxidative stres. *American Journal of Medicine,* Vol. 109, No. 1, (Jul 2000) pp. 33-44, ISSN 0002-9343

Bandt, M.D., Grossin, M., Driss, F., Pincemail, J., Babin-Chevaye, C. & Pasquier, C. (2002) Vitamin E uncouples joint destruction and clinical inflammation in a transgenic mouse model of rheumatoid arthritis. *Arthritis Rheumatism,* Vol. 46, No. 2, (February 2002) pp. 522-532, ISSN 1529-0131

Baskol, G., Demir, H., Baskol, M., Kilic, E., Ates, F., Kocer, D. & Muhtaroglu, S. (2005) Assessment of paraoxonase 1 activity and malondialdehyde levels in patients with rheumatoid arthritis. *Clinical Biochemistry,* Vol. 38, No. 10, (October 2005) pp. 951-955, ISSN 0009-9120

Baskol, G., Demir, H., Baskol, M., Kilic, E., Ates, F., Karakukcu, C. & Ustdal, M. (2006) Investigation of protein oxidation and lipid peroxidation in patients with rheumatoid arthritis. *Cell Biochemistry and Function,* Vol. 24, No. 4, (Jul-August 2006) pp. 307-311, ISSN 1099-0844

Bauerova, K. & Bezek, S. (1999) Role of reactive oxygen and nitrogen species in etiopathogenesis of rheumatoid arthritis. *General Physiology and Biophysics,* Vol. 18, (October 1999) pp. 15-20, ISSN 0231-5882

Bauerova, K., Neradova, B., Zitnanova, I., Horakova, L. & Stefek, M. (2002). Oxidative protein damage in rats with adjuvant arthritis. Comparison of carbonyl assay performed by ELISA and a spectrophotometricmethod. In J. Timko, J. Turna, & J. Pastorek (Eds.), Abstracts of the XVIII. Biochemical congress held in Vysoke Tatry, Stara Lesna, Slovakia, 10-13 September 2002, VEDA-Publishing House of Slovakcademy of Sciences, p. 256, Bratislava

Bauerova, K., Kucharska, J., Mihalova, D., Navarova, J., Gvozdjakova, A. & Sumbalova, Z. (2005a). Effect of coenzyme Q(10) supplementation in the rat model of adjuvant arthritis. *Biomedical papers of the Medical Faculty of the University Palacký, Olomouc, Czech Republic,* Vol. 149, No. 2, (December 2005) pp. 501-503, ISSN 1213-8118

Bauerova, K., Valentova, J., Ponist, S., Navarova, J., Komendova, D., Mihalova, D. (2005b) Effect of copper complexes on the development of adjuvant arthritis: Therapeutic and toxicological aspects. *Biologia,* Vol. 60, No. 17, (2005) pp. 65-68, ISSN 0006-3088

Bauerova, K., Ponist, S., Ondrejickova, O., Komendova, D. & Mihalova, D. (2006) Association between tissue gamma-glutamyl-transferase and clinical markers of adjuvant arthritis in Lewis rats. *Neuroendocrinology letters,* Vol. 27, No. 2, (December 2006) pp. 172-175, ISSN 0172-780X

Bauerova, K., Paulovicova, E., Mihalova, D., Komendova, D. & Ponist, S. (2007) Monitoring of pro-inflammatory cytokines in the development of adjuvant arthritis. *Chemické listy,* Vol. 101, (2007) pp. 166-167, ISSN 1213-7103

Bauerova, K., Kucharska, J., Ponist, S. & Gvozdjakova, A. (2008a) Coenzyme Q10 supplementation in adjuvant arthritis (pre-clinical study). In: *Mitochondrial medicine: mitochodrial metabolism, diseases,diagnosis and therapy.* Gvozdjakova, A., (eds), pp. 340-342, Springer, ISBN 9781402067143, Netherlands.

Bauerova, K., Ponist, S., Navarova, J., Dubnickova, M., Paulovicova, E., Pajtinka, M., Kogan, G. & Mihalova, D. (2008b) Glucomannan in prevention of oxidative stress and infammation occuring in adjuvant arthritis. *Neuroendocrinology letters,* Vol. 29, No. 5, (October 2008) pp. 691-696, ISSN 0172-780X

Bauerova, K., Paulovicova, E., Mihalova, D., Svik, K. & Ponist, S. (2009) Study of new ways of supplementary and combinatory therapy of rheumatoid arthritis with immunomodulators. Glucomannan and Imunoglukán in adjuvant arthritis. *Toxicology and Industrial Health,* Vol. 25, No 4-5, (May-Jun 2009) pp. 329-335, ISSN 1477-0393

Bauerova, K., Paulovicova, E., Mihalova, D., Drafi, F., Strosova, M., Mascia, C., Biasi, F., Rovensky, J., Kucharska, J., Gvozdjakova, A. & Ponist, S. (2010a) Combined methotrexate and coenzyme Q_{10} therapy in adjuvant-induced arthritis evaluated using parameters of inflammation and oxidative stress. *Acta Biochimica Polonica,* Vol. 57, No. 3, (September 2010) pp. 347-354, ISSN 0001-527X

Bauerova, K., Ponist, S., Drafi, F., Mihalova, D., Paulovičova, E., Jancinova, V. & Nosal, R. (2010b) Study of combination of pinosylvin and methotrexate in the model of adjuvant arthritis: beneficial effect on clinical and non-clinical parameters. *Interdisciplinary Toxicology,* Vol. 3, No. 3, (2010) pp. 32-33, ISSN 1337-9569

Bauerova, K., Ponist, S., Mihalova, D., Drafi, F. & Kuncirova, V. (2011) Utilization of adjuvant arthritis model for evaluation of new approaches in rheumatoid arthritis therapy focused on regulation of immune processes and oxidative stress. *Interdisciplinary Toxicology,* Vol. 4, No. 1, (March 2011) pp. 33-39, ISSN 1337-9569

Bendele, A., McComb, J., Gould, T., McAbee, T., Sennello, G., Chlipala, E. & Guy, M. (1999) Animal models of arthritis: relevance to human disease. *Toxicologic Pathology,* Vol. 27, No. 1, (January - February 1999) pp.134-142, ISSN 1533-1601

Biasi, F., Bosco, M., Lanfranco, G. & Poli G (1995) Cytolysis does not per se induce lipid peroxidation: Evidence in man. *Free Radical Biology and Medicine,* Vol. 18, No. 5, (May 1995) pp. 909–912, ISSN 0891-5849

Blake, D.R., Hall, N.D., Treby, D.A., Halliwell, B. & Gutteridge, J.M. (1981) Protection against superoxide and hydrogen peroxide in synovial fluid from rheumatoid patients. *Clinical Science,* Vol. 61, No. 4, (October 1981) pp. 483–486, ISSN 1470-8736

Bohanec, G.P., Logar, D., Tomsic, M., Rozman, B. & Dolzan, V. (2009) Genetic polymorphisms modifying oxidative stress are associated with disease activity in rheumatoid arthritis patients. *Disease Markers,* Vol. 26, No. 1, (March 2009) pp. 41–48, ISSN 0278-0240

Boldyrev, A.A. (1990) Retrospectives and perspectives on the biological activity of histidine-containing dipeptides. *International Journal of Biochemistry,* Vol. 22, No. 2, (1990) pp.129–132, ISSN 0020-711X.

Boldyrev, A. A. & Severin, S.E. (1990) The histidine-containing dipeptides, carnosine, and anserine: distribution, properties, and biological significance. *Advances in Enzyme Regulation,* Vol. 30, (1990) pp. 175–193, ISSN 0065-2571

Boldyrev, A.A., Yuneva, M.O., Sorokina, E.V., Kramarenko, G.G., Fedorova, T.N., Konovalova, G.G. & Lankin, V.Z. (2001) Antioxidant systems in tissues of senescence accelerated mice (SAM). *Biochemistry Moscow,* Vol. 66, No. 10, (October, 2001) pp.1157–1163, ISSN 1608-3040

Boldyrev, A. (2002) Carnosine as natural antioxidant and neuroprotector: biological functions and possible clinical use. In: *Free Radicals, Nitric Oxide, and Inflammation: Molecular, Biochemical, and Clinical Aspects.* Tomasi, A., Ozben, T. & Skulachev, V. (Eds), 202–217. IOS Press, ISBN 1-58603-198-8, Amsterdam

Boldyrev, A. (2005) Protection of Proteins from Oxidative Stress A New Illusion or a Novel Strategy? *Annals of the New York Academy of Sciences,* Vol.1057, (December 2005) pp. 193–205, ISSN 1749-6632

Brennan, M.L. & Hazen, S.L. (2003) Emerging role of myeloperoxidase and oxidant stress markers in cardiovascular risk assessment. *Current Opinion in Lipidology,* Vol. 14, No. 4, (August 2003) pp. 353–359, ISSN 1473-6535

Brown, R. K. & Kelly, F.J. (1996) Peroxides and other products, In: *Free Radicals, a Practical Approach.* Punchard, N.A. & Kelly, F.J., (eds) pp. 119–131, Oxford University Press, ISBN 0-19-963559-5, Oxford

Buss, H., Chan, T.P., Sluis, K.B., Domigan, N.M. & Winterbourn, C.C. (1997) Protein carbonyl measurement by a sensitive ELISA method. *Free Radical Biology and Medicine,* Vol. 23, No. 3, (1997) pp. 361–366, ISSN 0891-5849

Cardoso, S.M., Pereira, C. & Oliveira, C.R. (1999) Mitochondrial function is differently affected upon oxidative stress. *Free Radical Biology and Medicine,* Vol. 26, No. 1-2, (January 1999) pp. 3–13, ISSN 0891-5849

Carlisle, M.L., King, M.R. & Karp, D.R. (2003) Gamma-glutamyl transpeptidase activity alters the T cell response to oxidative stress and Fas-induced apoptosis. *International Immunology,* Vol. 15, No. 1, (January 2003) pp. 17–27, ISSN 1460-2377

Cedergren, J., Forslund, T., Sundqvist, T. & Skogh, T. (2007) Intracellular oxidative activation in synovial fluid neutrophils from patients with rheumatoid arthritis but not from other arthritis patients. *The Journal of Rheumatology,* Vol. 34, No. 11, (November 2007) pp. 2162-2170, ISSN 1499-2752

Chapman, A.P., Antoniw, P., Spitali, M., West, S., Stephens, S. & King, D. J. (1999) Therapeutic antibody fragments with prolonged in vivo half-lives. *Nature Biotechnology,* Vol 17, No. 8, (August 1999) pp. 780–783, ISSN 1087-0156

Cheng, J., Wang, F., Yu, D.F., Wu, P.F. & Chen, J.G. (2011) The cytotoxic mechanism of malondialdehyde and protective effect of carnosine via protein cross-linking/mitochondrial dysfunction/reactive oxygen species/MAPK pathway in neurons. *European Journal of Pharmacology,* Vol. 650, No. 1, (January 2011) pp. 184-94, ISSN 0014-2999

Comstock, G.W., Burke, A.E., Hoffman, S.C., Helzlsouer, K.J., Bendich, A., Masi, A.T., Norkus, E.P., Malament, R.L., & Gershwin, M.E. (1997) Serum concentrations of alpha-tocopherol, beta-carotene, and retinol proceeding the diagnosis of rheumatoid arthritis and systemic lupus erythematosus. *Annals of Rheumatic Disease,* Vol. 56, No. 5, (May 1997) pp. 323–325, ISSN 1468-2060

Connolly, K.M., Stecher, V.J., Danis, E., Pruden, D.J. & LaBrie, T. (1988) Alteration of interleukin-1 production and the acute phase response following medication of adjuvant arthritic rats with cyclosporin-A or methotrexate. *International Immunopharmacology,* Vol. 10, No. 6, (1988) pp. 717–728, ISSN 1878-1705

Cross, A., Barnes, T., Bucknall, R.C., Edwards, S.W. & Moots, R.J. (2006) Neutrophil apoptosis in rheumatoid arthritis is regulated by local oxygen tensions within joints. *Journal of Leukocyte Biology,* Vol. 80, No. 3, (September 2006) pp. 521–528, ISSN 0741-5400

Cuzzocrea, S., McDonald, M.C., Mota-Filipe, H., Mazzon, E., Costantino, G., Britti, D., Mazzullo, G., Caputi, A.P. & Thiemermann, C. (2000) Beneficial effects of tempol, a membrane-permeable radical scavenger, in a rodent model of collagen-induced arthritis. *Arthritis Rheumatism,* Vol. 43, No. 2, (February 2000) pp. 320-328, ISSN 1529-0131

Dalle-Donne, I., Rossi, R., Giustarini, D., Milzani, A., & Colombo, R. (2003). Protein carbonyl groups as biomarkers of oxidative stress. *Clinica Chimica Acta,* Vol. 329, No. 1-2, (March 2003) pp. 23–38, ISSN 0009-8981

Dallner, G. & Sindelar, P.J. (2000) Regulation of ubiquinone metabolism. *Free Radical Biology and Medicine,* Vol. 29, No. 3-4, (August 2000) pp. 285–294, ISSN 0891-5849

De Palma, L., Chillemi, C., Albanelli, S., Rapali, S. & Bertoni-Freddari, C. (2000) Muscle involvement in rheumatoid arthritis: an ultrastructural study. *Ultrastructural Pathology,* Vol. 24, No. 3, (May-Jun 2000) pp. 151–156, ISSN 1521-0758

Dinarello, C.A. & Moldawer, L.L. (2002) *Pro-infammatory and anti-infammatory cytokines in rheumatoid arthritis: a primer for clinicians.* 3rd ed., pp 351, Thousand Oaks, CA: Amgen

Drabikova, K., Perecko, T., Nosal, R., Bauerova, K., Ponist, S., Mihalova, D., Kogan, G. & Jancinova, V. (2009) Glucomannan reduces neutrophil free radical production in vitro and in rats with adjuvant arthritis. *Pharmacological Research,* Vol. 59, No. 6, (Jun 2009) pp. 399–403, ISSN 1096-1186

Drafi, F., Bauerova, K., Valachova, K., Poništ, S., Mihalova, D., Juranek, I., Boldyrev, A., Hrabarova, E. & Soltes, L. (2010). Carnosine inhibits degradation of hyaluronan induced by free radical processes in vitro and improves the redox imbalance in adjuvant arthritis in vivo. *Neuroendocrinology letters,* Vol. 31, No. 2, (2010) pp. 96–100, ISSN 0172-780X

Edmonds, S.E., Winyard, P.G., Guo, R., Kidd, B., Merry, P., Langrish-Smith, A., Hansen, C., Ramm, S. & Blake, D.R. (1997) Putative analgesic activity of repeated oral doses of vitamin E in the treatment of rheumatoid arthritis. Results of a prospective placebo controlled double blind trial. *Annals of the Rheumatic Diseases,* Vol. 56, No. 11, (November 1997) pp. 649-655, ISSN 1468-2060

Gambhir, J.K., Lali, P. & Jain, A.K. (1997) Correlation between blood antioxidant levels and lipid peroxidation in rheumatoid arthritis. *Clinical Biochemistry,* Vol. 30, No. 4, (Jun 1997) pp. 351–355, ISSN 0009-9120

Genestier, L., Paillot, R., Quemeneur, L., Izeradjene, K. & Revillard, J.P. (2000). Mechanisms of action of methotrexate. *Immunopharmacology,* Vol. 47, No. 2-3, (May 2000) pp. 247- 257, ISSN 0162-3109

Giustarini, D., Rossi, R., Milzani, A., Colombo, R. & Dalle-Donne, I. (2004) S-Glutathionylation: from redox regulation of protein functions to human diseases. *Journal of Cellular and Molecular Medicine,* Vol. 8, No. 2, (April-June 2004) pp. 201–212, ISSN 1582-4934

Guglielmotti, A., D'Onofrio, E., Coletta, I., Aquilini, L., Milanese, C. & Pinza, M. (2002) Amelioration of rat adjuvant arthritis by therapeutic treatment with bindarit, an inhibitor of MCP-1 and TNF-alpha production. *Inflammation Research,* Vol. 51, No. 5, (May 2002) pp. 252-258, ISSN 1420-908X.

Gvozdjakova, A., Kucharska, J., Tanaka , S., Neradova, B. & Bauerova, K. (2004) Coenzyme Q 10 supplementation differently modulated heart and skeletal muscle mitochondrial function induced by adjuvant arthritis. *Mitochondrion,* Vol. 4, (2004) pp. 20–21, ISSN 1567-7249

Gvozdjaková, A., Kucharska, J., Ponist, S. & Bauerova, K. (2007) Coenzyme Q 10 supplementation in an experimental model of adjuvant arthritis. Kobe, Japan, November 9–12,The fifth conference of the International Coenzyme Q 10 Association, p. 180

Hagfors, L., Leanderson, P., Skoldstam, L., Andersson, J. & Johansson, G. (2003) Antioxidant intake, plasma antioxidants and oxidative stress in a randomized, controlled, parallel, Mediterranean dietary intervention study on patients with rheumatoid arthritis. *Nutrition Journal,* Vol. 2, No. 5, (Jul 2003) p. 5, ISSN 1475-2891

Harmatha, J., Zídek, Z., Kmoníčková, E. & Šmidrkal, J. (2011) Immunobiological properties of selected natural and chemically modified phenylpropanoids. *Interdisc. Toxicol.,* Vol. 4, No. 1, p. 5-10, ISSN 1337-6853

Harris, E.D. (1993). Etiology and pathogenesis of rheumatoid arthritis. In: *Textbook of rheumatology,* Kelley, W.N., Harris, E.D., Ruddy, S., Sledge, C.B. (Ed.), pp. 833–873, WB Saunders, ISBN 9780721631554, Philadelphia

He, Y.H., Zhou J., Wang, Y.S., Xiao, C., Tong, Y., Tang, J.C., Chan, A.S., Lu, A.P. (2006) Anti-infammatory and anti-oxidative effects of cherries on Freund's adjuvant-induced arthritis in rats. *Scandinavian Journal of Rheumatology,* Vol. 35, No. 5, (September-October 2006) pp. 356–358, ISSN 1502-7732

Heliovaara, M., Knekt, P., Aho, K., Aaran, R.K., Alfthan, G. & Aromaa, A. (1994) Serum antioxidant and risk of rheumatoid arthritis. *Annals of the Rheumatic Diseases,* Vol. 53, No. 1, (January 1994) pp. 51–53, ISBN 1468-2060

Hetland, G., Lovik, M. &Wiker, H.G. (1998) Protective effect of beta-glucan against mycobacterium bovis, BCG infection in BALB/c mice. *Scandinavian Journal of Immunology,* Vol. 47, No. 6, (Jun 1998) pp. 548–553, ISSN 1365-3083.

Hetland, G. & Sandven, P. (2002) Beta-1,3-glucan reduces growth of Mycobacterium tuberculosis in macrophage cultures. *FEMS Immunology and Medical Microbiology,* Vol. 33, No. 1, (March 2002) pp. 41–45, ISSN 1574-695X.

Hipkiss, A.R., Worthington, V.C., Himsworth, D.T. & Herwig, W. (1998) Protective effect of carnosine against protein modification mediated by malondialdehyde and hypochlorite. *Biochimica et Biophysica Acta,* Vol. 1380, No. 1, (March 1998) pp. 46–54, ISSN 0005-2736

Hipkiss, A.R. & Brownson, C. (2000) Carnosine reacts with protein carbonyl groups: another possible role for the anti-ageing peptide? *Biogerontology,* Vol. 1, No. 3, (2000) pp. 217–223, ISSN 1573-6768

Hitchon, C.A. & El-Gabalawy, H.S. (2004) Oxidation in rheumatoid arthritis. *Arthritis Research and Therapy,* Vol. 6, No. 6, (October 2004) pp. 265-278, ISSN 1478-6362

Inoue, T., Yamashita, M. & Higaki, M. (2001) The new antirheumatic drug KE-298 suppresses monocyte chemoattractant protein (MCP)-1 and RANTES production in rats with adjuvant-induced arthritis and in IL-1beta-stimulated synoviocytes of patients with rheumatoid arthritis. *Rheumatology International,* Vol 20, No. 4, (May 2001) pp. 149-153, ISSN 1437-160X

Ishizuka, Y., Moriwaki, S., Kawahara-Hanaoka, M., Uemura, Y., Serizawa, I., Miyauchi, M., Shibata, S., Kanaya, T., Takata, T., Taniguchi, N. & Niida, S. (2007) Treatment with anti-gamma-glutamyl transpeptidase antibody attenuates osteolysis in collagen-induced arthritis mice. *Journal of Bone and Mineral Research,* Vol. 22, No. 12, (December 2007) pp. 1933-1942, ISSN 0884-0431

Itoh, K., Udagawa, N., Kobayashi, K., Suda, K., Li, X., Takami, M., Okahashi, N., Nishihara, T. & Takahashi, N. (2003) Lipopolysaccaride promotes the survival of osteoclasts via Tool-Like Receptor 4, but cytokine production of osteoclasts in response to lipopolysaccaride is different from that of macrophages. *Journal of Immunology,* Vol. 170, No. 7, (April 2003) pp. 3688–3695, ISSN 1550-6606

Jancinova, V., Perecko, T., Nosal, R., Kostalova, D., Bauerova, K. & Drabikova, K. (2009) Decreased activity of neutrophils in the presence of diferuloylmethane (curcumin) involves protein kinase C inhibition. *European Journal of Pharmacology,* Vol. 612, No. 1-3, (Jun 2009) pp. 161-6, ISSN 0014-2999

Jancinova, V., Nosal, R., Lojek, A., Ciz, M., Ambrozova, G., Mihalova, D., Bauerova, K., Harmatha, J. & Perecko, T. (2010). Formation of reactive oxygen and nitrogen species in the presence of pinosylvin - an analogue of resveratrol. *Neuroendocrinology letters,* Vol. 31, No. 2, (2010) pp. 79-83, ISSN 0172-780X

Jaswal, S., Mehta, H.C., Sood, A.K. & Kaur, J. (2003) Antioxidant status in rheumatoid arthritis and role of antioxidant therapy. *Clinica Chimica Acta,* Vol. 338, No. 1-2, (December 2003) pp. 123-129, ISSN 0009-898

Joe, B., Griffiths, M.M., Remmers, E.F. & Wilder, R.L. (1999) Animal models of rheumatoid arthritis and related inflammation. *Current Rheumatology Reports,* Vol. 1, No. 2, (December 1999) pp. 139-148, ISSN 1534-6307

Johansson, M.W., Patarroyo, M., Oberg, F., Siegbahn, A. & Nilsson, K. (1997) Myeloperoxidase mediates cell adhesion via the alpha M beta 2 integrin (Mac-1, CD11b/CD18). *Journal of Cell Science,* Vol. 110, No. 9, (May 1997) pp. 1133-1139, ISSN 0021-9533

Jurcovicova, J., Svik, K., Scsukova, S., Bauerova, K., Rovensky, J. & Stancikova, M. (2009) Methotrexate treatment ameliorated testicular suppression and anorexia related leptin reduction in rats with adjuvant arthritis. *Rheumatology International,* Vol. 29, No. 10, (August 2009) pp. 1187-1191, ISSN 1437-160X

Kalpakcioglu, B. & Senel, K. (2008) The interrelation of glutathione reductase, catalase, glutathione peroxidase, superoxide dismutase, and glucose-6-phosphate in the pathogenesis of rheumatoid arthritis. *Clinical Reumatology,* Vol. 27, No. 2, (February 2008) pp.141-145, ISSN 1434-9949

Knekt, P., Heliovaara, M., Aho, K., Alfthan, G., Marniemi, J. & Aromaa, A. (2000) Serum selenium, serum alpha-tocopherol, and the risk of rheumatoid arthritis. *Epidemiology,* Vol. 11, No. 4, (Jul 2000) pp. 402-405, ISSN 1531-5487

Kogan, G., Staško, A., Bauerova, K., Polovka, M., Šoltés, L., Brezova, V., Navarova, J., Mihalova, D. (2005). Antioxidant properties of yeast (1/3)-β-D-glucan studied by electron paramagnetic resonance spectroscopy and its activity in adjuvant arthritis. *Carbohydrate Polymers,* Vol. 61, (2005) pp.18-28, ISSN 0144-8617.

Koner, B.C., Banerjee, B.D. & Ray, A. (1997) Effects of stress on gamma glutamyl transpeptidase (GGT) activity in lymphoid system of rats: modulation by drugs. *Indian Journal of Experimental Biology,* Vol. 35, No. 3, (March 1997) pp. 222-224, ISSN 0019-5189

Kronek, J., Luston, J., Kronekova, Z., Paulovicova, E., Farkas, .P, Petrencikova, N., Paulovicova, L. & Janigov, I. (2010) Synthesis and bioimmunological efficiency of poly(2-oxazolines) containing a free amino group. *Journal of Materials Science: Materials in Medicine.* Vol 21, No. 3, (March 2009) pp. 879-86, ISSN 1573-4838

Kucharska, J., Gvozdjakova, A., Sumbalova, Z., Mihalova, D. & Bauerova, K. (2005) Can coenzyme Q10 supplementation protect heart and skeletal muscle mitochondrial function and antioxidants dysbalance in adjuvant arthritis? Los Angeles USA, Fourth Conference of the International Coenzyme Q10 Association, 2005, Abstr. p. 125

Kunsch, C.H., Sikorski, J.A. & Sundell, C.L. (2005) Oxidative stress and the use of antioxidants for the treatment of rheumatoid arthritis. *Current Medicinal Chemistry - Immunology, Endocrine & Metabolic Agents,* Vol. 5, No. 3, (June 2005) pp. 249–258, ISSN 1568-0134

Kurien, B.T., Hensley, K., Bachmann, M. & Scofeld, R.H. (2006) Oxidatively modifed autoantigens in autoimmune diseases. *Free Radical Biology and Medicine,* Vol. 41, No. 4, (August 2006) pp. 549–556, ISSN 0891-5849

Lefkowitz, D.L., Gelderman, M.P., Fuhrmann, S.R., Graham, S., Starnes, J.D. 3rd, Lefkowitz, S.S., Bollen, A. & Moguilevsky, N. (1999). Neutrophilic myeloperoxidase-macrophage interactions perpetuate chronic inflammation associated with experimental arthritis. *Clinical Immunology,* Vol. 91, No. 2, (May 1999) pp. 145–155, ISSN 1521-6616

Levine, R. L., Garland, D., Oliver, C. N., Amici, A., Climent, I., Lenz, A. G., Ahn, B.W., Shaltiel, S. & Stadtman, E.R. (1990). Determination of carbonyl content in oxidatively modified proteins. *Methods in Enzymology,* Vol. 186, (1990) pp. 464–478, ISSN 0076-6879

Littarru, G.P., Lippa, S., Oradei, A., Fiorni, R.M. & Mazzanti, L. (1991) Metabolic and diagnostic implications of blood CoQ10 levels. In: *Biomedical and clinical aspects of coenzyme Q.* Folkers, K., Yamagami, T. & Littarru, G.P.,(eds), pp. 167–178. Elsevier Science, ISBN 0444808019, Amsterdam.

Liu, Y., Xu, G. & Sayre, L.M. (2003) Carnosine inhibits (E)-4-hydroxy-2-nonenalinduced protein cross-linking: structural characterization of carnosine-HNE adducts. *Chemical Research in Toxicology,* Vol. 16, No. 12, (December 2003) pp. 1589–1597, ISSN 1520-5010

Luft, R. (1995) The development of mitochondrial medicine. *Biochimica et Biophysica Acta,* Vol. 1271, No. 1, (May 1995) pp. 1–6, ISSN 0005-2736

Lynn, W.A. & Golenbock, D.T. (1992) Lipopolysaccaride antagonists. *Immunology Today,* Vol. 13, No. 7, (Jul 1992) pp. 271–282, ISSN 0167-5699

Macdonald, J., Galley, H.F. & Webster, N.R. (2003) Oxidative stress and gene expression in sepsis. *British Journal of Anaesthesia,* Vol. 90, No. 2, (February 2003) pp. 221–232, ISSN 1471-6771.

Macickova, T., Drabikova, K., Nosal, R., Bauerova, K., Mihalova, D., Harmatha, J. & Pecivova, J. (2010) In vivo effect of pinosylvin and pterostilbene in the animal model of adjuvant arthritis. *Neuroendocrinology letters,* Vol. 31, No. 2, (2010) pp. 91-95, ISSN 0172-780X

Maini. R.N., Breedveld, F.C., Kalden, J.R., Smolen, J.S., Davis, D., Macfarlane, J.D., Antoni, C., Leeb, B., Elliott, M.J., Woody, J.N., Schaible, T.F. & Feldmann M. (1998) Therapeutic efficacy of multiple intravenous infusions of anti-tumor necrosis factor alpha monoclonal antibody combined with low-dose weekly methotrexate in rheumatoid arthritis. *Arthritis & Rheumatism,* Vol. 41, No. 9, (September 1998) pp. 1552-1563, ISSN 1529-0131

Maneiro, E., Martin, M.A., deAndres, M.C., Lopez-Armada, M.J., Fernandez-Sneiro, J.L., delHoyo, P., Galdo, F., Arenas, J. & Blanco, J. (2003) Mitochondrial respiratory activity is altered in osteoarthritic human articular chondrocytes. *Arthritis Rheumatism,* Vol. 48, No. 3, (March 2003) pp. 700–708, ISSN 1529-0130

Mazetti, I., Grigolo, B., Borzi, R.M., Meliconi, R. & Facchini, A. (1996) Serum copper/zinc superoxide dismutase levels in patients with rheumatoid arthritis. *International Journal of Clinical and Laboratory Research,* Vol. 26, No. 4, (1996) pp. 245–249, ISSN 1434-4467

McKendry, R.J. & Dale, P. (1993) Adverse effects of low dose methotrexate therapy in rheumatoid arthritis. *The Journal of Rheumatology,* Vol. 20, No. 11, (November 1993), pp. 1850-1856, ISSN 1499-2752

Miesel, R., Hartung, R. & Kroeger, H. (1996) Priming of NADPH oxidase by tumor necrosis factor alpha in patients with infammatory and autoimmune rheumatic diseases. *Infammation,* Vol. 20, No. 4, (August 1996) pp. 427–438, ISSN 1573-2576

Miesel, R., Murphy, M.P. & Kroger H (1996) Enhanced mitochondrial radical production in patients which rheumatoid arthritis correlates with elevated levels of tumor necrosis factor alpha in plasma. *Free Radical Research,* Vol. 25, No. 2, (August 1996) pp. 161–169, ISSN 1029-2470

Mihalova, D., Ponist, S., Kucharska, J., Komendova, D. & Bauerova, K. (2007) Total antioxidant status-systemic marker of oxidative stress in adjuvant arthritis. *Chemické listy,* Vol. 101, No. 14, (2007) pp. 225-226, ISSN 1215-7103

Miyata, T., Ishiguro, N., Yasuda, Y., Ito, T., Nangaku, M., Iwata, H. & Kurokawa, K. (1998) Increased pentosidine, an advanced glycation end product, in plasma and synovial fluid from patients with rheumatoid arthritis and its relation with inflammatory markers. *Biochemical and Biophysical Research Communications,* Vol. 244, No. 1, (March 1998) pp. 45–49, ISSN 1090-2104

Moreland, L.W., Heck, L.W. Jr & Koopman, W.J. (1997). Biologic agents for treating rheumatoid arthritis: concepts and progress. *Arthritis Rheumatism,* Vol. 40, No. 3, (March 1997) pp. 397–409, ISSN 1529-0131

Nosal, R., Jancinova, V., Petríkova, M., Ponist, S. & Bauerova, K. (2007) Suppression of oxidative burst of neutrophils with methotrexate in rat adjuvant arthritis. *Chemické Listy,* Vol. 101, (2007) pp. 243–244, ISSN 1215-7103

Novoselova, E.G., Lunin, S.M., Novoselova, T.V., Khrenov, M.O., Glushkova, O.V., Avkhacheva, N.V., Safronova, V.G. & Fesenko, E.E. (2009) Naturally occurring antioxidant nutrients reduce inflammatory response in mice. *European Journal of Pharmacology,* Vol. 615, No. 1-3, (August 2009) pp. 234-240, ISSN: 0014-2999

Ondrejickova, O., Ziegelhoeffer, A., Gabauer, I., Sotnikova, R., Styk, J., Gibala, P., Sedlak, J. & Horakova, L. (1993) Evaluation of ischemia-reperfusion injury by malondialdehyde, glutathione and gamma-glutamyl transpeptidase: lack of specifc local effects in diverse parts of the dog heart following acute coronary occlusion. *Cardioscience,* Vol. 4, No. 4, (December 1993) pp. 225–230, ISSN 1015-5007

Oppenheim, J.J., Zachariae, C.O., Mukaida, N. & Matsushima, K. (1991) Properties of the novel proinflammatory supergene "intercrine" cytokine family. *Annual Review of Immunology,* Vol. 9, (1991) pp. 617–48, ISSN 0732-0582.

Orlowski, M. & Meister, A. (1970) The γ-glutamyl cycle: a possible transport system for amino acids. *Proceedings of the National Academy of Sciences of the United States of America,* Vol. 67, No. 3, (November 1970) pp. 1248–1255, ISSN 1091-6490

Pavlov, A.R., Revina, A.A., Dupin, A.M., Boldyrev, A.A. & Yaropolov, A.I. (1993) The mechanism of interaction of carnosine with superoxide radicals in water solutions.

Biochimica et Biophysica Acta, Vol. 1157, No. 3, (Jun 1993) pp. 304– 312, ISSN 0006-3002

Perecko, T., Jancinova, V., Drabikova, K., Nosal, R. & Harmatha, J. (2008). Structure efficiency relationship in derivatives of stilbene. Comparison of resveratrol, pinosilvin and pterostilbene. *Neuroendocrinology letters,*Vol. 29, No. 5, (October 2008) pp. 802–805, ISSN 0172-780X

Poli, G., Leonarduzzi, G., Biasi, F. & Chiarpotto, E. (2004) Oxidative stress and cell signalling. *Current Medicinal Chemistry,* Vol. 11, No. 9, (May 2004) pp. 1163–1182, ISSN 0929-8673

Ponist, S., Kucharska, J., Gvozdjakova, A., Komendova, D., Mihalova, D. &Bauerova, K. (2007) Mitochondrial bioenergetics of skeletal musclestudied in adjuvant arthritis. *Chemicke Listy,* Vol. 101, (2007) pp. 256–257, ISSN 1213-7103

Ponist, S., Mihalova, D., Jancinova, V., Snirc, V., Ondrejickova, O., Mascia, C., Poli, G., Stancikova, M., Nosal, R. & Bauerová, K. (2010) Reduction of oxidative stress in adjuvant arthritis. Comparison of efficacy of two pyridoindoles: stobadine dipalmitate and SMe1.2HCl. *Acta Biochimica Polonica,* Vol. 57, No. 2, (Jun 2010) pp. 223-228, ISSN 0001-527X

Ponist, S., Drafi, F., Kuncirova, V., Mihalova, D., Ondrejickova, O., Trunova, O., Fedorova, T., Boldyrev, A., Bauerova, K. (2011) Anti-inflammatory effect of carnosine on rat adjuvant arthritis. International Congress on Carnosine in Exercise and Disease, July 10-12, 2011 Ghent (Belgium), Programme and abstract book p. 41

Prokopova, A., Kery, V., Stancikova, M., Grimova J., Capek, P., Sandula, J. & Orvisky E. (1993) Methyl-α- D -mannopyranoside, mannooligosaccharides and yeast mannans inhibit development of rat adjuvant arthritis. *Journal of Rheumatology,* Vol. 20, No. 4, (April 1993) pp. 673–677, ISSN 1499-2752

Rambabu, K., Ansari, A.A., Shaafe, I.A., Chelvam A.P., Ziu, M.M. (1990) Gamma-glutamyl transpeptidase in synovial fluid, serum, and urine of patients with rheumatoid arthritis. *Biochemical Medicine and Metabolic Biology,* Vol. 43, No. 3, (Jun 1990) pp. 183–192, ISSN 0885-4505

Requena, J.R., Fu, M.X., Ahmed, M.U., Jenkins, A.J., Lyons, T.J. & Thorpe, S.R. (1996) Lipoxidation products as biomarkers of oxidative damage to proteins during lipid peroxidation reactions. *Nephrology Dialysis Transplantation,* Vol. 11, No. 5, (1996) pp. 48–53, ISSN 1460-2385

Rollins, B.J. (1996) Monocyte chemoattractant protein 1: a potential regulator of monocyte recruitment in inflammatory disease. *Molecular Medicine Today,* Vol. 12, No. 5, (May 1996) pp. 198–204, ISSN 1357-4310

Rovensky, J., Stancikova, M., Svik, K., Uteseny, J., Bauerova, K. & Jurcovicova, J. (2009) Treatment of adjuvant-induced arthritis with the combination of methotrexate and probiotic bacteria Escherichia coli O83 (Colinfant). *Folia Microbiologica,* Vol. 54, No. 4, (2009) pp. 359–363, ISSN 1874-9356

Rovensky, J., Stancikova, M., Svik, K., Bauerova, K. & Jurcovicova, J. (2011) The effects of b-glucan isolated from Pleurotus ostreatus on methotrexate treatment in rats with adjuvant arthritis. *Rheumatology International,* Vol. 31, No. 4, (April 2011) pp.507-11, ISSN 1437-160X

Rowley, D., Gutteridge, M.C., Blake, D., Farr, M. & Halliwell, B. (1984) Lipid peroxidation in rheumatoid arthritis: thiobarbituric acid-reactive material and catalytic iron salts in synovial fluid from rheumatoid patients. *Clinical Science,* Vol. 66, No. 6, (Jun 1984) pp. 691-695, ISSN 1470-8736

Rubtsov, A.M., Schara, M., Sentjurc, M. & Boldyrev, A. (1991) Hydroxyl radical-scavenging activity of carnosine: a spin trapping study. *Acta pharmaceutica Jugoslavica.* Vol. 41, (1991) pp. 401-407, ISSN 0001-6667

Sarban, A., Kocyigit, A., Yazar, M. & Isikan, U.E. (2005) Plasma total antioxidant capacity, lipid peroxidation, and erythrocyte antioxidant enzyme activities in patients with rheumatoid arthritis and osteoarthritis. *Clinical Biochemistry,* Vol. 38, No. 11, (November 2005) pp. 981-986, ISSN 0009-9120

Schepetkin, I.A. & Quinn, M.T. (2006) Botanical polysaccharides: macrophage immunomodulation and therapeutic potential. *International Immunopharmacology,* Vol. 6, No. 3, (March 2006) pp. 317-333, ISSN 1878-1705

Shah, Z.A. & Vohora, S.B. (2002) Antioxidant/restorative effects of calcined gold preparations used in indian systems ofmedicine against global and focal models of ischaemia. *Pharmacology & Toxicology,* Vol. 90, No. 5, (May 2002) pp. 254-259, ISSN 1600-0773

Skoldstam, L., Hagfors, L. & Johansson, G. (2003) An experimental study of a Mediterranean diet intervention for patients with rheumatoid arthritis. *Annals of the Rheumatic Diseases,* Vol. 62, No. 3, (March 2003) pp. 208-214, ISSN 1468-2060

Smolen, J.S., Aletaha D., Bijlsma, J.W., Breedveld, F.C., Boumpas, D., Burmester, G., Combe, B., Cutolo, M., de Wit, M., Dougados, M., Emery, P., Gibofsky, A., Gomez-Reino, J.J., Haraoui, B., Kalden, J., Keystone, E.C., Kvien, T.K., McInnes, I., Martin-Mola, E., Montecucco, C., Schoels, M. & van der Heijde, D. (2010) Treating rheumatoid arthritis to target: recommendations of an international task force. *Annals of the Rheumatic Diseases,* Vol. 69, No. 4, (April 2010) pp. 631-637, ISSN 1468-2060

Sotnikova, R., Ponist S., Navarova, J., Mihalova, D., Tomekova, V., Strosova, M., & Bauerova, K. (2009) Effects of sesame oil in the model of adjuvant arthritis. *Neuroendocrinology letters,* Vol. 30, No. 1, (2009) pp. 22-24, ISSN 0172-780X

Stankovic, A., Slavic, V., Stamenkovic, B., Kamenov, B., Bojanovic, M. & Mitrovic, D.R. (2009) Serum and synovial fluid concentrations of CCL2 (MCP-1) chemokine in patients suffering rheumatoid arthritis and osteoarthritis reflect disease activity. *Bratislavské Lekárske Listy,* Vol. 110, No. 10, (2009) pp. 641-6, ISSN 1336-0345

Strosova, M., Tomaskova, I., Ponist, S., Bauerova, K., Karlovska J., Spickett, C.M. & Horakova, L. (2008) Oxidative impairment of plasma and skeletal muscle sarcoplasmic reticulum in rats with adjuvant arthritis - effects of pyridoindole antioxidants. *Neuroendocrinology letters,*Vol. 29, No. 5, (October 2008) pp. 706-711, ISSN 0172-780X

Strosova, M., Karlovska, J., Spickett, C. M., Orszaghova, Z., Ponist, S., Bauerova, K., Mihalova, D. & Horakova, L. (2009) Modulation of SERCA in the chronic phase of adjuvant arthritis as a possible adaptation mechanism of redox imbalance. *Free Radical Research,* Vol. 43, No. 9, (September 2009) pp. 852-864, ISSN 1029-2470

Smidrkal, J., Harmatha, J., Budesinsky, M., Vokac, K., Zidek, Z., Kmonickova, E., Merkl, R. & Filip, V. (2010) Modified approach for preparing (E)-stilbens related to resveratrol, and evaluation of their potential immunobiological effects. *Collection of Czechoslovak Chemical Communications,* Vol. 75, No. 2, p. 175-186, ISSN 0010-0765

Tastekin, N., Aydogdu, N., Dokmeci, D., Usta, U., Birtane, M., Erbas, H. &Ture, M. (2007) Protective effects of L-carnitine and alpha-lipoic acid in rats with adjuvant arthritis. *Pharmacological Research,* Vol. 56, No. 4, (October 2007) pp. 303–310, ISSN 1096-1186

Tsuchida, M., Miura, T., Mizutani, K. & Aibara, K. (1985) Fluorescent substances in mouse and human sera as a parameter of in vivo lipidperoxidation. *Biochimica et Biophysica Acta,* Vol. 834, No. 2, (April 1985) pp. 196–204, ISSN 0006-3002

Tuma, D.J. (2002) Role of malondialdehyde-acetaldehyde adducts in liver injury. *Free Radical Biology and Medicine,* Vol. 32, No. 4, (February 2002) pp. 303–308, ISSN 0891-5849

Tzianabos, A.O. (2000) Polysaccharide immunomodulators as therapeutic agents: structural aspects and biological function. *Clinical Microbiology Reviews,*Vol. 13, No. 4, (October 2000) pp. 523–533, ISSN 1098-6618

Vannier, E., Miller, M.C. & Dinarello, C.A. (1992) Coordinated anti-inflammatory effects of interleukin 4: interleukin 4 suppresses interleukon1 production but up regulates gene expression and synthesis of interleukin 1 receptor antagonist. *Proc Natl Acad Sci Unit States Am,* Vol. 89, No. 9, (May 1992) pp. 4076–4080, ISSN 1091-6490

Venkatraman, J.T. & Chu, W.C. (1999) Effects of dietary omega-3 and omega-6 lipids and vitamin E on serum cytokines, lipid mediators and anti-DNA antibodies in a mouse model for rheumatoid arthritis. *Journal of the American College of Nutrition,* Vol. 18, No 6, (December 1999) pp. 602-613, ISSN 1541-1087

Volejnikova, S., Laskari, M., Marks, S.C. Jr. & Graves, D.T. (1997) Monocyte recruitment and expression of monocyte chemoattractant protein-1 are developmentally regulated in remodeling bone in the mouse. *American Journal of Pathology,* Vol. 150, No. 5, (May 1997) pp. 1711-21, ISSN 1525-2191

Waage, A., Brandtzaeg, P., Espevik, T. & Halstensen, A. (1991) Current understanding of the pathogenesis of gram-negative shock. *Infectious Disease Clinics of North America,* Vol. 5, No. 4, (1991) pp. 781–791, ISSN 0891-5520

Weinblatt, M.E., Kremer, J.M., Bankhurst, A.D., Bulpitt, K.J., Fleischmann, R.M., Fox, R.I., Jackson, C.G., Lange, M. & Burge, D.J. (1999) A trial of etanercept, a recombinant tumor necrosis factor receptor:Fc fusion protein, in patients with rheumatoid arthritis receiving methotrexate. *The New England Journal of Medicine,* Vol. 340, No. 4, (January 1999) pp. 253-259, ISSN 1533-4406

Welles, W.L., Silkworth, J., Oronsky, A.L., Kerwar, S.S. & Galivan, J. (1985) Studies on the effect of low dose methotrexate in adjuvant arthritis. *Journal of Rheumatology,*Vol. 12, No. 5, (October 1985) pp. 904–906, ISSN 1499-2752

Wessels, J.A., Huizinga T.W., Guchelaar H.J. (2008) Recent insights in the pharmacological actions of methotrexate in the treatment of rheumatoid arthritis. *Rheumatology (Oxford),* Vol. 47, No. 3, pp. 249-55, ISSN 1462-0324.

Williams, H.J., Willkens, R.F., Samuelson, C.O. Jr., Alarcon, G.S., Guttadauria, M., Yarboro, C., Polisson, R.P., Weiner, S.R., Luggen, M.E., Billingsley, L.M., Dahl, S.L., Egger, M.J., Reading, J.C. & Ward, J.R. (1985). Comparison of low-dose oral pulse methotrexate and placebo in the treatment of rheumatoid arthritis: a controlled clinical trial. *Arthritis Rheumatism,* Vol. 28, No. 7, (Jul 1985) pp. 721–730, ISSN 1529-0131

Williams, R.O., Mauri, C., Mason, L.J., Marinova-Mutafchieva, L., Ross, S.E., Feldmann, M. & Maini, R.N. (1998) Therapeutic actions of cyclosporine and anti-tumor necrosis factor alpha in collagen-induced arthritis and the effect of combination therapy. *Arthritis & Rheumatism*, Vol. 41, No. 10, (October 1998) pp.1806-1812, ISSN 1529-0131

Yuneva, A.O., Kramarenko, G.G., Vetreshchak, T.V., Gallant, S. & Boldyrev, A.A. (2002) Effect of carnosine on Drosophila melanogaster lifespan. *Bulletin of Experimental Biology and Medicine,* Vol. 133, No. 6, (Jun 2002) pp. 559–561, ISSN 1573-8221

13

Resveratrol: A Candidate Drug for Treating Rheumatoid Arthritis

Tomoyuki Nishizaki and Takeshi Kanno
Division of Bioinformation, Department of Physiology, Hyogo College of Medicine
Japan

1. Introduction

Rheumatoid arthritis is a systemic autoimmune disease characterized by chronic inflammation of multiple joints, with disruption of joint cartilage. Accumulating evidence has pointed to inflammatory cytokines inducing hyperplasia of synovial cells in joints as an etiology for rheumatoid arthritis. High concentrations of cytokines such as tumor necrosis factor-α (TNF-α) and interleukin-1 (IL-1) are found in synovial fluid and plasma from patients with rheumatoid arthritis (Eastgate et al., 1988; Saxne et al., 1998) and those cytokines produce matrix metalloproteinases or activate osteoclasts, causing irreversible damage to soft tissues and bones (Olsen & Stein, 2004). Challenges for rheumatoid arthritis treatment, therefore, have been attempted using TNF-α inhibitors, anti-TNF antibodies, a soluble TNF receptor-fusion protein, or an IL-1 receptor antagonist. A concern with these therapies, however, are side effects such as serious infections and inducible malignant tumors (den Broeder et al., 2002).

Resveratrol (Fig. 8), a phytoalexin that is present in grape skin and red wine, exerts a variety of actions to reduce superoxides, suppress carcinogenesis and angiogenesis, prevent diabetes mellitus, inhibit inflammation, and prolong life span (Elliott & Jirousek, 2008). Furthermore, resveratrol decreases plaque formation relevant to neurodegenerative diseases such as Alzheimer's disease and Huntington's disease (Karuppagounder et al., 2009). Of particular interest is that resveratrol is a potent and specific inhibitor of NF-κB activation induced by TNF-α or IL-1β, and therefore, resveratrol might be a potential therapy for rheumatoid arthritis (Elmali et al., 2007; Molnar & Garai, 2005; Penberthy, 2007).

2. Materials and methods

2.1 Cell culture

MH7A human rheumatoid arthritis synovial cells were obtained from the Riken cell bank (Ibaraki, Japan). Cells were cultured in a culture medium; RPMI-1640 (Wako, Osaka, Japan) supplemented with 10% heat-inactivated fetal bovine serum (FBS), penicillin (final concentration, 100 U/ml), and streptomycin (final concentration, 0.1 mg/ml), in a humidified atmosphere of 5% CO_2 and 95% air at 37°C.

2.2 Cell viability

Cell viability was evaluated by the method of Mosmann (1983) using 3-(4,5-dimethyl-2-thiazolyl)-2,5-diphenyl-2H-tetrazolium bromide (MTT).

2.3 Terminal deoxynucleotidyl transferase-mediated dUTP nick end labeling (TUNEL) assay

MH7A cells were fixed with 4% paraformaldehyde. After inactivating endogenous peroxidase with methanol containing 0.3% H_2O_2, a Permeabilization Buffer (Takara Bio Inc., Otsu, Japan) was applied to cells and stood on ice for 5 min. Then, a Labeling Reaction Mixture (Takara Bio Inc.) was added and incubated in a humidified chamber at 37°C for 60 min. Reactive cells were stained with 3% methyl green and detected with a light microscope.

2.4 H2A phosphorylation assay

MH7A cells were incubated in a chemiluminescence detection assay kit (Upstate, Charlottesville, Virginia, USA) and reacted with an anti-phospho-H2A.X (Ser139) followed by an anti-mouse-HRP conjugate. Phosphorylation of H2A.X at Ser139 was identified by staining with chemiluminescent HRP substrate LumiGLO, and signals were detected with a microplate luminometer (ARVO mx/light, Perkinelmer, Waltham, MA, USA).

2.5 Assay of mitochondrial membrane potentials

Mitochondrial membrane potentials were measured using a DePsipher™ kit. MH7A cells were untreated and treated with resveratrol (100 μM) in the absence and presence of sirtinol (10 μM) for 24 h. After washing with cold phosphate-buffered saline (PBS), cells were incubated in a DePsipher™ solution at 37°C for 20 min. Then, cells were washed with 1 ml of a reaction buffer containing a stabilizer solution. The fluorescent signals were observed with a laser scanning microscopes (LSM 510, Carl Zeiss Co., Ltd, Germany) equipped with an epifluorescence device using a fluorescein long-pass filter (fluorescein and rhodamine) at an absorbance of 590 nm for red aggregations and at an absorbance of 530 nm for green aggregations.

2.6 Reverse transcription-polymerase chain reaction (RT-PCR)

Total RNAs of MH7A cells before and after treatment with resveratrol (100 μM) were purified by an acid/guanidine/thiocyanate/chloroform extraction method using a Sepasol-RNA I Super kit (Nacalai Tesque, Kyoto, Japan). After purification, total RNAs were treated with RNase free-DNase I (2 unit) at 37°C for 30 min to remove genomic DNAs, and 10 μg of RNAs were resuspended in water. Then, oligo dT primers, dNTP, 5 x First Strand buffer, and SuperScript III RNase H-Reverse Transcriptase were added to the RNA solution and incubated at 65°C for 5 min followed by 60°C for 1 min, 56°C for 60 min, 58°C for 60 min, 85°C for 5 min to synthesize the first strand cDNA. Subsequently, 1 μl of the reaction solution was diluted with water and mixed with 10 x PCR reaction buffer, dNTPs, $MgCl_2$, oligonucleotide, dimethylsulfoxide [final concentration, 5% (v/v)] and 1 unit of Taq polymerase (Fermentas, St. Leon-Roth, Germany) (final volume, 20 μl). RT-PCR was carried out with a Takara Thermal cycler Dice (Takara Bio Inc.) programmed as follows: the first one step, 94°C for 2 min and the ensuing 30 cycles, 94°C for 1 s, 62°C for 15 s, and 72°C for

30 s using primers shown in Table 1. PCR products were stained with ethidium bromide and visualized by 2% agarose electrophoresis.

Gene name	Sense primer	Anti-sense primer	Base pair
Bad	CTGGGGCTGTGGAGATCCGGAGTCGCC	TCACTGGGAGGGGGCGGAGCTTCCCC	320
Bak	GAGCCCATTCCCACCATTCTACCT	AGAGAGGAAGGGAGAGAACTGAGAGGAC	381
Bax	GGGAGACACCTGAGCTGACC	GGACTCCAGCCACAAAGATGG	404
Bcl-2	GAACTGGGGGAGGATTGTGGCC	TCGACGTTTTGCCTGAAGACTGTTAA	486
Bcl-X_L	AGGGAGGCAGGCGACGAGTTT	TGAAGAGTGAGCCCAGCAGAACCA	421
Sirtuin 1	ATTACTGAAAAACCTCCACGAACACAAAA	GCCTACTAATCTGCTCCTTTGCCACTCT	379

Table 1. Primers used for RT-PCR

2.7 Real-time RT-PCR

Total RNA was isolated from MH7A cells with Sepasol RNA I super kit (Nacalai Tesque, Kyoto, Japan). Total RNA (5 μg) was reverse-transcribed to cDNA using the High Capacity cDNA Reverse Transcription kit (Applied Biosystems, Tokyo, Japan), and quantitative real-time RT-PCR was performed with Applied Biosystems 7900HT real-time PCR system (Applied Biosystems, Foster City, CA, USA) using the SYBR Green realtime Master Mix (TOYOBO, Osaka, Japan) protocol. Primers used for real-time RT-PCR are shown in Table 2. The PCR cycling conditions were 95°C for 4 min, followed by 40 cycles at 95°C for 15 s and 62°C for 15 s and 72°C for 45 s. A standard curve was made by amplifying 0.5, 1, 2, 4, and 8 μl of the GAPDH mRNA diluted at 1:250. The mRNA quantity for each target gene was calculated from the standard curve using an SDS 2.1 Software (Applied Biosystems, Foster City, CA, USA).

Gene name	Sense primer	Anti-sense primer	Base pair
AIF	TCACAAAGACACTGCGATTCAAACAGT	GTTGCTGAGGTATTCGGGGAGGAT	491
FOXO-1	TATGGACACTTTGCGTTTCTTATTTAGGATAAC	GGCAGAAGGGAGAATGAGATGAAGTATG	366
FOXO-3	TGGATGCTGATGGGTTGGATTTTAA	TGGTGCTGAGGGGTGCTGTCC	415
P21	ACCGAGTGGGGGCATCATCAA	GGATGGGGTGGATGAGGAAGGTC	534
P27	CGTGGCTCGTCGGGGTCTGT	CCCTTCTCCACCTCTTGCCACTC	393
P53	GCCATCTACAAGCAGTCACAGCACAT	GGCACAAACACGCACCTCAAAGC	348
GAPDH	GACTTCAACAGCGACACCCACTCC	AGGTCCACCACCCTGTTGCTGTAG	128

Table 2. Primers used for real-time RT-PCR

2.8 Western blotting

After treatment with resveratrol (100 μM) for 6-24 h, MH7A cells were harvested and centrifuged at 600 x g for 10 min. After washing-out with 1 ml of PBS, the pellet was resuspended in 50 μl of buffer A (20 mM Hepes, 10 mM KCl, 1.5 mM $MgCl_2$, 1 mM EDTA, 1 mM EGTA, 1 mM dithiothreitol, 0.1 mM phenylmethylsulfonyl fluoride, 250 mM sucrose, pH 7.5) and homogenized. The lysate was centrifuged at 1000 x g for 10 min and the supernatant was further centrifuged at 10000 x g for 1 h. The pellet and supernatant were regarded as the mitochondria- and cytosol-enriched fractions, respectively. Each fraction was loaded on 12% sodium dodecylsulfate polyacrylamide gel electrophoresis (SDS-PAGE) and transferred to polyvinylidene difluoride membranes. Blotting membranes were blocked with TTBS (150 mM NaCl, 0.05% Tween20, and 20 mM Tris, pH 7.5) containing 5% BSA and subsequently reacted with an anti-cytochrome c antibody (1:400) (Chemicon, Billerica, MA, USA), followed by an HRP-conjugated goat anti-mouse IgG antibody. Immunoreactivity was detected with an ECL kit (GE Healthcare, NJ, USA) and visualized using a chemiluminescence detection system (FUJIFILM, Tokyo, Japan). Signal density was measured with Image Gauge software (FUJIFILM, Tokyo, Japan).

2.9 Enzymatic assay of caspase activity

Caspase activation was measured using a caspase fluorometric assay kit (Ac-Asp-Glu-Val-Asp-MCA for a caspase-3 substrate peptide; Ac-Ile-Glu-Thr-Asp-MCA for a caspase-8 substrate peptide; and Ac-Leu-Glu-His-Asp-MCA for a caspase-9 substrate peptide).

3. Results

3.1 Resveratrol induces MH7A cell apoptosis

In the MTT assay, resveratrol reduced MH7A cell viability in a concentration (1-200 μM)- and treatment time (24-72 h)-dependent manner (Fig. 1A), suggesting that resveratrol induces MH7A cell death.

Resveratrol increased TUNEL-positive cells in a concentration (100-200 μM)-dependent manner (Fig. 1B), indicating that resveratrol induces MH7A cell apoptosis. DNA damage or apoptosis is recognized to stimulate phosphorylation of histone H2A.X. Resveratrol (100 μM) significantly enhanced H2A.X phosphorylation, the extent reaching approximately 13 fold of control levels (Fig. 1C). This provides further evidence for resveratrol-induced MH7A cell apoptosis.

3.2 Resveratrol disrupts mitochondrial membrane potentials in a sirtuin 1-dependent manner

Resveratrol is shown to regulate mitochondrial functions or energy metabolism by interacting with NAD-dependent deacetylase sirtuin 1 (Kaeberlein et al., 2005; Lagouge et al., 2006). Interestingly, resveratrol-induced MH7A cell death was inhibited by sirtinol (10 μM), an inhibitor of sirtuin 1 (Fig. 2), suggesting that resveratrol induces MH7A cell death in a sirtuin 1-dependent manner. Moreover, the resveratrol effect was inhibited by tricostatin A (30 nM), an inhibitor of histone deacetylase (HDAC) (Fig. 2). This may account for the implication of sirtuin 1-regulated apoptosis-related gene transcription in the resveratrol effect.

To see whether resveratrol-induced MH7A cell apoptosis is mediated via the mitochondria, mitochondrial membrane potentials were monitored. For untreated cells, orange-red fluorescent signals alone were found (Fig. 3A,B). In contrast, resveratrol (100 μM) accumulated green fluorescent signals without orange-red fluorescent signal (Fig. 3C,D), indicating that resveratrol disrupts mitochondrial membrane potentials in MH7A cells. The resveratrol effect on mitochondrial membrane potentials was abolished by sirtinol (10 μM) (Fig. 3E,F). This implies that resveratrol disrupts mitochondrial membrane potentials in MH7A cells under the control of sirtuin 1. Taken together, these results indicate that resveratrol induces MH7A cell apoptosis by damaging the mitochondria in a sirtuin 1-dependent manner.

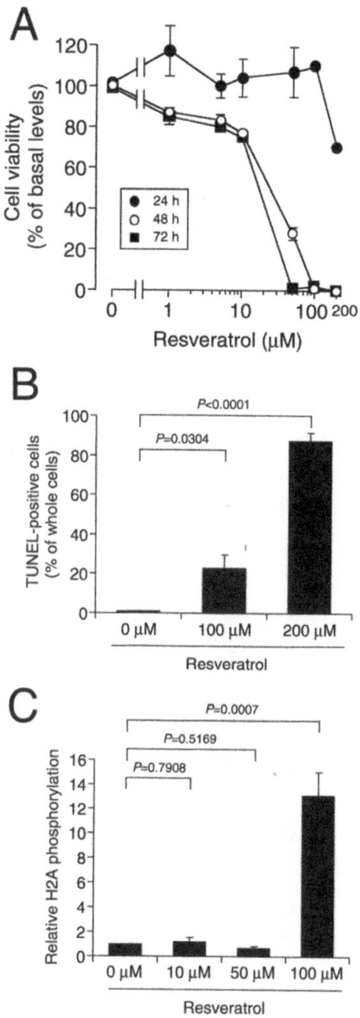

Fig. 1. Resveratrol induces apoptosis in MH7A cells. (**A**) MH7A cells were treated with resveratrol at concentrations as indicated for 24-72 h in serum-free culture medium, and cell viability was quantified with an MTT assay. In the graph, each point represents the mean (± SEM) percentage of basal levels (MTT intensities for cells untreated with resveratrol) (n=8). (**B**) Cells were treated with resveratrol at concentrations as indicated for 24 h in serum-free culture medium, and TUNEL-positive cells were counted. In the graph, each column represents the mean (± SEM) percentage of basal levels (TUNEL-positive cell numbers without resveratrol treatment) (n=3-6). *P* values, unpaired *t*-test. (**C**) Cells were treated with resveratrol at concentrations as indicated for 24 h in FBS-free culture medium, and H2A.X phosphorylation was quantified. In the graph, each column represents the mean (± SEM) ratio against basal levels (H2A.X phosphorylation without resveratrol treatment) (n=4). *P* values, unpaired *t*-test.

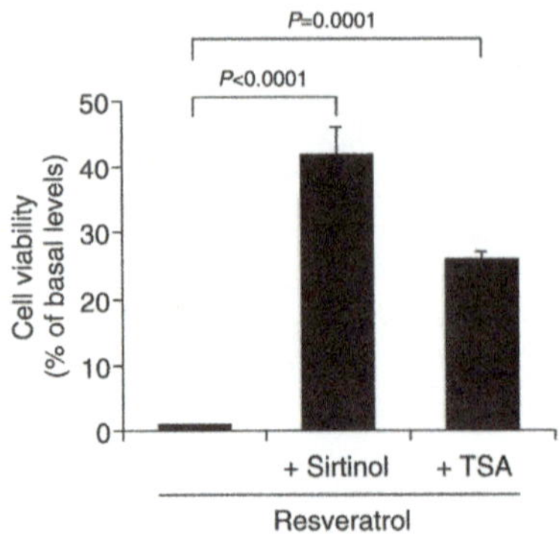

Fig. 2. Resveratrol-induced MH7A cell death is inhibited by a sirtuin 1 inhibitor or an HDAC inhibitor. MH7A cells were treated with resveratrol (100 μM) in the absence and presence of sirtinol (10 μM) or tricostatin A (TSA) (30 nM) for 48 h in serum-free culture medium, and cell viability was quantified with an MTT assay. In the graph, each column represents the mean (± SEM) percentage of basal levels (MTT intensities for cells untreated with any drug) (n=4). *P* values, unpaired *t*-test.

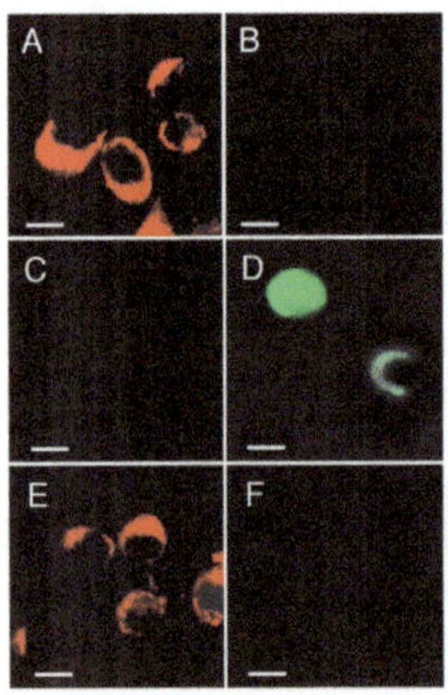

Fig. 3. Resveratrol disrupts mitochondrial membrane potentials in a sirtuin 1-dependent manner. MH7A cells were treated with resveratrol (100 μM) in the absence and presence of sirtinol (10 μM) for 24 h in serum-free culture medium, and mitochondrial membrane potentials were monitored. (**A,C,E**) Orange-red fluorescent images at an absorbance of 590 nm. (**B,D,F**) Green fluorescent images at an absorbance of 530 nm. Note that similar results were obtained with 3 independent experiments.

In the RT-PCR analysis, resveratrol (100 μM) increased expression of the sirtuin 1 mRNA in MH7A cells in a treatment time (20-60 min)-dependent manner (Fig. 4A). This points to sirtuin 1 being a significant target in resveratrol-induced MH7A cell death. Accumulating evidence has shown that resveratrol upregulates or downregulates expression of the Bcl-2 family that includes Bcl-2 and Bcl-X_L, to prevent from mitochondrial damage, and Bad, Bax, and Bak, to induce mitochondrial damage (Shakibaei et al., 2009). Resveratrol (100 μM) downregulated expression of the Bcl-X_L mRNA in MH7A cells from 1-h through 3-h treatment (Fig. 4C), while it had no effect on expression of mRNAs for Bcl-2 (Fig. 4B), Bad (Fig. 4D), Bax (Fig. 4E), and Bak (Fig. 4F). Collectively, resveratrol may disrupt mitochondrial membrane potentials by reducing Bcl-X_L expression through a pathway relevant to sirtuin 1-mediated transcription.

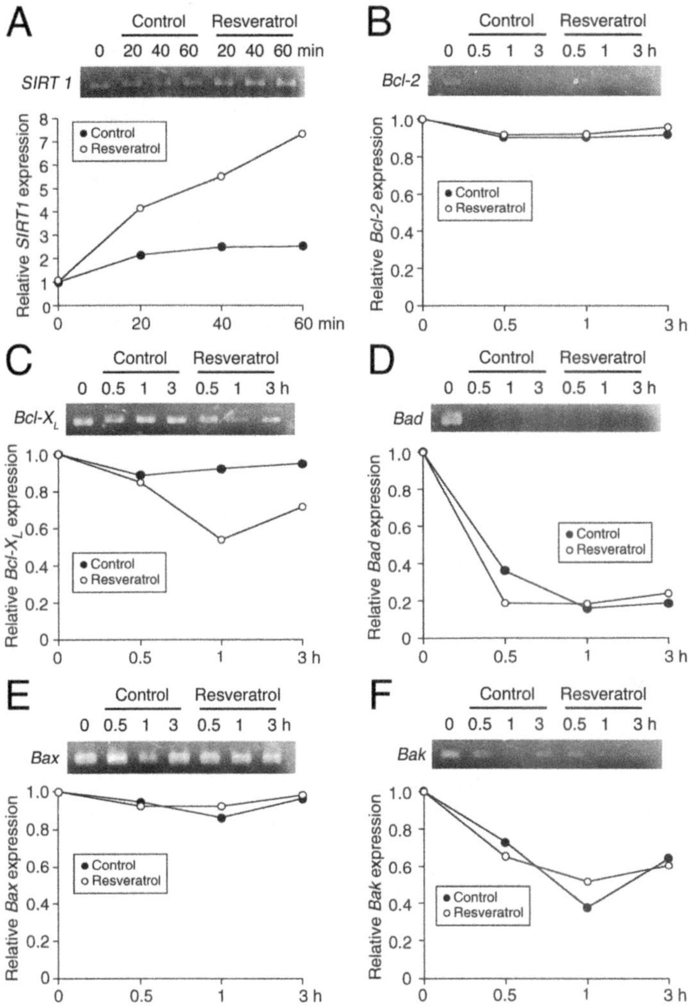

Fig. 4. Resveratrol upregulates expression of the sirtuin 1 mRNA and downregulates expression of the Bcl-X_L mRNA. MH7A cells were untreated (Control) and treated with resveratrol (100 μM) for 20-60 min or 0.5-3 h in serum-free culture medium, and then RT-PCR was carried out. In the graphs, each point represents the ratio against the intensity at 0 min/h regarded as 1. Note that similar results were obtained with 3 independent experiments.

3.3 Resveratrol activates caspase-3 and -9 through mitochondrial damage in a sirtuin 1-dependent manner

Mitochondrial damage allows release of apoptosis-related factors including cytochrome c. In the Western blot analysis using the mitochondrial and cytosolic component from MH7A cells, resveratrol (100 μM) increased presence of cytosolic cytochrome c in parallel with a treatment time (3-24 h)-dependent decrease in the presence of mitochondrial cytochrome c (Fig. 5). This suggests that resveratrol stimulates release of cytochrome c from the mitochondria into the cytosol.

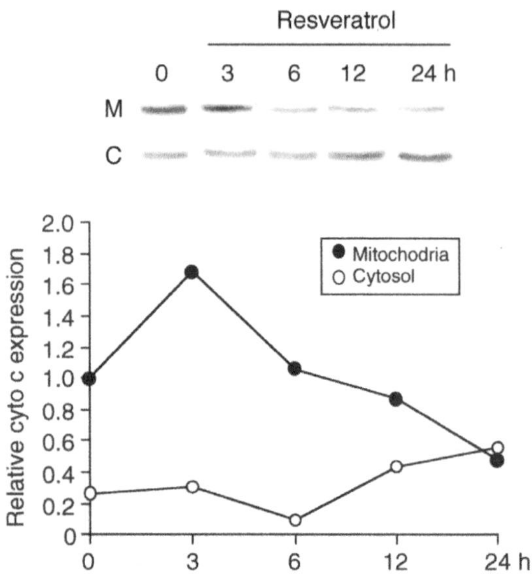

Fig. 5. Resveratrol stimulates cytochrome c release from the mitochondria. MH7A cells were treated with resveratrol (100 μM) for 3-24 h in serum-free culture medium, followed by fractionation into the mitochondrial (M) and cytosolic component (C), and Western blotting was carried out. In the graph, each point represents the ratio against the immunoreactive intensity at 0 h for the mitochondrial component regarded as 1. cyto c, cytochrome c. Note that similar results were obtained with 3 independent experiments.

In the enzymatic assay of caspase activity, resveratrol (100 μM) significantly activated caspase-3 and -9, but no activation of caspase-8 was obtained (Fig. 6). Resveratrol-induced activation of caspase-3 and -9 was inhibited by sirtinol (10 μM) (Fig. 6). Consequently, the results indicate that resveratrol activates caspase-9 and the effector caspase-3 in association with mitochondrial damage allowing cytochrome c release in a sirtuin-dependent manner, to induce MH7A cell apoptosis.

Overall, resveratrol appears to downregulate Bcl-X_L expression in a sirtuin 1-dependent manner, which promotes Bax-Bax complex, causing disruption of mitochondrial membrane potentials allowing cytochrome c release from the mitochondria. This is followed by activation of caspase-9 and the effector caspase-3, which, in turn, are responsible for apoptosis in MH7A human rheumatoid arthritis synovial cells (Nakayama et al., 2010) (Fig. 7).

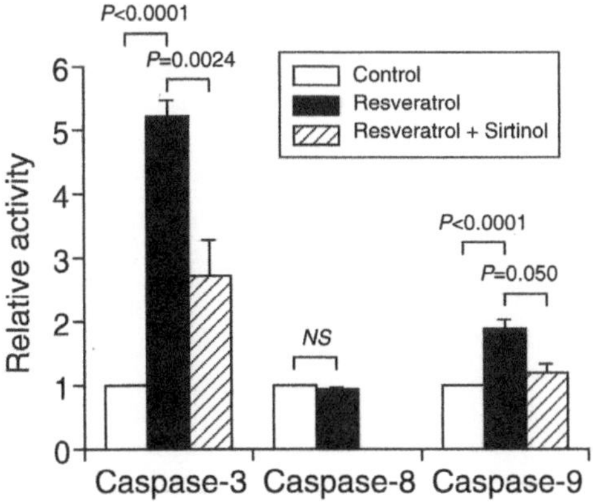

Fig. 6. Resveratrol activates caspase-3 and -9 in a sirtuin 1-dependent manner. MH7A cells were treated with resveratrol (100 μM) in the absence and presence of sirtinol (10 μM) for 24 h in serum-free culture medium, and caspase activities were assayed. In the graph, each column represents the mean (± SEM) ratio against basal levels (caspase activities for cells untreated with any drug) (n=4-6). *P* values, unpaired t-test. *NS*, not significant.

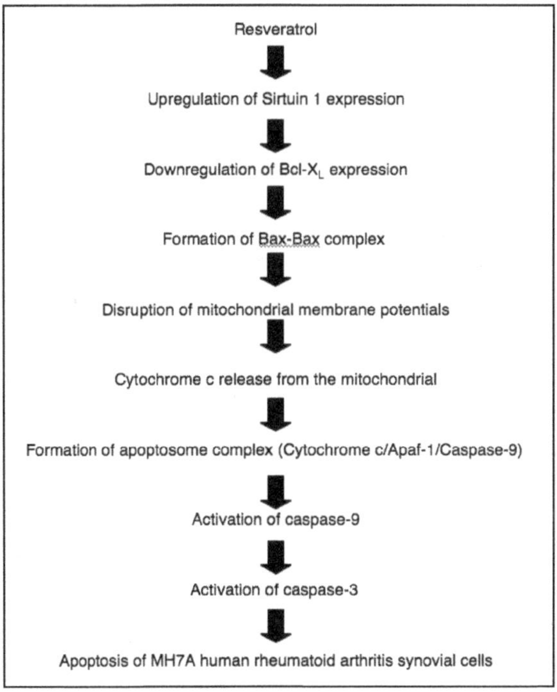

Fig. 7. Pathway underlying resveratrol-induced apoptosis in MH7A human rheumatoid arthritis synovial cells.

3.4 Resveratrol induces MH7A cell apoptosis with higher potency

We examined the effect of other polyphenols such as piceatannol, rhapontin, (-)-catechin, (+)-catechin, (-)-epicatechin, (-)-gallocatechin, (-)-epigallocatechin, (-)-catechin gallate, (-)-epicatechin gallate, (-)-gallocatechin gallate, and (-)-epigallocatechin gallate on MH7A cell death (Fig. 8). Of these, piceatannol, rhapontin, (-)-gallocatechin, (-)-epigallocatechin, (-)-catechin gallate, (-)-epicatechin gallate, (-)-gallocatechin gallate, and (-)-epigallocatechin gallate induced MH7A cell death in a concentration (10-100 μM)- and treatment time (24-72 h)-dependent manner, but with lesser potency than resveratrol, whilst no effect was observed for (-)-catechin, (+)-catechin, or (-)-epicatechin (Fig. 9). This indicates that resveratrol is capable of inducing apoptosis in MH7A human rheumatoid arthritis synovial cells, with much higher potency than other polyphenols.

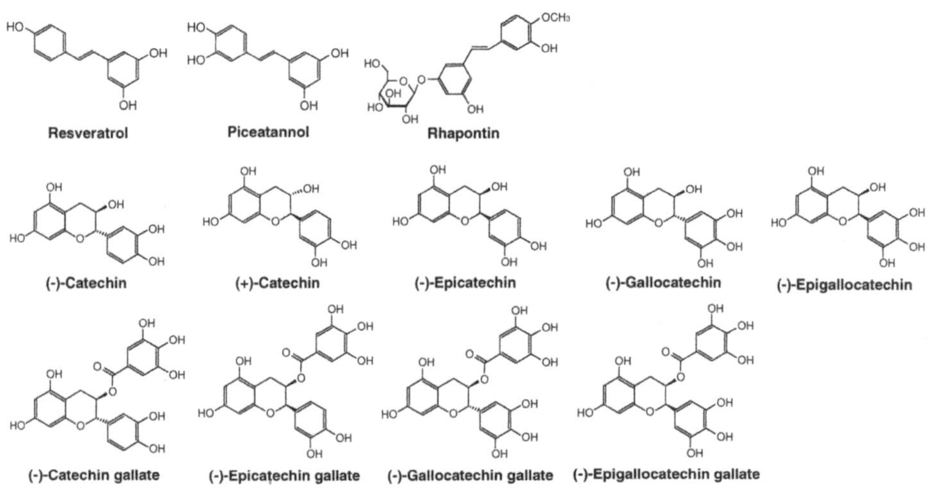

Fig. 8. Chemical structures of resveratrol and a variety of polyphenols.

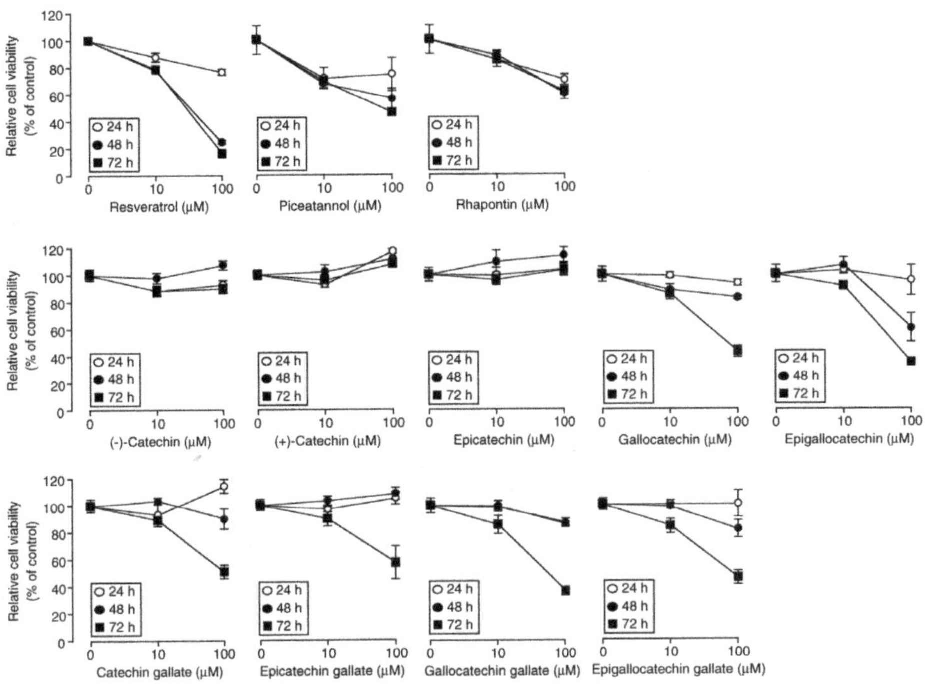

Fig. 9. Effects of resveratrol and a variety of polyphenols on MH7A cell death. MH7A cells were treated with resveratrol and polyphenols as indicated at concentrations ranging from 10-100 μM for 24-72 h in serum-free culture medium, and cell viability was quantified with an MTT assay. In the graphs, each point represents the mean (± SEM) percentage of basal levels (MTT intensities for cells untreated with resveratrol or polyphenols) (n=8).

3.5 Resveratrol increases expression of mRNAs for FOXO-1, FOXO-3, p21, p27, and AIF in MH7A cells

Sirtuin 1 regulates apoptosis-related gene transcription mediated by FOXO or NF-κB (Giannakou & Partridge, 2004; Salminen & Kaarniranta, 2009). In support of this, resveratrol induces growth arrest and apoptosis by activating FOXO in prostate cancer cells (Chen et al., 2010). In the real-time RT-PCR analysis, resveratrol (100 μM) increased expression of mRNAs both for FOXO-1 and FOXO-3 in MH7A cells in a bell-shaped treatment time (20-60 min)-dependent manner, with the peak at 20-min treatment (Fig. 10A), indicating involvement of FOXO in resveratrol-induced MH7A cell apoptosis.

Lines of studies have shown that resveratrol induces apoptosis in a variety of cells by activating p53 (Huang et al., 1999; Kuo et al., 2002; She et al., 2001). Resveratrol (100 μM) here, however, had no effect on expression of the p53 mRNA in MH7A cells (Fig. 10B). This suggests that resveratrol induces MH7A cell apoptosis in a p53-independent manner.

Resveratrol is shown to upregulate expression of p21 and p27 (Ganapathy et al., 2010; Ragione et al., 2003). Resveratrol (100 μM) increased expression of mRNAs both for p21 and p27 still in MH7A cells in a bell-shaped treatment time (20-60 min)-dependent manner, with the peak at 40-min treatment (Fig. 10B). This raises the possibility that resveratrol could suppress MH7A cell proliferation and growth by inhibiting cyclin-dependent protein kinases (Cdks) via control of p21 and p27.

Apoptosis-inducing factor (AIF) is released from damaged mitochondria and causes chromatin condensation and large-scale (~50 kbp) DNA fragmentation, leading to caspase-independent apoptosis. Interestingly, resveratrol induces apoptosis in human lung adenocarcinoma ASTC-a-1 cells through mitochondria-mediated AIF release (Zhang et al., 2011). In the present study, a huge increase in the expression of the AIF mRNAs in MH7A cells was found after 40-min treatment with resveratrol (100 μM) (Fig. 10C), suggesting that AIF also participates in resveratrol-induced MH7A cell apoptosis.

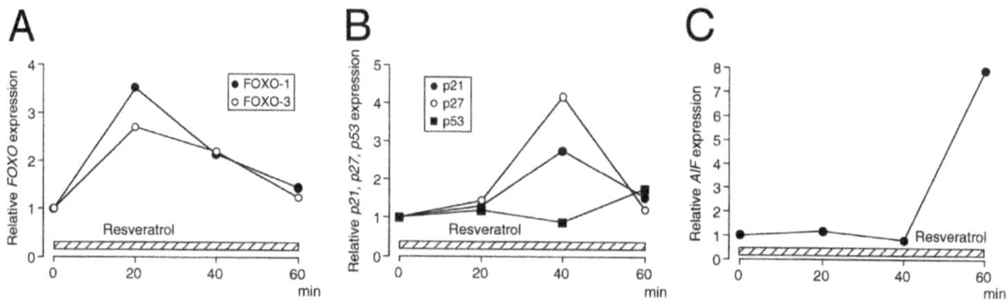

Fig. 10. Effects of resveratrol on mRNAs for FOXO-1, FOXO-3, p21, p27, p53, and AIF. MH7A cells were treated with resveratrol (100 μM) for periods as indicated in serum-free culture medium, and then real-time RT-PCR was carried out. The mRNA quantity for each gene was calculated from the standard curve made by amplifying different amounts of the GAPDH mRNA, and normalized by regarding the average of independent basal mRNA quantity at 0 h as 1. In the graphs, each point represents the mean (± SEM) ratio (n=3 independent experiments).

4. Discussion

Accumulating evidence has shown that resveratrol induces apoptosis or suppresses cell growth and proliferation by interacting with FOXO, NF-kB, and p53 involving wide-range of gene transcriptions such as those for apoptosis-related proteins, p21, p27, and AIF (Chen et al., 2010; Ganapathy et al., 2010; Huang et al., 1999; Kuo et al., 2002; Ragione et al., 2003; She et al., 2001). Notably, resveratrol is shown to increase expression of sirtuin 1, a mammalian NAD^+-dependent deacetylase (class III HDAC) (Franco et al., 2010). In the present study, resveratrol upregulated expression of mRNAs for FOXO-1, FOXO-3, p21, p27, AIF, and sirtuin 1 in MH7A cells but otherwise downregulated expression of the Bcl-X_L mRNA, without affecting expression of mRNAs for p53, Bcl-2, Bad, Bax, or Bak. FOXO belongs to the O subclass of the forkhead family of transcription factors, which includes FOXO-1, FOXO-3, FOXO-4, and FOXO-6. Evidence has pointed to the role of sirtuin 1 in the regulation of apoptosis-related gene transcription mediated by FOXO or NF-κB (Giannakou & Partridge, 2004; Salminen & Kaarniranta, 2009). FOXO and/or sirtuin 1, therefore, may be a primary target of resveratrol-regulated apoptosis-related gene transcription.

Resveratrol induced MH7A cell apoptosis in a concentration (1-200 μM)- and treatment time (24-72 h)-dependent manner. Two major pathways for apoptosis are well-recognized, i.e., oxidative stress-induced mitochondria-mediated apoptotic pathway and endoplasmic reticulum (ER) stress-induced apoptotic pathway. For the former pathway, the Bcl-2 family such as Bcl-2, Bcl-X_L, Bad, and Bax plays a central role; Bcl-2 and Bcl-X_L protect the mitochondria by capturing Bax, but Bad otherwise disrupts mitochondrial membrane potentials by releasing Bax from a Bcl-2/Bax complex or a Bcl-X_L/Bax complex. Oxidative stress disrupts mitochondrial membrane potentials by making a Bax/Bax pore, thereby damaging the mitochondria to allow release of apoptosis-related proteins such as cytochrome c, AIF, Smac/DIABLO, Omi/HtrA2, and endonuclease G into the cytosol (Wang, 2001). Subsequently, released cytochrome c activates caspase-3 by forming an apoptosome complex together with apoptosis proteases activating factor-1 (Apaf-1) and caspase-9, leading to apoptosis (Wang, 2001). Resveratrol disrupted mitochondrial membrane potentials, stimulated cytochrome c release from the mitochondria into the cytosol, and activated caspase-3 and -9 in MH7A cells. This, taken together with the finding that resveratrol downregulated the Bcl-X_L mRNA, accounts for mitochondria-mediated caspase-dependent pathway in resveratrol-induced MH7A cell apoptosis. Of particular interest is that resveratrol-induced MH7A cell apoptosis, mitochondrial damage, and caspase-3/-9 activation were prevented by a sirtuin 1 inhibiter or an HDAC inhibitor. This confirms that sirtuin 1 is required for resveratrol-induced MH7A cell apoptosis.

Findings by Byun et al. (2008) suggest that resveratrol induces apoptosis in fibroblast-like synoviocytes derived from patients with rheumatoid arthritis by activating caspase-8 as a primary target, which cleaves Bid, causing mitochondrial damage that triggers activation of caspase-9 and the effector caspase-3, without affecting the levels of Bax, Bcl-X_L, and Bcl-2. This observation contrasts with our finding that resveratrol does not activate caspase-8 in MH7A cells (Nakayama et al., 2010). Thus, resveratrol-induced MH7A cell apoptosis may be mediated via a novel apoptotic pathway.

In contrast, resveratrol upregulated expression of the AIF mRNA in MH7A cells. AIF induces apoptosis by causing chromatin condensation and DNA fragmentation. This suggests that resveratrol could induce MH7A cell apoptosis via an additional pathway, i.e., mitochondria-mediated caspase-independent pathway.

Resveratrol also increased expression of the p21 and p27 mRNAs in MH7A cells. p21 and p27 are recognized to inhibit cyclin E/Cdk2 that proceeds cell growth at the G_1 phase of cell cycling. Resveratrol, consequently, could suppress MH7A cell growth by inhibiting cyclin E/Cdk2 under the control of p21 and/or p27.

Like resveratrol, some other polyphenols induced apoptosis in MH7A human rheumatoid arthritis synovial cells. Of polyphenols examined here resveratrol induced MH7A cell apoptosis with the highest potency. This implies that, of the polyphenols, resveratrol could be the best target for the development of new drugs for treating rheumatoid arthritis.

In summary, the results of the present study show that resveratrol upregulates expression of FOXO and suirtuin 1 relevant to apoptosis-related gene transcription and its regulation in MH7A human rheumatoid arthritis synovial cells. Resveratrol downregulates expression of the Bcl-X_L mRNA, possibly mediated by FOXO, which causes disruption of mitochondrial membrane potentials, allowing cytochrome c release from the mitochondria into the cytosol, leading to activation of caspase-9 and the effector caspase-3 in a sirtuin 1-dependent manner. This represents a mitochondria-mediated caspase-dependent apoptotic pathway. Upregulation of the AIF mRNA by resveratrol, alternatively, suggests resveratrol-induced MH7A cell apoptosis via a mitochondria-mediated caspase-independent pathway. Moreover, upregulation of the p21 and p27 mRNAs by resveratrol may account for resveratrol-induced inhibition of MH7A cell growth.

5. Conclusion

Resveratrol induces apoptosis in MH7A human rheumatoid arthritis synovial cells, and does so with much higher potency than other polyphenols. It achieves this effect by decreasing Bcl-X_L expression, which disrupts mitochondrial membrane potentials, allowing cytochrome c release from the mitochondria into the cytosol, thereby activating caspase-9 and the effector caspase-3 in a sirtuin 1-dependent manner, which induces apoptosis. In addition, AIF, p21, and p27 may also participate in resveratrol-induced MH7A cell apoptosis and growth inhibition. These findings imply that resveratrol may be capable of preventing hyperplasia of synovial cells in human rheumatoid arthritis. Resveratrol, thus, could be developed as a promising drug for treatment of rheumatoid arthritis.

6. References

Byun, H.S., Song, J.K., Kim, Y.R., Piao. L., Won, M., Park, K.A., Choi, B.L., Lee, H., Hong, J.H., Park, J., Seok, J.H., Lee, Y.J., Kang, S.W. & Hur, G.M. (2008). Caspase-8 has an essential role in resveratrol-induced apoptosis of rheumatoid fibroblast-like synoviocytes. Rheumatology 47:301-308.

den Broeder, A., van de Putte, L., Rau, R., Schattenkirchner, M., Van Riel, P., Sander, O., Binder, C., Fenner, H., Bankmann, Y., Velagapudi, R., Kempeni, J. & Kupper, H. (2002). A single dose, placebo controlled study of the fully human anti-tumor necrosis factor-antibody adalimumab (D2E7) in patients with rheumatoid arthritis. The Journal of Rheumatology 9:2288-2298.

Chen, Q., Ganapathy, S., Singh, K.P., Shankar, S. & Srivastava, R.K. (2010). Resveratrol induces growth arrest and apoptosis through activation of FOXO transcription factors in prostate cancer cells. PLoS One 5(12):e15288.

Eastgate, J.A., Symons, J.A., Wood, N.C., Grinlinton, F.M., di Giovine, F.S. & Duff, G.W. (1988). Correlation of plasma interleukin-1 levels with disease activity in rheumatoid arthritis. Lancet 2:706-709.

Elmali, N., Baysal, O., Harma, A., Esenkaya, I. & Mizrak, B. (2007). Effects of resveratrol in inflammatory arthritis. Inflammation 30:1-6.

Elliott, P.J. & Jirousek, M. (2008). Sirtuins: Novel targets for metabolic disease. Current Opinion in Investigational Drugs 9:371-378.

Franco, J.G., de Moura1, E.G., Koury, J.C., Trotta1, P.A., Cordeiro, A., Souza, L.L., Almeida, N.A., Lima, N.daS., Pazos-Moura, C.C., Lisboa, P.C. & Passos, M.C. (2010). Resveratrol reduces lipid peroxidation and increases sirtuin 1 expression in adult animals programmed by neonatal protein restriction. The Journal of Endocrinology 207:319-328.

Ganapathy, S., Chen, Q., Singh, K.P., Shankar, S. & Srivastava, R.K. (2010). Resveratrol enhances antitumor activity of TRAIL in prostate cancer xenografts through activation of FOXO transcription factor. PLoS One 5(12):e15627.

Giannakou, M.E. & Partridge, L. (2004). The interaction between FOXO and SIRT1: tipping the balance towards survival. Trends in Cell Biology 14:408-412.

Huang, C., Ma, W.-ya., Goranson, A. & Dong, Z. (1999). Resveratrol suppresses cell transformation and induces apoptosis through a p53-dependent pathway. Carcinogenesis 20:237–242.

Kaeberlein, M., McDonagh, T., Heltweg, B., Hixon, J., Westman, E.A., Caldwell, S.D., Napper, A., Curtis, R., DiStefano, P.S., Fields, S., Bedalov, A. & Kennedy, B.K. (2005). Substrate-specific activation of sirtuins by resveratrol. The Journal of Biological Chemistry 280:17038-17045.

Karuppagounder, S.S., Pinto, J.T., Xu, H., Chen, H.L., Beal, M.F. & Gibson, G.E. (2009). Dietary supplementation with resveratrol reduces plaque pathology in a transgenic model of Alzheimer's disease. Neurochemistry International 54:111-118.

Kuoa, P.L., Chiangb, L.C. & Lin, C.C. (2002). Resveratrol- induced apoptosis is mediated by p53-dependent pathway in Hep G2 cells. Life Sciences 72:23–34.

Lagouge, M., Argmann, C., Gerhart-Hines, Z., Meziane, H., Lerin, C., Daussin, F., Messadeq, N., Milne, J., Lambert, P., Elliott, P., Geny, B., Laakso, M., Puigserver, P. & Auwerx, J. (2006). Resveratrol improves mitochondrial function and protects against metabolic disease by activating SIRT1 and PGC-1α. Cell 127:1109-1122.

Molnar, V. & Garai, J. (2005). Plant-derived anti-inflammatory compounds affect MIF tautomerase activity. International Immunopharmacology 5:849-856.

Mosmann T. (1983). Rapid colorimetric assay for cellular growth and survival: Application to proliferation and cytotoxicity assays. Journal of Immunological Methods 65:55-63.

Nakayama, H., Yaguchi, T., Yoshiya, S. & Nishizaki, T. (2010). Resveratrol induces apoptosis MH7A human rheumatoid arthritis synovial cells in a sirtuin 1-dependent manner. Rheumatology International DOI 10.1007/s00296-010-1598-8.

Olsen, N.J. & Stein, C.B. (2004). New drugs for rheumatoid arthritis. The New England Journal of Medicine 350:2167-2179.

Penberthy, W.T. (2007). Pharmacological targeting of IDO-mediated tolerance for treating autoimmune disease. Current Drug Metabolism 8:245-266.

Ragione, F.D., Cucciolla, V., Criniti, V., Indaco, S., Borriello, A. & Zappia, V. (2003). p21Cip1 gene expression is modulated by Egr1: a novel regulatory mechanism involved in the resveratrol antiproliferative effect. The Journal of Biological Chemistgry 278:23360–23368.

Salminen, A. & Kaarniranta, K. (2009). Regulation of the aging process by autophagy. Trends in Molecular Medicine 15:217-224.

Saxne, T., Palladino, M.A.Jr., Heinegard, D., Talal, N. & Wollheim, F.A. (1998). Detection of tumor necrosis factor-α but not tumor necrosis factor-β in rheumatoid arthritis synovial fluid and serum. Arthritis & Rheumatism 31:1041-1044.

Shakibaei, M., Harikumar, K.B. & Aggarwal, B.B. (2009). Resveratrol addiction: to die or not to die. Molecular Nutrition & Food Research 53:115-128.

She, Q.B., Bode A.M., Ma, W.Y., Chen, N.Y. & Dong, Z. (2001). Resveratrol-induced activation of p53 and apoptosis is mediated by extracellular-signal-regulated protein kinases and p38 kinase. Cancer Research 61:1604–1610.

Wang, X. (2001). The expanding role of mitochondria in apoptosis. Genes & Development 15:2922-2933.

Zhang, W., Wang, X. & Chen, T. (2011). Resveratrol induces mitochondria-mediated AIF and to a lesser extent caspase-9-dependent apoptosis in human lung adenocarcinoma ASTC-a-1 cells. Molecular and Cellular Biochemistry DOI: 10.1007/s11010-011-0802-9.

Part 4

Exercise and Alternative Therapies

14

Molecular Effects of Exercise in Rheumatoid Arthritis

Daniel J. Leong and Hui B. Sun
Department of Orthopaedic Surgery and Radiation Oncology, Oncophysics Research Institute, Albert Einstein College of Medicine/Montefiore Medical Center, New York USA

1. Introduction

Rheumatoid arthritis (RA) is an autoimmune disorder that affects approximately 1% of adults in the United States (Alamanos and Drosos 2005). Clinically, RA is manifested by pain and swelling of joints, disability, and diminished overall patient well-being (Scott et al. 2010). The etiology of RA remains enigmatic, but a range of genetic and environmental factors closely associated with RA have been identified over the past two decades. It is now known that the pathogenic process of RA involves the initiation and establishment of autoimmunity, followed by an inflammatory response, angiogenesis to maintain the chronic inflammatory state, and tissue degradation of the joint (Scott et al. 2010).

Despite the advances in the pharmacological therapies of RA over the past years, most patients (85-90%) do not achieve full remission, with up to 15% showing little clinical improvement in outcomes (Geborek et al. 2002; van der Woude et al. 2009). Accumulating studies have demonstrated the effectiveness of non-drug treatment modalities, e.g. exercise and physical activity, as an adjunct to drug therapy in patients with RA (Stenstrom and Minor 2003; Lundberg and Nader 2008). As a result, physical training is now a standard part of treatment for RA patients.

This chapter will first review results from randomized clinical trials which investigated the effects of exercise on RA disease activity. In RA patients, exercise was demonstrated to improve physical performance, cardiorespiratory fitness and muscle strength without worsening joint inflammation (Ekblom et al. 1975). Subsequent clinical studies have not only shown that exercise leads to meaningful effects on physical performance and fitness, but exercise can also reduce RA disease activity, measured by the number of swollen or tender joints (Stenstrom and Minor 2003). At the systemic level, there are several reports indicating a reduction in circulating levels of inflammatory biomarkers following long-term physical exercise (Dekker et al. 2007; Olson et al. 2007). These beneficial effects of exercise have been observed following different types of physical activity, after short-term and long-term (>2 years) exercise programs, at different phases of the disease course, and even in patients with high disease activity (van den Ende et al. 2000; Stenstrom and Minor 2003).

Next, by focusing on the effects of exercise, delivered in the form of physiologically relevant mechanical loading, this review will provide updated insights into exercise at both the systemic and local (e.g. cartilage and synovium) levels. Studies indicate that exercise activates an anti-rheumatologic response which includes an inhibition of pro-inflammatory cytokines such as tumor necrosis factor-alpha (TNF-α) in healthy and diabetic patients (Lundberg and Nader 2008). There is also evidence regarding the potential beneficial effects of exercise in preventing or suppressing the destructive consequences of inflammation in joint tissues (Ferretti et al. 2005; Ferretti et al. 2006). Clearly, the mechanical loading component of the exercise stimulus might be one of the mechanisms by which exercise exerts a protective anti-inflammatory effect at the local tissue level by preventing the expression of pro-inflammatory molecules. For example, studies have shown that moderate mechanical loading *in vitro* and *in vivo* upregulate production of anti-inflammatory cytokines interleukin (IL)-4 and IL-10, and suppress expression of IL-1β (Millward-Sadler and Salter 2004; Ferretti et al. 2005).

This will be followed by a discussion of how anti-inflammatory cytokines may work in concert with the anti-catabolic nature of physiologic biomechanical signals to mediate the protective effects of exercise. Elevated levels of pro-inflammatory cytokines such as IL-1β and TNF-α stimulate production of proteolytic enzymes matrix metalloproteinases (MMPs) and A Disintegrin and Metalloproteinase with Thrombospondin Motifs (ADAMTS) which mediate the cartilage destruction process in RA (Sun 2010). Studies have demonstrated physiological loading suppresses MMP and ADAMTS expression in both inflamed and non-inflamed joints to exert protective effects on the synovium and articular cartilage (Ferretti et al. 2005; Ferretti et al. 2006; Leong et al. 2010). The most recent progress on these mechanotransduction pathways which regulate the loading-induced anti-inflammatory and anti-catabolic responses will be presented, as well as possible crosstalk between these two pathways.

The chapter will conclude with perspectives on how identification of the signaling pathways activated by exercise will lead to the discovery of new treatment targets and development of novel treatment strategies which may have significant clinical potential in treating rheumatoid arthritis.

2. Exercise in rheumatoid arthritis treatment

The primary goals of RA treatment are to suppress inflammation and limit or prevent joint damage, while relieving pain and improving the patients' quality of life (Kowh et al. 2002). There is currently no cure for rheumatoid arthritis and treatment strategies involve a combination of drugs as well as non-pharmacologic treatments such as exercise and physical therapy (Smolen et al. 2010). As soon as the diagnosis for RA is established, prescribed medications include disease-modifying antirheumatic drugs (DMARDs), non-steroidal anti-inflammatory drugs, glucocorticoids, and TNF-α inhibitors (Deighton et al. 2009; Bijlsma 2010).

Although drug treatment helps improve disease outcome, exercise is still a vital part of rheumatoid arthritis treatment. For the general adult population, the American College of Sports Medicine and the Heart Association recommends at least 30 minutes of moderate-intensity exercise five days a week (Haskell et al. 2007). The benefits of regular exercise for healthy adults are well accepted, and include reducing the risk of coronary artery disease and improving cardiovascular health (Muller-Riemenschneider et al. 2011), reducing adiposity (Brukner and Brown 2005), and increasing muscle strength (Brentano and Martins Kruel 2011; Peterson and Gordon 2011). Randomized clinical trials have reported that the health benefits of exercise are also obtained in patients with RA without adverse effects on disease activity (van den Ende et al. 2000; de Jong et al. 2003; Bilberg et al. 2005; Melikoglu et al. 2006; van den Berg et al. 2006; Neuberger et al. 2007; Baillet et al. 2009; Lemmey et al. 2009). Furthermore, exercise at a high intensity, but within a physiologic range, was more effective in increasing physical function when compared to low intensity exercise (van den Ende et al. 2000; Lemmey et al. 2009).

2.1 Description of prescribed exercises

Based on the beneficial effects of physical activity in RA clinical trials, exercise programs for people with RA typically involve a combination of stretching exercises, aerobic training, and strength training (Stenstrom and Minor 2003; Cairns and McVeigh 2009; Forestier et al. 2009; Hurkmans et al. 2009; Baillet et al. 2010; Metsios et al. 2010). Table 1 summarizes commonly prescribed modes of exercise and their recommended doses (Resnick 2001; Medicine et al. 2009). Exercise programs are initially prescribed and supervised by an experienced professional, who tailors the program according to the patient's disease activity and symptoms (de Jong and Vliet Vlieland 2005). Since many RA patients have severe disability and a below average physical capacity, the intensity of training is initially low and gradually increased. If pain or swelling appears during exercise, patients are advised to reduce exercise intensity and/or duration until the pain or swelling subsides.

Daily stretching is recommended to decrease joint stiffness and maintain or increase pain-free range of motion (ROM). Patients with RA should begin their exercise programs with two to three daily repetitions of each stretching and ROM exercise, and eventually progress to 10 repetitions daily (Nieman 2000; Medicine et al. 2009). Range of motion exercises should be performed slowly with appropriate support, and should not be attempted in a rapid manner with bouncing movements (Resnick 2001).

Walking, cycling, rowing, swimming, water aerobics, and dance are examples of aerobic exercises prescribed to RA patients. Regular brisk walking in previously sedentary adults improved aerobic fitness and reduced cardiovascular risk in healthy adults (Murphy et al. 2002). Cycling at 70-80% predicted maximum heart rate significantly improved aerobic capacity, muscle strength, and joint mobility in RA individuals when compared to patients who only performed ROM exercises (van den Ende et al. 1996). Hydrotherapy, which combines elements of warm water immersion and exercise, was reported to improve the physical and emotional states of RA patients. Specifically, there was a reduction in joint tenderness and an improvement in knee range of motion, and emotional and physiological well-being (Hall et al. 1996). Moderately intensive pool exercise therapy in patients with RA did not improve aerobic capacity, but there were significant improvements in the muscle endurance in the lower and upper extremities (Bilberg et al. 2005). Although dance programs are not well-studied in the RA population, one study did report that female participants in a four week dance-based exercise program involving slow body movements exhibited significant improvements in locomotor ability (Moffet et al. 2000).

Loss of muscle mass and strength is a common characteristic in RA patients (Pedersen and Saltin 2006), and therefore muscle strengthening exercises are often recommended. These high-intensity training exercises include the leg press, chest press, leg extension, seated rowing, leg curl, triceps extension, standing calf raises, and bicep curl (Lemmey et al. 2009). Progressive resistance training (PRT) programs involving the large muscle groups as well as hand exercises have demonstrated improvements in physical function, increase in muscle mass, and reduction in fat mass (Hakkinen et al. 2005; Marcora et al. 2005; Lemmey et al. 2009). Early RA patients who enrolled in a two year strength training program exhibited significant improvements not only in muscle strength, but also showed reductions in systemic inflammation, pain, and disease activity (Hakkinen et al. 2001). With continued training, these gains in muscle strength can be maintained (de Jong et al. 2009).

Class of Exercise	Type of exercise	Recommended intensity/frequency/duration
Flexibility	Stretching Range of motion	Daily, before and after aerobic exercise. Hold stretch for 10-30 seconds, 3-5 repetitions Full range of motion for all joints daily
Aerobic	Walking Cycling Rowing Swimming Water aerobics Dance	60-80% maximum heartrate Up to 30 minutes/session 3-5 days/week
Strength	Free weights Weight machines Elastic bands	At least 1 set of 2-3 reps (up to 3 sets of 10 reps) at 80% of the 1-repetition maximum (the maximum load lifted for each of the prescribed exercises) 2-3 days/week

Table 1. Exercise management guidelines for the treatment of RA (Resnick 2001; Lemmey et al. 2009; Medicine et al. 2009)

2.2 Beneficial effects of exercise in RA

Many RA patients suffer from cachexia, which is characterized by a decrease in muscle mass along with an increase in fat mass. This is unlike the cachexia associated with conditions such as HIV-AIDS, cancers, chronic obstructive pulmonary disease (COPD), and old age, which is defined by significant muscle wasting alone, and is usually characterized by weight loss (Roubenoff et al. 1992). These changes in body composition may increase the risk of developing diabetes and cardiovascular disease (Roubenoff et al. 1992; Lavie et al. 2009), as well as lead to muscle weakness, decreased physical activity, pain, and fatigue, which together further adversely affect skeletal health (Hakkinen 2004). Muscle strengthening is important not only to regain normal physical function, but it is also necessary for joint stability, which may protect against the development of osteoarthritis (Sun 2010). Exercise has been demonstrated to significantly improve many of the symptoms of rheumatoid arthritis, including disability, pain, joint stiffness and fatigue (Hakkinen 2004; Marcora et al. 2005; Neill et al. 2006; Brorsson et al. 2009; Lemmey et al. 2009). Progressive resistance training was reported to increase muscle mass, improve physical function, and reduce disabilities associated with RA (Marcora et al. 2005; Lemmey et al. 2009). High intensity resistance exercise also has been reported to reverse RA cachexia by restoring muscle mass (Marcora et al. 2005).

Because of RA cachexia, it was hypothesized that patients with RA were resistant to the anabolic effects of exercise (Rall et al. 1996). However, no differences in the physiological properties of muscle that determine force, including contractile properties, voluntary activation capacity, and contraction velocity, were found between cachectic RA patients and healthy controls (Matschke et al. 2010). Recent clinical trials have found that the muscle of RA patients respond in similar manner to that of muscle in healthy individuals. The strengthening effects of PRT in RA patients (Lemmey et al. 2009) are similar to those observed in healthy middle-aged subjects (Morse et al. 2007). Studies which directly compared RA patients with age-matched healthy patients reported similar findings. Following resistance and aerobic exercise training, comparable increases in strength and thigh muscle cross-section, and decreases in thigh fat thickness were found in both RA and healthy female patients (Hakkinen et al. 2005). Together, these studies demonstrate that exercise training increases muscle mass, strength, and improves physical function in a similar manner in patients with RA and in healthy individuals. In fact, the inclusion of high-intensity PRT is recommended in RA treatment strategies to counteract the effects of rheumatoid cachexia (Pedersen and Saltin 2006; Lemmey et al. 2009).

2.3 Anti-inflammatory effects of exercise

Regular exercise, such as endurance training, can reduce basal levels of many inflammatory mediators/markers (King et al. 2003). Consequently, exercise has been recommended as an anti-inflammatory therapy in chronic inflammatory disorders such as RA (Kowh et al. 2002), and its effects are observed on the systemic and local levels.

2.3.1 Systemic effects

Physical inactivity, a common consequence of RA symptoms, leads to the accumulation of visceral fat and activation of inflammatory pathways (Walsh et al. 2011). Chronic inflammation can also drive the development of insulin resistance and atherosclerosis (Handschin and Spiegelman 2008). Increased physical activity has been reported to reduce inflammation in non-RA patients, as indicated by a downregulation of inflammation markers/mediators (Petersen and Pedersen 2005). In another demonstration of the anti-inflammatory effects of exercise, a model of low grade inflammation was established in healthy volunteers through the administration of a low dose of E. coli endotoxin. While circulating levels of TNF-α were increased in resting individuals, this increase was blocked in subjects who exercised prior to the endotoxin administration (Starkie et al. 2003), suggesting exercise may inhibit the production of TNF-α. Together, it is possible the anti-inflammatory effects of exercise are due to a decrease in visceral fat mass as well as the production of anti-inflammatory factors.

With exercise, there is a release of inflammatory-related cytokines from muscle into the circulation. IL-6 is the first cytokine released during exercise. Levels of circulating IL-6 increase exponentially after exercise and then decline post-exercise (Petersen and Pedersen 2006, Walsh et al. 2011). It is unclear whether this acute elevation in IL-6 modulates inflammatory processes during physical activity. Although IL-6 is a pro-inflammatory cytokine in the rheumatic joint, recent studies suggest the transient response of IL-6 may play a metabolic, rather than an immunological role (Walsh et al. 2011). Following the increase of IL-6 in response to exercise in healthy individuals, IL-10 and IL-1 receptor antagonist (IL-1ra) are released into the circulation (Petersen and Pedersen 2006). Notably, an infusion of IL-6 enhanced plasma levels of IL-1ra and IL-10, (Steensberg et al. 2003). This suggests that the anti-inflammatory effect of exercise can be attributed, at least in part, to the induction of IL-6 and the creation of an anti-inflammatory environment (Table 2). Of note, no changes in serum IL-6 were detected in RA patients after exercise, but this might be attributable to a less strenuous exercise regimen when compared to healthy individuals (Knudsen et al. 2008). It is also possible that the anti-inflammatory effect of exercise is blunted in patients with RA, but this requires further study.

Type of exercise	Beneficial effect on health
Aerobic exercise (humans)	Increase plasma levels of IL-10, IL-1ra (Walsh et al. 2011)
Cycling (humans)	Suppress endotoxin-induced TNF-α (Starkie et al. 2003)
Strength training (humans)	Increase IL-15 (Pedersen and Febbraio 2008)
Continuous passive motion (rabbits)	Suppression of proteoglycan loss Downregulation of MMP-1 Upregulation of IL-10 (Ferretti et al. 2005; Ferretti et al. 2006)
Continuous passive motion (rats)	Suppression of proteoglycan loss Downregulation of MMP-1, -3 (Leong et al. 2010; Leong et al. 2011)

Table 2. Anti-inflammatory and anti-catabolic effects of exercise

2.3.2 Local effects on cartilage

Clinical trials investigating the anti-inflammatory effect of exercise in the articular cartilage of RA patients are lacking, but results from clinical studies of osteoarthritis patients and animal models of RA suggest that moderate exercise has an anti-inflammatory effect on cartilage. Following acute resistance exercise, a significant increase in IL-10 was observed in the intra-articular and synovial spaces of subjects who exercised when compared to a non-exercise group (Helmark et al. 2010). Increases in IL-10 expression were also reported in chondrocytes in antigen-induced arthritis, an animal model of rheumatoid arthritis, after two weeks of continuous passive motion when compared to immobilized joints (Ferretti et al. 2005; Ferretti et al. 2006). Continuous passive motion also suppressed expression of IL-1β and inflammatory mediator COX-2 (Ferretti et al. 2006). Together, these data suggest that physiologic loading has the potential to generate anti-inflammatory biomechanical signals in cartilage, at least in part, by inducing IL-10.

To test the direct effect of IL-10 on rheumatic activity, collagen-induced arthritis mice were treated with recombinant IL-10, which resulted in a mild, but significant suppression of arthritic phenotype/symptoms (Johansson et al. 2001). Endogenous IL-10 plays a pivotal role in the regulation of antigen (streptococcal cell wall)-induced arthritis (Lubberts et al. 1998), since the blocking of endogenous IL-10 with anti-IL-10 antibodies resulted in a sustained arthritis with denser synovial infiltrates as well as enhanced cartilage damage. Adding exogenous IL-10 further enlarged the suppressive effect of endogenous IL-10. However, these findings require further investigation in human clinical trials of RA patients.

2.4 Anti-catabolic effects of exercise on cartilage

Considering cartilage destruction is a hallmark of RA, the role of exercise in maintaining cartilage matrix integrity is of great importance (Table 2) (Maini and Feldmann 2004). Articular cartilage functions as a nearly frictionless bearing surface while uniformly transferring loads on underlying bone and preventing high stress concentrations. Cartilage consists of one cell type, the chondrocyte, embedded in an extracellular matrix of mainly type II collagen and proteoglycans (Milner 2008). Physiologic loading of the cartilage tissue is required to maintain tissue homeostasis, while non-physiologic loading (disuse and overuse) promotes its degradation (Sun 2010). Intensive dynamic and weight-bearing exercises were originally considered detrimental for patients with RA due to concerns of exacerbating disease, (van den Ende et al. 1996), but studies have shown such exercise does not cause an increase in the rate of damage to either large (de Jong et al. 2003) or small joints (de Jong et al. 2004). There were no significant differences in the rate of damage of large joints 18 months following the end of a high-intensity program between RA patients who discontinued exercise and those who were still exercising (de Jong et al. 2009). Furthermore, levels of cartilage oligomeric matrix protein (COMP), a measure of cartilage damage were unchanged after 3 months of exercise in RA patients, suggesting exercise did not cause significant damage to the cartilage matrix (de Jong et al. 2008). Exercise may also enhance joint lubrication, further acting to promote the health of the RA joint. During joint movement, synovial fluid is squeezed out from between the two surfaces of the joint, resulting in fluid film lubrication (Isenberg et al. 2004). Lubricin, a mucinous glycoprotein secreted by synovial fibroblasts, is the factor responsible for lubrication (Jay et al. 2001), and reduced levels of this protein found in RA patients may increase joint friction and promote cartilage degradation (Jay et al. 2004; Elsaid et al. 2007). However, whether exercise increases lubricin expression in patients with RA has not yet been determined. Exercise also promotes adequate strength of the muscles and surrounding joint soft tissues, providing optimal joint stability, alignment and attenuation of impact and compressive forces (Sun 2010).

After vigorous exercise in patients with moderate disease activity, a reduction in the number of diseased joints is observed (Minor et al. 1989; van den Ende et al. 1996). Animal studies have demonstrated physiologic loading of joints exerts beneficial effects by suppressing the activity of proteolytic enzymes in healthy and arthritic rats. Passive joint motion prevented cartilage destruction due to inactivity and downregulated MMPs 1 and 3 (Leong et al. 2010; Leong et al. 2011). In antigen-induced rabbits, passive motion prevented proteoglycan loss and suppressed expression of MMP-1 (Ferretti et al. 2005; Ferretti et al. 2006).

3. Mechanisms of exercise in rheumatoid arthritis treatment

Although the beneficial effects of exercise for rheumatoid arthritis patients are well documented, the mechanisms are still largely unclear. As detailed previously, the effects of exercise are commonly characterized as anti-inflammatory and anti-catabolic. Each of these components is mediated by distinct signalling pathways and evidence indicates crosstalk between these pathways (see Figure 1 for hypothesized pathways/mechanisms).

3.1 Anti-inflammatory signaling

One of the first evidences of anti-inflammatory signalling in chondrocytes was the elucidation of the α5β1 integrin/IL-4 pathway. In this pathway, mechanical stimulation of normal chondrocytes acts through the α5β1 integrin to release IL-4, which acts in an autocrine/paracrine manner. Following IL-4 release, there is a decrease in MMP-3 and an increase in aggrecan mRNA, resulting in a net increase in cartilage extracellular matrix production (Millward-Sadler and Salter 2004). The transcription factor Signal Transducer and Activator of Transcription 6 (STAT6) plays a principal role in IL-4 signaling as demonstrated in mice lacking STAT6 that show a similar phenotype as mice lacking the IL-4 receptor alpha (IL-4Rα) (Takeda et al. 1996). IL-4 stimulates intracellular signaling pathways including the recruitment of STAT6 to the IL-4Rα. STAT6 binds to specific phosphotyrosine residues within the IL-4Rα (Ryan et al. 1998). In this complex, STAT6 is quickly phosphorylated by a JAK-dependent mechanism. After phosphorylation, STAT6 leaves the receptor, dimerizes, and migrates to the nucleus where it binds to specific DNA sequences in the promoter of genes (Darnell 1997). It is believed that STAT6 is tightly regulated, because in the absence of IL-4 stimulation, STAT6 is quickly deactivated (Andrews et al. 2002). Methylation of STAT6 is a regulator of STAT6 activity, necessary for optimal STAT6 phosphorylation, nuclear translocation, and DNA-binding activity (Chen et al. 2004). Accumulating evidence suggests that IL-4 STAT6 is a central anti-rheumatoid signaling pathway because it upregulates three factors known to antagonize the actions of specific pro-inflammatory agents implicated in RA: (1) soluble IL-1 receptor antagonist (sIL-1ra); (2) tristetraprolin (TTP), which antagonizes TNF-α; and (3) the β_3 integrin, which was shown to antagonize the angiogenic actions of vascular endothelial growth factor (VEGF) (Vannier et al. 1992; McHugh et al. 2001; Suzuki et al. 2003).

While the mechanisms underlying the anti-inflammatory effects of IL-10 are largely unknown in chondrocytes, studies which overexpress IL-10 provide insight on the downstream targets of IL-10. IL-10 treatment in an antigen-induced arthritis animal model resulted in a marked reduction of TNF-α levels (Lubberts et al. 1998). In human chondrocytes treated with TNF-α, IL-10 overexpression ssuppressed MMP-13 levels and antagonized the TNF-α-mediated suppression of aggrecan (Muller et al. 2008). It has been hypothesized that IL-10 may exert its effects by stimulating the production of endogenous TNF-α inhibitors such as soluble TNF-α receptors (Fernandes et al. 2002).

3.2 Anti-catabolic signaling

In vivo, motion-based therapies have been demonstrated to mitigate joint inflammation in animal models of antigen-induced arthritis. Mechanical signals generated from these passive joint motion therapies were reported to be potent inhibitors of pro-inflammatory gene induction and inhibit expression of catabolic mediators, e.g., IL-1β, COX-2, and MMP-1 (Ferretti et al. 2005; Ferretti et al. 2006). At low magnitudes *in vitro,* biomechanical signals inhibit IL-1β- or TNF-α-induced transcriptional activation of COX-2, MMPs, IL-1β, and other pro-inflammatory molecules (Chowdhury et al. 2003; Agarwal et al. 2004; Ferretti et al. 2005; Chowdhury et al. 2006; Deschner et al. 2006).

Exposure of meniscal or articular chondrocytes to proinflammatory cytokines (e.g. IL-1β and TNF-α) is reported to result in the expression of cyclo-oxygenase 2, inducible nitric oxide synthase, and genes involved in cartilage catabolism, such as matrix metalloproteinases 9 and 13 (Gassner et al. 1999). By contrast, when cells are subjected to mechanical stimuli in the form of cyclic tensile strain, they display a blunted response to cytokine exposure, thereby antagonizing the proinflammatory and catabolic effects of these cytokines (Ferretti et al. 2006; Madhavan et al. 2006). Interestingly, this anti-catabolic response seems to be mediated by inhibition of nuclear translocation of Nuclear factor-kappa B (NF-κB) and modulation of upstream signaling events associated with NF-κB, suggesting that mechanical activity can act at multiple points within the proinflammatory signaling network to counteract cytokine-induced proinflammatory gene expression (Dossumbekova et al. 2007).

NF-κB transcription factors regulate a wide range of pro-inflammatory and anti-apoptotic genes, and are involved in both acute and chronic inflammatory responses. NF-κB is a rapid response, multiple-stimuli inducible transcription factor that is controlled by sequential signal activation cascades (Seguin and Bernier 2003). In the classical NF-κB signaling pathway, binding of pro-inflammatory mediators, such as IL-1β, TNF-*a*, and/or LPS to their cognate receptors leads to activation of a series of receptor-associated signaling molecules leading to activated NF-κB, which translocates to the nucleus, where it binds to the consensus sequences of several genes including pro-inflammatory cytokines and mediators (Ghosh and Karin 2002; Hoffmann et al. 2002; Liacini et al. 2003). Mechanical signals of low/physiological magnitudes block the IL-1β-induced transcriptional activity of NF-κB by intercepting multiple steps in the NF-κB signaling cascade. In chondrocytes, cyclic tensile strain of low magnitudes does not appear to inhibit IL-1β, TNF-α, or LPS receptor-mediated pro-inflammatory gene induction (Agarwal et al. 2004; Dossumbekova et al. 2007; Madhavan et al. 2007). These findings suggest that mechanical signals use specific target sites to trigger NF-κB signaling.

Another transcriptional regulator which plays a critical role in cartilage homeostasis is CBP/p300-interacting transactivator with ED-rich tail 2 (CITED2). CITED2 expression is increased by moderate flow shear (5 dyn/cm^2), intermittent hydrostatic pressure (1-5 MPa), and joint motion (Yokota et al. 2003; Leong et al. 2011). The induction of CITED2 *in vivo* by joint motion loading was correlated with the downregulation of MMP-1 and the maintenance of cartilage matrix integrity (Leong et al. 2011), suggesting it plays a key role in mediating the anti-catabolic effects of moderate loading. The induction of CITED2 by physiologic loading was mediated by mitogen-activated protein kinase (MAPK) p38δ, and CITED2 regulated the transcription of MMPs (ie. MMP-1) by competing with MMP transactivator ETS-1 for binding to limiting amounts of co-activator p300 (Leong et al. 2011).

3.3 Crosstalk between anti-inflammatory and anti-catabolic responses

There is also evidence of crosstalk between the anti-inflammatory and anti-catabolic pathways. CITED2, induced by p38δ, has also been demonstrated to be upregulated in response to IL-4 (Sun et al. 1998), raising the possibility these two pathways could work in synergy. Furthermore, treatment strategies involving gene transfer of IL-4 or IL-10 combined with mechanical stimulation may augment the chondroprotective effects of exercise. However, these hypotheses still require further investigation.

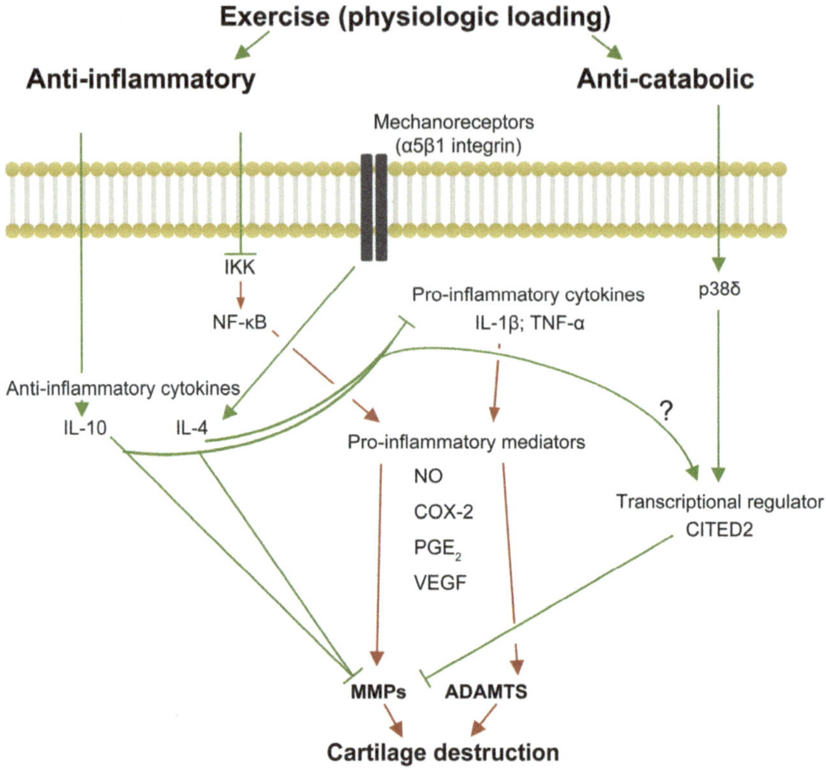

Fig. 1. Hypothesized anti-inflammatory and anti-catabolic mechanisms underlying the effects of exercise in suppressing cartilage destruction in arthritis.

4. Conclusion

Compelling evidence suggests that physiologic exercise exerts beneficial effects in rheumatoid arthritis patients that not only increases quality of life but also suppresses disease activity. The beneficial effects are dependent on the mechanical nature of exercise, including the loading intensity, frequency, and duration. Exercise regimens may have varying effects with age and stage of disease. Furthermore, elucidating mechanisms underlying these beneficial effects of exercise may lead to the development of novel therapeutic strategies to prevent joint destruction in rheumatoid arthritis.

5. Acknowledgment

The authors thank Dr. John Hardin for his critical reading of the manuscript and the National Institutes of Health for funding this work (AR52743 and AR47628-04).

6. References

Agarwal, S., J. Deschner, P. Long, A. Verma, C. Hofman, C. H. Evans, & N. Piesco (2004). Role of NF-kappaB transcription factors in antiinflammatory and proinflammatory actions of mechanical signals. *Arthritis Rheum* Vol.50, No.11, (Nov 2004), pp. (3541-8), ISSN 0004-3591 (Print), 0004-3591 (Linking)

Alamanos, Y., & A. A. Drosos (2005). Epidemiology of adult rheumatoid arthritis. *Autoimmun Rev* Vol.4, No.3, (Mar 2005), pp. (130-6), ISSN 1568-9972 (Print), 1568-9972 (Linking)

Andrews, R. P., M. B. Ericksen, C. M. Cunningham, M. O. Daines, & G. K. Hershey (2002). Analysis of the life cycle of stat6. Continuous cycling of STAT6 is required for IL-4 signaling. *J Biol Chem* Vol.277, No.39, (Sep 2002), pp. (36563-9), ISSN 0021-9258 (Print), 0021-9258 (Linking)

Baillet, A., E. Payraud, V. A. Niderprim, M. J. Nissen, B. Allenet, P. Francois, L. Grange, P. Casez, R. Juvin, & P. Gaudin (2009). A dynamic exercise programme to improve patients' disability in rheumatoid arthritis: a prospective randomized controlled trial. *Rheumatology (Oxford)* Vol.48, No.4, (Apr 2009), pp. (410-5), ISSN 1462-0332 (Electronic), 1462-0324 (Linking)

Baillet, A., N. Zeboulon, L. Gossec, C. Combescure, L. A. Bodin, R. Juvin, M. Dougados, & P. Gaudin (2010). Efficacy of cardiorespiratory aerobic exercise in rheumatoid arthritis: meta-analysis of randomized controlled trials. *Arthritis Care Res (Hoboken)* Vol.62, No.7, (Jul 2010), pp. (984-92), ISSN 2151-4658 (Electronic)

Bijlsma, J. W. (2010). Optimal treatment of rheumatoid arthritis: EULAR recommendations for clinical practice. *Pol Arch Med Wewn* Vol.120, No.9, (Sep 2010), pp. (347-53), ISSN 1897-9483 (Electronic), 0032-3772 (Linking)

Bilberg, A., M. Ahlmen, & K. Mannerkorpi (2005). Moderately intensive exercise in a temperate pool for patients with rheumatoid arthritis: a randomized controlled study. *Rheumatology (Oxford)* Vol.44, No.4, (Apr 2005), pp. (502-8), ISSN 1462-0324 (Print), 1462-0324 (Linking)

Brentano, M. A., & L. F. Martins Kruel (2011). A review on strength exercise-induced muscle damage: applications, adaptation mechanisms and limitations. *J Sports Med Phys Fitness* Vol.51, No.1, (Mar 2011), pp. (1-10), ISSN 0022-4707 (Print), 0022-4707 (Linking)

Brorsson, S., M. Hilliges, C. Sollerman, & A. Nilsdotter (2009). A six-week hand exercise programme improves strength and hand function in patients with rheumatoid arthritis. *J Rehabil Med* Vol.41, No.5, (Apr 2009), pp. (338-42), ISSN 1651-2081 (Electronic), 1650-1977 (Linking)

Brukner, P. D., & W. J. Brown (2005). 3. Is exercise good for you? *Med J Aust* Vol.183, No.10, (Nov 2005), pp. (538-41), ISSN 0025-729X (Print), 0025-729X (Linking)

Cairns, A. P., & J. G. McVeigh (2009). A systematic review of the effects of dynamic exercise in rheumatoid arthritis. *Rheumatol Int* Vol.30, No.2, (Dec 2009), pp. (147-58), ISSN 1437-160X (Electronic), 0172-8172 (Linking)

Chen, W., M. O. Daines, & G. K. Hershey (2004). Methylation of STAT6 modulates STAT6 phosphorylation, nuclear translocation, and DNA-binding activity. *J Immunol*

Vol.172, No.11, (Jun 2004), pp. (6744-50), ISSN 0022-1767 (Print), 0022-1767 (Linking)

Chowdhury, T. T., D. L. Bader, & D. A. Lee (2003). Dynamic compression counteracts IL-1 beta-induced release of nitric oxide and PGE2 by superficial zone chondrocytes cultured in agarose constructs. *Osteoarthritis Cartilage* Vol.11, No.9, (Sep 2003), pp. (688-96), ISSN 1063-4584 (Print), 1063-4584 (Linking)

Chowdhury, T. T., D. L. Bader, & D. A. Lee (2006). Anti-inflammatory effects of IL-4 and dynamic compression in IL-1beta stimulated chondrocytes. *Biochem Biophys Res Commun* Vol.339, No.1, (Jan 2006), pp. (241-7), ISSN 0006-291X (Print), 0006-291X (Linking)

Darnell, J. E., Jr. (1997). STATs and gene regulation. *Science* Vol.277, No.5332, (Sep 1997), pp. (1630-5), ISSN 0036-8075 (Print), 0036-8075 (Linking)

de Jong, Z., M. Munneke, L. M. Jansen, K. Ronday, D. J. van Schaardenburg, R. Brand, C. H. van den Ende, T. P. Vliet Vlieland, W. M. Zuijderduin, & J. M. Hazes (2004). Differences between participants and nonparticipants in an exercise trial for adults with rheumatoid arthritis. *Arthritis Rheum* Vol.51, No.4, (Aug 2004), pp. (593-600), ISSN 0004-3591 (Print), 0004-3591 (Linking)

de Jong, Z., M. Munneke, H. M. Kroon, D. van Schaardenburg, B. A. Dijkmans, J. M. Hazes, & T. P. Vliet Vlieland (2009). Long-term follow-up of a high-intensity exercise program in patients with rheumatoid arthritis. *Clin Rheumatol* Vol.28, No.6, (Jun 2009), pp. (663-71), ISSN 1434-9949 (Electronic), 0770-3198 (Linking)

de Jong, Z., M. Munneke, V. Vilim, A. H. Zwinderman, H. M. Kroon, H. K. Ronday, W. F. Lems, B. A. Dijkmans, F. C. Breedveld, T. P. Vliet Vlieland, J. M. Hazes, & J. Degroot (2008). Value of serum cartilage oligomeric matrix protein as a prognostic marker of large-joint damage in rheumatoid arthritis--data from the RAPIT study. *Rheumatology (Oxford)* Vol.47, No.6, (Jun 2008), pp. (868-71), ISSN 1462-0332 (Electronic), 1462-0324 (Linking)

de Jong, Z., M. Munneke, A. H. Zwinderman, H. M. Kroon, A. Jansen, K. H. Ronday, D. van Schaardenburg, B. A. Dijkmans, C. H. Van den Ende, F. C. Breedveld, T. P. Vliet Vlieland, & J. M. Hazes (2003). Is a long-term high-intensity exercise program effective and safe in patients with rheumatoid arthritis? Results of a randomized controlled trial. *Arthritis Rheum* Vol.48, No.9, (Sep 2003), pp. (2415-24), ISSN 0004-3591 (Print), 0004-3591 (Linking)

de Jong, Z., & T. P. Vliet Vlieland (2005). Safety of exercise in patients with rheumatoid arthritis. *Curr Opin Rheumatol* Vol.17, No.2, (Mar 2005), pp. (177-82), ISSN 1040-8711 (Print), 1040-8711 (Linking)

Deighton, C., R. O'Mahony, J. Tosh, C. Turner, & M. Rudolf (2009). Management of rheumatoid arthritis: summary of NICE guidance. *BMJ* Vol.338, 2009), pp. (b702), ISSN 1468-5833 (Electronic), 0959-535X (Linking)

Dekker, M. J., S. Lee, R. Hudson, K. Kilpatrick, T. E. Graham, R. Ross, & L. E. Robinson (2007). An exercise intervention without weight loss decreases circulating interleukin-6 in lean and obese men with and without type 2 diabetes mellitus. *Metabolism* Vol.56, No.3, (Mar 2007), pp. (332-8), ISSN 0026-0495 (Print), 0026-0495 (Linking)

Deschner, J., B. Rath-Deschner, & S. Agarwal (2006). Regulation of matrix metalloproteinase expression by dynamic tensile strain in rat fibrochondrocytes. *Osteoarthritis Cartilage* Vol.14, No.3, (Mar 2006), pp. (264-72), ISSN 1063-4584 (Print), 1063-4584 (Linking)

Dossumbekova, A., M. Anghelina, S. Madhavan, L. He, N. Quan, T. Knobloch, & S. Agarwal (2007). Biomechanical signals inhibit IKK activity to attenuate NF-kappaB transcription activity in inflamed chondrocytes. *Arthritis Rheum* Vol.56, No.10, (Oct 2007), pp. (3284-96), ISSN 0004-3591 (Print), 0004-3591 (Linking)

Ekblom, B., O. Lovgren, M. Alderin, M. Fridstrom, & G. Satterstrom (1975). Effect of short-term physical training on patients with rheumatoid arthritis. a six-month follow-up study. *Scand J Rheumatol* Vol.4, No.2, (1975), pp. (87-91), ISSN 0300-9742 (Print), 0300-9742 (Linking)

Elsaid, K. A., G. D. Jay, & C. O. Chichester (2007). Reduced expression and proteolytic susceptibility of lubricin/superficial zone protein may explain early elevation in the coefficient of friction in the joints of rats with antigen-induced arthritis. *Arthritis Rheum* Vol.56, No.1, (Jan 2007), pp. (108-16), ISSN 0004-3591 (Print), 0004-3591 (Linking)

Fernandes, J. C., J. Martel-Pelletier, & J. P. Pelletier (2002). The role of cytokines in osteoarthritis pathophysiology. *Biorheology* Vol.39, No.1-2, (2002), pp. (237-46), ISSN 0006-355X (Print), 0006-355X (Linking)

Ferretti, M., R. Gassner, Z. Wang, P. Perera, J. Deschner, G. Sowa, R. B. Salter, & S. Agarwal (2006). Biomechanical signals suppress proinflammatory responses in cartilage: early events in experimental antigen-induced arthritis. *J Immunol* Vol.177, No.12, (Dec 2006), pp. (8757-66), ISSN 0022-1767 (Print), 0022-1767 (Linking)

Ferretti, M., A. Srinivasan, J. Deschner, R. Gassner, F. Baliko, N. Piesco, R. Salter, & S. Agarwal (2005). Anti-inflammatory effects of continuous passive motion on meniscal fibrocartilage. *J Orthop Res* Vol.23, No.5, (Sep 2005), pp. (1165-71), ISSN 0736-0266 (Print), 0736-0266 (Linking)

Forestier, R., J. Andre-Vert, P. Guillez, E. Coudeyre, M. M. Lefevre-Colau, B. Combe, & M. A. Mayoux-Benhamou (2009). Non-drug treatment (excluding surgery) in rheumatoid arthritis: clinical practice guidelines. *Joint Bone Spine* Vol.76, No.6, (Dec 2009), pp. (691-8), ISSN 1778-7254 (Electronic), 1297-319X (Linking)

Gassner, R., M. J. Buckley, H. Georgescu, R. Studer, M. Stefanovich-Racic, N. P. Piesco, C. H. Evans, & S. Agarwal (1999). Cyclic tensile stress exerts antiinflammatory actions on chondrocytes by inhibiting inducible nitric oxide synthase. *J Immunol* Vol.163, No.4, (Aug 1999), pp. (2187-92), ISSN 0022-1767 (Print), 0022-1767 (Linking)

Geborek, P., M. Crnkic, I. F. Petersson, & T. Saxne (2002). Etanercept, infliximab, and leflunomide in established rheumatoid arthritis: clinical experience using a structured follow up programme in southern Sweden. *Ann Rheum Dis* Vol.61, No.9, (Sep 2002), pp. (793-8), ISSN 0003-4967 (Print), 0003-4967 (Linking)

Ghosh, S., & M. Karin (2002). Missing pieces in the NF-kappaB puzzle. *Cell* Vol.109 Suppl, Apr 2002), pp. (S81-96), ISSN 0092-8674 (Print), 0092-8674 (Linking)

Hakkinen, A. (2004). Effectiveness and safety of strength training in rheumatoid arthritis. *Curr Opin Rheumatol* Vol.16, No.2, (Mar 2004), pp. (132-7), ISSN 1040-8711 (Print), 1040-8711 (Linking)

Hakkinen, A., A. Pakarinen, P. Hannonen, H. Kautiainen, K. Nyman, W. J. Kraemer, & K. Hakkinen (2005). Effects of prolonged combined strength and endurance training on physical fitness, body composition and serum hormones in women with rheumatoid arthritis and in healthy controls. *Clin Exp Rheumatol* Vol.23, No.4, (Jul-Aug 2005), pp. (505-12), ISSN 0392-856X (Print), 0392-856X (Linking)

Hakkinen, A., T. Sokka, A. Kotaniemi, & P. Hannonen (2001). A randomized two-year study of the effects of dynamic strength training on muscle strength, disease activity, functional capacity, and bone mineral density in early rheumatoid arthritis. *Arthritis Rheum* Vol.44, No.3, (Mar 2001), pp. (515-22), ISSN 0004-3591 (Print), 0004-3591 (Linking)

Hall, J., S. M. Skevington, P. J. Maddison, & K. Chapman (1996). A randomized and controlled trial of hydrotherapy in rheumatoid arthritis. *Arthritis Care Res* Vol.9, No.3, (Jun 1996), pp. (206-15), ISSN 0893-7524 (Print), 0893-7524 (Linking)

Handschin, C., & B. M. Spiegelman (2008). The role of exercise and PGC1alpha in inflammation and chronic disease. *Nature* Vol.454, No.7203, (Jul 2008), pp. (463-9), ISSN 1476-4687 (Electronic), 0028-0836 (Linking)

Haskell, W. L., I. M. Lee, R. R. Pate, K. E. Powell, S. N. Blair, B. A. Franklin, C. A. Macera, G. W. Heath, P. D. Thompson, & A. Bauman (2007). Physical activity and public health: updated recommendation for adults from the American College of Sports Medicine and the American Heart Association. *Med Sci Sports Exerc* Vol.39, No.8, (Aug 2007), pp. (1423-34), ISSN 0195-9131 (Print), 0195-9131 (Linking)

Helmark, I. C., U. R. Mikkelsen, J. Borglum, A. Rothe, M. C. Petersen, O. Andersen, H. Langberg, & M. Kjaer (2010). Exercise increases interleukin-10 levels both intraarticularly and peri-synovially in patients with knee osteoarthritis: a randomized controlled trial. *Arthritis Res Ther* Vol.12, No.4, (2010), pp. (R126), ISSN 1478-6362 (Electronic), 1478-6354 (Linking)

Hoffmann, A., A. Levchenko, M. L. Scott, & D. Baltimore (2002). The IkappaB-NF-kappaB signaling module: temporal control and selective gene activation. *Science* Vol.298, No.5596, (Nov 2002), pp. (1241-5), ISSN 1095-9203 (Electronic), 0036-8075 (Linking)

Hurkmans, E., F. J. van der Giesen, T. P. Vliet Vlieland, J. Schoones, & E. C. Van den Ende (2009). Dynamic exercise programs (aerobic capacity and/or muscle strength training) in patients with rheumatoid arthritis. *Cochrane Database Syst Rev* Vol.No.4, (2009), pp. (CD006853), ISSN 1469-493X (Electronic), 1361-6137 (Linking)

Isenberg, D., A. Bull, A. Unsworth, & A. Amis (2004). Biomechanics of articulations and derangements in disease, In: *Oxford Textbook of Rheumatology,* D. Isenberg, P. J. Maddison, P. Woo, D. Glass and F. Breedveld, pp. (379-386), Oxford University Press, Oxford.

Jay, G. D., K. A. Elsaid, J. Zack, K. Robinson, F. Trespalacios, C. J. Cha, & C. O. Chichester (2004). Lubricating ability of aspirated synovial fluid from emergency department patients with knee joint synovitis. *J Rheumatol* Vol.31, No.3, (Mar 2004), pp. (557-64), ISSN 0315-162X (Print), 0315-162X (Linking)

Jay, G. D., U. Tantravahi, D. E. Britt, H. J. Barrach, & C. J. Cha (2001). Homology of lubricin and superficial zone protein (SZP): products of megakaryocyte stimulating factor (MSF) gene expression by human synovial fibroblasts and articular chondrocytes localized to chromosome 1q25. *J Orthop Res* Vol.19, No.4, (Jul 2001), pp. (677-87), ISSN 0736-0266 (Print), 0736-0266 (Linking)

Johansson, A. C., A. S. Hansson, K. S. Nandakumar, J. Backlund, & R. Holmdahl (2001). IL-10-deficient B10.Q mice develop more severe collagen-induced arthritis, but are protected from arthritis induced with anti-type II collagen antibodies. *J Immunol* Vol.167, No.6, (Sep 2001), pp. (3505-12), ISSN 0022-1767 (Print), 0022-1767 (Linking)

King, D. E., P. Carek, A. G. Mainous, 3rd, & W. S. Pearson (2003). Inflammatory markers and exercise: differences related to exercise type. *Med Sci Sports Exerc* Vol.35, No.4, (Apr 2003), pp. (575-81), ISSN 0195-9131 (Print), 0195-9131 (Linking)

Knudsen, L. S., I. J. Christensen, T. Lottenburger, M. N. Svendsen, H. J. Nielsen, L. Nielsen, K. Horslev-Petersen, J. E. Jensen, G. Kollerup, & J. S. Johansen (2008). Pre-analytical and biological variability in circulating interleukin 6 in healthy subjects and patients with rheumatoid arthritis. *Biomarkers* Vol.13, No.1, (Feb 2008), pp. (59-78), ISSN 1354-750X (Print), 1354-750X (Linking)

Kowh, C., L. Anderson, J. Greene, D. Johnson, J. O'Dell, M. Robbins, W. Roberts Jr, R. Simms, & R. Yood (2002). Guidelines for the management of rheumatoid arthritis: 2002 Update. *Arthritis Rheum* Vol.46, No.2, (Feb 2002), pp. (328-46), ISSN 0004-3591 (Print), 0004-3591 (Linking)

Lavie, C. J., R. J. Thomas, R. W. Squires, T. G. Allison, & R. V. Milani (2009). Exercise training and cardiac rehabilitation in primary and secondary prevention of coronary heart disease. *Mayo Clin Proc* Vol.84, No.4, (Apr 2009), pp. (373-83), ISSN 1942-5546 (Electronic), 0025-6196 (Linking)

Lemmey, A. B., S. M. Marcora, K. Chester, S. Wilson, F. Casanova, & P. J. Maddison (2009). Effects of high-intensity resistance training in patients with rheumatoid arthritis: a randomized controlled trial. *Arthritis Rheum* Vol.61, No.12, (Dec 15 2009), pp. (1726-34), ISSN 0004-3591 (Print), 0004-3591 (Linking)

Leong, D. J., X. I. Gu, Y. Li, J. Y. Lee, D. M. Laudier, R. J. Majeska, M. B. Schaffler, L. Cardoso, & H. B. Sun (2010). Matrix metalloproteinase-3 in articular cartilage is upregulated by joint immobilization and suppressed by passive joint motion. *Matrix Biol* Vol.29, No.5, (Jun 2010), pp. (420-6), ISSN 1569-1802 (Electronic), 0945-053X (Linking)

Leong, D. J., Y. H. Li, X. I. Gu, L. Sun, Z. Zhou, P. Nasser, D. M. Laudier, J. Iqbal, R. J. Majeska, M. B. Schaffler, M. B. Goldring, L. Cardoso, M. Zaidi, & H. B. Sun (2011). Physiological loading of joints prevents cartilage degradation through CITED2. *FASEB J* Vol.25, No.1, (Jan 2011), pp. (182-91), ISSN 1530-6860(Electronic), 0892-6638 (Linking)

Liacini, A., J. Sylvester, W. Q. Li, W. Huang, F. Dehnade, M. Ahmad, & M. Zafarullah (2003). Induction of matrix metalloproteinase-13 gene expression by TNF-alpha is mediated by MAP kinases, AP-1, and NF-kappaB transcription factors in articular chondrocytes. *Exp Cell Res* Vol.288, No.1, (Aug 2003), pp. (208-17), ISSN 0014-4827 (Print), 0014-4827 (Linking)

Lubberts, E., L. A. Joosten, M. M. Helsen, & W. B. van den Berg (1998). Regulatory role of interleukin 10 in joint inflammation and cartilage destruction in murine streptococcal cell wall (SCW) arthritis. More therapeutic benefit with IL-4/IL-10 combination therapy than with IL-10 treatment alone. *Cytokine* Vol.10, No.5, (May 1998), pp. (361-9), ISSN 1043-4666 (Print), 1043-4666 (Linking)

Lundberg, I. E., & G. A. Nader (2008). Molecular effects of exercise in patients with inflammatory rheumatic disease. *Nat Clin Pract Rheumatol* Vol.4, No.11, (Nov 2008), pp. (597-604), 1745-8390 (Electronic), ISSN 1745-8390 (Linking)

Madhavan, S., M. Anghelina, B. Rath-Deschner, E. Wypasek, A. John, J. Deschner, N. Piesco, & S. Agarwal (2006). Biomechanical signals exert sustained attenuation of proinflammatory gene induction in articular chondrocytes. *Osteoarthritis Cartilage* Vol.14, No.10, (Oct 2006), pp. (1023-32), ISSN 1063-4584 (Print), 1063-4584 (Linking)

Madhavan, S., M. Anghelina, D. Sjostrom, A. Dossumbekova, D. C. Guttridge, & S. Agarwal (2007). Biomechanical signals suppress TAK1 activation to inhibit NF-kappaB transcriptional activation in fibrochondrocytes. *J Immunol* Vol.179, No.9, (Nov 2007), pp. (6246-54), ISSN 0022-1767 (Print), 0022-1767 (Linking)

Maini, R., & M. Feldmann (2004). Rheumatoid arthritis: immunopathgenesis of rheumatoid arthritis, In: *Oxford Textbook of Rheumatology,* D. Isenberg, P. J. Maddison, P. Woo, D. Glass and F. Breedveld, pp. Oxford University Press, Oxford.

Marcora, S. M., A. B. Lemmey, & P. J. Maddison (2005). Can progressive resistance training reverse cachexia in patients with rheumatoid arthritis? Results of a pilot study. *J Rheumatol* Vol.32, No.6, (Jun 2005), pp. (1031-9), ISSN 0315-162X (Print), 0315-162X (Linking)

Matschke, V., P. Murphy, A. B. Lemmey, P. Maddison, & J. M. Thom (2010). Skeletal muscle properties in rheumatoid arthritis patients. *Med Sci Sports Exerc* Vol.42, No.12, (Dec 2010), pp. (2149-55), ISSN 1530-0315 (Electronic), 0195-9131 (Linking)

McHugh, K. P., S. Kitazawa, S. L. Teitelbaum, & F. P. Ross (2001). Cloning and characterization of the murine beta(3) integrin gene promoter: identification of an interleukin-4 responsive element and regulation by STAT-6. *J Cell Biochem* Vol.81, No.2, (Mar 2001), pp. (320-32), ISSN 0730-2312 (Print), 0730-2312 (Linking)

Medicine, A. C. o. S., L. Durstine, G. Moore, P. Painter, & S. Roberts (2009). *ACSM's Exercise Management for Persons with Chronic Diseases and Disabilities-3rd Edition* Human Kinetics, 0736074333, Champaign.

Melikoglu, M. A., S. Karatay, K. Senel, & F. Akcay (2006). Association between dynamic exercise therapy and IGF-1 and IGFBP-3 concentrations in the patients with rheumatoid arthritis. *Rheumatol Int* Vol.26, No.4, (Feb 2006), pp. (309-13), ISSN 0172-8172 (Print), 0172-8172 (Linking)

Metsios, G. S., A. Stavropoulos-Kalinoglou, A. Sandoo, J. J. van Zanten, T. E. Toms, H. John, & G. D. Kitas (2010). Vascular function and inflammation in rheumatoid arthritis: the role of physical activity. *Open Cardiovasc Med J* Vol.4, (2010), pp. (89-96), ISSN 1874-1924 (Electronic)

Millward-Sadler, S. J., & D. M. Salter (2004). Integrin-dependent signal cascades in chondrocyte mechanotransduction. *Ann Biomed Eng* Vol.32, No.3, (Mar 2004), pp. (435-46), ISSN 0090-6964 (Print), 0090-6964 (Linking)

Milner, C. E. (2008). *Functional Anatomy for Sport and Exercise; Quick Reference* Routledge, Oxfordshire.

Minor, M. A., J. E. Hewett, R. R. Webel, S. K. Anderson, & D. R. Kay (1989). Efficacy of physical conditioning exercise in patients with rheumatoid arthritis and osteoarthritis. *Arthritis Rheum* Vol.32, No.11, (Nov 1989), pp. (1396-405), ISSN 0004-3591 (Print), 0004-3591 (Linking)

Moffet, H., L. Noreau, E. Parent, & M. Drolet (2000). Feasibility of an eight-week dance-based exercise program and its effects on locomotor ability of persons with functional class III rheumatoid arthritis. *Arthritis Care Res* Vol.13, No.2, (Apr 2000), pp. (100-11), ISSN 0893-7524 (Print), 0893-7524 (Linking)

Morse, C. I., J. M. Thom, O. S. Mian, K. M. Birch, & M. V. Narici (2007). Gastrocnemius specific force is increased in elderly males following a 12-month physical training programme. *Eur J Appl Physiol* Vol.100, No.5, (Jul 2007), pp. (563-70), ISSN 1439-6319 (Print), 1439-6319 (Linking)

Muller-Riemenschneider, F., C. Meinhard, K. Damm, C. Vauth, A. Bockelbrink, W. Greiner, & S. N. Willich (2011). Effectiveness of nonpharmacological secondary prevention of coronary heart disease. *Eur J Cardiovasc Prev Rehabil* Vol.17, No.6, (Dec 2011), pp. (688-700), ISSN 1741-8275 (Electronic), 1741-8267 (Linking)

Muller, R. D., T. John, B. Kohl, A. Oberholzer, T. Gust, A. Hostmann, M. Hellmuth, D. Laface, B. Hutchins, G. Laube, R. W. Veh, S. K. Tschoeke, W. Ertel, & G. Schulze-Tanzil (2008). IL-10 overexpression differentially affects cartilage matrix gene expression in response to TNF-alpha in human articular chondrocytes in vitro. *Cytokine* Vol.44, No.3, (Dec 2008), pp. (377-85), ISSN 1096-0023 (Electronic), 1043-4666 (Linking)

Murphy, M., A. Nevill, C. Neville, S. Biddle, & A. Hardman (2002). Accumulating brisk walking for fitness, cardiovascular risk, and psychological health. *Med Sci Sports Exerc* Vol.34, No.9, (Sep 2002), pp. (1468-74), ISSN 0195-9131 (Print), 0195-9131 (Linking)

Neill, J., I. Belan, & K. Ried (2006). Effectiveness of non-pharmacological interventions for fatigue in adults with multiple sclerosis, rheumatoid arthritis, or systemic lupus erythematosus: a systematic review. *J Adv Nurs* Vol.56, No.6, (Dec 2006), pp. (617-35), ISSN 0309-2402 (Print), 0309-2402 (Linking)

Neuberger, G. B., L. S. Aaronson, B. Gajewski, S. E. Embretson, P. E. Cagle, J. K. Loudon, & P. A. Miller (2007). Predictors of exercise and effects of exercise on symptoms, function, aerobic fitness, and disease outcomes of rheumatoid arthritis. *Arthritis Rheum* Vol.57, No.6, (Aug 2007), pp. (943-52), ISSN 0004-3591 (Print), 0004-3591 (Linking)

Nieman, D. (2000). Exercise Soothes Arthritis Joint Effects. *ACSM's Health and Fitness Journal* Vol.4, No.3, (2000), pp. (20-27), ISSN 1091-5397 (Print)

Olson, T. P., D. R. Dengel, A. S. Leon, & K. H. Schmitz (2007). Changes in inflammatory biomarkers following one-year of moderate resistance training in overweight women. *Int J Obes (Lond)* Vol.31, No.6, (Jun 2007), pp. (996-1003), ISSN 0307-0565 (Print), 0307-0565 (Linking)

Pedersen, B. K., & M. A. Febbraio (2008). Muscle as an endocrine organ: focus on muscle-derived interleukin-6. *Physiol Rev* Vol.88, No.4, (Oct 2008), pp. (1379-406), ISSN 0031-9333 (Print), 0031-9333 (Linking)

Pedersen, B. K., & B. Saltin (2006). Evidence for prescribing exercise as therapy in chronic disease. *Scand J Med Sci Sports* Vol.16 Suppl 1, (Feb 2006), pp. (3-63), ISSN 0905-7188 (Print), 0905-7188 (Linking)

Petersen, A. M., & B. K. Pedersen (2005). The anti-inflammatory effect of exercise. *J Appl Physiol* Vol.98, No.4, (Apr 2005), pp. (1154-62), ISSN 8750-7587 (Print), 0161-7567 (Linking)

Petersen, A. M., & B. K. Pedersen (2006). The role of IL-6 in mediating the anti-inflammatory effects of exercise. *J Physiol Pharmacol* Vol.57 Suppl 10, (Nov 2006), pp. (43-51), ISSN 1899-1505 (Electronic), 0867-5910 (Linking)

Peterson, M. D., & P. M. Gordon (2011). Resistance exercise for the aging adult: clinical implications and prescription guidelines. *Am J Med* Vol.124, No.3, (Mar 2011), pp. (194-8), ISSN 1555-7162 (Electronic), 0002-9343 (Linking)

Rall, L. C., S. N. Meydani, J. J. Kehayias, B. Dawson-Hughes, & R. Roubenoff (1996). The effect of progressive resistance training in rheumatoid arthritis. Increased strength without changes in energy balance or body composition. *Arthritis Rheum* Vol.39, No.3, (Mar 1996), pp. (415-26), ISSN 0004-3591 (Print), 0004-3591 (Linking)

Resnick, B. (2001). Managing arthritis with exercise. *Geriatr Nurs* Vol.22, No.3, (May-Jun 2001), pp. (143-50), ISSN 0197-4572 (Print), 0197-4572 (Linking)

Roubenoff, R., R. A. Roubenoff, L. M. Ward, S. M. Holland, & D. B. Hellmann (1992). Rheumatoid cachexia: depletion of lean body mass in rheumatoid arthritis. Possible association with tumor necrosis factor. *J Rheumatol* Vol.19, No.10, (Oct 1992), pp. (1505-10), ISSN 0315-162X (Print), 0315-162X (Linking)

Ryan, J. J., L. J. McReynolds, H. Huang, K. Nelms, & W. E. Paul (1998). Characterization of a mobile Stat6 activation motif in the human IL-4 receptor. *J Immunol* Vol.161, No.4, (Aug 1998), pp. (1811-21), ISSN 0022-1767 (Print), 0022-1767 (Linking)

Scott, D. L., F. Wolfe, & T. W. Huizinga (2010). Rheumatoid arthritis. *Lancet* Vol.376, No.9746, (Sep 2010), pp. (1094-108), ISSN 1474-547X (Electronic), 0140-6736 (Linking)

Seguin, C. A., & S. M. Bernier (2003). TNFalpha suppresses link protein and type II collagen expression in chondrocytes: Role of MEK1/2 and NF-kappaB signaling pathways. *J Cell Physiol* Vol.197, No.3, (Dec 2003), pp. (356-69), ISSN 0021-9541 (Print), 0021-9541 (Linking)

Smolen, J. S., R. Landewe, F. C. Breedveld, M. Dougados, P. Emery, C. Gaujoux-Viala, S. Gorter, R. Knevel, J. Nam, M. Schoels, D. Aletaha, M. Buch, L. Gossec, T. Huizinga, J. W. Bijlsma, G. Burmester, B. Combe, M. Cutolo, C. Gabay, J. Gomez-Reino, M. Kouloumas, T. K. Kvien, E. Martin-Mola, I. McInnes, K. Pavelka, P. van Riel, M. Scholte, D. L. Scott, T. Sokka, G. Valesini, R. van Vollenhoven, K. L. Winthrop, J. Wong, A. Zink, & D. van der Heijde (2010). EULAR recommendations for the management of rheumatoid arthritis with synthetic and biological disease-modifying antirheumatic drugs. *Ann Rheum Dis* Vol.69, No.6, (Jun 2010), pp. (964-75), ISSN 1468-2060 (Electronic), 0003-4967 (Linking)

Starkie, R., S. R. Ostrowski, S. Jauffred, M. Febbraio, & B. K. Pedersen (2003). Exercise and IL-6 infusion inhibit endotoxin-induced TNF-alpha production in humans. *FASEB J* Vol.17, No.8, (May 2003), pp. (884-6), ISSN 1530-6860 (Electronic), 0892-6638 (Linking)

Steensberg, A., C. P. Fischer, C. Keller, K. Moller, & B. K. Pedersen (2003). IL-6 enhances plasma IL-1ra, IL-10, and cortisol in humans. *Am J Physiol Endocrinol Metab* Vol.285, No.2, (Aug 2003), pp. (E433-7), ISSN 0193-1849 (Print), 0193-1849 (Linking)

Stenstrom, C. H., & M. A. Minor (2003). Evidence for the benefit of aerobic and strengthening exercise in rheumatoid arthritis. *Arthritis Rheum* Vol.49, No.3, (Jun 2003), pp. (428-34), ISSN 0004-3591 (Print), 0004-3591 (Linking)

Sun, H. B. (2010). Mechanical loading, cartilage degradation, and arthritis. *Ann N Y Acad Sci* Vol.1211, (Nov 2010), pp. (37-50), ISSN 1749-6632 (Electronic), 0077-8923 (Linking)

Sun, H. B., Y. X. Zhu, T. Yin, G. Sledge, & Y. C. Yang (1998). MRG1, the product of a melanocyte-specific gene related gene, is a cytokine-inducible transcription factor with transformation activity. *Proc Natl Acad Sci U S A* Vol.95, No.23, (Nov 1998), pp. (13555-60), ISSN 0027-8424 (Print), 0027-8424 (Linking)

Suzuki, K., H. Nakajima, K. Ikeda, Y. Maezawa, A. Suto, H. Takatori, Y. Saito, & I. Iwamoto (2003). IL-4-Stat6 signaling induces tristetraprolin expression and inhibits TNF-alpha production in mast cells. *J Exp Med* Vol.198, No.11, (Dec 2003), pp. (1717-27), ISSN 0022-1007 (Print), 0022-1007 (Linking)

Takeda, K., T. Tanaka, W. Shi, M. Matsumoto, M. Minami, S. Kashiwamura, K. Nakanishi, N. Yoshida, T. Kishimoto, & S. Akira (1996). Essential role of Stat6 in IL-4 signalling. *Nature* Vol.380, No.6575, (Apr 1996), pp. (627-30), ISSN 0028-0836 (Print), 0028-0836 (Linking)

van den Berg, M. H., H. K. Ronday, A. J. Peeters, S. le Cessie, F. J. van der Giesen, F. C. Breedveld, & T. P. Vliet Vlieland (2006). Using internet technology to deliver a home-based physical activity intervention for patients with rheumatoid arthritis: A randomized controlled trial. *Arthritis Rheum* Vol.55, No.6, (Dec 2006), pp. (935-45), ISSN 0004-3591 (Print), 0004-3591 (Linking)

van den Ende, C. H., F. C. Breedveld, S. le Cessie, B. A. Dijkmans, A. W. de Mug, & J. M. Hazes (2000). Effect of intensive exercise on patients with active rheumatoid arthritis: a randomised clinical trial. *Ann Rheum Dis* Vol.59, No.8, (Aug 2000), pp. (615-21), ISSN 0003-4967 (Print), 0003-4967 (Linking)

van den Ende, C. H., J. M. Hazes, S. le Cessie, W. J. Mulder, D. G. Belfor, F. C. Breedveld, & B. A. Dijkmans (1996). Comparison of high and low intensity training in well controlled rheumatoid arthritis. Results of a randomised clinical trial. *Ann Rheum Dis* Vol.55, No.11, (Nov 1996), pp. (798-805), ISSN 0003-4967 (Print), 0003-4967 (Linking)

van der Woude, D., A. Young, K. Jayakumar, B. J. Mertens, R. E. Toes, D. van der Heijde, T. W. Huizinga, & A. H. van der Helm-van Mil (2009). Prevalence of and predictive factors for sustained disease-modifying antirheumatic drug-free remission in rheumatoid arthritis: results from two large early arthritis cohorts.

Arthritis Rheum Vol.60, No.8, (Aug 2009), pp. (2262-71), ISSN 0004-3591 (Print), 0004-3591 (Linking)

Vannier, E., L. C. Miller, & C. A. Dinarello (1992). Coordinated antiinflammatory effects of interleukin 4: interleukin 4 suppresses interleukin 1 production but up-regulates gene expression and synthesis of interleukin 1 receptor antagonist. *Proc Natl Acad Sci U S A* Vol.89, No.9, (May 1992), pp. (4076-80), ISSN 0027-8424 (Print), 0027-8424 (Linking)

Walsh, N. P., M. Gleeson, R. J. Shephard, J. A. Woods, N. C. Bishop, M. Fleshner, C. Green, B. K. Pedersen, L. Hoffman-Goetz, C. J. Rogers, H. Northoff, A. Abbasi, & P. Simon (2011). Position statement. Part one: Immune function and exercise. *Exerc Immunol Rev* Vol.17, 2011), pp. (6-63), ISSN 1077-5552 (Print), 1077-5552 (Linking)

Yokota, H., M. B. Goldring, & H. B. Sun (2003). CITED2-mediated regulation of MMP-1 and MMP-13 in human chondrocytes under flow shear. *J Biol Chem* Vol.278, No.47, (Nov 2003), pp. (47275-80), ISSN 0021-9258 (Print), 0021-9258 (Linking)

15

Perceptions Relating to Exercise in Rheumatoid Arthritis

Rebecca-Jane Law, David Markland,
Peter Maddison and Jeanette M. Thom
School of Sport, Health and Exercise Sciences, Bangor University, Wales, United Kingdom

1. Introduction

Historically, the recommendation of exercise for patients with rheumatoid arthritis (RA) has been avoided by clinicians due to fears that such activity may contribute to joint damage and result in worsening of disease. Hence, previous treatment of active RA has included bed rest and splinting of the affected joints (Partridge & Duthie, 1962). Over recent decades however, the numerous physiological advantages of exercise have become well-established and include improved cardiovascular health, increased muscular hypertrophy and increased bone mineral density. Enhanced physical function and psychosocial advantages have also been shown in followers of a continued exercise programme (Baillet et al., 2009; Bilberg et al., 2005; de Jong et al, 2003, 2004; Hakkinen et al., 2001; Lemmey et al., 2009; Marcora et al., 2005; Melikoglu et al., 2006; Van Den Berg et al., 2006; van den Ende et al., 1996, 2000). Importantly, it has also been found that high-intensity exercise training is of superior effectiveness, with no detrimental effect on disease activity. This has been confirmed in patients with controlled (Ekdahl et al., 1990; Lemmey et al., 2009; van den Ende et al., 1996) and active RA (van den Ende et al., 2000). Furthermore, as advances in pharmacological treatment work to effectively control disease, this patient group are now able to tolerate regular, progressive and intensive exercise (Lemmey, 2011). A recent systematic review also provides further information as to the benefits, effectiveness and safety of exercise in RA (Hurkmans et al., 2009).

Patients with RA are also at an increased risk for cardiovascular disease (Metsios et al., 2008), cachexia (Walsmith & Roubenoff, 2002) and osteoporotic fracture (Van Staa et al., 2006). Therefore, the aforementioned improvements associated with exercise are vital in limiting the negative consequences inherent to the disease. Furthermore, physical activity has been found to be a significant predictor of the number of hospital admissions and the length of hospitalisation in RA (Metsios et al., 2011). In light of this evidence, exercise is now considered an essential component within the management of this condition. However, despite this it is apparent that RA patients are less physically active than the general population (Sokka et al., 2008), and greater medical costs are coupled with this inactivity (Wang et al., 2001). Therefore it is important for those involved in the care of RA patients to be aware of factors that may positively and negatively affect the uptake and maintenance of an exercise prescription for this patient group.

This chapter will discuss the perceptions of patients and health professionals in relation to exercising with RA, alongside the implications and recommendations for patient care. Many of these issues have been highlighted as part of our continuing research and it is the findings from these novel investigations, alongside others, which form the basis of this chapter. Illustrative quotes from patients and practitioners have been included to facilitate description of these issues.

2. Patient perceptions relating to exercise in RA

Understanding the perceptions of people with RA regarding exercise is vital to assist in the initiation of and adherence to effective exercise training (Cooney et al., 2011). Primarily, a positive mindset regarding exercise prescription is necessary in order to challenge the long-standing opinion that exercise exacerbates disease (Gecht et al., 1996). However, many patients harbour concerns relating to the potential detrimental effects of exercise and perceive specific barriers to uptake and participation. Furthermore, due to uncertainties about which exercises to do and how to do them without causing harm, many patients feel they are unable to exercise at all. Encouragingly however, qualitative research has revealed that patients with arthritis believe exercise to be an important factor in treatment (Lambert et al., 2000; Law et al., 2010).

Qualitative research methods, including the analysis of focus group discussions and one-to-one interviews, have been successfully utilised in the clinical setting. These methods allow the researcher to gather rich, plentiful data and enable an in-depth description of experiences, thought-processes and beliefs (Kitzinger, 1995; Ong & Coady, 2006). In patients with osteoarthritis, a qualitative study following the onset of disease revealed a subgroup of patients who had previously exercised but had stopped because of their symptoms and because they believed exercise was damaging their joints (Hendry et al., 2006). As may be expected of a condition that presents with similar symptoms (i.e. joint pain, swelling and stiffness), comparable perceptions have been confirmed in RA patients (Law et al., 2010). This study involved four moderated focus groups of RA patients (n = 18) and included both males and females of varied ages and disease duration, thus incorporating a broad range of experiences. Systematic content analysis of the discussion transcripts formed the basic meaning units for analysis. These quotes were then categorized, smaller constructs or sub-themes were grouped, and the following main themes were identified: 'Health professionals showing a lack of exercise knowledge', 'Not knowing what exercise should be done', 'Not wanting to exercise as joints hurt', 'Worry about causing harm to joints' and 'Having to exercise because it is helpful'. Following discussion and comprehensive data interrogation, an analytical model was then developed (Figure 1). These themes were then used to develop a questionnaire to collect analogous quantitative data. Preliminary results (n = 247) from this questionnaire offer confirmatory findings of the prevalence of these issues in a larger population (Law et al., manuscript in preparation).

2.1 Perceived benefits of exercise

Although RA patients appear to be insufficiently active (Sokka et al., 2008), research suggests they are aware that exercise is a beneficial and necessary aspect of their disease management (Lambert et al., 2000, Law et al., 2010). This notion is reflected in the theme that emerged from focus group research; **'Having to exercise because it is helpful'**, indicating

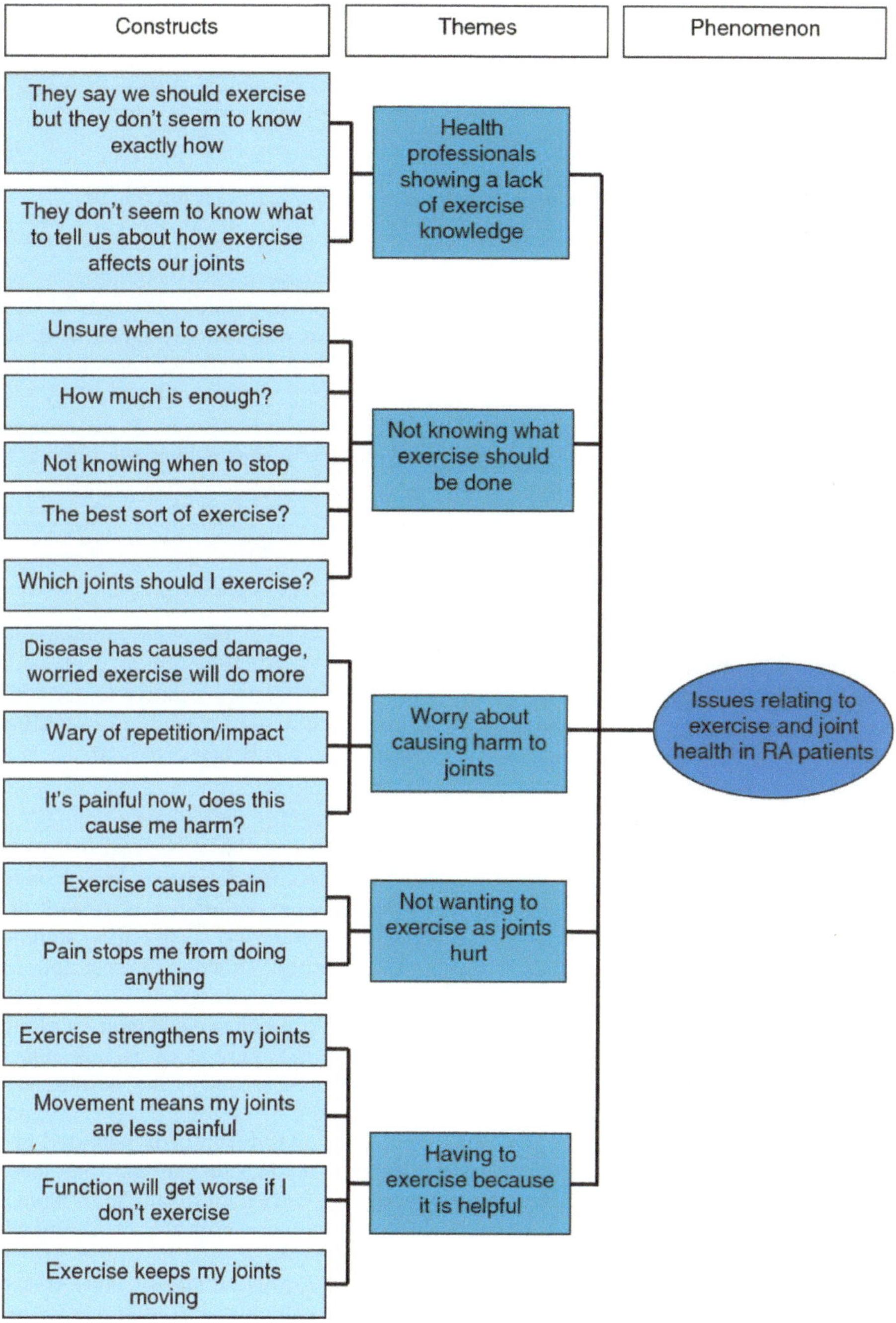

Fig. 1. Analytical model of the issues relating to exercise and joint health in RA patients (Law et al., 2010).

that patients felt they needed to exercise in order for strength, mobility, pain relief and functional benefits to occur. Example quotes are shown below:

'I only do it [exercise] because I know it benefits me. I don't do it because I enjoy it.' (65 year old female)

'If you're strong where the muscles are, it helps to take the weight off the joint.' (74 year old male)

'....it [the exercise] improved the pain and it improved the mobility.' (65 year old female)

'I'm frightened that if I don't get up every morning, if I stay in bed it will become progressive.' (66 year old female)

Additionally, the notion of having to exercise because it is helpful was upheld in our questionnaire study. Over two thirds of patients either agreed or strongly agreed with items relating to this theme. These items included statements such as 'Exercise helps to keep my joints moving' and 'I feel exercise relieves joint pain'.

However, it is important to note that not all patients considered exercise as advantageous and some felt that exercise is not 'helpful' as it causes pain or makes their condition worse. This is shown by the following quotes:

'...you come back to this exercise business and you come back, exercise is painful...' (67 year old male)

'I actually find if you push yourself it makes it [RA] worse.' (56 year old female)

These negative perceptions, alongside other barriers, will be discussed in more detail throughout this chapter. Overall however, it is apparent that patients do perceive that exercise will be of benefit. Yet, if the perception that exercise as a positive feature of RA treatment is to supersede any negative connotations, continual emphasis and education of the benefits is critical (de Jong et al., 2004, Gecht et al., 1996; Neuberger et al., 2007).

2.2 Barriers to exercise

Within the general population, numerous barriers to exercise have been shown to exist (Trost et al., 2002). These barriers are broad and also affect the RA population. However, there are additional barriers that exist within the RA population, arising as a result of the local and systemic characteristics of the disease. Psychosocial aspects also make significant contribution. Concerns relating to joint health and limitations in exercise prescription are also key issues and are discussed in following sections.

Specific barriers to exercise in the RA population include musculoskeletal pain and fatigue. Medications and physical capabilities have also been highlighted as factors affecting patients' exercise behaviour, alongside complications associated with additional co-morbidities. Time constraints brought about by lifestyle and other commitments are factors common to both the general and RA patient population, often further compounded by the distance necessary to travel to an exercise facility, alongside limited methods of transportation. Barriers such as a lack of enjoyment, motivation and confidence have also been identified, and especially for those on a limited income, concerns about cost and a lack of adequate insurance are also prevalent amongst non-exercisers (Gyursik et al., 2009; Hutton et al., 2010; Law et al., 2010; Neuberger et al., 2007; Shutzer & Graves, 2004; Wilcox et al., 2006). Table 1 displays a summary of these barriers, highlighting in bold those that are specific to arthritis. Examples relating to enjoyment, access and fatigue are provided here; quotes relating to pain will be provided later:

'Even on days when I do have time, I think I'd rather be doing something else' (65 year old female)

'You want something there [somewhere to exercise], something you can access easily.' (58 year old female)

'...you get very tired with this. Sometimes in a week you might feel exhausted, doing nothing'. (46 year old female)

Physical	Psychological/ behavioural	Social	Environmental
Pain before exercise	Lack of time	Lack of encouragement	**No arthritis-specific facilities**
Pain during exercise	Lack of enjoyment	**Lack of acknowledgement of arthritis**	Weather/surfaces
Pain after exercise	Not a priority	Lack of information from healthcare provider	Cost
Fatigue	Feeling that 'physically can't'	Nobody to exercise with	Transportation
Impaired mobility	Lacking in skills	Competing roles and responsibilities	
Co-morbid conditions	**Fear of a flare-up**		
Joint swelling/ stiffness	Stress		
Muscle/joint pain	Perceived negative outcomes		
	Perceived lack of positive outcomes **Worry about putting health at risk**		

Table 1. Summary of barriers to exercise in arthritis (adapted from der Anian et al., 2006; Gyursik et al., 2009; Hutton et al., 2010; Law et al., 2010; Wilcox et al., 2006;). Those specific to arthritis are shown in bold.

This summary table has been created based upon our focus group research and the work of four other groups exploring barriers to exercise in patients with arthritis. Wilcox et al., (2006) conducted twelve focus groups including 68 adults with arthritis and described differences in barriers to exercise between 'exercisers' and 'non-exercisers'. Various barriers to exercise were identified, many of which were similar to those that have been described by the general population (Trost et al., 2002). However, as shown in bold in Table 1, others were unique to people with a chronic disease such as arthritis. Those patients who were already exercising indicated barriers similar to those who were not, but these did not prevent them from exercising. This was mainly because they felt able to make modifications and accommodate physical limitations.

Research by der Anian et al., (2006) also investigated barriers to exercise amongst individuals with arthritis and included a subgroup of patients who were defined as 'insufficiently active'. These patients felt that they could not perform any more exercise because of their pain and because they did not know which exercises were safe or appropriate to do. In addition, they appeared to lack the knowledge necessary to modify exercise routines. It was also more common for these 'insufficiently active' individuals to express the need for more detailed advice.

The Obstacles to Action study (New Zealand) (Hutton et al., 2010) used a questionnaire to investigate factors influencing exercise participation for individuals with self-reported arthritis. These authors also compared participants defined as 'active' with those who were 'insufficiently active'. Arthritis, fatigue, and discomfort were ranked by both groups as the top three barriers. Further confirming the findings by Wilcox et al., (2006), the active participants reported significantly lower impact scores for these barriers than the inactive group, with these findings persisting after adjustments for occupational status, body mass index, and co-morbidities. They also revealed that active people with arthritis believed more strongly in the benefits of physical activity, reported significantly higher levels of encouragement from others, and had greater overall levels of self-efficacy when compared with the less active participants.

Gyursik et al., (2009) used a web-based survey to explore the frequency of barrier occurrence and extent of limitation brought about by barriers to exercise. Arthritis-specific personal barriers such as pain (reported by 50% of the sample) and fatigue (reported by nearly 40% of the sample), were more commonly reported than generic barriers (e.g. lack of time, bad weather). Interestingly, barrier frequency did not predict physical activity, further suggesting that it is the individual perception of the impact of the particular barriers and the ability to overcome these that is important. Coping strategies, such as thinking about the disease-specific health benefits and activity modification, were also reported in this study.

The barriers to exercise that exist in the general population also affect individuals with RA. However, our qualitative research highlighted further barriers specific to this patient group, including those relating to joint health, limited exercise prescription and pain. Similar to that of previous researchers, it appears that those patients who were attendees of a specialised exercise class perceived these barriers to exercise as less of a hindrance (Law et al., 2010). Nevertheless, and especially for those patients with no prior exercise experience, methods of overcoming these barriers are essential to ascertain and implement. This will be discussed in later sections.

2.3 Perceptions relating to exercise and joint health

RA is often associated with impaired joint health, including joint inflammation, pain and damage, and it appears that these physical manifestations create additional barriers to exercise for RA patients. Corresponding with this, the perception that exercise may have detrimental effects on joint health has been found to exist in many patients with RA (Law et al., 2010). In particular, joint pain has been highlighted as a definitive barrier and has also been perceived as a prominent factor in determining patients' exercise behaviour (der Anian et al., 2006; Gyursik et al., 2009; Hutton et al., 2010; Wilcox et al., 2006;). The negative influence of pain on patients' exercise behaviour was also described during our focus groups, forming the theme '**Not wanting to exercise as joints hurt'.** This was discussed in terms of disease-related pain before, during and after exercise. Example quotes are shown below:

'There's only one word that affects my exercise behaviour and that's pain.' (66 year old female)

'I mean you can't exercise if you are in pain can you. You can't really do anything.' (57 year old female)

'...if it hurts you don't want to move.' (46 year old female)

This patient described how she felt in terms of her RA in the days after exercising:

'Immediately it would ache for a bit, then ease off and then the day after, it would still be, I know that was what aggravated it.' (40 year old female)

An interesting contrast is also provided with regards to this theme, with some patients (especially those who had previously been involved in exercise), suggesting that they would continue exercising even if it was painful as they felt it was *'worth the risk'* (69 year old male). Furthermore and as previously mentioned, perceptions indicating that patients have experienced feelings of reduced pain have been noted (Wilcox et al., 2006). This was also indicated in our focus group research, as shown by the following quote:

'...best way to relieve pain is to do something and it [exercise] seems to soothe it and it goes away.' (67 year old male)

As became clear in our focus group study, it is evident that patients with RA have concerns about the effects of exercise on joint health. Empirical evidence from a randomised controlled trial investigating the effects of a 2 year, high-intensity exercise programme also brought attention to this issue (de Jong & Vliet Vlieland, 2005). Whilst there was no evidence of further damage to the small joints of the hands and feet (de Jong et al., 2003), radiological evidence from a subgroup of exercisers indicated accelerated progression in large joints which had extensive, pre-existing damage (Munneke et al., 2005). However, the authors have since retracted this conclusion after a follow-up study at eighteen months was not able to confirm this trend (de Jong et al., 2009). Nonetheless, apprehension felt by patients in our focus groups regarding joint damage as a consequence of exercise was reflected in the theme **'Worry about causing harm to joints'**. The dialogue below provides an example:

'The worry is whether you are damaging yourself really.' (66 year old male)

'Yeah.' (44 year old female)

'Am I going to be worse as a result of it?' (73 year old male)

'That's a significant anxiety for me.' (66 year old male)

As highlighted in the following quotes, it also became clear that previous damage and pain provoked additional concern:

'You can do all the exercises out, it won't affect what's at the back of your head saying, if I do that, will I do any damage to what's already been damaged?' (67 year old male)

'...if you do something and it's that painful, it must be doing your joints some damage.' (66 year old female)

On the other hand, qualitative research has revealed that some patients *feel* that their joints benefit from exercise, with quotes indicating the view that joints are 'lubricated' as a result of movement and patients have expressed that they feel more agile (Kamwendo et al., 1999; Law et al., 2010). This is demonstrated by the quote below:

'...it helps to keep them lubricated doesn't it. It helps keep you moving, exercise. If you don't they seize up...' (65 year old female)

Overall, however, as factors salient to individual beliefs regarding the effects of exercise, patient perceptions relating to joint health, pain and damage are important to consider when addressing the issue of exercise for this population. Moreover, just under half of the patients involved in our follow-up questionnaire study indicated agreement with items relating to the themes 'worry about causing harm to joints' and 'not wanting to exercise as joints hurt' (Law et al., manuscript in preparation). Therefore, it is evident that RA patients need continued reassurance and encouragement that exercise is a vital part of disease management and that the aforementioned benefits are achievable *without* unfavourable effects for joint health or disease activity.

2.4 Perceptions relating to exercise prescription

The pharmacological treatment of RA involves a clear and specific prescription for medication. However, despite recommendations by the British Society for Rheumatology (BSR; Luqmani et al., 2006; 2009), National Institute of Health and Clinical Excellence (NICE, 2009), European League Against Rheumatism (EULAR; Combe et al., 2007) and the American College of Sports Medicine (ACSM; Nelson et al., 2007), that exercise should be incorporated into the treatment of people with RA, specific recommendations are less clear. Corresponding with this limited clarity, research suggests that a perceived uncertainty about which exercises to do, and how to do them, may be inhibiting patients from participating in regular exercise (Lambert et al. 2000, Law et al. 2010). Emerging from our focus group research, the theme **'Not knowing what exercise should be done'** reflects patients' concerns about not knowing enough about exercise with respect to their disease. Patients discussed doubts about the best forms of exercise to undertake and were unclear how much exercise they should do. Discussion relating to sufficient exercise intensity and heart rate also took place, with questions arising as to whether fast walking would be enough, and how breathless they should feel. Example quotes are provided below:

'If you do it fast it does raise your heart rate. And how much do you need to raise your heart rate, you don't know how much. Do you raise your heart rate until you can't breathe?' (65 year old female)

'...It's just the type of exercise that you do. Obviously not something too strenuous, but sometimes you need reassurance as well before you do something. You think well, is that good for me or is that bad for me?' (23 year old female)

'Do you think you have to do different exercises for muscle to joints?' (65 year old female)

'Do you know, I haven't got a clue' (56 year old female)

Furthermore, patients also showed concern about the possibility that they might do something wrong. This is demonstrated by the following quotes:

'Yeah, it's, what is the exercise about. How do I do it, will it affect my worse little bits. You've got to go through the bit about it, you've got to read what the exercise is, you've got to look at what the exercise is, will I be alright with it ... ' (67 year old male)

'It's difficult to know where to draw the line between 'oh for goodness sake, give it a bit of effort'... or 'you know this is harmful, it's time to stop.' (57 year old female)

'Only if you do too much I think.' (62 year old male)

'Or if you do the wrong thing as well, I think you could easily do the wrong thing.' (46 year old female)

Furthermore, repetitive, impact-based exercise and pain provoked additional concern as shown in the quotes below:

'.... got to be careful of a repetitive move.' (58 year old female)

'I think impact is really disastrous...' (66 year old female)

'.... I don't think weight impact, I don't think that would be very helpful.' (62 year old male)

As previously mentioned, high-intensity exercise is now considered to provide the greatest benefit. However, in a study by Munneke et al., (2003), the outcome expectations of patients for a high-intensity exercise programme were found to be significantly less positive when compared to a conventional exercise programme. In this study, conventional exercise was described as 'calmly performed exercises for the joints not leading to tiredness, e.g. bending and stretching of the arm' and high-intensity exercise as 'individually tailored and supervised physical fitness and strength training exercises for the whole body leading to tiredness'. As will be discussed later, it was found that health professionals also held the view that conventional exercise was preferable for a patient with RA. Despite this however, the majority of patients indicated that they thought an intensive exercise programme would be attainable for at least half of their patient group.
An additional theme that emerged from our focus groups offered further insight into patient perceptions relating to exercise prescription. The theme **'Health professionals showing a lack of exercise knowledge'** reflected patient perceptions that, while health professionals advocated exercise, there were uncertainties regarding the specifics of exercise prescription. Furthermore, when exploring this issue on a larger scale, our questionnaire study revealed that less than 20% of patients agreed that health professionals showed exercise knowledge. Patients were also unsure whether or not current disease state (i.e. pain and fatigue levels) affected the overall benefit of exercise. As previously mentioned, further uncertainties were perceived in relation to concerns within the health profession about exercise and joint health. These views are demonstrated in the following extract:

'... if I do that sort of thing and I get pain, I can go on doing it, now my next question [to a health professional] is am I doing myself harm if I get pain? (66 year old male)

'...mmmm' (73 year old male)

'Yeah' (44 year old female)

'[The health professional] can't tell me, right' (66 year old male)

'No, that's what worries me' (65 year old female)

'Nobody knows' (66 year old male)

These perceptions relating to exercise prescription suggest that patients require education to include specific exercise recommendations that are of sufficient intensity to provide beneficial effects. Furthermore, there is a perception amongst patients that health professionals lack clarity and certainty regarding exercise, especially in relation to joint health. This perception of health professionals is also an important area to explore in order to determine if and where uncertainties exist, alongside the best way to deliver a clear and consistent message to the patient population. It may be that a firm and assertive approach to recommending exercise is important when prescribing exercise to people with RA.

3. The impact of the health professional

The health professional has an important role when prescribing exercise to a patient with RA. Due to the nature of their condition, RA patients are in frequent contact with their healthcare team and place great value on the information they provide (Lambert et al., 2000; Kamwendo et al., 1999). Hence, this regular contact forms an integral part of patient perceptions relating to exercise. However, evidence suggests that this is not a source from which they consistently get appropriate information (Lambert et al., 2000; Law et al., 2010). For example:

'I would really like to know what they call exercise and whether or not it conforms to what I think is exercise' (66 year old male).

On the other hand, health professionals are increasingly involved in conducting or referring to an exercise programme and those focus group patients who attended a specialised exercise class (an 8-week circuit-based exercise programme of 8–12 stations) demonstrated more experiential and education-derived knowledge of the types of exercise they could do. This is also consistent with findings comparing the views of active and inactive people with arthritis, with the active patients found to have additional exercise knowledge and the ability to draw from past experiences (Wilcox et al., 2006). An example is provided in a quote from a 65 year old female patient:

'There are lots of exercises that you can do at home…I'll go to the stairs and spend 10 minutes as fast as I can up one step down, up down. Just that little exercise that we did.' (65 year old female patient)

In contrast, the knowledge of non-attendees appeared to be mainly speculative. Nonetheless, whilst exercise class attendees did not highlight disadvantages to the same extent, queries relating to pain and its link with harm were still expressed, especially regarding exercises of a higher intensity. Therefore, it remains necessary that health professionals address these concerns, even with those who are currently exercising or have done so in the past.

It is also important to note further ways in which the health professional may impact upon patient perceptions and exercise behaviour. Unfortunately, interventions designed to provide advice and support for increasing physical activity levels have been largely unsuccessful in increasing long-term participation (Hillsden et al., 2002; van der Bij et al., 2002). Iversen et al. (2004a) examined the predictors of exercise behaviour in RA patients at six months following consultation with their rheumatologist and found that patients were more likely to be engaged in exercise if their rheumatologist was currently performing aerobic exercise themselves. This research also concluded that discussions about exercise were four times more likely to occur when the rheumatologist initiated exercise discussion (Iversen et al., 2004a). These findings draw attention to the significance of health professionals and the influence they have on the exercise perceptions of this patient group.

3.1 Perceptions of health professionals

When working towards a successful exercise prescription, it is important to consider the perceptions of health professionals involved in the care of people with RA. Common barriers cited for a lack of exercise-based intervention have included a lack of time during the patient visit, limited reimbursement, lack of training and perceived ineffectiveness as a behavioural counsellor (Calfas et al., 1996). In the study by Iversen et al. (1999), many rheumatologists felt that exercise prescription would take more time than they had available and also doubted their patients' interest in and ability to comply with an exercise programme. Further research by this group indicated that only 51% of rheumatologists reported feeling confident that they knew *when* exercises were appropriate for their patients with RA with only 22% reporting that they felt confident to instruct patients as to appropriate exercises (Iversen et al., 2004b).

The perceptions of health professionals in relation to exercise type may also be limiting recommendation and consequent uptake of exercise. Rheumatologists have reported negative attitudes towards aerobic exercise, with 29% of the belief that aerobic exercises were *rarely* useful in the management of RA (Iversen et al., 1999; 2004a). Furthermore and as previously mentioned, the outcome expectations of rheumatologists and physiotherapists for high intensity exercise have been found to be significantly less positive than those for a conventional exercise programme. Despite this, the majority of rheumatologists (and patients) felt that a high-intensity exercise programme would be attainable. Interestingly, the physiotherapists in this study were even more conservative than rheumatologists regarding high-intensity exercise with only a minority of physiotherapists of the view that intensive exercise would be attainable for half of all RA patients (Munneke et al., 2004).

Limitations within the existing literature may partially explain these perceptions as reservations regarding exercise and joint health were in existence (Munneke et al., 2005). However, as previously discussed, the most recent study by de Jong and colleagues (2009) refuted this, offering further substantiation of the earlier studies that showed no exacerbation of joint damage with prolonged, high-intensity exercise (Hakkinen et al., 1994; 2001; 2004; Nordemar et al., 1981;). Consequently, it may be that supplementary education for health professionals involved in the treatment of patients with RA is necessary to ensure they are sufficiently informed with respect to current scientific evidence (Munneke et al., 2004). Furthermore, it appears that further research and information dissemination, with the aim of addressing deficiencies in knowledge of specific exercise prescription for this population is required. As shown in the quotes below, our ongoing research investigating the perceptions of health professionals with regards to exercise has given an initial insight into the difficulties of providing an exercise prescription to individuals with RA.

'I don't know specific recommendations for aerobic exercise in RA because journal articles on this never specify or describe exactly what exercise was prescribed…' (Rheumatologist)

'...patients are given a lot of conflicting advice and I am not sure how good the evidence is for advising exercise or exercise avoidance. It would be good to have clear advice/evidence/guidelines...exercise is good for RA patients especially when inflammation is controlled but I expect that it is much more difficult when disease is active' (Rheumatologist)

'...never prescribe, often recommend.' (Rheumatologist)

The following quote demonstrates some of the considerations when deciding how to approach an exercise prescription for this patient group:

'...The amount of pain a patient is in, whether synovitis is present and if there is joint damage will all affect the type, duration and number of 'reps' of exercise I would prescribe.' (Physiotherapist)

Despite the superior effectiveness of intensive exercise (de Jong et al., 2003; Ekdahl et al., 1990; Hakkinen et al., 2001; Lemmey, 2009; van den Ende et al., 1996, 2000;) and a lack of detrimental consequences for disease activity and progression (deJong et al., 2003; Hakkinen et al., 2001; Lemmey et al., 2009; Strenstrom & Minor, 2003), it appears that health professionals may still struggle with the concept of recommending high-intensity exercise to patient with RA. Considering the increased risks to this population in terms of cardiovascular health, bone mineral density and rheumatoid cachexia, it is important to foster positive perceptions for both strength and aerobic-based exercise amongst health professionals. Thus, improved education is necessary to overcome any existing negative perceptions and enhance overall confidence to make a worthwhile exercise recommendation for health.

4. Recommendations for improving patient perceptions

It is evident that perceptions relating to exercise need to be improved in order to increase physical activity levels amongst RA patients and enhance the success of exercise recommendations. At present however, overall exercise education is insufficient and further support is required to overcome the physical, psychological, social and environmental barriers common to this patient group. The model previously discussed (Figure 1) presents the issues indicated by patients in relation to exercising with RA and Table 1 summarises the barriers to exercise for this patient group. On the other hand, Table 2 summarises the and factors that could be used encourage patients with arthritis to exercise. In addition to the pivotal role of the rheumatologist in influencing exercise prescription (Iversen et al., 1999; 2004a and 2004b), these implications are also relevant to other health professionals involved in the treatment of RA patients (i.e. nurse specialists, physiotherapists, occupational therapists).

Continual emphasis and communication of the known benefits of exercise for RA patients is necessary. It is also important to acknowledge the challenges that are faced by patients when attempting to exercise appropriately. For example, especially at the onset of their disease, it is important for patients to understand and feel able to make decisions about how to modify their exercise according to their fluctuating symptoms (Iversen et al., 1999). It is also important to consider methods of overcoming potential barriers when promoting the maintenance of an exercise programme. For example, working towards strengthening patient beliefs that they are able to continue exercise outside of the healthcare environment may be valuable (Swardh et al., 2008).

Physical	Psychological/ behavioural	Social	Environmental
Reduced pain	Increased independence	Enjoyment of exercising with others	Water exercise
Reduced stiffness	Experiencing positive emotion	Encouragement	Programmes for people with arthritis
Increased energy	Increased enjoyment	Motivated by someone to exercise with	Low cost
Improved mobility and function	Goal-setting/self-motivation	Want others to approve	Available equipment
Easier activities of daily living	Making exercise a priority		
Improved strength and flexibility			
Increasing muscle mass, reducing fat mass			

Table 2. Summary of benefits and factors encouraging a patient to exercise in arthritis (adapted from der Anian et al., 2006; Gyursik et al., 2009; Hutton et al., 2010; Law et al., 2010; Wilcox et al., 2006).

Factors encouraging patients to exercise are also important considerations. Low cost, easy access, and weight reduction have been highlighted, alongside receiving assistance from instructors and the opportunity for social interaction. Examples quotes are provided from our focus group research:

'...that for me was the secret. Was to find a good instructor and be in the company of others...' (58 year old female)

'...there's a lot of people at the moment complaining of the cost...' (65 year old female)

'That's another thing it [exercise] does, it helps you to keep the weight off.' (62 year old male)

It is also evident from our research that difficulties arise as a result of incomplete information being provided, with health professionals advising exercise but lacking a definitive explanation of how to do so. It is also important that efforts are made to ensure that a consistent message is given. For example, during our focus group study, patients were introduced to the quote 'Many people are afraid to exercise because they believe that it will cause further damage to their joints'. The discussion extract below was from a patient in response to this:

'...a symptom of misinformation and no information. That's why people believe that. They are not educated on Day 1 to believe that things are possible with the right help ... ' (58 year old female).

This highlights the importance of emphasising the benefits of exercise and giving specific exercise recommendations early in treatment. Furthermore, within the Obstacles to Action study (Hutton et al., 2010) 'insufficient advice from a healthcare provider' was a theme for the insufficiently active individuals, with queries relating to the type, frequency, and intensity of appropriate exercise. These correspond with recommendations by the American College of Sports Medicine, who describe exercise prescription using the 'FITT' principle (Swain, 2010). This incorporates the following: how often per week the patient should exercise (Frequency), how energetically or vigorously the patient should exercise (Intensity), how long the patient should exercise to obtain benefits (Time) and what type of exercises should be prescribed to the patient (Type) (Tancred & Tancred, 1996). This acronym offers a useful and simple framework upon which to base an exercise prescription.

An interesting point also stems from the quote below, indicating that means of continuing assessment and feedback may benefit patients.

'...I would love to have some measurement that shows me that it's doing me some good.' (66 year old male)

However, whilst working to develop these areas would be worthwhile, barriers for the health professional also exist. As previously mentioned, limited knowledge may hinder their ability and confidence to discuss the topic of exercise. Moreover, the time constraint of a standard appointment often means that medication and symptom control is prioritised (Calfas et al., 1996). In a study by Podl et al. (1999) involving family physicians, it was highlighted that an average of 45 seconds of consultation time involved conversation about exercise. This lack of consultation time was confirmed by Iversen et al., (1999) who found that when a medical regime was more complicated, there was less talk about exercise. Therefore, quick and effective means of prescribing exercise and providing continual follow-up and feedback would be of benefit. Future direction could also include referral to a trained clinical exercise physiologist, who would possess the skills to make physiological assessments and prescribe exercise. Additionally, as local communities vary widely in the availability of resources and programmes for individuals with arthritis (Wilcox et al., 2006), incorporating home-based recommendations may be of value.

In summary, clear exercise guidelines and prescription advice is necessary to address the fact that RA patients are often faced with ambiguous and incomplete information. This may mean that further information for those health professionals involved in the care of this patient group is necessary to instil the confidence and allegiance required to positively shape the perceptions of this patient group.

5. Conclusions

The benefits of continued, regular exercise of a sufficient intensity for RA patients are clear. Furthermore, it appears that many patients are aware that exercise forms an advantageous part of their disease management. However, negative perceptions relating to joint health, pain and the clarity of exercise prescription for this patient group add to the barriers to exercise uptake that already exist in the general population. Therefore, to improve patient perceptions, the benefits require continual emphasis and the additional concerns regarding joint health, pain symptoms the specificity of exercise recommendations need to be acknowledged and addressed. Initiation of exercise discussion by the health professional alongside a motivational and assertive approach to exercise prescription is also important to implement.

Further research and use of evidence-based practice within the health profession will address limitations in current exercise knowledge. The most effective method of enhancing transfer of this information and educating patients and health professionals in this area needs to be utilised, an area which may also require further investigation. With more specific exercise information and an effectual method of education and delivery, exercise can become akin to a medical prescription. Working to build upon perceptions that exercise is an essential part of disease management and lifelong health promotion will facilitate this process.

6. Acknowledgment

The authors would like to thank Dr. Jeremy Jones, Mrs. Anne Breslin, Dr. Emily Oliver, Lauren Mawn and Serena Halls for their valued contributions.

7. References

Baillet, A, Payraud, E, Niderprim, V-A, Nissen, MJ, Allenet, B, Francois, P, Grange, L, Casez, P, Juvin R & Gaudin, P. (2009). A dynamic exercise programme to improve patients' disability in rheumatoid arthritis: a prospective randomized controlled trial. *Rheumatology*, vol. 48, no. 4, pp. 410–415.

Bilberg, A, Ahlmen, M, Mannerkorpi, K. (2005). Moderately intensive exercise in a temperate pool for patients with rheumatoid arthritis: a randomized controlled study. *Rheumatology*, vol. 44, no. 4, pp. 502–508.

Calfas KJ, Long BJ, Sallis JF, Wooten, WJ, Pratt, M & Patrick, K. (1996). A controlled trial of physician counseling to promote the adoption of physical activity. *Preventative Medicine*, vol. 25, pp. 225–33.

Combe, B, Landewe, R, Lukas, C, Bolosiu, HD, Breedveld, F, Dougados, M, Emery, P, Ferraccioli, G, Hazes, JMW, Klareskog, L, Machold, K, Martin-Mola, E, Nielsen, H, Silman, A, Smolen, J & Yazici H. (2007). EULAR recommendations for the management of early arthritis: report of a task force of the European Standing Committee for International Clinical Studies Including Therapeutics (ESCISIT). *Annals of the Rheumatic Diseases*, vol. 66, pp. 34-45

Cooney, JK., Law, R-J, Matschke, V, Lemmey, AB, Moore, JP, Ahmad, Y, Jones, JG, Maddison, P & Thom, J. (2011). Benefits of Exercise in Rheumatoid Arthritis. *Journal of Aging Research*, Vol. 2011, available at:

de Jong Z & Vliet Vlieland TPM. (2005). Safety of exercise in patients with rheumatoid arthritis. *Current Opinion in Rheumatology*, Vol. 17, pp. 177-182.

de Jong, Z, Munneke, M, Jansen, LM, Ronday, K, van Schaardenburg, DJ, Brand, R, van den Ende, CHM, Vliet Vlieland, TPM, Zuijderduin, WM & Hazes, JMW. (2004). Differences between participants and nonparticipants in an exercise trial for adults with rheumatoid arthritis. *Arthritis Care & Research*, vol. 51, No. 4, pp. 593-600.

de Jong, Z, Munneke, M, Kroon, HM, van Schaardenburg, D, Dijkmans, BAC, Hazes, JMW & Vliet Vlieland, TPM. (2009). Long-term follow-up of a high-intensity exercise program in patients with rheumatoid arthritis. *Clinical Rheumatology*, vol. 28, no. 6, pp. 663–671.

de Jong, Z, Munneke, M, Lems, WF, Zwinderman, AH, Kroon, HM, Pauwels, EKJ, Jansen, A, Ronday, KH, Dijkmans, BAC, Breedveld, FC, Vliet Vlieland, TPM & Hazes, JMW. 2004. Slowing of bone loss in patients with rheumatoid arthritis by long-term high-intensity exercise: Results of a randomized, controlled trial. *Arthritis & Rheumatism*, Vol. 50, No. 4, pp. 1066–1076.

de Jong, Z, Munneke, M, Zwinderman, A, Kroon, H, Jansen, A, Ronday, K, Van Schaardenburg, D, Dijkmans, BAC, Van den Ende, CH, Breedveld FC, Vliet Vlieland, TPM & Hazes, JMW. (2003). Is a long-term high-intensity exercise program effective and safe in patients with rheumatoid arthritis? Results of a randomized controlled trial. *Arthritis & Rheumatism*, vol. 48, No. 9, pp. 2415-2424.

der Ananian D, Wilcox S, Saunders R, Watkins K & Evans A. (2006). Factors that influence exercise among adults with arthritis in three activity levels. Preventing Chronic Disease, Vol. 3, No. 3, pp. 1-16.

Ekblom B, Lövgren O, Alderin M, Fridström M & Sätterström G. (1975). Effect of Short-Term Physical Training on Patients with Rheumatoid Arthritis. *Scandinavian Journal of Rheumatology*, Vol. 4, No. 2, pp. 80-86.

Ekdahl, C, Andersson, SI, Moritz, U & Svensson, B. (1990). Dynamic versus Static Training in Patients with Rheumatoid Arthritis. *Scandinavian Journal of Rheumatology*, Vol. 19, No. 1, pp. 17-26.

Forestier, R, André-Vert, J, Guillez, P, Coudeyre, E, Lefevre-Colau M-M , Combeg B & Mayoux-Benhamouh M-A. (2009) Non-drug treatment (excluding surgery) in rheumatoid arthritis: Clinical practice guidelines. *Joint Bone Spine*, Vol. 76, No. 6, pp. 691–698.

Gecht MR, Connell, KJ, Sinacore, JM & Prohaska, TR. (1996). A Survey of Exercise Beliefs and Exercise Habits Among People with Arthritis. *Arthritis Care & Research*, Vol. 9, No. 2, pp. 82-8.

Gyurcsik NC, Brawley LR, Spink KS, Brittain DR, Fuller DL & Chad K. (2009). Physical activity in women with arthritis: Examining perceived barriers and self-regulatory efficacy to cope. *Arthritis Care & Research*, Vol. 61, No. 8, pp. 1087-1094.

Häkkinen A, Hannonen P, Nyman K, Lyyski T & Häkkinen K. (2003). Effects of concurrent strength and endurance training in women with early or longstanding rheumatoid arthritis: Comparison with healthy subjects. *Arthritis Care & Research*, Vol. 49, pp. 789-797.

Häkkinen A, Sokka T, Kotaniemi A & Hannonen P. (2001). A randomized two-year study of the effects of dynamic strength training on muscle strength, disease activity, functional capacity, and bone mineral density in early rheumatoid arthritis. *Arthritis & Rheumatism*, Vol. 44, No. 3, pp. 515-522.

Hakkinen, A, Hakkinen, K & Hannonen, P. (1994). Effects of strength training on neuromuscular function and disease-activity in patients with recent-onset inflammation arthritis. *Scandinavian journal of rheumatology*, Vol. 23, No. 5, pp. 237-242.

Hakkinen, A, Sokka, T, Kautiainen, H, Kotaniemi, A & Hannonen P. (2004). Sustained maintenance of exercise induced muscle strength gains and normal bone mineral density in patients with early rheumatoid arthritis: a 5 year follow up. *Annals of the Rheumatic Diseases*, Vol. 63, No. 8, pp. 910-6.

Hansen, TM, Hansen, G, Langgaard, AM & Rasmussen, JO (1993). Longtermphysical training in rheumatoid arthritis. A randomized trial with different training programs and blinded observers. *Scandinavian Journal of Rheumatology*, vol. 22, No. 3, pp. 107–112.

Harkcom, TM, Lampman, RM, Banwell, BF & Castor, CW. (1985). Therapeutic value of graded aerobic exercise training in rheumatoid arthritis. *Arthritis and Rheumatism*, Vol. 28, No. 1, pp. 32–39.

Hendry M, Williams NH, Markland D, Wilkinson C & Maddison P. (2006). Why should we exercise when our knees hurt? A qualitative study of primary care patients with osteoarthritis of the knee. *Family Practice*, Vol. 23, No. 5, pp. 558-567. http://www.ncbi.nlm.nih.gov/pmc/articles/PMC3042669/pdf/JAR2011-681640. pdfCairns AP & McVeigh JG. (2009). A systematic review of the effects of dynamic exercise in rheumatoid arthritis. *Rheumatology Internation*, vol. 30, pp. 147–158. http://www.nice.org.uk/nicemedia/pdf/CG79NICEGuideline.pdf

Hurkmans, E, van der GieseN, FJ, Vliet Vlieland, TPM, Schoones, J, Van den Ende, ECHM. (2009). Dynamic exercise programs (aerobic capacity and/or muscle strength training) in patients with rheumatoid arthritis. *Cochrane Database of Systematic Reviews*, No. 4. Art. No.: CD006853. DOI: 10.1002/14651858.CD006853.pub2.

Hutton, I, Gamble, G, McLean, G, Butcher, H, Gow, P & Dalbeth, N. (2010). What is associated with being active in arthritis? Analysis from the obstacles to action study. *Internal Medicine Journal*, Vol. 40, No. 7, pp. 512–520.

Iversen MD, Eaton HM & Daltroy LH. (2004a). How Rheumatologists and Patients with Rheumatoid Arthritis Discuss Exercise and the Influence of Discussions on Exercise Prescriptions. *Arthritis & Rheumatism (Arthritis Care & Research)*, Vol. 51, No. 1, pp. 63-72.

Iversen MD, Fossel AH, Ayers K, Palmsten A, Wang HW & Daltroy LH. (2004b). Predictors of Exercise Behaviour in Patients With Rheumatoid Arthritis 6 Months Following a Visit With Their Rheumatologist. *Physical Therapy*, Vol. 84, No. 8, pp. 706-716.

Iversen, MD, Fossel, AH & Daltroy, LH. (1999). Rheumatologist-Patient communication about exercise and physical therapy in the management of rheumatoid arthritis. *Arthritis Care & Research*, Vol. 12, No. 3, pp. 180-192.

Kamwendo, K, Askenbom, M & Wahlgren, C (1999). Physical activity in the life of the patient with rheumatoid arthritis. *Physiotherapy Research International*, Vol. 4, No. 4, pp. 278–292.

Kitzinger, J. (1995). Qualitative Research: Introducing focus groups. *British Medical Journal*, Vol. 311, No. 7000, pp. 299-302.

Lambert, BL, Butin, DN, Moran, D, Zhao, SZ, Carr, BC, Chen, C & Kizis, FJ. (2000). Arthritis care: comparison of physicians' and patients' views. *Seminars in Arthritis and Rheumatism*, Vol. 30, No. 2, pp. 100–110.

Law R-J, Breslin A, Oliver EJ, Mawn, L, Markland, DA, Maddison, P & Thom, JM. (2010). Perceptions of the effects of exercise on joint health in rheumatoid arthritis patients. *Rheumatology*, Vol. 49, No. 12, pp. 2444–2451.

Lemmey AB, Marcora, SM, Chester, K, Wilson, S, Casanova, F & Maddison, PJ. (2009). Effects of high-intensity resistance training in patients with rheumatoid arthritis: a randomized controlled trial. *Arthritis Care and Research*, Vol. 61, No. 12, pp. 1726–1734.

Lemmey, A. (2011). Efficacy of progressive resistance training for patients with rheumatoid arthritis and recommendations regarding its prescription. International Journal of Clinical Rheumatololgy, Vol. 6, No. 2. ISSN 1758-4272.

Luqmani, R, Hennell, S, Estrach, C, Birrell, F, Bosworth, A, Davenport, G, Fokke, C, Goodson, N, Jeffreson, P, Lamb, E, Mohammed, R, Oliver, S, Stableford, Z, Walsh, D, Washbrook, C & Webb, F. (2006). British Society for Rheumatology and British Health Professionals in Rheumatology Guideline for the Management of Rheumatoid Arthritis (the first two years). *Rheumatology*, Vol. 45, No. 9, pp. 1167–1169

Luqmani, R. Hennell, S. Estrach, C. Basher, D, Birrell, F, Bosworth, A, Burke, F, Callaghan, C, Candal-Couto, J, Fokke, C, Goodson, N, Homer, D, Jackman, J, Jeffreson, P, Oliver, S, Reed, M, Sanz, L, Stableford, Z, Taylor, P, Todd, N, Warburton, L, Washbrook C & Wilkinson, M. (2009). British Society for Rheumatology and British Health Professionals in Rheumatology guideline for the management of rheumatoid arthritis (after the first 2 years). *Rheumatology*, Vol. 48, No. 4, pp. 436–439.

Marcora SM, Lemmey AB & Maddison PJ. (2005). Can progressive resistance training reverse cachexia in patients with rheumatoid arthritis? Results of a pilot study. *Journal of Rheumatology*, Vol. 32, No. 6, pp. 1031-9.

Melikoglu, MA, Karatay, S, Senel, K & Akcay,F. (2006). Association between dynamic exercise therapy and IGF-1 and IGFBP-3 concentrations in the patients with rheumatoid arthritis. *Rheumatology International*, Vol. 26, No. 4, pp. 309–313.

Metsios, GS, Stavropoulos-Kalinoglou, A, Treharne, GJ, Nevill, AM, Sandoo, A, Panoulas, VF, Toms, TE, Koutedakis, Y & Kitas, GD. (2011). Disease activity and low physical activity associate with number of hospital admissions and length of hospitalisation in patients with rheumatoid arthritis. *Arthritis Research & Therapy*, Vol. 13, No. 3, doi:10.1186/ar3390. Available at: http://arthritis-research.com/content/pdf/ar3390.pdf

Metsios, GS, Stavropoulos-Kalinoglou, A, Veldhuijzen van Zanten, J JCS, Treharne, GJ, Panoulas, VF, Douglas, KMJ, Koutedakis, Y & Kitas, GD. (2008). Rheumatoid arthritis, cardiovascular disease and physical exercise: a systematic review. *Rheumatology*, Vol. 47, pp. 239–248.

Munneke, M, de Jong, Z, Zwinderman, AH, Ronday, HK, van den Ende, CHM, Vliet Vlieland, TPM, Hazes, JMW. (2004). High intensity exercise or conventional exercises for patients with rheumatoid arthritis? Outcome expectations of patients, rheumatologists, and physiotherapists. *Annals of the Rheumatic Diseases*, Vol. 63, No. 7, pp. 804–808.

National Institute for Health and Clinical Excellence. (2009). Rheumatoid arthritis: The management of rheumatoid arthritis in adults. *National Collaborating Centre for Chronic Conditions,* Guideline 79, Available from:

Nelson, ME, Rejeski, WJ, Blair, SN, Duncan, PW, Judge, JO, King, AC, Macera, CA & Castaneda-Sceppa, C. (2007). Physical Activity and Public Health in Older Adults: Recommendation from the American College of Sports Medicine and the American Heart Association. *Circulation*, Vol. 116, pp. 1094-1105.

Neuberger GB, Aaronson LS, Gajewski B, Embretson SE, Cagle PE, Loudon JK, Miller, PA. (2007). Predictors of exercise and effects of exercise on symptoms, function, aerobic fitness, and disease outcomes of rheumatoid arthritis. *Arthritis Care & Research*, Vol. 57, No. 6, pp. 943-952.

Nordemar, R. (1981). Physical training in rheumatoid arthritis: a controlled long-term study. II. Functional capacity and general attitudes. *Scandinavian Journal of Rheumatology*, Vol. 10, No. 1, pp. 25–30.

Ong, BN & Coady, DA. Qualitative research. Its relevance and use in musculoskeletal medicine. *Topical reviews: an overview of current research and practice in rheumatic disease*. Chesterfield: Arthritis Research Campaign, 2006; Series 5: Number 9:1–8.

Partridge, REH & Duthie, JR. (1963). Controlled trial of the effect of complete immobilization of the joints in rheumatoid arthritis. *Annals of Rheumatic Diseases*, Vol. 22, pp. 91-99.

Podl, TR, Goodwin, MA, Kikano, GE & Stange, KC. (1999). Direct observation of exercise counseling in community family practice. *American Journal of Preventive Medicine*, Vol. 17, No. 3, pp. 207-210

Schutzer, KA & Graves, BS. (2004). Barriers and motivations to exercise in older adults. *Preventive Medicine*, vol. 39, no. 5, pp. 1056–1061.

Sokka T, Häkkinen A, Kautiainen H, Maillefert JF, Toloza S, Hansen TM, Calvo-Alen, J, Oding, R, Liveborn, M, Huisman, M, Alten, R, Pohl, C, Cutolo, M, Immonen, K, Woolf, A, Murphy, E, Sheehy, C, Quirke, E, Celik, S, Yazici, Y, Tlustochowicz, W, Kapolka, D, Skakic, V, Rojkovich, B, Müller, R, Stropuviene, S, Andersone, D, Drosos, AA, Lazovskis, J, Pincus, T. (2008). Physical inactivity in patients with rheumatoid arthritis: Data from twenty-one countries in a cross-sectional, international study. *Arthritis Care and Research*, Vol. 59, No. 1, pp. 42-50.

Staa TPV, Geusens P, Bijlsma JWJ, Leufkens HGM, Cooper C. Clinical assessment of the long-term risk of fracture in patients with rheumatoid arthritis. Arthritis & Rheumatism 2006; 54(10):3104-12.

Stenstrom, CH & Minor, MA. (2003). Evidence for the Benefit of Aerobic and Strengthening Exercise in Rheumatoid Arthritis. *Arthritis & Rheumatism (Arthritis Care & Research)*, Vol. 49, No. 3, pp. 428–434.

Swain, DP. (2010). Cardiorespiratory exercise prescription. In Ehrman JK ed. *ACSM's resource manual for Guidelines for Exercise Testing and Prescription*. 6th Edition. Philadelphia: Lippincott Williams and Wilkins, pp. 448-462.

Swardh, E, Biguet, G & Opava, CH. (2008).Views on exercise maintenance: variations among patients with rheumatoid arthritis. *Physical Therapy*, Vol. 88, No. 9, pp. 1049–1060.

Tancred B & Tancred G. (1996). Implementation of Exercise Programmes for Prevention and Treatment of Low Back Pain. Physiotherapy 1996;82(3):168-173.

Trost, SG, Owen, N, Bauman, A, Sallis, J & Brown, W. (2002). Correlates of adults' participation in physical activity: review and update. *Medicine & Science in Sports & Exercise*, Vol. 34, No. 12, pp. 1996-2001.

van den Berg, MH, Ronday, HK, Peeters, AJ, Le Cessie, SF, Van Der Giesen, J, Breedveld, FC & Vliet Vlieland TPM. (2006). Using internet technology to deliver a home-based physical activity intervention for patients with rheumatoid arthritis: a randomized controlled trial. *Arthritis Care and Research*, Vol. 55, No. 6, pp. 935–945.

van den Ende CH, Hazes JM, le Cessie S, Mulder WJ, Belfor DG, Breedveld FC, et al. Comparison of high and low intensity training in well controlled rheumatoid arthritis. Results of a randomised clinical trial. Ann Rheum Dis 1996;55(11):798-805.

van den Ende CHM, Breedveld FC, le Cessie S, Dijkmans BAC, de Mug AW, Hazes JMW. Effect of intensive exercise on patients with active rheumatoid arthritis: a randomised clinical trial. Ann Rheum Dis 2000; 59(8):615-621.

van der Bij, AK, Laurant, MGH & Wensing, M. (2002). Effectiveness of physical activity interventions for older adults: a review. *American Journal of Preventive Medicine*, Vol. 22, No. 2, pp. 120-133.

Walsmith J, Roubenoff R. Cachexia in rheumatoid arthritis. International Journal of Cardiology 2002;85(1):89-99.

Wang G, Helmick, C G, Macera, C, Zhang, P and Pratt, M. Inactivity-associated medical costs among US adults with arthritis', . Arthritis Care and Research 2001;45:439-445.

Wilcox S, Ananian C, Abbott J, Vrazel J, Ramsey C, Sharpe P, Brady T. Perceived exercise barriers, enablers, and benefits among exercising and nonexercising adults with arthritis: Results from a qualitative study. *Arthritis Care & Research* 2006;55(4):616-627.

16

Resistance Training for Patients with Rheumatoid Arthritis: Effects on Disability, Rheumatoid Cachexia, and Osteoporosis; and Recommendations for Prescription

Andrew B. Lemmey
School of Sport, Health and Exercise Sciences, Bangor University
U.K

1. Introduction

Rheumatoid arthritis (RA) is characterised by disability, cachexia, and obesity, and features exacerbated risk of both cardiovascular disease (CVD) and osteoporosis. To deal with RA generally and these associated conditions specifically, the World Health Organisation (WHO, 2008) and various national health authorities (e.g. American College of Rheumatology, ACR, 2002, 2006; European League Against Rheumatism, EULAR, Combe et al., 2007; American College of Sports Medicine, ACSM, 2010a, 2010b, 2010c, 2010d; American Heart Association, AHA, Williams et al., 2007) have advocated progressive resistance training (PRT; i.e. systematic weight training) as adjunct therapy. Additionally, two Cochrane Reviews (Hurkmans et al., 2009; van den Ende et al., 2000) have supported inclusion of this form of exercise in the routine management of RA patients. However, despite this weighty advocacy regular PRT is rarely prescribed for or undertaken by RA patients.

In this chapter, the efficacy and safety of PRT as a treatment for RA will be discussed, with training recommendations and considerations outlined.

2. Disability, rheumatoid cachexia and osteoporosis in RA patients

2.1 Disability

Despite advances in the pharmaceutical treatment of RA, disability remains a feature of the disease. In a recent report from the British Society for Rheumatology Biologics Register (Lunt et al., 2010), the median (interquartile range) Health Assessment Questionnaire (HAQ) scores for large samples of patients receiving anti-tumor necrosis factor (anti-TNF) treatment (n=12,672) or standard disease modifying anti-rheumatic drugs (DMARD's; n=3,522) were 2.1 (1.8-2.5) and 1.6 (0.9-2.1), respectively; which are levels indicative of moderate to severe disability. Such widespread disability, as well as causing enormous suffering and reduction of Quality of Life (QoL) on a personal level, also has huge social and economic costs (Verstappen et al., 2004; Yelin, 1996). For example, within 10 years of RA diagnosis a prevalence of 35% for work disability is currently reported for both US and European populations (Allaire et al., 2008; Eberhardt et al., 2007).

Whilst the causes of disability in RA are multifactorial (Escalante & del Rincon, 1999, 2002), Giles et al. (2008) has shown that it is strongly associated with adverse changes in body composition, with HAQ scores inversely related to appendicular lean mass (ALM; a surrogate measure of muscle mass) and directly related to total and appendicular fat masses. Subsequently, Stavropoulos-Kalinoglou et al. (2009) have also shown that obesity is significantly and independently associated with disability in RA patients. Such links between body composition and physical function are not surprising as they reflect those observed in the general elderly population, whereby classification as either muscle-wasted (sarcopenic) or obese significantly exacerbates the likelihood of disability, whilst the co-incidence of both conditions (sarcopenic-obesity) increases disability risk 12-fold in women and 9-fold in men (Morley et al., 2001).

2.2 Rheumatoid cachexia

Unfortunately, both reduced muscle mass and elevated adiposity, termed "rheumatoid cachexia" (Roubenoff et al., 1992), are characteristic of RA. Muscle wasting due to RA was first observed by Sir James Paget in 1873 and has been consistently reported in recent decades (see Summers et al., 2008 for a review); most prolifically and notably by Ronenn Roubenoff's group (Rall & Roubenoff, 1996, 2004; Rall et al., 1996a, 2002; Roubenoff, 2000; Roubenoff et al., 1992, 1994, 2002; Walsmith & Roubenoff, 2002; Walsmith et al., 2004). Using a definition of significant muscle loss as being below the 50th percentile for arm muscle circumference of a reference population, Roubenoff et al. (1994) found that 67% of their RA patients were cachectic. Whilst Munro and Capell (1997), employing the more stringent cut-off of the 10th percentile, concluded that 50% of their British RA sample was muscle wasted. More recently, in a series of studies, mostly featuring patients who volunteered for high intensity exercise training (Marcora et al., 2005a, 2005b; Lemmey et al., 2009; Elamanchi et al. and Lemmey et al., manuscripts in preparation), we have identified that 2/3's of our stable RA patients are muscle wasted according to the whole-body dual-energy x-ray absorptiometry (DXA) definitions of Baumgartner et al. (1998; i.e. ALM (kg) / height^2 (m^2) more than two standard deviations below the mean of a young reference group). Interestingly, using the same methodology we found a similar incidence of rheumatoid cachexia in treatment-naïve, recent-onset RA patients (<6 months since diagnosis), suggesting that the loss of lean body mass (LBM) occurs early in the course of the disease (Marcora et al., 2006).

The magnitude of this loss in LBM is reported by Roubenoff's group (using the potassium-40 method) to be 14-16% in RA patients with controlled disease (Rall et al., 2002; Roubenoff et al., 1994, 2002); which agrees with the ≈15% loss we observe in stable RA patients relative to age- and sex-matched healthy sedentary controls (Lemmey et al., unpublished observations). Given this magnitude of muscle loss, it is not surprising that RA patients have substantially reduced muscle strength, with values ranging from 30-80% of normal being reported (Ekblom et al., 1974; Ekdahl & Broman, 1992; Ekdahl et al., 1989; Hakkinen et al., 1995; Madsen et al., 1998; Nordesjo et al., 1983). Also consistent with expectations is the very strong relationship Stucki et al. (1998) revealed between muscle weakness and disability in RA patients. In this study, HAQ was significantly correlated with muscle strength index (MSI), disease activity, morning stiffness, pain, and joint damage. However, when analysing the effect of change in these predictors with change in HAQ, only MSI and pain remained significantly associated. Thus confirming the importance of strength's, and by extension - muscle mass's, association with disability in RA.

The degree and prevalence of cachexia typically present in RA patients is alarming since it represents in excess of a third of the maximal loss of body cell mass or LBM that is compatible with survival (i.e. 40%; Walsmith & Roubenoff, 2002). Additionally, as in other catabolic diseases, muscle loss as well as causing weakness and disability is associated with osteoporosis, low aerobic capacity, impaired immune and pulmonary function, glucose intolerance, depression, loss of independence, compromised QoL, and increased mortality (see Kotler, 2000 for a review).

2.3 Obesity

Muscle depletion associated with RA, however, is generally undiagnosed (and consequently, untreated) as a concomitant increase in fat mass (FM) masks the decrease in muscle mass when bodyweight is measured. Thus, for a given body mass index (BMI), Stavropoulos-Kalinoglou et al. (2007) found that RA patients had on average 4.3% more body fat than matched, healthy controls. Alternatively, for a given body fat percentage (%BF), RA patients have a BMI almost 2kg/m^2 lower than members of the general population. Consequently, these authors have proposed that the BMI cut-offs for defining "overweight" and "obesity" in RA patients should be reduced to 23kg/m^2 and 28kg/m^2, respectively (Stavropoulos-Kalinoglou et al., 2007). This recommendation is supported by comparisons of BMI and %BF values reported for RA patients. Mean BMI's usually reported for RA patients (25.2-29.1 kg/m^2) (Gordon et al., 2002; Marcora et al., 2005a, 2005b; Saravana & Gillot, 2004; Stavropoulos-Kalinoglou et al., 2007) are consistent with that of the entire adult UK population (27.1 kg/m^2) (Craig et al., 2009), suggesting that RA patients, like the overall population, are generally merely overweight. However, when body composition is assessed (Elkan et al., 2009; Lemmey et al., 2009; Marcora et al., 2005a, 2005b; Stavropoulos-Kalinoglou et al., 2007, 2009; Westhovens et al., 1997) RA patients are revealed to be significantly fatter than the overall population, with a mean %BF of around 40% and a prevalence of obesity (using the criteria of 38%BF or more for women, and 27%BF or more for men; Baumgartner et al., 1999) of approximately 80% (Lemmey et al., 2009; Marcora et al., 2005a, 2005b; Stavropoulos-Kalinoglou et al., 2009). Using a stricter criteria, Elkan et al. (2009a) found that 33% of female and >50% of male RA patients had a FM index above the 90th percentile for the whole population. As with muscle loss, this high prevalence of obesity is evident in recently diagnosed RA patients (Marcora et al., 2006), again indicating that the body composition perturbations characteristic of rheumatoid cachexia occur early in the disease.

Disturbingly, as well as favouring accumulation of higher total fat, RA appears to preferentially predispose to central obesity (Elkan et al., 2009b; Giles et al., 2010; Inaba et al., 2007; Westhovens et al., 1997). In the general population, obesity, and in particular central obesity, is a well established, independent risk factor for CVD and many of the classical CVD risk factors (e.g. Mahabadi et al., 2009; Rosito et al., 2008). Similarly in RA patients, central obesity is linked with hypertension, elevated fasting glucose levels, and metabolic syndrome (Giles et al., 2010), and arterial thickening and stiffening (Inaba et al., 2007). As there is an increased risk of CVD in RA patients, with rates of both CVD events and mortality increased approximately 50% relative to non-RA controls (Avina-Zubieta et al., 2008; Naranjo et al., 2008), one would assume that loss of fat, particularly trunk fat, would be highly beneficial for the CV health of this population.

2.4 Osteoporosis

Another feature of RA is secondary osteoporosis. RA patients have greater incidence of osteoporosis and osteoporotic fractures than matched non-RA controls (e.g. Frank & Gottwalt, 2009; Huusko et al., 2001; Sinigaglia et al., 2006); with this increase attributed to the disease itself (systemic inflammation), treatment with high dose oral glucocorticoids, and sedentary lifestyle (Cantley et al., 2009; Frank & Gottwalt, 2009; Huusko et al., 2001; Sinigaglia et al., 2006;). Interestingly, after high-dose steroid therapy, the reduced bone mineral density (BMD) in RA patients has been found to be most strongly associated with low strength (quadriceps and handgrip) and poor physical function (Huusko et al., 2001; Madsen et al., 1998, 2001).

2.5 Treatments for rheumatoid cachexia

Clearly, interventions capable of reversing cachexia in RA patients (i.e. increasing muscle mass and decreasing FM, especially trunk FM) have the potential to improve physical function and thus decrease disability, prolong independence, improve QoL, reduce comorbidities, and perhaps increase life expectancy. Such an intervention would also significantly reduce the huge economic impact of RA (half of which results from production losses caused by functional impairment (McIntosh, 1996)). Several anabolic agents, such as recombinant human GH and anabolic steroids, have been proposed for increasing muscle mass in sarcopenic/cachectic states (e.g. Bross et al., 1999; Johansen et al., 1999, 2006; Macdonald et al., 2007). However, GH therapy is expensive and may cause carpal tunnel syndrome and insulin resistance, whilst anabolic steroids are associated with side effects such as liver disorders, masculinisation in women, and prostate cancer and testicular atrophy in men (Bhasin, 2003; Johansen et al., 1999; Korkia & Stimson, 1997; Macdonald et al., 2007). Furthermore, when used alone, despite increasing lean mass, these drugs often fail to improve physical function (Bross et al., 1999; Johansen et al., 2006; Macdonald et al., 2007; Rodriguez-Arnao et al., 1999). Consistent with these findings, are the findings of an unpublished randomised controlled trial we conducted (Elamanchi et al., manuscript in preparation), in which nandrolone decanoate (ND), an anabolic steroid, was administered (i.m. injection, 100mg/wk) for 6 months to 20 male RA patients with stable disease Despite inducing substantial increases in mean ALM (≈1.5kg), administration of ND failed to improve any of the objective measures of physical function assessed.

As rheumatoid cachexia has been attributed to cytokine (principally TNF-α) driven muscle catabolism by Roubenoff group (Rall & Roubenoff, 2004; Rall et al., 1996a; Roubenoff et al., 1994, 2002), it was anticipated that treatment with anti-TNF drugs could restore a healthier body composition to RA patients. However, Marcora et al. (2006) found that treatment of recently diagnosed RA patients for 6 months with etanercept (anti-TNF agent) had no effect on body composition relative to treatment with methotrexate ("standard DMARD"). This lack of effect of anti-TNF's on LBM in RA patients has subsequently been confirmed by Metsios et al. (2007). Of concern was their additional observation of increased trunk fat in established RA patients following 3 months on anti-TNF's. These findings are further supported by a recent report (Engvall et al., 2010), which observed increased FM in recent-onset RA patients treated with anti-TNF's for 21 months relative to DMARD treated patients (mean±sd; +3.4±1.4kg, $p<0.05$), and no changes in LBM for either treatment.

3. Efficacy of progressive resistance training

The most, perhaps the only, effective, safe and economical intervention known to increase both muscle and bone mass and also improve strength and physical function in subjects of various ages is progressive resistance training (PRT) (see Kraemer et al., 1996 for a review).

3.1 Effects on function

The efficacy of resistance training for improving strength in RA patients (Table 1) was first demonstrated by Machover and Sopecky in 1966. In this pioneering study, 11 male RA patients performed maximal isometric contractions of the quadriceps 3 times a day, 5 days/week for 7 weeks, for an average strength gain of 23%. Since then, significant improvements in strength in RA patients have been elicited by a variety of resistance training regimes (Table 1). The only exception identified being the home-based intervention of Komatireddy et al. (1997).

Consistent with the increases in strength are reports of improvements in physical function assessed objectively (e.g. walk tests, stair climbing, bench stepping, balance/coordination, hand-grip strength, timed up and go, vertical jump, 30-sec arm curl test, chair test, aerobic capacity; Ekdahl et al., 1990; Hakkinen et al., 1994, 1999, 2003, 2004a, 2005; Hoenig et al., 1993; Komatireddy et al., 1997; Lemmey et al., 2009; Lyngberg et al., 1994; Marcora et al., 2005a; McMeeken et al., 1999; Nordemar et al., 1976, 1981; Rall et al., 1996b; van den Ende et al., 1996, 2000) and subjectively (e.g. 100-point truth-value scale, study generated questionnaire, self reported fatigue, HAQ, McMaster Toronto Arthritis (MACTAR) Patient Preference Disability Questionnaire; Ekdahl et al., 1990; Hakkinen et al., 1994, 2001, 2004a; Komatireddy et al., 1997; Lyngberg et al., 1994; Marcora et al., 2005a; McMeeken et al., 1999; van den Ende et al., 2000) (Table 1). Although it is notable that improvements in physical function are usually not observed when it is subjectively assessed by the HAQ (de Jong et al., 2003; Hakkinen et al., 1999, 2003, 2004b, 2005; Lemmey et al., 2009; van den Ende et al., 1996). The general inability of HAQ scores to reflect objectively assessed improvements in physical function is probably due to the insensitivity of this instrument in detecting performance gains in mildly disabled patients i.e. the type of patient likely to feature in exercise intervention studies. This lack of sensitivity is evident in findings from the Rheumatoid Arthritis Patients in Training (RAPIT) program (de Jong et al., 2003) which showed improvements in patients' self-reported physical function following high intensity exercise training when assessment was by the MACTAR Questionnaire, but not when the HAQ was used. The unsuitability of the HAQ for detecting improvements in function following exercise therapy has been highlighted by van den Ende et al. (1997), who advocate objective measures related to performing activities of daily living (ADL's) as measures of efficacy.

As concluded by the 2 Cochrane Reviews conducted to date (Hurkmans et al., 2009; van den Ende et al., 2000), the efficacy of resistance training programs in improving strength and physical function in RA patients is clear. In fact, with appropriate training it is not unreasonable to expect that patients with established, controlled RA can achieve levels of physical function at least as good as sedentary, healthy individuals of the same age and sex. In the RCT conducted by our group (Lemmey et al., 2009), patients with established RA (11

Study (author/year/ref)	Intervention group † (n)	Exercise type	Training frequency & duration	Intensity % max ‡	Volume (sets/reps)	Control Ψ	Strength	Function	Body composition	Disease activity
Ekdahl et al., 1990	17	RT + aerobic + balance	2/wk, 6 wks	_	_	**RCT** ROM, isom	↑	↑	_	↔↓
Hoenig et al., 1993	30	Hand RT	14/wk, 12 wks	_	_	**RCT** ROM, NC	↑	↑	_	↓
Hakkinen et al., 1994, 1997	21	PRT	2-3/wk, 6 mths	70-80	3 sets of 6-12 reps	**RCT** NC	↑	↑	↑LM*	↓
van den Ende et al., 1996	25	PRT + aerobic + circuits	3/wk, 12 wks	_	_	**RCT** ROM, isom	↑	↑	_	↔
Komatireddy et al., 1997	25	PRT	3/wk, 12 wks	"low intensity"	2-3 sets of 12-15 reps	**RCT** NC	↔	↑	_	↓
McMeeken et al., 1999	17	Leg PRT	14 sessions over 6 wks	70	4 sets of 5 reps	**RCT** NC	↑	↑	_	_
Hakkinen et al., 1999, 2001, 2004[a,b]	32	PRT	2/wk, 24 mths	50-70	2 sets of 8-12 reps	**RCT** ROM	↑	↑	_	↓
van den Ende et al., 2000	34	PRT + aerobic	5/wk, 4 wks	_	_	**RCT** ROM, isom	↑	↑	_	↓
de Jong et al., 2003, 2009	150	RT + aerobic	2/wk, 24 mths	_	8-15 reps	**RCT** NC	↑	↑	_	↔
Lemmey et al., 2009	13	PRT	2/wk, 24 wks	80	3 sets of 8 reps	**RCT** ROM	↑	↑	↑LM, ↓FM	↔
Machover & Sapecky, 1966	11	Unilateral leg isometric RT	15/wk, 7 wks	100	3 reps	contralateral leg	↑	_	_	↔
Nordemar et al., 1976	10	Leg RT + aerobic	5/wk, 6 wks	_	_	none	↑	↑	↑ fibre x-sect area	↔
Nordemar et al., 1981	23	Leg RT + aerobic	1/fortnight, 4-8 yrs	_	_	RA	↑	↑	_	↓
Lyngberg et al., 1994	9	PRT; isom	3/wk, 3 wks for each leg	50	48 reps; 24 reps	none	↑	↑	_	↔
Rall et al., 1996b	8	PRT	2/wk, 12 wks	80	3 sets of 8 reps	HC	↑	↑	↔	↔
Hakkinen et al., 2003	23	PRT + aerobic	3/fortnight, 21 wks	50-80	4-6 sets of 3-12 reps	HC	↑	↑	_	↔
Hakkinen et al., 2005	23	PRT + aerobic	3/fortnight, 21 wks	50-80	3-5 sets of 5-12 reps	HC	↑	↑	↑LM*, ↓FM*	↔
Marcora et al.,	10	PRT	3/wk, 12 wks	80	3 sets of 8 reps	RA	↑	↑	↑LM, ↓FM	↔

† = exercise group or, if multiple exercise groups, the highest intensity exercise group. PRT = progressive resistance training, RT = resistance training, isom = isometric strength exercises, aerobic = aerobic training e.g. cycling, walking, swimming etc, balance = balance training. ‡ = % 1-repetition maximum. **Ψ RCT** = randomised controlled trial, ROM = range of movement exercises, NC = normal care, RA = non-randomised rheumatoid arthritis patients, HC = healthy controls. ↑ = improved strength/function, ↔ = no change. ↑LM = increased total lean mass, ↓FM = decreased total/trunk fat mass, ↑LM* = increased quadriceps LM, ↓FM* = decreased quadriceps subcutaneous fat, ↑ fibre x-sect area = increase in vastus lateralis fibre cross-sectional area. ↓ = decreased disease activity. _ = not assessed +/or reported.

Table 1. Summary of interventions and effects of resistance training programs women, 2 men; age 55.6±8.3 years; disease duration 74±76 months) whose objectively measured physical function at baseline was poor relative to population norms, were able to achieve or exceed these performance norms following 24 weeks of high-intensity PRT. Restoration of normal levels of strength and function in RA patients following PRT has also been observed in the studies of Hakkinen et al. (2003, 2005) which featured healthy, age- and sex-matched control subjects, and in our uncontrolled pilot study (Marcora et al., 2005). In a point that will be pursued later, it should be noted that the only investigation that did not report significant increases in strength in RA patients following resistance training utilised a very low training intensity (Komatireddy et al., 1997).

3.2 Effects on rheumatoid cachexia (body composition)

The effects of resistance training on body composition in RA are less well reported (Table 1). In 1976, Nordemar et al. observed increased cross-sectional area of type I and especially type II fibres in 10 RA patients following 6 weeks of cycling, walking and quadriceps strength training. Similarly, Hakkinen et al. (1994) observed increases in quadriceps muscle cross-sectional area in RA patients following 6 months PRT. However, when Rall et al. (1996b) reported no changes in whole-body composition (DXA assessed) in 8 RA subjects following 12 weeks PRT (despite significant improvements in strength), the conclusion was that RA patients are resistant to the anabolic effects of exercise. This concern has subsequently been refuted by methodologically more robust trials. Initially, we (Marcora et al., 2005a) reported significant increases in (DXA assessed) LBM, ALM and estimated total body protein (TBP), and reductions in %BF, with a trend toward reduced trunk fat (-0.75kg) following 12 weeks of high-intensity PRT. Subsequently, these effects were confirmed by our RCT (Lemmey et al., 2009); LBM, ALM (≈1.2kg), and TBP were all significantly increased (p's=0.002-0.006) and total and especially trunk FM (-2.5kg, i.e. 18%) were substantially reduced following 24 weeks of PRT. Additionally, Hakkinen et al. (2005) have reported quadriceps femoris hypertrophy ($p<0.001$) and reduced quadriceps subcutaneous fat thickness ($p<0.001$) in female RA patients following 21 weeks of combined PRT and aerobic training.

Whilst aerobic exercise training, by increasing daily energy expenditure, has been shown to be an effective adjunct to restricted energy intake for weight loss in young adults, its efficacy in middle aged and elderly individuals is questionable. This is because sedentary individuals of this aged are usually so deconditioned that they are unable to perform exercise of sufficient intensity and duration to significantly elevate daily energy expenditure (Evans, 1999). In contrast, in elderly men and women an elevation of approximately 15% in resting metabolic rate (RMR) has been observed following 12 weeks PRT as a consequence of increased LBM (Campbell et al., 1994). An increase in RMR of this magnitude is very relevant as RMR typically accounts for 60-75% of 24 hr energy expenditure.

In our PRT studies (Lemmey et al., 2009; Marcora et al., 2005a), the elicited increases in muscle mass were significantly associated with improvements in objectively assessed physical function (i.e. 30 sec arm curl, 30 sec sit-to-stand, 50′ walk, hand-grip strength, and knee extensor strength; tests taken from the Senior Fitness Test (Rikli & Jones, 2001), and designed to reflect the ability to perform ADL's). Interestingly, the increased muscle mass and reduced fat mass in the PRT subjects in our RCT (Lemmey et al., 2009) caused a reclassification of the body types of many of these patients. Wherein, whereas at baseline, 9 (out of 13) were classified as cachectic, 10 as obese, and 5 as both (i.e. "cachectic-obese"), after 24 weeks of PRT the number of patients in these high disability risk categories (Morley et al., 2001) were reduced to 4, 7 and 2, respectively. Given the reported links between adverse body composition and physical disability in RA patients (Giles et al., 2008) and the general elderly population (Morley et al., 2001), the positive effects of PRT on function in RA patients are anticipated. To emphasise the crucial role played by training intensity, in our RCT study (Lemmey et al., 2009) range-of-movement (ROM) exercises (i.e. the form of exercise most commonly prescribed for RA patients) were performed by the control group. Despite good compliance to the intervention, this low intensity exercise failed to have any effect on the various measures of body composition or objective physical function.

3.3 Impact on mechanisms of rheumatoid cachexia

As mentioned earlier, the precise mechanisms underlying rheumatoid cachexia have not been clarified. However, an additional insight was provided by Lemmey et al's RCT (2009). In this study diminished muscle levels of insulin-like growth factor-I (mIGF-I) were identified in our RA patients. This finding is consistent with reports of reduced mIGF-I levels in other conditions characterised by muscle wasting: chronic heart failure (CHF) (Hambrecht et al., 2005), chronic obstructive pulmonary disease (COPD) (Vogiatzis et al., 2007), chronic renal failure (Macdonald et al., 2004, 2005), and advanced aging (Fiatarone Singh et al., 1999); and with the proposed role of mIGF-I in regulating the maintenance of adult skeletal muscle (Adams, 2002). Following 24 weeks PRT, along with muscle hypertrophy, mIGF-I levels were observed to increase 50% in our RA patients. Again, this finding of coincident increases in mIGF-I levels and muscle mass in cachectic individuals following exercise training is consistent with responses in COPD (Vogiatzis et al., 2007) and dialysis (Macdonald et al., 2005) patients, and the frail elderly (Fiatarone Singh et al., 1999); and the pivotal role put forward for mIGF-I in muscle's hypertrophic response to loading (Adams, 2002).

3.4 Responsiveness of RA patients to PRT

The magnitude of effects of PRT on strength and body composition observed in RA patients are similar to those reported for healthy middle-aged or older individuals (e.g. Frontera et al., 1991; Morse et al., 2007; Nichols et al., 1993; Pedersen & Saltin, 2006). The study by Hakkinen et al. (2005) described previously provides a direct comparison of training responses. This investigation featured female RA patients and age-matched healthy women who completed the same 21 week combined resistance and aerobic exercise training program, and noted remarkably similar improvements in strength and body composition (with regard to both absolute and relative increases in quadriceps femoris cross-section and reductions in quadriceps femoris subcutaneous fat thickness) following training. This similarity in training response is consistent with recent reports that muscle quality (muscle force per size) is not compromised in RA patients (Matschke et al., 2010a, 2010b). In these studies, a range of skeletal muscle parameters (e.g. specific force, muscle architecture, co-activation of antagonist muscles, voluntary activation capacity) were observed to be the same for well controlled RA patients, including those classified as cachectic, as for matched healthy subjects. This finding that rheumatoid muscle is normal both qualitatively and in its response to resistance training is important for health professionals involved in prescribing exercise for people with RA.

3.5 Effects on bone

The benefit of weight-bearing and strengthening exercise in maximising and maintaining BMD, and reducing the risk of falling by improving strength and balance is well accepted in the general population (ACSM, 2010a). With specific reference to RA, a sedentary lifestyle confers a relative risk of 1.6 for low BMD in RA patients, and even moderate physical activity has been shown to reduce this risk by 50% (Tourinho et al., 2008). Additionally, de Jong et al. (2004) showed that bone loss at the hip was reduced in RA patients participating in the 2 year, high-intensity RAPIT exercise program (median -1.1% vs -1.9% for non-exercising controls, $p<0.05$). Further analysis revealed that these changes in BMD were significantly and independently associated with changes in strength and aerobic power, and that the high-intensity training had a benefit comparable to that of biphosphonate treatment. This finding led the investigators to conclude that intense weight-bearing exercise, including PRT, is essential for improving BMD in RA patients. Similar conclusions were made by Hakkinen et al. following their RCT (1999, 2001, 2004a). In this trial, twelve months PRT by RA patients resulted in mean BMD gains of +1.10% at the femoral head and +0.19% at the lumbar spine in contrast to losses of -0.03% and -1.14%, respectively, in the ROM controls (Hakkinen et al., 1999). Following a further 12 months PRT, the mean differences between the groups increased with the changes in BMD at the femoral head and the lumbar spine now +0.51% and +1.17% for the training group and -0.70% and -0.91%, respectively, for the controls (Hakkinen et al., 2001). These observed trends in BMD were noted again at a 3 year follow-up (Hakkinen et al., 2004a). Whilst the differences between the groups were not statistically significant, except for the femoral head at 24 months, it was suggested by the authors that such an effect would be substantial and of clinical significance if PRT was prolonged and its impact on BMD given longer to accrue.

Treatments for osteopenia or osteoporosis are judged on their ability to increase BMD, or failing that, to minimise bone loss. Thus, although the evidence from RA patients is limited, PRT appears to be as efficacious in this population as it is generally (e.g. Dornemann et al., 1997; Nelson et al., 1994; Rhodes et al., 2000).

In RCT's conducted to evaluate the effect of PRT on BMD in the general population, the evidence is compelling that intensity (i.e. loading) is the key variable (see Layne and Nelson, 2001 for a review). This is consistent with Wolff's law which states that the magnitude of the stress or mechanical load applied to bone via muscles and tendons directly determines the osteogenic response (Chamay & Tschantz, 1972). The results of Kerr et al. (1996) serve to illustrate this. In this study, post-menopausal women (aged 51-62 years) were randomised to either high-intensity (HI) "strength" PRT (high load, low repetitions i.e. 3 sets of 8 repetitions) or low-intensity (LI) "endurance" PRT (low load, high repetitions i.e. 3 sets of 20 repetitions). After training 3x's/week for 12 months, the HI group had increased femoral head and distal radial BMD significantly more than the LI group; with the site-specific gains in BMD significantly correlated to the site-specific strength increases. In patients recovering from surgery, strength training has also been shown to be effective in countering glucocorticoid-induced bone loss (Braith et al., 1996). However, as for the general population, the greatest benefit of PRT in reducing osteoporotic fractures in RA patents is likely to be a consequence of lowering the incidence of falling due to improved strength and balance (Layne and Nelson, 2001; Nelson et al., 1994; Vanderhoek et al., 2000). With regards to the suitability of high-intensity PRT for individuals with low BMD; Vanderhoek et al. (2000) specifically chose osteopenic or osteoporotic elderly women (mean±sd; age = 69.0±1.3

years) for 32 weeks of HI PRT in which they performed 3 sets of 8 repetitions at 75-80% of 1-repetition maximum (1-RM, i.e. the maximum load that can be correctly lifted for a given exercise) for each exercise. As anticipated, this high intensity PRT resulted in substantial, and correlated, improvements in strength and balance. More importantly, it also proved to be well tolerated and safe with no compression fractures or other training related injuries observed.

3.6 Safety of PRT for RA patients

For many years, intensive weight-bearing exercise was considered inappropriate for RA patients due to concern that this unaccustomed stress on the joints would exacerbate inflammation, pain, and joint damage (e.g. Sutej & Hadler, 1991). Even today, many rheumatologists and their multidisciplinary teams retain these anachronistic beliefs and advise patients to avoid strenuous physical pursuits in order to protect their joints and conserve their energy (i.e. the strategy of "pacing") (for further discussion on this see Metsios et al., 2007; Munneke et al., 2004). This is despite the unanimity of research findings that exercise training, including resistance training (Table 1), irrespective of the intensity employed, is safe in RA patients. In fact, although most studies report no changes in disease activity following resistance training, findings of improvements are not uncommon; e.g. reductions in: erythrocyte sedimentation rate (ESR; Hakkinen et al., 1994, 1997, 1999), morning stiffness (Ekdahl et al., 1990), number of tender and swollen joints (Ritchie articular index; Ekdahl et al., 1990; Hakkinen et al., 1994, 1997; van den Ende et al., 1996), self-reported joint count (Komatireddy et al., 1997), pain (Komatireddy et al., 1997; McMeeken et al., 1999; Rall et al., 1996b), and Disease Activity Score (DAS28, DAS4; Hakkinen et al., 1999, 2001, 2004a). High-intensity exercise even appears to be safe in patients with active disease; van den Ende et al. (2000) randomly allocated RA patients admitted to hospital for RA flares to perform either HI exercise (isokinetic and isometric strength training) or LI exercise (ROM and isometric exercises). After 24 weeks of training (3x's/week), improvements in DAS were observed for both groups with a trend toward greater improvement in the HI patients.

Adherence to PRT over prolonged periods also provides no cause for concern. Hakkinen et al. (2001) in an RCT comparing 2 years of strength training to conventional physiotherapy (ROM exercises), found that although DAS28 improved significantly for both groups, the strength training group enjoyed greater benefit. Similarly, de Jong et al. (2003) in their 2 year RCT (the RAPIT trial) also identified reductions in disease activity (DAS4) in their HI exercise (including strength training) group; albeit, this time with no difference between the exercise and control ("usual care") groups.

In a broader investigation of immune responses to PRT in RA patients, Rall et al. (1996c) detected no effects of 12 weeks HI training on peripheral blood mononuclear (PBMC) subpopulations, or stimulated proliferation of TNF-α, interleukin (IL)-1β, IL-2, IL-6, or prostaglandin E_2, or delayed type hypersensitivity skin response.

Although reassuring effects on joint counts, systemic inflammation, pain, and more generalised disease activity are provided by studies of strength training interventions in RA patients, relatively few studies have assessed the effects of training on radiographic joint damage. An exception to this was the RAPIT trial. Initially, reports from this investigation (de Jong et al., 2003; Munneke et al., 2005) raised concerns by suggesting that high intensity exercise exacerbated joint damage progression in large joints with extensive pre-existing damage. Results from an 18 month follow-up study (de Jong et al., 2009), however, have seen the investigators retract this conclusion. Instead, they are now confident that long-term, intense weight-bearing exercise does not cause further damage to large joints, even those already extensively damaged. This revised interpretation thus accords with the verdict they had previously made with regard to the small joints of the hands and feet (de Jong et al., 2003). This general conclusion of training not increasing radiological progression of joint damage agrees with the findings of others (Hakkinen et al., 1994, 2001, 2004b; Nordemar et al., 1981). In the earliest of these studies, Nordemar et al. (1981) found that RA patients who had performed 4-8 years of resistance exercises for the legs had reduced joint damage in these limbs relative to non-exercising disease-matched controls. Whilst in the other studies, all by Hakkinen's group (1994, 2001, 2004b), no acceleration in joint damage was detected by x-ray in RA patients performing long-term (up to 5 years; Hakkinen et al., 2004b), regular, HI PRT relative to patients receiving standard care.

4. Fundamentals of PRT prescription for RA patients

"The key factor to successful resistance training at any level of fitness or age is appropriate program design" (Kraemer & Ratamess, 2004); and this requires that specific needs and goals are addressed. For RA patients generally, the needs a PRT program should address are: counteracting rheumatoid cachexia by restoring muscle mass and reducing adiposity (especially central stores); augmenting strength and thus improving physical function and the ability to perform ADL's; and lowering osteoporotic fracture risk by stabilizing or increasing bone mass and reducing the likelihood of falling by enhancing strength and balance. In specifying these aims, the intention is not to ignore the numerous generic benefits of exercise training such as reduced CVD risk, improved insulin-sensitivity, decreased risk of specific cancers, enhanced mood and mental health etc., but to concentrate on those aspects of RA-specific health for which PRT is particularly appropriate. Additionally, individuals may also have personal goals and these should be taken into account when designing the training program. Since untrained individuals readily respond physiologically to most protocols, it is unnecessary to devise complicated or advanced programs.

To maximise the health and performance benefits, and to best ensure safety, it is important that appropriately qualified professionals are involved in designing the PRT program and, for the initial weeks at least, in supervising training. The following training recommendations are all consistent with guidelines provided by the ACR (2022, 2006), EULAR (Combe et al., 2007), ACSM (1998, 2010a-e) and AHA (Williams et al., 2007) either for RA specifically or for the co-morbid conditions common in RA, and by the WHO (2008) "for promoting and maintaining health" in the general population. As with most exercise programs, these guidelines are based on the FITT principle: frequency, intensity, time (or volume), and type (or modality) (ACSM, 2010e).

4.1 Frequency

It is generally recommended that strength training is performed 2-3 days a week with at least 48 hours rest between sessions (Evans, 1999; Hass et al., 2001; Kraemer & Ratamess, 2004). Training on alternate days allows adequate time for recovery and adaptation, and this is particularly important for untrained and/or elderly individuals (Hakkinen, 1995). Whilst there are benefits for highly trained individuals in training more frequently (e.g. daily), for the previously untrained there is insufficient additional training gain to justify the reduction in the recovery period and the additional time commitment (ACSM, 1998; Demichele et al., 1997). For example, Demichele et al. (1997) found that training twice a week elicited 80-90% of the strength gain achieved when training more frequently. In addition to facilitating recovery, limiting PRT sessions to 2-3 times per week should also enhance adherence to the training program, as "insufficient time" is a common reason for not commencing or dropping out of exercise programs (Dishman, 1994).

In healthy individuals it appears that once the training effects of PRT have been established (after 8-12 weeks training), that training once per week, perhaps even once fortnightly is sufficient to maintain these benefits (Graves et al., 1990). A similar maintenance training frequency seems to be appropriate for RA patients, as in the RAPIT study (de Jong et al., 2009), strength gains following 2 years of twice weekly HI training (including strength training) were maintained by patients who continued exercising once/week for the subsequent 18 months, but completely lost by those who stopped exercising. .

4.2 Intensity

To maximise improvements in strength and muscle hypertrophy, it is necessary to recruit the maximal number of motor unit; and since the high-threshold motor units may not be activated by light-to-moderate loads, it is essential to use heavy loads to ensure activation of all motor units. Thus, maximal or near maximal loads elicit the greatest gains in strength and muscle mass (Fleck & Kraemer, 1997). Additionally, as mentioned previously bone also responds most favourably to heavy loading (e.g. Chamay & Tschantz, 1972; Kerr et al., 1996).

In resistance training, intensity is determined by the percentage of the 1-RM a load (weight) corresponds to. Although improvements in strength and muscle mass in previously untrained subjects have been demonstrated following training with loads of 50% 1-RM, multiple studies have shown that loads of ≥ 80% 1-RM are optimal for increasing strength and inducing muscle hypertrophy (e.g. ACSM, 1998; Evans, 1999; Hass et al., 2001; Kraemer & Ratamess, 2004). For untrained subjects and clinical populations aiming to enhance strength and muscle mass, an intensity of 80% 1-RM is generally prescribed, with higher intensities usually the preserve of competition athletes. For 80% 1-RM, 6-12 repetitions or lifts are usually possible. If less than 6 repetitions can be performed then the weight is too heavy, and if more than 12 repetitions can be achieved then the weight is too light. It should be noted that even when the relative intensity is fixed (e.g. 80% 1-RM), the maximum number of repetitions that can be performed varies both between individuals and for a given individual performing different exercises (Hoeger et al., 1987).

It is absolutely crucial that for untrained individuals, intensity at the commencement of PRT, should start low and progress slowly to allow the musculo-skeletal system sufficient time to adapt to the (unaccustomed) demands of training. For example, in our RCT (Lemmey et al., 2009), although the aim was for patients to eventually perform 3 sets of 8-12 repetitions at 80% 1-RM, (primarily to reduce muscle soreness) training was initially performed at much lower intensities. Thus, one set of 15 repetitions at 60% 1-RM was performed for each exercise in the first week, increasing to 2 sets at the same intensity in the second week and 3 sets at the same intensity in the third week. Intensity then increased to 70% 1-RM (12 repetitions per set) for weeks 4-6. Before finally progressing to 8 repetitions per set at 80% 1-RM for weeks 7-24 (note: to ensure maintenance of relative intensities, 1-RM's were reassessed every 4 weeks). By adhering to this protocol substantial training benefits were gained (e.g. increased LM and improvements of 119% in training specific strength), with no occurrences of training related injuries or dropouts from the program.

4.3 Time (volume)

With PRT, training volume is defined as the product of: number of exercises x number of sets per exercise x number of repetitions per set. Thus, training volume can be manipulated by altering any of these variables. It needs to be stated that there is no "magic number" for any of these variables; and if there was it would no doubt vary from individual to individual, and vary again within an individual for each exercise performed.

With regard to the number of exercises; to maximise muscle hypertrophy and to facilitate improvement in the performance of ADL's, resistance training should involve the whole-body. Thus, 6-10 exercises each involving large muscle groups are usually prescribed (e.g. 1) leg press; 2) chest press; 3) leg extension; 4) seated rowing; 5) leg curl; 6) triceps extensions; 7) abdominal crunches/curls; 8) standing calf raises; 9) bicep curl (Lemmey et al., 2009; Marcora et al., 2005a).

Numerous studies have tried to determine the optimal number of sets per exercise, with comparisons of all permutations from one to 6 sets made, but no single number has consistently emerged as the best (e.g. Campos et al., 2002; Kraemer, 1997). When enhanced health and general function is the principle aim of training, for both healthy and clinical populations, 2 or 3 sets are usually prescribed (e.g. ACR, 2002, 2006; ACSM, 2010a-d; Combe et al., 2007; WHO, 2008, Williams et al., 2007). And for novice trainers, both 2 and 3 sets are very effective in eliciting training effects, with controversy persisting as to whether performing 3 sets delivers substantially better returns than performing 2 sets (Ostrowski et al., 1997). Of recent interest is the efficacy of single-set programs. In a number of studies one set of 8-12 repetitions performed to voluntary failure has, in previously untrained subjects, produced training gains comparable to those of conventional multiple set programs (ACSM, 1998); although there is disagreement with this finding (Paulsen et al., 2003), particularly in trained individuals (Kraemer, 1997). Even if single-set protocols are marginally less effective than multi-set programs, the time efficiency of the former may result in better training compliance, as programs that require in excess of 1 hour per session have higher dropout rates (Pollock, 1988). Thus, if time constraint is an important consideration, and especially if the patient wants to additionally perform aerobic training, the use of single-set protocols should be considered as, provided the intensity is sufficient, these will certainly produce beneficial responses (Hass et al., 2001).

Another variable that can be manipulated is the duration of the rest period between sets. Researchers have found that short rest periods (≤1 min) elicit more pronounced muscle hypertrophy (Kraemer, 1997) whilst longer rest periods (2-5 min) produce greater strength gains (ACSM, 2002). These differing effects have been attributed to the extent of ATP-PC (phosphagen system) repletion (Kraemer & Ratamess, 2004); hence, for maximal strength gains complete restoration of ATP-PC is required to enable maximal lifts, whereas incomplete restoration results in metabolic, hormonal, and CV responses that facilitate hypertrophy (Kraemer, 1997; Kraemer et al., 1987, 1991). Not surprisingly, body builders favour programs which feature short rest periods, whilst strength and power athletes generally employ longer rest intervals. Whether these differential effects of rest period duration also operate in middle-aged and elderly previously untrained exercisers is unclear. As such, and given that training benefit is unlikely to be significantly compromised but training time will be markedly reduced if short rest periods are preferred to long rest periods, allocation of 1-2 min rest between sets appears optimal.

4.4 Type (modality)

For safety, training on resistance machines with incremental weight stacks rather than using free weights is recommended (ACR, 2002; Pollock et al., 2000). Machines are also easier and quicker to set up. On the other hand, free weights allow more variety in the exercises performed and are better able to simulate ADL's. As mentioned previously, an optimal PRT program will feature exercises that collectively involve all the major joints and muscle groups. Such whole-body programs, as well as being more effective in increasing overall strength and muscle hypertrophy, also produce significant improvements in aerobic capacity (VO_2max) and endurance performance. For example, Vincent et al. (2000) noted that 6 months whole-body PRT increased peak VO_2 by 22% and treadmill time to exhaustion by 26% in elderly (60-85 years) men and women. Similarly, 10-12 weeks of HI PRT has been shown to improve time to exhaustion while cycling (47%), running (12%) and walking (38%) (Ades et al., 1996; Hickson et al., 1980).

Exercises should be performed rhythmically, in a slow, controlled movement (≈2 secs to lift and ≈4 secs to lower the weight) and, to avoid a Valsalva's manoeuvre and the resultant rises in blood pressure (BP), breathing should be continuous. When proper technique is observed, systolic BP during weight lifting is considerably lower than it is during aerobic exercise of similar intensity, and CV stress is minimal (Pollock et al., 2000). Naturally, with RA patients attention to affected joints is essential and joint pain, instability, poor proprioception, or reduced ROM may necessitate modification or substitution of prescribed exercises (ACSM, 2010c).

4.5 Progression

Gains in strength are usually rapid and substantial following commencement of PRT, with 10-15% increases in strength typically observed each week for the first 8 weeks of training in healthy, previously untrained individuals (Evans, 1999). Initially these improvements are due to enhanced neural factors i.e. improved motor unit recruitment, firing rate and synchronisation (Sale, 2003), with muscle hypertrophy contributing from about week 4 onwards (Sale, 2003). In order to maintain the maximal muscle fibre recruitment necessary for optimal increases in strength and muscle hypertrophy to occur, progressively higher loads need to be lifted. This increase in resistance (in accordance with increases in strength) to maintain a constant relative intensity is termed "progressive overload", and is a fundamental principle of all exercise training regimes.

Whilst marked responses to training are expected in untrained or deconditioned individuals, after an extended period of training the "law of diminishing returns" applies i.e. as an individual's fitness improves and he/she approaches their genetic ceiling it becomes harder to achieve further fitness gains. Consequently, when PRT is prolonged, plateaus in training response should be anticipated. The usual way of dealing with this situation is to manipulate the training program variables (types of exercises, training intensity, number of sets and/or repetitions, rest period between sets), so that the body is challenged by an unfamiliar training stimulus.

4.6 Exclusion criteria and further recommendations

As discussed previously, appropriately designed PRT is safe, and well tolerated by males and females of all ages and most conditions, including RA (ACSM, 1998). In the recommendations made by the AHA regarding resistance training for patients with and without CVD (Pollock et al., 2000), the contraindications to PRT are: unstable angina, uncontrolled hypertension (≥160/100 mm Hg), recent and untreated episodes of congestive heart failure, uncontrolled dysrhythmias, severe stenotic or regurgitant valvular disease, and hypertrophic cardiomyopathy. Additionally, for low to moderate risk cardiac patients wanting to participate in PRT programs, they suggest preliminary aerobic exercise training for 2-4 weeks (Pollock et al., 2000). Overall, however, they concluded that "resistance training exercise is strongly recommended for implementation in primary and secondary cardiovascular disease-prevention programs" and "…is particularly beneficial for improving the function of most cardiac, frail, and elderly patients"(Pollock et al., 2000). In part, this is because increased strength reduces the myocardial demands (i.e. heart rate and BP) when patients perform ADL's because the task requires a lower percentage of functional capacity (McCartney et al., 1993).

Caution must be taken when prescribing PRT to severely osteoporotic patients, with high-intensity exercise to be avoided (ACSM, 2010a). In the case of these patients, specialist advice with regard to exercise should be sought.

Despite the apparently beneficial consequences of training during acute flares shown by Van den Ende et al. (2000), we discourage training during flares. Similarly, as healthy individuals should be advised, we also discourage training during illness (e.g. colds, influenza etc), and tell patients to only resume training when health is restored. Upon resumption of training, loads should be adjusted to account for loss of strength due to detraining. Under these circumstances, pre-illness strength levels are usually rapidly regained. To underline the safety of and tolerance to PRT for RA patients, in our high intensity PRT intervention studies (Lemmey et al., 2009; Marcora et al., 2005a), mean compliance to training sessions (i.e. sessions attended as a % of those scheduled) was around 80%. Thus, even when advised to avoid training when unwell, patients training compliance was similar to that expected of healthy individuals.

5. Conclusion

This chapter has described important consequences of RA which are usually untreated (i.e. diminished muscle mass and high fat mass, particularly central obesity; rheumatoid cachexia) or are still prevalent despite enhanced pharmaceutical treatment (disability, CVD, osteoporotic fractures), and then reviewed the research into the efficacy and safety of PRT in treating these conditions. The evidence indicates that PRT is an appropriate adjunct therapy for RA patients. In particular, its efficacy in positively affecting body composition and physical function is almost unique, particularly when accessibility and the lack of negative side effects are considered. As such, rheumatologists and allied health professionals overseeing the management of RA patients should be encouraging them to undertake PRT, ideally in conjunction with aerobic training. To better inform clinicians in their exercise advice, the fundamental principles of PRT program design have been outlined, with particular reference made to experiences with the RA population.

6. References

Adams GR: Invited Review: Autocrine/paracrine IGF-I and skeletal muscle adaptation. *J. Appl. Physiol.* 93, 1159-67 (2002).

Ades PA, Ballor DL, Ashikaga T, Utton JL, Nair KS: Weight training improves walking endurance in healthy elderly persons. *Ann. Intern. Med.* 124, 568-572 (1996).

Allaire S, Wolfe F, Niu J, Lavalley MP: Contemporary prevalence and incidence of work disability associated with rheumatoid arthritis in the US. *Arthritis Rheum.* 59(4), 474-480 (2008).

American College of Sports Medicine: Exercise prescription for other clinical populations: osteoporosis. In: *ACSM's guidelines for exercise testing and prescription, 8th Edition.* Lippincott, Williams & Wilkins, Baltimore, MA., USA, 193-203 (2010a).

American College of Sports Medicine: Exercise prescription for other clinical populations. In: *ACSM's guidelines for exercise testing and prescription, 8th Edition.* Lippincott, Williams & Wilkins, Baltimore, MA., USA, 248-250 (2010b).

American College of Sports Medicine: Exercise prescription for other clinical populations: Arthritis. In: *ACSM's guidelines for exercise testing and prescription, 8th Edition.* Lippincott, Williams & Wilkins, Baltimore, MA., USA, 225-228 (2010c).

American College of Sports Medicine: Exercise prescription for other clinical populations: Cardiac Disease. In: *ACSM's guidelines for exercise testing and prescription, 8th Edition.* Lippincott, Williams & Wilkins, Baltimore, MA., USA, 212-213 (2010d).

American College of Sports Medicine: General principles of exercise prescription. In: *ACSM's guidelines for exercise testing and prescription*, 8th ed. Lippincott, Williams & Wilkins, Baltimore, MA., USA, 152-182 (2010e).

American College of Sports Medicine position stand: the recommended quantity and quality of exercise for developing and maintaining cardiorespiratory and muscular fitness and flexibility in healthy adults. *Med. Sci. Sports Exerc.* 30, 975-991 (1998).

American College of Sports Medicine: Position stand: progression models in resistance training for healthy adults. *Med. Sci. Sports Exerc.* 34, 364-380 (2002).

American College of Rheumatology Subcommittee on Rheumatoid Arthritis Guidelines: Guidelines for the management of rheumatoid arthritis: 2002 update. *Arthritis Rheum.* 46, 328-346 (2002).

American College of Rheumatology: ACR: Exercise and Arthritis. (2006) www.rheumatology.org/public/factsheets/diseases_and _conditions/exercise.asp

Avina-Zubieta JA, Choi HK, Sadatsafavi M, Etminan M, Esdaile JM, Lacaille D: Risk of cardiovascular mortality in patients with rheumatoid arthritis: a meta-analysis of observational studies. *Arthritis Rheum* 59, 1690-1697 (2008).

Baumgartner RN, Koehler KM, Gallagher D *et al.*: Epidemiology of sarcopenia among the elderly in New Mexico. *Am. J. Epidemiology* 147, 755-763 (1998).

Bhasin S: Testosterone supplementation for aging-associated sarcopenia. *J. Gerontol. A. Biol. Sci. Med. Sci.* 58, 1002-1008 (2003).

Braith RW, Mills RM, Welsh MA, Keller JW, Pollock ML: Resistance exercise training restores bone mineral density in heart transplant recipients. *J. Am. Coll. Cardiol.* 28, 1471-1477 (1996).

Bross R, Javanbakht M, Bhasin S: Anabolic interventions for aging-associated Sarcopenia. *J. Clin. Endocrinol. Metab.* 84, 3420-3430 (1999).

Campbell WW, Crim MC, Young VR, Evans WJ: Increased energy requirements and body composition changes with resistance training in older adults. *Am. J. Clin. Nutr.* 60, 167-175 (1994).

Campos GER, Lubcke TJ, Wendeln HK: Muscular adaptations in response to three different training regimens: specificity of repetition training zones. *Eur. J. Appl. Physiol.* 88, 50-60 (2002).

Cantley MD, Smith MD, Haynes DR: Pathogenic bone loss in rheumatoid arthritis: mechanisms and therapeutic approaches. *Int. J. Clin. Rheumatol.* 4(5), 561-582 (2009).

Chamay A, Tschantz P: Mechanical influences in bone remodelling. Experimental research on Wolff's law. *J. Biochem.* 5, 173-180 (1972).

Combe B, Landewe R, Lukes C *et al.*: EULAR recommendations for the management of early arthritis: report of a task force of the European Standing Committee for International Clinical Studies Including Therapeutics (ESCISIT). *Ann. Rheum. Dis.* 66, 34-45 (2007).

Craig R, Mindell J, Hirani V: *Health survey for England 2008 Volume 1. Physical Activity and Fitness.* The Health and Social Care Information Center, London, UK (2009).

Demichele PD, Pollock ML, Graves JE et al.: Effect of training frequency on the development of isometric torso rotation strength. *Arch. Phys. Med. Rehabil.* 27, 64-69 (1997).

de Jong Z, Munneke M, Kroon HM *et al.*: Long-term follow-up of a high-intensity exercise program in patients with rheumatoid arthritis. *Clin. Rheumatol.* 28, 663-671 (2009).

de Jong Z, Munneke M, Lems WF *et al.:* Slowing of bone loss in patients with rheumatoid arthritis by long-term high-intensity exercise. *Arthritis Rheum.* 50, 1066-1076 (2004).

de Jong Z, Munneke M, Zwinderman AH *et al.*: Is a long-term high-intensity exercise program effective and safe in patients with rheumatoid arthritis? Results of a randomized controlled trial. *Arthritis Rheum.* 48, 2415-2424 (2003).

Dishman RK (Ed.): *Exercise adherence: Its impact on public health,* 2nd ed. Human Kinetics, Champaign, IL., USA (1994).

Dornemann TM, McMurray RG, Renner JB, Anderson JJB: Effects of high-intensity resistance exercise on bone mineral density and muscle strength on 40-50-year-old women. *J. Sports Med. Phys. Fitness* 37, 246-251 (1997).

Eberhardt K, Larsson BM, Nived K, Lindqvist E: Work disability in rheumatoid arthritis: development over 15 years and evaluation of predictive factors over time. *J. Rheumatol.* 34, 481-487 (2007).

Ekblom B, Lovgren O, Alderin M, Fridstrom M, Satterstrom G: Physical performance in patients with rheumatoid arthritis. *Scand. J. Rheumatol.* 3, 121-125 (1974).

Ekdahl C, Andersson SI, Moritz U, Svensson B: Dynamic versus static training in patients with rheumatoid arthritis. *Scand. J. Rheumatol.* 19, 17-26 (1990).

Ekdahl C, Andersson SI, Svensson B: Muscle function of the lower extremities in rheumatoid arthritis and osteoarthritis: A descriptive study of patients in a primary care district. *J. Clin. Epidemiol.* 42, 947-954 (1989).

Ekdahl C, Broman G: Muscle strength, endurance, and aerobic capacity in rheumatoid arthritis patients: a comparative study with healthy subjects. *Ann. Rheum. Dis.* 51, 35-40 (1992).

Elkan AC, Engvall IL, Cederholm T, Hafstrom I: Rheumatoid cachexia, central obesity and malnutrition in patients with low-active rheumatoid arthritis: feasibility of anthropometry, Mini Nutritional Assessment and body composition techniques. *Eur. J. Nutr.* 48, 315-322 (2009a).

Elkan AC, Hakansson N, Frostegard J, Cederholm T, Hafstrom I: Rheumatoid cachexia is associated with dyslipidemia and low levels of atheroprotective natural antibodies against phosphorylchlorine but not with dietary fat in patients with rheumatoid arthritis: a cross sectional study. *Arthritis Res. Therapy* 11, R37 (2009b).

Engvall I-L, Trengstrand B, Brismar K, Hafstrom I: Infliximab therapy increases body fat mass in early rheumatoid arthritis independently of changes in disease activity and levels of leptin and adiponectin: a randomised study over 21 months. *Arthritis Res. Therapy* 12, R197 (2010).

Escalante A, del Rincon I: How much disability in rheumatoid arthritis is explained by rheumatoid arthritis? *Arthritis Rheum.* 42(8), 1712-1721 (1999).

Escalante A, del Rincon I: The disablement process in rheumatoid arthritis. *Arthritis Rheum.* 47(3), 333-342 (2002).

Evans WJ: Exercise training guidelines for the elderly. *Med. Sci. Sports Exerc.* 31, 12-17 (1999).

Fiatarone Singh MA, Ding W, Manfredi TJ *et al.*: Insulin-like growth factor I in skeletal muscle after weight-lifting exercise in frail elders. *Am. J. Physiol. (Endocrinol. Metab.)* 277, 135-43 (1999).

Fleck SJ, Kraemer WJ: *Designing resistance training programs,* 2nd ed. Human Kinetics, Champaign, IL., USA (1997).

Franck H, Gottwalt J: Peripheral bone density in patients with rheumatoid arthritis. *Clin. Rheumatol.* 28, 1141-1145 (2009).

Frontera WR, Hughes VA, Lutz KJ, Evans WJ: A cross-sectional study of muscle strength and mass in 45- to 78-yr-old men and women. *J. Appl. Physiol.* 71, 644-650 (1991).

Giles JT, Allison M, Blumenthal RS *et al.*: Abdominal adiposity in rheumatoid arthritis. Association with cardiometabolic risk factors and disease characteristics. *Arthritis Rheum.* 62, 3173-3182 (2010).

Giles JT, Bartlett SJ, Andersen RE, Fontaine KR, Bathon JM: Association of body composition with disability in rheumatoid arthritis: Impact of appendicular fat and lean tissue mass. *Arthritis Rheum.* 59(10), 1407-1415 (2008).

Gordon MM, Thomson EA, Madhok R, Capell HA: Can intervention modify adverse lifestyle variables in a rheumatoid population? Results of a pilot study. *Ann. Rheum. Dis.* 61, 66-69 (2002).

Graves JE, Pollock ML, Foster D *et al.*: Effect of training frequency and specificity on isometric lumbar extension strength. *Spine* 15, 504-509 (1990).

Hakkinen A, Hakkinen K, Hannonen P: Effects of strength training on neuromuscular function and disease activity in patients with recent-onset inflammatory arthritis. *Scand. J. Rheumatol.* 23, 237-242 (1994).

Hakkinen A, Hannonen P, Hakkinen K: Muscle strength in healthy people and in patients suffering from recent-onset inflammatory arthritis. *Br. J. Rheumatol.* 34, 355-360 (1995).

Hakkinen A, Hannonen P, Nyman K, Lyyski T, Hakkinen K: Effects of concurrent strength and endurance training in women with early or longstanding rheumatoid arthritis: Comparison with healthy subjects. *Arthritis Rheum.* 49, 789-797 (2003).

Hakkinen A, Malkia E, Hakkinen K, Jappinen I, Laitinen L, Hannonen P: Effects of detraining subsequent to strength training on neuromuscular function in patients with inflammatory arthritis. *Br. J. Rheumatol.* 36, 1075-1081 (1997).

Hakkinen A, Pakarinen A, Hannonen P *et al.*: Effects of prolonged combined strength and endurance training on physical fitness, body composition and serum hormones in women with rheumatoid arthritis and in healthy controls. *Clin. Exp. Rheumatol.* 23, 505-512 (2005).

Hakkinen A, Sokka T, Hannonen P: A home-based two-year strength training period in early rheumatoid arthritis led to good long-term compliance: A five-year follow-up. *Arthritis Rheum.* 51, 56-62 (2004).

Hakkinen A, Sokka T, Kautiainen H, Kotaniemi A, Hannonen P: Sustained maintenance of exercise induced muscle strength gains and normal bone mineral density in patients with early rheumatoid arthritis: a 5 year follow up. *Ann. Rheum. Dis.* 63, 910-916 (2004).

Hakkinen A, Sokka T, Kotaniemi A, Hakkinen K, Jappinen I, Laitinen L, Hannonen P: Dynamic strength training in patients with early rheumatoid arthritis increases muscle strength but not bone mineral density. *J. Rheumatol.* 26, 1257-1263 (1999).

Hakkinen A, Sokka T, Kotaniemi A, Hannonen P: A randomized two-year study of the effects of dynamic strength training on muscle strength, disease activity, functional capacity, and bone mineral density in early rheumatoid arthritis. *Arthritis Rheum.* 44, 515-522 (2001).

Hakkinen K: Neuromuscular fatigue and recovery in women at different ages during heavy resistance loading. *Electromyogr. Clin. Neurophysiol.* 35, 403-413 (1995).

Hambrecht R, Schulze PC, Gielen S *et al.*: Effects of exercise training on insulin-like growth factor-I expression in the skeletal muscle of non-cachectic patients with chronic heart failure. *Eur. J. Cardiovasc. Prev. Rehabil.* 12, 401-6 (2005).

Hass CJ, Feigenbaum MS, Franklin BA: Prescription of resistance training for healthy populations. *Sports Med.* 31, 953-964 (2001).

Hickson RC, Rosenkoetter MA, Brown MM: Strength training effects on aerobic power and short-term endurance. *Med. Sci. Sports Exerc.* 12, 336-339 (1980).

Hoeger WW, Barette SL, Hale DF, Hopkins DR: Relationship between repetitions and selected percentages of one repetition maximum. *J. Appl. Sports Sci. Res.* 1, 11-13 (1987).

Hoenig H, Groff G, Pratt K, Goldberg E, Franck W: A randomised controlled trial of home exercise on the rheumatoid hand. *J. Rheumatol.* 20, 785-789 (1993).

Hurkmans E, van der Giesen FJ, Vliet Vlieland TPM, Schoones J, Van den Ende ECHM: Dynamic exercise programs (aerobic capacity and/or muscle strength training) in patients with rheumatoid arthritis (Review). *Cochrane Database of Systematic Reviews* Issue 4 (2009).

Huusko TM, Korpela M, Karppi P, Avikainen V, Kautiainen H, Sulkava R: Threefold increased risk of hip fractures with rheumatoid arthritis in Central Finland. *Ann. Rheum. Dis.* 60, 521-522 (2001).

Inaba M, Tanaka K, Goto H *et al.*: Independent association of increased trunk fat with increased arterial stiffening in postmenopausal patients with rheumatoid arthritis. *J. Rheumatol.* 34, 290-295 (2007).

Johansen KL, Mulligan K, Schambelan M: Anabolic effects of nandrolone decanoate in patients receiving dialysis: a randomized controlled trial. *JAMA* 281, 1275-1281 (1999).

Johansen KL, Painter PL, Sakkas GK, Gordon P, Doyle J, Shubert T: Effects of resistance exercise training and nandrolone decanoate on body composition and muscle function among patients who receive hemodialysis: A randomized, controlled trial. *J. Am. Soc. Nephrol.* 17, 2307-2314 (2006).

Kerr D, Morton A, Dick I, Prince R: Exercise effects on bone mass in postmenopausal women are site-specific and load-dependant. *J. Bone Miner. Res.* 11, 218-225 (1996).

Komatireddy GR, Leitch RW, Cella K, Browning G, Minor M: Efficacy of low load resistive muscle training in patients with rheumatoid arthritis functional class II and III. *J. Rheumatol.* 24, 1531-1539 (1997).

Korkia P, Stimson GV: Indications of prevalence, practice and effects of anabolic steroid use in Great Britain. *Int. J. Sports Med.* 18, 557-562 (1997).

Kotler DP: Cachexia. *Ann. Internal Med.* 133, 622-634 (2000).

Kraemer WJ: A series of studies - the physiological basis for strength training in American Football: fact over philosophy. *J. Strength Cond. Res.* 11, 131-142 (1997).

Kraemer WJ, Fleck SJ, Evans WJ: Strength and power training: physiological mechanisms of adaptation. *Exerc. Sport Sci. Reviews* 24, 363-97 (1996).

Kraemer WJ, Gordon SE, Fleck SJ *et al.*: Endogenous anabolic hormonal and growth factor responses to heavy resistance exercise in males and females. *Int. J. Sports Med.* 12, 228-235 (1991).

Kraemer WJ, Noble BJ, Clark MJ, Culver BW: Physiologic responses to heavy-resistance exercise with very short rest periods. *Int. J. Sports Med.* 8, 247-252 (1987).

Kraemer WJ, Ratamess NA: Fundamentals of resistance training: Progression and exercise prescription. *Med. Sci. Sports Exerc.* 36, 674-688 (2004).

Layne JE, Nelson ME: Resistance training for the prevention of osteoporosis. In: *Resistance training and health rehabilitation.* Graves JE, Franklin BA (Eds.), Human Kinetics, Champaign, IL., USA, 385-404 (2001).

Lemmey AB, Marcora SM, Chester K, Wilson S, Casanova F, Maddison PJ: Effects of high-intensity resistance training in patients with rheumatoid arthritis: A randomised controlled trial. *Arthritis Rheum.* 61, 1726-1734 (2009).

Lunt M, Watson KD, Dixon WG, Symmons DPM, Hyrich KL: No evidence of association between anti-tumor necrosis factor treatment and mortality in patients with rheumatoid arthritis. Results from the British Society for Rheumatology Biologics Register. *Arthritis Rheum.* 62(11), 3145-3153 (2010).

Lyngberg KK, Ramsing BU, Nawrocki A, Harreby M, Dannskiold-Samsoe B: Safe and effective isokinetic knee extensor training in rheumatoid arthritis. *Arthritis Rheum.* 37, 623-628 (1994).

Macdonald JH, Marcora SM, Jibani MM, Kumwenda MJ, Ahmed W, Lemmey AB: Nandrolone decanoate as anabolic therapy in chronic kidney disease: A randomised phase II dose finding study. *Nephron Clin. Prac.* 106, 125-135 (2007).

MacDonald JH, Phanish MK, Marcora SM, Jibani M, Bloodworth LO, Holly JMP, Lemmey AB: Muscle insulin-like growth factor status, body composition, and functional capacity in hemodialysis patients. *J. Renal Nutr.* 14, 248-52 (2004).

MacDonald JH, Phanish MK, Marcora SM, Jibani M, Holly JMP, Lemmey AB: Intradialytic exercise as anabolic therapy in haemodialysis patients - a pilot study. *Clin. Physiol. Funct. Imaging* 25, 113-8 (2005).

Machover S, Sapecky AJ: Effect of isometric exercise on the quadriceps muscle in patients with rheumatoid arthritis. *Arch. Phys. Med. Rehab.* 47, 737-741 (1966).

Madsen OR, Egsmose C, Hansen B, Sorensen OH: Soft tissue composition, quadriceps strength, bone quality and bone mass in rheumatoid arthritis. *Clin. Exp. Rheumatol.* 16, 27-32 (1998).

Madsen OR, Sorensen OH, Egsmose C: Bone quality and bone mass as assessed by quantitative ultrasound and dual energy x ray absorptiometry in women with rheumatoid arthritis: Relationships with quadriceps strength. *Ann. Rheum. Dis.* 61, 325-329 (2001).

Mahabadi AA, Massaro JM, Rosito GA *et al.*: Association of pericardial fat, intrathoracic fat, and visceral abdominal fat with cardiovascular disease burden: the Framingham Heart Study. *Eur. Heart J.* 30, 850-856 (2009).

Marcora SM, Lemmey AB, Maddison PJ: Can progressive resistance training reverse cachexia in patients with rheumatoid arthritis? Results of a pilot study. *J. Rheumatol.* 32, 1031-1039 (2005a).

Marcora SM, Lemmey AB, Maddison PJ: Dietary treatment of rheumatoid cachexia with ß-hydroxy-ß-methylbutyrate, glutamine and arginine: a randomised controlled trial. *Clin. Nutr.* 24, 442-454 (2005b).

Marcora SM, Chester KR, Mittal G, Lemmey AB, Maddison PJ: Randomised phase 2 trial of anti-tumor necrosis factor therapy for cachexia in patients with early rheumatoid arthritis. *Am. J. Clin. Nutr.* 84, 1463-1472 (2006).

Matschke V, Murphy P, Lemmey AB, Maddison PJ, Thom JM: Muscle quality, architecture, and activation in cachectic patients with rheumatoid arthritis. *J. Rheumatol.* 37, 282-284 (2010a).

Matschke V, Murphy P, Lemmey AB, Maddison PJ, Thom JM: Skeletal muscle properties in rheumatoid arthritis patients. *Med. Sci. Sports Exerc.* 42, 2149-2155 (2010b).

McCartney N, McKelvie RS, Martin J, Sale DG, MacDougall JD: Weight-training-induced attenuation of the circulatory response of older males to weight lifting. *J. Appl. Physiol.* 74, 1056-1060 (1993).

McIntosh E: The cost of rheumatoid arthritis. *Br. J. Rheumatol.* 35, 781-790 (1996).

McMeeken J, Stillman B, Story I, Kent P: The effects of knee extensor training and flexor muscle training on the timed-up-and-go test in individuals with rheumatoid arthritis. *Physiotherapy Res. Int.* 4, 55-67 (1999).

Metsios GS, Stavropoulos-Kalinoglou A, Douglas KM *et al.*: Blockade of tumor necrosis factor alpha in rheumatoid arthritis: effects on components of rheumatoid cachexia. *Rheumatology* 46, 1824-1827 (2007).

Metsios GS, Stavropoulos-Kalinoglou A, Veldhuijzen van Zanten JJCS *et al.*: Rheumatoid arthritis, cardiovascular disease and physical exercise: a systematic review. *Rheumatology* 47(3), 239-248 (2007).

Morley JE, Baumgartner RN, Roubenoff R, Mayer J, Nair KS: From the Chicago meetings: Sarcopenia. *J. Lab. Clin. Med.* 137, 231-243 (2001).

Morse CI, Thom JM, Mian OS, Birch KM, Narici MV: Gastrocnemius specific force is increased in elderly males following a 12-month physical training programme. *Eur. J. Appl. Physiol.* 100, 563-570 (2007).

Munneke M, de Jong Z, Zwinderman AH *et al.*: High intensity exercise or conventional exercise for patients with rheumatoid arthritis? Outcome expectations of patients, rheumatologists, and physiotherapists. *Ann. Rheum. Dis.* 63, 804-808 (2004).

Munneke M, de Jong Z, Zwinderman AH *et al.*: Effect of a high-intensity weight-bearing exercise program on radiologic damage progression of the large joints in subgroups of patients with rheumatoid arthritis. *Arthritis Rheum.* 53, 410-417 (2005).

Munro R, Capell H: Prevalence of low body mass in rheumatoid arthritis: association with the acute phase response. *Ann. Rheum. Dis.* 56, 326-329 (1997).

Naranjo A, Sokka T, Descalzo MA *et al.*: Cardiovascular disease in patients with rheumatoid arthritis: results from the QUEST-RA study. *Arthritis Res. Therapy* 10, R30 (2008).

Nelson ME, Fiatarone MA, Morganti CM, Trice I, Greenberg RA, Evans WJ: Effects of high-intensity strength training on multiple risk factors for osteoporotic fractures. A randomised controlled trial. *JAMA* 272, 1909-1914 (1994).

Nichols JF, Omizo DK, Peterson KK, Nelson KP: Efficacy of heavy-resistance training for active women over sixty: Muscular strength, body composition, and program adherence. *J. Am. Geriatr. Soc.* 41, 205-210 (1993).

Nordemar R, Edstrom L, Ekblom B: Changes in muscle fibre size and physical performance in patients with rheumatoid arthritis after short-term physical training. *Scand. J. Rheumatol.* 5, 70-76 (1976).

Nordemar R, Ekblom B, Zachrisson, Lundqvist K: Physical training in rheumatoid arthritis: A controlled long-term study. I. *Scand. J. Rheumatol.* 10, 17-23 (1981).

Nordesjo LO, Nordgren B, Wigren A, Kolstad K: Isometric strength and endurance in patients with severe rheumatoid arthritis or osteoarthritis in knee joints. *Scand. J. Rheumatol.* 12, 152-156 (1983).

Ostrowski KJ, Wilson GJ, Weatherby R, Murphy PW, Lyttle AD: The effect of weight training volume on hormonal output and muscular size and function. *J. Strength Cond. Res.* 11, 148-154 (1997).

Pajet SJ: Nervous mimicry of organic diseases. *Lancet* 2, 727-729 (1873).

Paulsen G, Myklestad D, Raastad T: The influence of volume of exercise on early adaptations to strength training. *J. Strength Cond. Res.* 17, 113-118 (2003).

Pedersen BK, Saltin B: Evidence for prescribing exercise as therapy in chronic disease. *Scand. J. Med. Sci. Sports* 16, 3-63 (2006).

Pollock ML: Prescribing exercise for fitness and adherence. In: *Exercise adherence: its impact on public health.* Dishman RK (Ed.), Human Kinetics, Champaign, IL., USA, 259-282 (1988).

Pollock ML, Franklin BA, Balady GJ *et al.*: Resistance exercise in individuals with and without cardiovascular disease. Benefits, rationale, safety, and progression. An advisory from the Committee on Exercise, Rehabilitation, and Prevention, Council on Clinical Cardiology, American Heart Association. *Circulation* 101, 828-833 (2000).

Rall LC, Meydani SN, Kehayias JJ, Dawson-Hughes B, Roubenoff R: The effect of progressive resistance training in rheumatoid arthritis. Increased strength without changes in energy balance or body composition. *Arthritis Rheum.* 39, 415-426 (1996b).

Rall LC, Rosen CJ, Dolnikowski G *et al.*: Protein metabolism in rheumatoid arthritis and aging. Effects of muscle strength training and tumor necrosis factor α. *Arthritis Rheum.* 39 1115-1124 (1996a).

Rall LC, Roubenoff R: Body composition, metabolism, and resistance exercise in patients with rheumatoid arthritis. *Arthritis Care Res.* 9, 151-156 (1996)

Rall LC, Roubenoff R: Rheumatoid cachexia: metabolic abnormalities, mechanisms and interventions. *Rheumatology (Oxford)* 43, 1219-1223 (2004).

Rall LC, Roubenoff R, Cannon JG, Abad LW, Dinarello CA, Meydani SN: Effects of progressive resistance training on immune response in aging and chronic inflammation. *Med. Sci. Sports Exerc.* 28, 1356-1365 (1996c).

Rall LC, Walsmith JM, Snydman L *et al.*: Cachexia in rheumatoid arthritis is not explained by decreased growth hormone secretion. *Arthritis Rheum.* 46, 2574-2577 (2002).

Rhodes EC, Martin AD, Taunton JE, Donnelly M, Warren J, Elliot J: Effects of one year of resistance training on the relation between muscular strength and bone density in elderly women. *Br. J. Sports Med.* 34, 18-22 (2000).

Rikli RE, Jones CJ: *Senior fitness test manual.* Human Kinetics, Champaign, IL., USA (2001).

Rodriguez-Arnao J, Jabbar A, Fulcher K, Besser GM, Ross RJ: Effects of growth hormone replacement on physical performance and body composition in GH deficient adults. *Clin. Endocrinol.* 51, 53-60 (1999).

Rosito GA, Massaro JM, Hoffmann U *et al.*: Pericardial fat, visceral abdominal fat, cardiovascular disease risk factors, and vascular calcification in a community-based sample: the Framingham Heart Study. *Circulation* 117, 605-613 (2008).

Roubenoff R: Sarcopenic obesity: does muscle loss cause fat gain? Lessons from rheumatoid arthritis and osteoarthritis. *Ann. N.Y. Acad. Sci.* 904, 553-557 (2000).

Roubenoff R, Roubenoff RA, Cannon JG *et al.*: Rheumatoid cachexia: cytokine-driven hypermetabolism accompanying reduced body cell mass in chronic inflammation. *J. Clin. Invest.* 93, 2379-2386 (1994).

Roubenoff R, Roubenoff RA, Ward LM, Holland SM, Hellmann DB: Rheumatoid cachexia: Depletion of lean body mass in rheumatoid arthritis. Possible association with tumor necrosis factor. *J. Rheumatol.* 19, 1505-1510 (1992).

Roubenoff R, Walsmith J, Lundgren N, Snydman L, Dolnikowski G, Roberts S: Low physical activity reduces total energy expenditure in women with rheumatoid arthritis: implications for dietary intake recommendations. *Am. J. Clin. Nutr.* 76, 774-779 (2002).

Sale DG: Neural adaptations to strength training. In: *Strength and power in sports*, 2nd ed. Komi PV (Ed.), Blackwell Science, Malden, MA., USA, 281-314 (2003).

Saravana S, Gillott T: Ischaemic heart disease in rheumatoid arthritis patients. *Rheumatology (Oxford)* 43, 113-114 (2004).

Sinigaglia L, Varenna M, Girasole G, Bianchi G: Epidemiology of osteoporosis in rheumatic diseases. *Rheum. Dis. Clin. North Am.* 32, 631-658 (2006).

Sokka T, Hakkinen A, Kautiainen H *et al.*: Physical inactivity in patients with rheumatoid arthritis: Data from twenty-one countries in a cross-sectional, international study. *Arthritis Rheum.* 59, 42-50 (2008).

Stavropoulos-Kalinoglou A, Metsios G, Koutedakis Y *et al.*: Redefining overweight and obesity in rheumatoid arthritis patients. *Ann. Rheum. Dis.* 66, 1316-1321 (2007).

Stavropoulos-Kalinoglou A, Metsios G, Panoulas VF *et al.*: New resting energy expenditure prediction equations for patients with rheumatoid arthritis. *Rheumatology (Oxford)* 47, 500-506 (2008).

Stavropoulos-Kalinoglou A, Metsios G, Panoulas VF *et al.*: Underweight and obese states both associate with worse disease activity and physical function in patients with established rheumatoid arthritis. *Clin. Rheumatol.* 28, 439-444 (2009).

Stucki G, Bruhlmann S, Stucki S, Michel BA: Isometric muscle strength is an indicator of self-reported physical functional disability in patients with rheumatoid arthritis. *Br. J. Rheumatol.* 37, 643-648 (1998).

Summers GD, Deighton CM, Rennie MJ, Booth AH: Rheumatoid cachexia: a clinical perspective. *Rheumatology (Oxford)* 47, 1124-1131 (2008).

Sutej PG, Hadler NM: Current principles of rehabilitation for patients with rheumatoid arthritis. *Clin. Orthop.* 265, 116-124 (1991).

Tourinho TF, Capp E, Brenol JC, Stein A: Physical activity prevents bone loss in premenopausal women in rheumatoid arthritis: a cohort study. *Rheumatol. Int.* 28, 1001-1007 (2008).

van den Ende CHM, Breedveld FC, le Cessie S, Dijkmans BAC, de Mug AW, Hazes JMW: Effect of intensive exercise on patients with active rheumatoid arthritis : a randomised clinical trial. *Ann. Rheum. Dis.* 59, 615-621 (2000).

van den Ende CHM, Breedveld FC, Dijkmans BAC, Hazes JMW: The limited value of the Health Assessment Questionnaire as an ouotcome measure in short term exercise trials. *J. Rheumatol.* 24, 1972-1977 (1997).

van den Ende CHM, Hazes JMW, le Cessie S *et al.*: Comparison of high and low intensity training in well controlled rheumatoid arthritis. Results of a randomised clinical trial. *Ann. Rheum. Dis.* 55, 798-805 (1996).

van den Ende ECHM, Vliet Vlieland TPM, Munneke M, Hazes JMW: Dynamic exercise therapy for treating rheumatoid arthritis (review). *Cochrane Database of Systematic Reviews* Issue 2 (1998).

Vanderhoek KJ, Coupland DC, Parkhouse WS: Effects of 32 weeks of resistance training on strength and balance in older osteopenic/osteoporotic women. *Clin. Exerc. Physiol.* 2(2), 77-83 (2000).

Verstappen SM, Bijlsma JW, Verkleij H *et al.*, on behalf of the Utrecht Rheumatoid Arthritis Cohort Study Group: Overview of work disability in rheumatoid arthritis patients as observed in cross-sectional and longitudinal surveys (review). *Arthritis Rheum.* 51, 488-497 (2004).

Vincent KR, Vincent HK, Braith R *et al.*: Effects of 6 months of resistance exercise on lipid peroxidation in older adults. *Med. Sci. Sports Exerc.* 32, S105 (2000).

Vogiatzis I, Stratakos G, Simoes DC *et al.*: Effects of rehabilitative exercise on peripheral muscle TNF-alpha, IL-6, IGF-I and MyoD expression in patients with COPD. *Thorax* 62, 950-6 (2007).

Walsmith J, Abad L, Kehayias J, Roubenoff R: Tumor necrosis factor-α production is associated with less body cell mass in women with rheumatoid arthritis. *J. Rheumatol.* 31, 23-29 (2004).

Walsmith J, Roubenoff R: Cachexia in rheumatoid arthritis. *Int. J. Cardiol.* 85, 89-99 (2002).

Westhovens R, Nijs J, Taelman V, Dequeker J: Body composition in rheumatoid arthritis. *Br. J. Rheumatol.* 36, 444-448 (1997).

Williams MA, Haskell WL, Ades PA, *et al.*: American Heart Association Council on Nutrition, Physical Activity, and Metabolism. Resistance exercise in individuals with and without cardiovascular disease: 2007 update. A scientific statement from the American Heart Association Council on Clinical Cardiology and Council on Nutrition, Physical Activity, and Metabolism. *Circulation* 116, 572-584 (2007).

WHO: Recommended Amount of Physical Exercise. (2008) www.who.int/dietphysicalactivity/factsheet_recommendations/en/index.html

Yelin E: The costs of rheumatoid arthritis: absolute, incremental, and marginal estimates. *J. Rheumatol.* 44 (Suppl), 47-51 (1996).

17

Complementary and Alternative Medicine in the Treatment of Rheumatoid Arthritis

Chenchen Wang
Tufts Medical Center/ Tufts University School of Medicine
USA

1. Introduction

Treatment of rheumatoid arthritis, a systemic, diverse and dynamic disorder, has made major progress over the past few decades. Early active treatment with disease-modifying anti-rheumatic drugs and biological agents can be highly beneficial for controlling inflammatory activity and preventing disability in many patients. However, the most effective new drugs are expensive and many patients with rheumatoid arthritis continue to have significant pain, restricted mobility, reduced muscle strength and low endurance. In addition, it is increasingly recognized that co-morbid conditions play a pivotal role in rheumatoid arthritis outcomes. For example, cardiovascular complications are the leading contributor to mortality in rheumatoid arthritis, accounting for approximately one half of all deaths. Osteoporosis, resulting in bone fractures, also represents a major source of morbidity in rheumatoid arthritis. Complementary and alternative medicine treatment and lifestyle behavioral modification may play a role in preventing rheumatoid arthritis-associated comorbidities and their complications.

Rheumatoid arthritis is characterized by synovial inflammation that leads to joint destruction, resulting in substantial long-term disability and a significantly shorter life expectancy. Many patients with rheumatoid arthritis experience high levels of pain, functional impairment, psychological distress and negative emotions, but these symptoms have limited pharmacological therapeutic options. Given the complexity of the therapeutic armamentarium used in rheumatoid arthritis, non-pharmacological therapies are increasingly attractive to those with chronic rheumatic pain conditions. Recently, complementary and alternative medicine therapies for arthritis have been heavily advertised and increasing numbers of chronic pain patients report utilizing alternative therapies. At the same time, clinical trials and observational studies have provided encouraging evidence that Acupuncture, Mind-body Therapy, Chinese herbs and Tibetan Medicine have some benefits for patients with rheumatoid arthritis. Indeed, integrative approaches combine the best of conventional medicine and the wisdom of complementary and alternative medicine. Thus, this chapter synthesizes the current body of knowledge on the therapeutic benefits of several types of Complementary and Alternative Medicine on pain and symptom relief in patients with rheumatoid arthritis to better inform clinical decision-making for our patients.

2. Acupuncture for rheumatoid arthritis

2.1 Acupuncture therapeutics

Acupuncture, originating in China more than 3,000 years ago, is one of the most popular sensory stimulation therapies. It is an ancient technique of inserting and manipulating fine needles to stimulate specific anatomic points, also known as acupuncture points or meridian points. There have been extensive investigations into the biological mechanisms of acupuncture (Cho et al., 1998; Darras et al., 1992; Dhond et al., 2008; Gao et al., 1997; Han & Terenius, 1982; Han, 1997; Harris et al., 2009; Hui et al., 2000; Hui et al., 2005; Kaptchuk, 2002; Kovacs et al., 1992; Langevin et al., 2001a; Langevin et al., 2001b; Langevin et al., 2007; Li et al., 2007; Napadow et al., 2005; Napadow et al., 2007; Napadow et al., 2008; Pariente et al., 2005; Wu et al., 1999; Zhang et al., 2005). Some of the best evidence is in relation to treatment of pain. Three previous systematic reviews examined the efficacy of acupuncture in patients with rheumatoid arthritis and reported that acupuncture has conflicting evidence for treatment of RA in the placebo-controlled trials (Casimiro et al., 2005; Lee et al., 2008; Wang et al., 2008a). Another narrative review examined 63 Chinese studies with a variation of acupuncture therapies in patients with rheumatoid arthritis and concluded that acupuncture is helpful for rheumatoid arthritis (Suzuki et al., 2005). However, in addition to the complexities revealed by an evaluation of this sort of intervention, many of these prior studies have methodological concerns that limit their interpretation. Therefore, this section performs an updated review of all currently available data, including Chinese publications.

2.2 Clinical evidence

Explanatory mechanisms from eastern and western biological theory provide a supposed rationale for the effectiveness of acupuncture to treat the chronic inflammatory nature of rheumatoid arthritis (Han et al., 1986; Han, 2004; Wang et al., 1985; Zijlstra et al., 2003). Considerable evidence has shown that acupuncture analgesia may be imitated by stimulation of nerves, which, in turn, trigger endogenous opioid mechanisms. Recent functional magnetic resonance imaging studies also demonstrated that acupuncture has regionally specific, quantifiable effects on relevant structures of the human brain (Hsieh et al., 2001; Hui et al., 2000; Napadow et al., 2005; Pariente et al., 2005; Wu et al., 1999; Yoo et al., 2004). However, clinical research into the effects of acupuncture on chronic pain is challenged by methodological concerns, including finding appropriate inactive controls. For example, the larger literature on clinical trials of acupuncture on pain has failed to show a significant improvement over sham acupuncture (Brinkhaus et al., 2006; Linde et al., 2006; Melchart et al., 2005). Indeed, there are troublesome findings of non-superiority of acupuncture over shams.

To update the current clinical evidence regarding the effects of acupuncture on rheumatoid arthritis, a comprehensive search of 10 western and Chinese databases and reference lists was performed based on our previous work (Wang et al., 2008a). The review included clinical trials with pain as an endpoint being measured by tender joint count or a pain scale. The effects of acupuncture on morning stiffness, erythrocyte sedimentation rate and C-reactive protein were also reported. Nine studies met eligibility criteria with a total of 597 subjects. There were 4 placebo-controlled trials and 5 active-controlled trials (**Table 1**). The average study duration was 11 weeks. Mean (SD) numbers of acupuncture points and sessions were 11 (8) and 42 (62), respectively. The average duration of needle insertion was 24 minutes. Eight trials used traditional acupuncture (TA) (Cui et al., 2001; David et al.,

1999; Jiang & Fan, 2003; Liu et al., 2003; Tam et al., 2007; Wang, 2002; Zanette Sde et al., 2008; Zhou & Zhu, 2000), two used electroacupuncture, (EA) (Man & Baragar, 1974; Tam et al., 2007) and one used both (Tam et al., 2007). Four trials used placebo needles (sham acupuncture or incorrectly placed needles) as the control (David et al., 1999; Man & Baragar, 1974; Tam et al., 2007; Zanette Sde et al., 2008). The other five studies published in China used a variety of active interventions in the control groups, including methotrexate, topical Votalin ointment, and non-steroidal anti-inflammatory drugs.

2.1.1 Placebo-controlled trials

The four placebo-controlled trials involved 160 participants. Of those, two had optimal quality and two had moderate quality (David et al., 1999; Man & Baragar, 1974; Tam et al., 2007; Zanette Sde et al., 2008). Two high quality double-blind randomized, placebo-controlled trials and two moderate quality trials evaluated the effects of either traditional or electroacupuncture versus sham acupuncture. Tam et al (2007) conducted a trial in Hong Kong among 36 patients with RA and a disease duration of 9.3 years. Patients were randomly assigned to three groups: traditional acupuncture (TA), electroacupuncture (EA), and sham acupuncture (placebo needles). Patients received a total of 20 sessions for 10 weeks using six acupuncture points. The authors found that tender joint count improved for both EA and TA groups compared with the control group (tender joint count ↓5.5 vs. ↓0.5, $p<0.05$ and tender joint count ↓ 4 vs. ↓ 0.5, $p<0.05$, respectively). Physician's global score significantly improved for the EA group while patient's global score significantly improved for the TA group. Of note, the pain score remained unchanged in all three groups. The ACR core disease measures and DAS 28 score were not achieved at week 10.

In a contemporaneous high quality study conducted by Zanette Sde et al (2008), 40 patients with long-standing RA were randomized to traditional acupuncture or a control group using superficial acupuncture at non-acupuncture points. All participants received a total of 10 sessions, twice a week for five consecutive weeks. Tender joint count improved for the TA group compared with the control group (tender joint count ↓8.35 vs. ↓2.45, $p=0.145$). There was no significant difference between groups regarding ACR 20 improvement criteria (primary outcome) after the 5th and 10th sessions. At the last visit, there was a trend in favor of the acupuncture intervention compared with the control group (40% vs. 10% of each group achieved ACR20 criteria, $p=0.07$, respectively). In addition, there was a significant difference favoring the TA group on physician's global assessment of the treatment ($p=0.012$), and patient's ($p=0.003$) and physician's global assessment of disease activity ($p=0.011$), but there was no difference for other endpoints. The authors concluded that the negative result could be related to the small sample size, selection of patients, type of acupuncture protocol applied, and difficulties in establishing an appropriate control group.

A double-blind randomized placebo-controlled trial conducted by David et al (1999) used a six-week crossover design comparing traditional acupuncture with sham acupuncture in 64 patients. There was a total of five weekly sessions. After a washout period of six weeks, participants were crossed-over into the other intervention arm (acupuncture or control) for an additional five weeks. The tender joint count, swollen joints count, pain scale, patient's and physician's global assessments, modified DAS, ESR, and C-reactive protein were assessed at baseline and at the end of both intervention periods. The authors found no significant differences between the intervention and control groups for any of the endpoints at the end of both intervention periods and at the follow-up assessment.

An early RCT conducted by Man & Baragar (1974) used a parallel design among 20 participants with seropositive RA. Patients were randomly assigned to either electroacupuncture or control groups. The pain was assessed with a pain scale ranging from 0 to 4 at 24 hours after treatment. The authors reported that EA had a significant moderate and marked decrease in knee pain for 80% of the participants (60% and 20%, respectively) compared with no pain reduction in the control group. At three months, 70% of the participants in the EA group reported a significant minimal or moderate decrease in pain compared with no pain reduction in the control group. However, as no baseline data was reported, we estimated the following percentage improvements on the pain scale from the published figure (51% and 23%, at 24 hours and 3 months, respectively) for the EA group compared with no change in the control group (Man & Baragar, 1974).

2.1.2 Active-controlled trials

Since 2000, five active drug-controlled Chinese studies of modest quality have been conducted in China and include 468 subjects (Cui et al., 2001; Jiang & Fan, 2003; Liu et al., 2003; Wang, 2002; Zhou & Zhu, 2000). The mean study duration was 7 weeks, with 14 to 180 sessions. The number of acupuncture points varied from 8 to 24. In the control groups, two studies used indomethacin (25 mg tid for 4 weeks) (Jiang & Fan, 2003; Zhou & Zhu, 2000), one study used indomethacin (50 mg tid) plus triptolide (20 mg tid) for three weeks (Wang, 2002), one study used methotrexate (5 mg/week 1, 10 mg/week 2, 15 mg/week 3) and diclofenac (20 mg bid for 3 months) (Liu et al., 2003), and one study compared acupuncture with topical Votalin ointment (bid) (Cui et al., 2001), which may be considered as an NSAID. All five Chinese publications consistently reported that acupuncture treatment was associated with a significant decrease in pain (tender joint count mean change: -3.9) compared with controls. Three studies reported a significant reduction in morning stiffness (mean change: - 29 minutes) compared with controls (Jiang & Fan, 2003; Liu et al., 2003; Zhou & Zhu, 2000). In addition, three studies observed a reduction in ESR (mean change: -5.5 mm/hour) (Jiang & Fan, 2003; Liu et al., 2003; Zhou & Zhu, 2000) and 2 noted a C-reactive protein reduction (mean change: -3.0 mg/dl) (Jiang & Fan, 2003; Zhou & Zhu, 2000), but only one showed a significant difference for ESR and C-reactive protein (Jiang & Fan, 2003). No dropouts were reported. Although these trials concluded that acupuncture was effective in relieving symptoms of RA, the long-term benefits remain unknown.

2.1.3 Summary of clinical evidence

Collectively, seven studies reported a decrease in pain for acupuncture compared with controls, and five showed a statistically significant improvement (Cui et al., 2001; Jiang & Fan, 2003; Liu et al., 2003; Tam et al., 2007; Zhou & Zhu, 2000). Compared with controls, the mean or median changes of acupuncture-decreased tender joint count pain ranged from 1.5 to 6.5. In addition, four studies reported a significant reduction in morning stiffness (mean change -29 minutes) but the difference was non-significant compared with controls (Jiang & Fan, 2003; Liu et al., 2003; Zanette Sde et al., 2008; Zhou & Zhu, 2000). With regards to inflammatory markers, five studies observed a reduction in ESR (mean -3.9 mm/hour) (Jiang & Fan, 2003; Liu et al., 2003; Tam et al., 2007; Zanette Sde et al., 2008; Zhou & Zhu, 2000) and three noted a reduction in C-reactive protein (mean -2.9 mg/dl) (Jiang & Fan,

2003; Zanette Sde et al., 2008; Zhou & Zhu, 2000); but only 1 study showed a significant difference for both erythrocyte sedimentation rate and C-reactive protein (Jiang & Fan, 2003).

Three decades worth of cumulative literature on acupuncture for the treatment of RA have been evaluated in both Chinese and western populations. Despite some favorable results in one placebo-controlled and 5 active-controlled trials, conflicting evidence remains regarding the efficacy of acupuncture for RA in the placebo-controlled trials. While an early RCT reported that compared to sham, 1 EA session significantly improved knee pain in 20 patients with seropositive RA (Man & Baragar, 1974), a later randomized crossover study with 56 patients with RA reported no significant differences between traditional and sham acupuncture in pain relief or inflammation (David et al., 1999). A recent systematic review which utilized these two trials in their analysis concluded that the evidence was limited due to methodological considerations, such as the type of acupuncture (acupuncture vs. electroacupuncture), the site of intervention and the small sample size of the studies included (Casimiro et al., 2005).

All five active comparator trials published in China concluded that acupuncture treatment was associated with a significant decrease in tender joint count and was effective in relieving other symptoms of RA compared with controls. However, the methodological limitations of the Chinese studies included inappropriate control interventions (non-comparable), no double-blind interventions, inadequate description of the randomization process, and scarce use of validated outcome measures. The Chinese studies also used active drugs in place of placebo acupuncture, which makes comparisons across studies difficult.

Accurate quantitative estimates of treatment effects were not obtained due to the heterogeneity of the studies, as well as differences in acupuncture interventions, including dose/intensity and treatment duration. For instance, the number of acupuncture points ranged from 1 to 24, the duration of needle insertion ranged from 4 to 40 minutes, and the number of sessions varied from 1 to 180. The time elapsed between sessions also fluctuated.

For all these reasons, the evidence for the efficacy of acupuncture for pain relief in RA is modest and uncertain. Furthermore, the long-term benefits remain unknown. Because it is difficult to compare such divergent trials and there is a lack of standardized treatment protocols, future studies should focus on the optimum dose for acupuncture therapy in persons with RA, such as effective evidence-based dose/intensity , and number of acupuncture points, duration of needle insertion, frequency of acupuncture sessions, and intervention duration. It is possible that some studies, while designed correctly from a western scientific approach, do not have the correct Chinese medical approach (i.e. inappropriate dose/intensity and duration of acupuncture, insufficient expertise of acupuncturist leading to inappropriate needle insertion and manipulation techniques, or inappropriate acupuncture point selection by a standardized protocol that may neglect the individualized Chinese medical diagnosis). These reasons might explain why no specific effects were observed in western studies.

This comprehensive review of acupuncture for rheumatoid arthritis illustrates the need for methodologically rigorous acupuncture study designs that adhere to both the high standards of western scientific randomized controlled trials and accommodate the correct Chinese medical approach. Further research is needed to understand the effects of acupuncture on RA and how patients may or may not benefit from its inclusion in their treatment.

Ref.	RA Patients	Duration (weeks)	Acupuncture	Control*	Findings [a]
Placebo-controlled Randomized Controlled Trials					
Tam, 2007 Hong Kong	Active RA, mean disease duration 9.3 years N= 36 Age= 58	10	Group 1: EA Group 2: TA (20 sessions) Needle insertion time: 30 min	Sham acupuncture Placebo needles (20 sessions)	EA: ↓ 5.5 TA: ↓ 4 Control group: ↓ 0.5 Difference between groups at week 10: EA vs. control: ↓ 5.0 TA vs. control: ↓ 3.5
Zanette Sde, 2007 Brazil	RA for at least 6 months with stable drug treatment for at least 1 month N= 40 Age>50	9	TA (10 sessions) Needle insertion time: 20 min	Superficial acupuncture at non-acupuncture points (10 sessions)	TA: ↓ 8.35 Control group: ↓ 2.45 Difference between groups: ↓ 5.9
David, 1999 UK	RA, mean disease duration 10 years. N= 64 Age=18-75	22	TA (5 sessions) Needle insertion time: 4 min	Placebo needles (5 sessions)	Treatment effect: ↑ 0.5 (-1, 1.5)**
Man, 1974 Canada	Patients with seropositive RA for ≥ 5 years, for whom bilateral knee pain was a major problem N= 64 Age=18-75	16	EA (3 AP/ 1 session) Needle insertion time: 15 min	Placebo needles (1 session)	EA (24h): 51% improvement EA (3 months): 23% improvement Control group: 0% improvement in pain scale (0-4)
Randomized Controlled Trials Compared to Active Comparators					
Liu, 2003 China	RA with mean disease duration 3.6 years. N= 240 Age=42	12	TA (180 sessions) Needle insertion time: 30 min	Methotrexate IM injection - week 1: 5 mg - week 2: 10 mg - week 3: 15 mg + Diclofenac (20 mg/day)	TA: ↓ 16.6 Control group: ↓ 10.1 Difference between groups: ↓ 6.5
Jiang, 2003 China	Functional class 1 and 2 patients with RA with	4	TA (15 sessions)	Indomethacin (25 mg tid)	TA: ↓ 5.1 Control group: + 0.6

	mean disease duration 4.5 years. N= 60 Age=45		Needle insertion time: 30 min		Difference between groups: ↓ 4.5
Wang, 2002 China	RA with mean disease duration 10 years. N= 61 Age=ND	3	TA (14 sessions) Needle insertion time: 30 min	Indomethacin (50 mg tid) plus triptolide (20 mg tid)	Significant improvement of total effective rate
Cui, 2001 China	RA (1987 ACR criteria and no data for disease duration. N= 60 Age=ND	12	TA (90 sessions) Needle insertion time: 20-30min	Votalin ointment (bid)[b]	TA: ↓ 8.3 Control group: ↓ 6.8 Difference between groups: ↓ 1.5
Zhou, 2000 China	Functional class 1 and 2 patients with RA, with mean disease duration 3 years N= 45 Age=18-65	4	TA (15 sessions) Needle insertion time: 40 min	Indomethacin (25 mg tid)	TA: ↓ 7.1 Control group: 4.0 Difference between groups: ↓ 3.1

Abbreviations: EA= electro acupuncture; TA= traditional acupuncture; ND= No data; RA=Rheumatoid arthritis;
[a]Mean or median difference or improvement was calculated between groups and confidence interval cannot be calculated from published data. [b]Votalin ointment components not reported.*Sham acupuncture: needles inserted up to 2 mm, shorter insertion duration, and minimal needle stimulation. **Median difference.

Table 1. Randomized Controlled Trials Evaluating the Effect of Acupuncture on RA

3. Mind-body therapy for rheumatoid arthritis

3.1 Tai Chi mind-body therapeutics

In the past two decades, the literature has consistently recognized the potential therapeutic benefits of Tai Chi mind-body exercise. Significant improvements have been reported in balance, strength, flexibility, cardiovascular and respiratory function, mood, depression and anxiety, self-efficacy, pain reduction and health-related quality of life in diverse eastern and western populations for a variety of chronic conditions (Wang et al., 2004). Several recent reviews have further suggested that Tai Chi appears to improve a variety of medical conditions (Adler & Roberts, 2006; Jahnke et al., 2010; Rogers et al., 2009; Wang et al., 2010a; Yeh et al., 2009).

Tai Chi, a traditional Chinese mind-body exercise, has grown in popularity in the United States. According to the 2007 National Health Interview Survey, around 2.5 million

Americans have practiced Tai Chi for health reasons and that number is increasing (Barnes et al., 2009). Furthermore, individuals with musculoskeletal conditions are more likely to practice Tai Chi (Birdee et al., 2009). It is clear that our patients with rheumatic disease are interested in seeking this type of complementary and alternative treatment. Thus, it is important to examine the evidence base for mind-body medicine to provide the clinician with an overview of these new sources of knowledge for the best care for our rheumatic patients.

3.2 Scientific evaluation of Tai Chi for rheumatoid arthritis

One early publication by Kirsteins and colleagues reported on two non-randomized controlled trials of 47 and 28 rheumatoid arthritis patients with 10 weeks Tai Chi training. Disease activity (joint tenderness, number of swollen joints), 50 foot walks, handgrip strength, a written functional assessment, and exacerbation of joint symptoms were measured. The studies showed that Tai Chi appears to be safe for rheumatoid arthritis patients and may serve as a suitable weight-bearing exercise with the additional potential advantages of stimulating bone growth and strengthening connective tissue (Kirsteins et al., 1991).

Two randomized controlled trials were recently published in Korea. A study of 31 patients reported by Lee showed that compared with a usual care group, 6 weeks of Tai Chi training significantly improved mood and sleep disturbance (Lee, 2005). Another trial of 61 patients showed that 50 minutes per week of Tai Chi training for 12 weeks significantly decreased pain and fatigue compared to usual care controls (Lee & Jeong, 2006).

To obtain preliminary data on the effects of Tai Chi on rheumatoid arthritis, the author's research group conducted a pilot randomized controlled trial (Wang, 2008b). Twenty patients with functional Class I or II rheumatoid arthritis were randomly assigned to Tai Chi or attention control in twice-weekly sessions for 12 weeks. The American College Rheumatology 20 response criteria, functional capacity, health-related quality of life and the depression index were assessed. At 12 weeks, 5/10 patients (50%) randomized to Tai Chi achieved an American College Rheumatology 20% response compared with 0/10 (0%) in the control ($p= 0.03$). Tai Chi had greater improvement in the Disability Index ($p = 0.01$), Vitality subscale of the SF-36 ($p = 0.01$) and the Depression Index ($p = 0.003$). Similar trends to improvement were also observed for disease activity, functional capacity and health related quality of life. No adverse events were observed and no patients withdrew from the study, suggesting that Tai Chi is safe and may be beneficial for Functional Class I or II rheumatoid arthritis.

A subsequent study of Tai Chi in rheumatoid arthritis patients by Uhlig and colleagues, however, has produced inconsistent results. A with-in group comparison study involving 15 female patients with rheumatoid arthritis aged 40-70 years, participating in 8-week Tai Chi training showed no improvements in disease activity, muscle strength, flexibility, balance and health status (Uhlig et al., 2005). The second study from the same group of investigators overcame the previous limitations, using a 12-week Tai Chi program for another 15 patients. They found that Tai Chi improved lower-limb muscle function and endurance at 12 weeks follow-up (Uhlig et al., 2010). A Cochrane review, examining the evidence from 4 clinical trials, suggested that Tai Chi does not exacerbate symptoms of rheumatoid arthritis and has some benefits on lower extremity range of motion for people with rheumatoid arthritis, in particular ankle range of motion (Han et al., 2004).

Chronic pain in rheumatoid arthritis is commonly accompanied by psychosocial stress, anxiety and depression. Therapeutic approaches with psychological and behavioral impact, such as Tai Chi mind-body therapy, could better patients' emotional health outcomes (Bradley & Alberts, 1999).

The author's group systematically reviewed the evidence of the effects of Tai Chi on stress, anxiety, depression and mood disturbance in various eastern and western populations (Wang et al., 2010a). Specifically, the results of 33 randomized and nonrandomized trials suggest that regular Tai Chi practice is significantly associated with improvements in psychological well-being including reduced stress (effect size, 0.66; 95% confidence interval [CI], 0.23 to 1.09), anxiety (effect size, 0.66; 95% CI, 0.29 to 1.03), depression (effect size, 0.56; 95% CI, 0.31 to 0.80), and mood disturbance (effect size, 0.45; 95% CI, 0.20 to 0.69) in healthy participants and patients with chronic conditions. Seven observational studies with relatively large sample sizes reinforced the beneficial association between Tai Chi practice and psychological health. Notably, the review found that Tai Chi tended to reduce depression compared to various controls among individuals with osteoarthritis (Fransen et al., 2007; Wang et al., 2009), rheumatoid arthritis (Wang, 2008b) fibromyalgia (Taggart et al., 2003; Wang et al., 2010b), depression disorders (Chou et al., 2004), sedentary obese women (Dechamps et al., 2009), and elderly participants with cardiovascular disease risk factors (Taylor-Piliae et al., 2006). This positive result was associated with improvement in symptoms and physical function in patients with rheumatoid arthritis and other chronic conditions. Interestingly, the benefits were also associated with an improvement in the immune respons. A 50% improvement in varicella zoster virus-specific cell-mediated immunity (T cell-dependent response) after 15 and 25 weeks of Tai Chi in healthy elderly Americans (Irwin et al., 2003; Irwin et al., 2007) was observed.

However, the vast majority of the studies suffer from less rigorous designs with only two studies reporting results on participants diagnosed with clinical depression. Nevertheless, the potential mental health benefits of Tai Chi mind-body therapy support its inclusion as a key component of a multidisciplinary medical approach to promote psychological health, treat chronic pain, and better inform clinical decision-making for rheumatoid arthritis.

As a chronic disorder characterized by inflammation leading to joint destruction, rheumatoid arthritis has increased clinically important comorbidities including cardiovascular complications and osteoporosis. Numerous studies have evaluated the effects of Tai Chi on cardiovascular and respiratory function (Lai et al., 1993; Lai et al., 1995; Lan et al., 1996; Lan et al., 1998; Lan et al., 1999). Since 1979, results related to the effect of Tai Chi on cardiovascular and pulmonary function have been reported in 43 eastern and western publications (Wang et al., 2004; Yeh et al., 2008; Yeh et al., 2009). Among them, one study (Zhuo et al., 1984) reported that the metabolic intensity of the activity seems insufficient to generate improvements of cardiorespiratory fitness in healthy young adults. Yet, all other studies suggested that regular Tai Chi practice may preserve cardiorespiratory function in older individuals and may be prescribed as a suitable exercise for older adults. Our systematic reviews of literature have shown that Tai Chi can reduce blood pressure and increase cardiovascular exercise capacity (Yeh et al., 2008; Yeh et al., 2009). A very recent large single-blind, multisite, randomized controlled trial evaluated a 12 week Tai Chi exercise in patients with heart failure (Yeh et al., 2011). At completion of the study, patients in the Tai Chi group had greater improvements in quality of life ($P=0.02$), exercise self-efficacy ($P<0.001$) and mood ($P=0.01$). The authors concluded that Tai Chi exercise, a multi-component mind-body training modality that is safe and has good rates of adherence, may provide value in improving daily exercise, quality of life, mood, and exercise self-efficacy in patients with chronic heart failure. Thus, encouraging evidence suggests that Tai Chi may be a safe and beneficial adjunctive therapy to conventional care for patients with rheumatoid arthritis-associated cardiovascular disease and related complications.

Taken together, these trials show that Tai Chi may provide some important components in the treatment of Rheumatoid Arthritis. Further research should focus on ideal dose and duration of intervention to provide valuable information about how Tai Chi may be best used in clinical practice.

4. Benefit of tripterygium wilffordii hook F in patients with rheumatoid arthritis

4.1 Tripterygium wilffordii hook F therapeutics

In traditional Chinese medicine, extracts of the roots of Tripterygium Wilffordii Hook F (TwHF, *Lei Gong Teng*) has been widely used for the treatment of autoimmune and inflammatory disease in China. Several clinical trials have examined the therapeutic effects of TwHF in patients with rheumatoid arthritis (Cibere et al., 2003; Goldbach-Mansky et al., 2009; Tao et al., 2001; Tao et al., 2002; Vitetta et al., 2008). In an early nonrandomized controlled clinical trial, Tao and colleagues evaluated 13 patients with established rheumatoid arthritis who received a maximum dosage of 180 mg/day of TwHF. There were no adverse effects or disease improvements observed at that dosage and nine patients tolerated the extract up to a dosage of 570 mg/day. Eight of the nine patients who received the extract at doses over 360 mg/day experienced improvement in both clinical manifestations and laboratory findings and one patient met American College of Rheumatology criteria for remission (Tao et al., 2001). The results of this small trial suggested that the ethyl acetate extract of the Chinese herbal remedy was safe with tolerable side effects for most patients with rheumatoid arthritis who achieved clinical benefits. Subsequently, the same group of investigators used a prospective, double-blind, placebo-controlled trial for another 35 patients and found that eight patients in the 20-week low-dose (180 mg/day) group and four patients in the high-dose (360 mg/day) group met criteria for clinical response. The authors also concluded that the ethanol/ethyl acetate extract of TwHF, at a dosage of 360 mg/day, appeared to be safe in patients with rheumatoid arthritis (Tao et al., 2002). Another Chinese randomized double-blind placebo-controlled trial of 61 patients with rheumatoid arthritis suggested that six weeks of TwHF significantly improves American College of Rheumatology 20% response rate compared with placebo (TwHF 58% vs placebo 20%; P=0.002) (Cibere et al., 2003).

Recently, to compare the benefits and side effects of TwHF extract with those of sulfasalazine, a large randomized, controlled trial of 121 patients with active rheumatoid arthritis used TwHF extract 60mg, three times daily or sulfasalazine 1g, twice daily. Patients could continue stable doses of oral prednisone and non-steroidal anti-inflammatory drugs but not disease-modifying antirheumatic drugs. Among patients who continued treatment for 24 weeks, achievement of 20% improvement in American College of Rheumatology criteria was greater with TwHF than with sulfasalazine. Adverse event rates were similar. Also, patients receiving TwHF had significantly higher response rates for American College of Rheumatology 50% and American College of Rheumatology 70% criteria. In the TwHF group, significant improvement was demonstrated in all individual components of the American College of Rheumatology response, including the Health Assessment Questionnaire score. Interleukin-6 levels rapidly and significantly decreased in the TwHF group (Goldbach-Mansky et al., 2009).

The long-term effects and toxicities of TwHF and the potential combination of TwHF with other antirheumatic therapies need to be further investigated. However, evidence demonstrates that treatment with a standardized extract from the peeled roots of the

Chinese herbal remedy TwHF administered from four weeks to over 24 weeks may be both effective and safe in treating patients with active rheumatoid arthritis.

5. Tibetan Five Nectar Formula medicated bath therapy for pain relief in patients with RA

Tibetan Five Nectar Formula is derived from five types of plants and has been considered to have anti-inflammatory and immunomodulating effects for rheumatoid arthritis when used as bath therapy. To understand the beneficial effect of Tibetan Five Nectar Formula Medicated-Bath Therapy on patients with rheumatoid arthritis, the author's research group has recently conducted a comprehensive review of the literature of Tibetan Five Nectar Formula Medicated-Bath Therapy on patients with rheumatoid arthritis (Jacobson et al., 2010).

Eighty-seven potentially relevant studies were identified. Nine non-randomized controlled trials of 757 subjects met eligibility criteria (Jacobson et al., 2010). All the trials were conducted in the Tibetan area of China and used the Five Nectar formula in the Tibetan Medicated-Bath. Bath temperatures were of 35-46 ^{0}C for 10-15 min, once or twice a day. Mean treatment duration ranged from 7-30 days per course, for 1-3 courses. Two studies stopped some or all western medications during treatment. The 9 studies also used supplemental oral Tibetan herbal therapy. The effect of the Tibetan Five Nectar Formula Medicated-Bath Therapy on clinical symptoms was measured with Physician-assessed composite outcomes. All studies reported a positive association between the Tibetan Five Nectar Formula Medicated-Bath Therapy and improved clinical pain symptoms within group comparisons. In addition, three studies reported an improvement in immune function. There are discordant trial designs and lack of reported qualitative outcomes measure were among other methodological limitations. The overall study quality was poor with no controls or randomization, blinding or reports of dropout rates. However, these studies suggest that Tibetan Five Nectar Formula Medicated-Bath Therapy may be helpful in the treatment of pain symptoms due to rheumatoid arthritis. However, they are of only weak evidentiary value due to uniformly poor methodological quality. Future studies with more rigorous design and adequate statistical analysis are warranted.

6. Conclusion

In summary, as a complex immunologically mediated disorder, rheumatoid arthritis is still a therapeutically challenging chronic condition to control. Emerging evidence from clinical trials reviewed here support that evidence-based complementary and alternative medicine or integrative medicine therapies may offer effective treatments for patients with Rheumatoid Arthritis. Integrative approaches combine the best of conventional medicine and the wisdom of complementary and alternative medical approaches. These modalities may lead to the development of better lifestyle modifying strategies, while mind-body medicine such as Tai Chi exercise could affect progression of disease and decrease morbidity and mortality among individuals with rheumatoid arthritis. While existing evidence regarding complementary and alternative medicine on rheumatoid arthritis remains limited and inconclusive, the promising results suggest that these complementary and alternative medicine treatments may be a safe adjunctive therapy for rheumatoid arthritis and warrant further exploration.

7. References

Adler, P.A. & Roberts, B.L. (2006). The use of Tai Chi to improve health in older adults. *Orthopaedic Nursing*, 25, 2, 122-6.

Barnes, P.M., Bloom, B. & Nahin, R.L. (2009). Complementary and alternative medicine use among adults and children: United States, 2007. *National Health Status Report*, 1-23.

Birdee, G.S., Wayne, P.M., Davis, R.B., Phillips, R.S. & Yeh, G.Y. (2009). T'ai chi and qigong for health: patterns of use in the United States. *Journal of Alternative and Complementary Medicine*, 15, 9, 969-73.

Bradley, L.A. & Alberts, K.R. (1999). Psychological and behavioral approaches to pain management for patients with rheumatic disease. *Rheumatic Disease Clinics of North America*, 25, 1, 215-32, viii.

Brinkhaus, B., Witt, C.M., Jena, S., Linde, K., Streng, A., Wagenpfeil, S., Irnich, D., Walther, H.U., Melchart, D. & Willich, S.N. (2006). Acupuncture in patients with chronic low back pain: a randomized controlled trial. *Archives of Internal Medicine*, 166, 4, 450-7.

Casimiro, L., Barnsley, L., Brosseau, L., Milne, S., Robinson, V.A., Tugwell, P. & Wells, G. (2005). Acupuncture and electroacupuncture for the treatment of rheumatoid arthritis. *Cochrane Database of Systematic Reviews*, 4, CD003788.

Cho, Z.H., Chung, S.C., Jones, J.P., Park, J.B., Park, H.J., Lee, H.J., Wong, E.K. & Min, B.I. (1998). New findings of the correlation between acupoints and corresponding brain cortices using functional MRI. *Proceedings of the National Academy of Sciences of the United States of America*, 95, 5, 2670-3.

Chou, K.L., Lee, P.W., Yu, E.C., Macfarlane, D., Cheng, Y.H., Chan, S.S. & Chi, I. (2004). Effect of Tai Chi on depressive symptoms amongst Chinese older patients with depressive disorders: a randomized clinical trial. *International Journal of Geriatric Psychiatry*, 19, 11, 1105-7.

Cibere, J., Deng, Z., Lin, Y., Ou, R., He, Y., Wang, Z., Thorne, A., Lehman, A.J., Tsang, I.K. & Esdaile, J.M. (2003). A randomized double blind, placebo controlled trial of topical Tripterygium wilfordii in rheumatoid arthritis: reanalysis using logistic regression analysis. *Journal of Rheumatology*, 30, 3, 465-7.

Cui, L., Guo, R. & Gen, W. (2001). The effect of acupuncture on reducing the pain of patients with rheumatoid arthritis. *Analysis of Acupuncture*, 3, 185-6.

Darras, J.-C., Vernejoul, P. & Albararede, P. (1992). Nuclear medicine and acupuncture: A study on the migration of radioactive tracers after injection at acupoints. *American Journal of Acupuncture*, 20, 245-256.

David, J., Townsend, S:, Sathanathan, R., Kriss, S. & Dore, C.J. (1999). The effect of acupuncture on patients with rheumatoid arthritis: a randomized, placebo-controlled cross-over study. *Rheumatology (Oxford)*, 38, 9, 864-9.

Dechamps, A., Gatta, B., Bourdel-Marchasson, I., Tabarin, A. & Roger, P. (2009). Pilot study of a 10-week multidisciplinary Tai Chi intervention in sedentary obese women. *Clinical Journal of Sports Medicine*, 19, 1, 49-53.

Dhond, R.P., Yeh, C., Park, K., Kettner, N. & Napadow, V. (2008). Acupuncture modulates resting state connectivity in default and sensorimotor brain networks. *Pain*, 136, 3, 407-18.

Fransen, M., Nairn, L., Winstanley, J., Lam, P. & Edmonds, J. (2007). Physical activity for osteoarthritis management: a randomized controlled clinical trial evaluating hydrotherapy or Tai Chi classes. *Arthritis & Rheumatism*, 57, 3, 407-14.

Gao, M., Wang, M., Li, K. & He, L. (1997). Changes of mu opiod receptor binding sites in rat brain following electoacupuncture. *Acupuncture & Electrotherapies Research*, 22, 161-6.

Goldbach-Mansky, R., Wilson, M., Fleischmann, R., Olsen, N., Silverfield, J., Kempf, P., Kivitz, A., Sherrer, Y., Pucino, F., Csako, G., Costello, R., Pham, T.H., Snyder, C., van der Heijde, D., Tao, X., Wesley, R. & Lipsky, P.E. (2009). Comparison of Tripterygium wilfordii Hook F versus sulfasalazine in the treatment of rheumatoid arthritis: a randomized trial. *Annals of Internal Medicine*, 151, 4, 229-40, W49-51.

Han, A., Robinson, V., Judd, M., Taixiang, W., Wells, G. & Tugwell, P. (2004). Tai chi for treating rheumatoid arthritis. *Cochrane Database of Systematic Reviews*, 3, CD004849.

Han, J. (1997). Physiology of acupuncture: review of thirty years of research. *Journal of Alternative and Complementary Medicine*, (Suppl 1), S101-8.

Han, J.S. & Terenius, L. (1982). Neurochemical basis of acupuncture analgesia. *Annual Review of Pharmacology and Toxicology*, 22, 193-220.

Han, J.S., Ding, X.Z. & Fan, S.G. (1986). Cholecystokinin octapeptide (CCK-8): antagonism to electroacupuncture analgesia and a possible role in electroacupuncture tolerance. *Pain*, 27, 1, 101-15.

Han, J.S. (2004). Acupuncture and endorphins. *Neuroscience Letters*, 361, 1-3, 258-61. Harris, R.E., Zubieta, J.K., Scott, D.J., Napadow, V., Gracely, R.H. & Clauw, D.J. (2009).

Traditional Chinese acupuncture and placebo (sham) acupuncture are differentiated by their effects on mu-opioid receptors (MORs). *Neuroimage*, 47, 3, 1077-85.

Hsieh, J.C., Tu, C.H., Chen, F.P., Chen, M.C., Yeh, T.C., Cheng, H.C., Wu, Y.T., Liu, R.S. & Ho, L.T. (2001). Activation of the hypothalamus characterizes the acupuncture stimulation at the analgesic point in human: a positron emission tomography study. *Neuroscience Letters*, 307, 2, 105-8.

Hui, K.K., Liu, J., Makris, N., Gollub, R.L., Chen, A.J., Moore, C.I., Kennedy, D.N., Rosen, B.R. & Kwong, K.K. (2000). Acupuncture modulates the limbic system and subcortical gray structures of the human brain: evidence from fMRI studies in normal subjects. *Human Brain Mapping*, 9, 1, 13-25.

Hui, K.K., Liu, J., Marina, O., Napadow, V., Haselgrove, C., Kwong, K.K., Kennedy, D.N. & Makris, N. (2005). The integrated response of the human cerebro-cerebellar and limbic systems to acupuncture stimulation at ST 36 as evidenced by fMRI. *Neuroimage*, 27, 3, 479-96.

Irwin, M.R., Pike, J.L., Cole, J.C. & Oxman, M.N. (2003). Effects of a behavioral intervention, Tai Chi Chih, on varicella-zoster virus specific immunity and health functioning in older adults. *Psychosomatic Medicine*, 65, 5, 824-30.

Irwin, M.R., Olmstead, R. & Oxman, M.N. (2007). Augmenting immune responses to varicella zoster virus in older adults: a randomized, controlled trial of Tai Chi. *Journal of the American Geriatrics Society*, 55, 4, 511-7.

Jacobson, E., Yangga, T., McAlindon, T. & Wang, C. (2010) Effect of Tibetan Medicated-Beth Therapy on Rheumatoid Arthritis: A Systematic Review, *Proceedings of The 2010 International Congress on Complementary Medicine Research*, Norway, 2010, the Online Supplement

Jahnke, R., Larkey, L., Rogers, C., Etnier, J. & Lin, F. (2010). A comprehensive review of health benefits of qigong and tai chi. *American Journal of Health Promotion*, 24, 6, e1-e25.

Jiang, S. & Fan, F. (2003). Clinical observation on 40 cases of atrophic arthritis treated by acupuncture and moxibustion. *Hunan Guiding Journal of Traditional Chinese Medicine and Pharmacology*, 9, 41-2.

Kaptchuk, T.J. (2002). Acupuncture: theory, efficacy, and practice. *Annals of Internal Medicine*, 136, 5, 374-83.

Kirsteins, A.E., Dietz, F. & Hwang, S.M. (1991). Evaluating the safety and potential use of a weight-bearing exercise, Tai-Chi Chuan, for rheumatoid arthritis patients. *American Journal of Physical Medicine & Rehabilitation*, 70, 3, 136-41.

Kovacs, F.M., Gotzens, V., Garcia, A., Garcia, F., Mufraggi, N., Prandi, D., Setoain, J. & San Roman, F. (1992). Experimental study on radioactive pathways of hypodermically injected technetium-99m. *Journal of Nuclear Medicine*, 33, 3, 403-7.

Lai, J.S., Wong, M.K., Lan, C., Chong, C.K. & Lien, I.N. (1993). Cardiorespiratory responses of Tai Chi Chuan practitioners and sedentary subjects during cycle ergometry. *Journal of the Formosan Medical Association*, 92, 10, 894-9.

Lai, J.S., Lan, C., Wong, M.K. & Teng, S.H. (1995). Two-year trends in cardiorespiratory function among older Tai Chi Chuan practitioners and sedentary subjects. *Journal of the American Geriatrics Society*, 43, 11, 1222-7.

Lan, C., Lai, J.S., Wong, M.K. & Yu, M.L. (1996). Cardiorespiratory function, flexibility, and body composition among geriatric Tai Chi Chuan practitioners. *Archives of Physical Medicine and Rehabilitation*, 77, 6, 612-6.

Lan, C., Lai, J.S., Wong, M.K. & Yu, M.L. (1998). 12-month Tai Chi training in the elderly: its effect on health fitness. *Medicine and Science in Sports and Exercise*, 30, 3, 345-51.

Lan, C., Chen, S.Y., Lai, J.S. & Wong, M.K. (1999). The effect of Tai Chi on cardiorespiratory function in patients with coronary artery bypass surgery. *Medicine and Science in Sports and Exercise*, 31, 5, 634-8.

Langevin, H.M., Churchill, D.L. & Cipolla, M.J. (2001a). Mechanical signaling through connective tissue: a mechanism for the therapeutic effect of acupuncture. *The FASEB Journal*, 15, 12, 2275-82.

Langevin, H.M., Churchill, D.L., Fox, J.R., Badger, G.J., Garra, B.S. & Krag, M.H. (2001b). Biomechanical response to acupuncture needling in humans. *Journal of Applied Physiology*, 91, 6, 2471-8.

Langevin, H.M., Bouffard, N.A., Churchill, D.L. & Badger, G.J. (2007). Connective tissue fibroblast response to acupuncture: dose-dependent effect of bidirectional needle rotation. *Journal of Alternative and Complementary Medicine*, 13, 3, 355-60.

Lee, E.O. (2005). Effects of a Tai-Chi Program on Pain, Sleep Disturbance, Mood and Fatigue in Rheumatoid Arthritis Patients. *Journal of Muscle and Joint Health*, 12, 1, 57-68.

Lee, K.Y. & Jeong, O.Y. (2006). The effect of Tai Chi movement in patients with rheumatoid arthritis. *Taehan Kanho Hakhoe Chi*, 36, 2, 278-85.

Lee, M.S., Shin, B.C. & Ernst, E. (2008). Acupuncture for rheumatoid arthritis: a systematic review. *Rheumatology (Oxford)*, 47, 12, 1747-53.

Li, A., Zhang, R.X., Wang, Y., Zhang, H., Ren, K., Berman, B.M., Tan, M. & Lao, L. (2007). Corticosterone mediates electroacupuncture-produced anti-edema in a rat model of inflammation. *BMC Complementary and Alternative Medicine*, 7, 27.

Linde, K., Streng, A., Hoppe, A., Brinkhaus, B., Witt, C.M., Hammes, M., Irnich, D., Hummelsberger, J., Willich, S.N. & Melchart, D. (2006). Treatment in a randomized multicenter trial of acupuncture for migraine (ART migraine). *Forschende Komplementarmedizin*, 13, 2, 101-8.

Liu, W., Liu, B., Wang, Y., Zhang, L. & Shi, X. (2003). Observation on the therapeutic effect of acupuncture and moxibustion in 120 cased of rheumatoid arthritis. *Chinese Acupuncture & Moxibustion*, 23, 577-8.

Man, S. & Baragar, F. (1974). Preliminary clinical study of acupuncture in rheumatoid arthritis. *Journal of Rheumatology*, 1, 1, 126-9.

Melchart, D., Streng, A., Hoppe, A., Brinkhaus, B., Witt, C., Wagenpfeil, S., Pfaffenrath, V., Hammes, M., Hummelsberger, J., Irnich, D., Weidenhammer, W., Willich, S.N. &

Linde, K. (2005). Acupuncture in patients with tension-type headache: randomised controlled trial. *British Medical Journal*, 331, 7513, 376-82.

Napadow, V., Makris, N., Liu, J., Kettner, N.W., Kwong, K.K. & Hui, K.K. (2005). Effects of electroacupuncture versus manual acupuncture on the human brain as measured by fMRI. *Human Brain Mapping*, 24, 3, 193-205.

Napadow, V., Liu, J., Li, M., Kettner, N., Ryan, A., Kwong, K.K., Hui, K.K. & Audette, J.F. (2007). Somatosensory cortical plasticity in carpal tunnel syndrome treated by acupuncture. *Human Brain Mapping*, 28, 3, 159-71.

Napadow, V., Ahn, A., Longhurst, J., Lao, L., Stener-Victorin, E., Harris, R. & Langevin, H.M. (2008). The status and future of acupuncture mechanism research. *Journal of Alternative and Complementary Medicine*, 14, 7, 861-9.

Pariente, J., White, P., Frackowiak, R.S. & Lewith, G. (2005). Expectancy and belief modulate the neuronal substrates of pain treated by acupuncture. *Neuroimage*, 25, 4, 1161-7.

Rogers, C.E., Larkey, L.K. & Keller, C. (2009). A review of clinical trials of tai chi and qigong in older adults. *Western Journal of Nursing Research*, 31, 2, 245-79.

Suzuki, S., Tian, W. & Li, X.W. (2005). Advances of clinical studies of acupuncture and moxibustion for treatment of rheumatoid arthritis. *Zhongguo Zhen Jiu*, 25, 2, 147-50.

Taggart, H.M., Arslanian, C.L., Bae, S. & Singh, K. (2003). Effects of T'ai Chi exercise on fibromyalgia symptoms and health-related quality of life. *Orthopaedic Nursing*, 22, 5, 353-60.

Tam, L.S., Leung, P.C., Li, T.K., Zhang, L. & Li, E.K. (2007). Acupuncture in the treatment of rheumatoid arthritis: a double-blind controlled pilot study. *BMC Complementary and Alternative Medicine*, 7, 35.

Tao, X., Cush, J.J., Garret, M. & Lipsky, P.E. (2001). A phase I study of ethyl acetate extract of the chinese antirheumatic herb Tripterygium wilfordii hook F in rheumatoid arthritis. *Journal of Rheumatology*, 28, 10, 2160-7.

Tao, X., Younger, J., Fan, F.Z., Wang, B. & Lipsky, P.E. (2002). Benefit of an extract of Tripterygium Wilfordii Hook F in patients with rheumatoid arthritis: a double-blind, placebo-controlled study. *Arthritis & Rheumatism*, 46, 7, 1735-43.

Taylor-Piliae, R.E., Haskell, W.L., Waters, C.M. & Froelicher, E.S. (2006). Change in perceived psychosocial status following a 12-week Tai Chi exercise programme. *Journal of Advanced Nursing*, 54, 3, 313-29.

Uhlig, T., Larsson, C., Hjorth, A.G., Odegard, S. & Kvien, T.K. (2005). No improvement in a pilot study of tai chi exercise in rheumatoid arthritis. *Annals of the Rheumatic Diseases*, 64, 3, 507-9.

Uhlig, T., Fongen, C., Steen, E., Christie, A. & Odegard, S. (2010). Exploring Tai Chi in rheumatoid arthritis: a quantitative and qualitative study. *BMC Musculoskeletal Disorders*, 11, 43.

Vitetta, L., Cicuttini, F. & Sali, A. (2008). Alternative therapies for musculoskeletal conditions. *Best Practice & Research Clinical Rheumatology*, 22, 3, 499-522.

Wang, C., Collet, J.P. & Lau, J. (2004). The effect of Tai Chi on health outcomes in patients with chronic conditions: a systematic review. *Archives of Internal Medicine*, 164, 5, 493-501.

Wang, C., de Pablo, P., Chen, X., Schmid, C. & McAlindon, T. (2008a). Acupuncture for pain relief in patients with rheumatoid arthritis: a systematic review. *Arthritis & Rheumatism*, 59, 9, 1249-56.

Wang, C. (2008b). Tai Chi improves pain and functional status in adults with rheumatoid arthritis: results of a pilot single-blinded randomized controlled trial. *Medicine and Sport Science*, 52, 218-29.

Wang, C., Schmid, C.H., Hibberd, P.L., Kalish, R., Roubenoff, R., Rones, R. & McAlindon, T. (2009). Tai Chi is effective in treating knee osteoarthritis: a randomized controlled trial. *Arthritis & Rheumatism*, 61, 11, 1545-53.

Wang, C., Bannuru, R., Ramel, J., Kupelnick, B., Scott, T. & Schmid, C.H. (2010a). Tai Chi on psychological well-being: systematic review and meta-analysis. *BMC Complementary and Alternative Medicine*, 10, 23.

Wang, C., Schmid, C., Rones, R., Kalish, R., Yinh, J., Goldenberg, D., Lee, Y. & McAlindon, T. (2010b). A randomized trial of Tai Chi for fibromyalgia. *New England Journal of Medicine*, 363, 743-54.

Wang, K.M., Yao, S.M., Xian, Y.L. & Hou, Z.L. (1985). A study on the receptive field of acupoints and the relationship between characteristics of needling sensation and groups of afferent fibres. *Scientia Sinica Series B*, 28, 9, 963-71.

Wang, Y. (2002). Combined acupuncture and west medication treating 109 cases of rheumatoid arthritis. *Hunan Guiding Journal of Traditional Chinese Medicine and Pharmacology*, 8, 769-70.

Wu, M.T., Hsieh, J.C., Xiong, J., Yang, C.F., Pan, H.B., Chen, Y.C., Tsai, G., Rosen, B.R. & Kwong, K.K. (1999). Central nervous pathway for acupuncture stimulation: localization of processing with functional MR imaging of the brain--preliminary experience. *Radiology*, 212, 1, 133-41.

Yeh, G.Y., Wang, C., Wayne, P.M. & Phillips, R.S. (2008). The effect of tai chi exercise on blood pressure: a systematic review. *Preventative Cardiology*, 11, 2, 82-9.

Yeh, G.Y., Wang, C., Wayne, P.M. & Phillips, R. (2009). Tai chi exercise for patients with cardiovascular conditions and risk factors: A SYSTEMATIC REVIEW. *Journal of Cardiopulmonary Rehabilitation and Prevention*, 29, 3, 152-60.

Yeh, G.Y., McCarthy, E.P., Wayne, P.M., Stevenson, L.W., Wood, M.J., Forman, D., Davis, R.B. & Phillips, R.S. (2011). Tai chi exercise in patients with chronic heart failure: a randomized clinical trial. *Archives of Internal Medicine*, 171, 8, 750-7.

Yoo, S.S., Teh, E.K., Blinder, R.A. & Jolesz, F.A. (2004). Modulation of cerebellar activities by acupuncture stimulation: evidence from fMRI study. *Neuroimage*, 22, 2, 932-40.

Zanette Sde, A., Born, I.G., Brenol, J.C. & Xavier, R.M. (2008). A pilot study of acupuncture as adjunctive treatment of rheumatoid arthritis. *Clinical Rheumatology*, 27, 5, 627-35.

Zhang, R.X., Lao, L., Wang, X., Fan, A., Wang, L., Ren, K. & Berman, B.M. (2005). Electroacupuncture attenuates inflammation in a rat model. *Journal of Alternative and Complementary Medicine*, 11, 1, 135-42.

Zhou, J. & Zhu, Q. (2000). Effects of acupuncture on the rheumatoid arthritis. *Chinese Journal of Rheumatology*, 4, 3, 169-171.

Zhuo, D., Shephard, R.J., Plyley, M.J. & Davis, G.M. (1984). Cardiorespiratory and metabolic responses during Tai Chi Chuan exercise. *Canadian Journal of Applied Sport Sciences*, 9, 1, 7-10.

Zijlstra, F.J., van den Berg-de Lange, I., Huygen, F.J. & Klein, J. (2003). Anti-inflammatory actions of acupuncture. *Mediators of Inflammation*, 12, 2, 59-69.

Permissions

The contributors of this book come from diverse backgrounds, making this book a truly international effort. This book will bring forth new frontiers with its revolutionizing research information and detailed analysis of the nascent developments around the world.

We would like to thank Dr. Andrew B. Lemmey, for lending his expertise to make the book truly unique. He has played a crucial role in the development of this book. Without his invaluable contribution this book wouldn't have been possible. He has made vital efforts to compile up to date information on the varied aspects of this subject to make this book a valuable addition to the collection of many professionals and students.

This book was conceptualized with the vision of imparting up-to-date information and advanced data in this field. To ensure the same, a matchless editorial board was set up. Every individual on the board went through rigorous rounds of assessment to prove their worth. After which they invested a large part of their time researching and compiling the most relevant data for our readers. Conferences and sessions were held from time to time between the editorial board and the contributing authors to present the data in the most comprehensible form. The editorial team has worked tirelessly to provide valuable and valid information to help people across the globe.

Every chapter published in this book has been scrutinized by our experts. Their significance has been extensively debated. The topics covered herein carry significant findings which will fuel the growth of the discipline. They may even be implemented as practical applications or may be referred to as a beginning point for another development. Chapters in this book were first published by InTech; hereby published with permission under the Creative Commons Attribution License or equivalent.

The editorial board has been involved in producing this book since its inception. They have spent rigorous hours researching and exploring the diverse topics which have resulted in the successful publishing of this book. They have passed on their knowledge of decades through this book. To expedite this challenging task, the publisher supported the team at every step. A small team of assistant editors was also appointed to further simplify the editing procedure and attain best results for the readers.

Our editorial team has been hand-picked from every corner of the world. Their multi-ethnicity adds dynamic inputs to the discussions which result in innovative outcomes. These outcomes are then further discussed with the researchers and contributors who give their valuable feedback and opinion regarding the same. The feedback is then collaborated with the researches and they are edited in a comprehensive manner to aid the understanding of the subject.

Apart from the editorial board, the designing team has also invested a significant amount of their time in understanding the subject and creating the most relevant covers. They scrutinized every image to scout for the most suitable representation of the subject and create an appropriate cover for the book.

The publishing team has been involved in this book since its early stages. They were actively engaged in every process, be it collecting the data, connecting with the contributors or procuring relevant information. The team has been an ardent support to the editorial, designing and production team. Their endless efforts to recruit the best for this project, has resulted in the accomplishment of this book. They are a veteran in the field of academics and their pool of knowledge is as vast as their experience in printing. Their expertise and guidance has proved useful at every step. Their uncompromising quality standards have made this book an exceptional effort. Their encouragement from time to time has been an inspiration for everyone.

The publisher and the editorial board hope that this book will prove to be a valuable piece of knowledge for researchers, students, practitioners and scholars across the globe.

List of Contributors

Alper Okyar
Istanbul University Faculty of Pharmacy Department of Pharmacology, Beyazıt- Istanbul

Yıldız Özsoy and Sevgi Güngör
Istanbul University Faculty of Pharmacy Department of Pharmaceutical Technology, Beyazıt- Istanbul, Turkey

Hussein Al-Mossawi and John R. Kirwan
Academic Rheumatology Unit, Bristol Royal Infirmary, Bristol, UK

Sarah K. Brode and Theodore K. Marras
University of Toronto, Canada

Koichiro Komiya and Nobuki Terada
Department of Orthopaedic Surgery, Fujita Health University Second Hospital, Japan

Yoshikazu Mizoguchi
Department of Pathology, Fujita Health University Second Hospital, Japan

Harumoto Yamada
Department of Orthopaedic Surgery, Fujita Health University, Japan

Yasuhiko Hirabayashi
Hikarigaoka Spellman Hospital, Japan
Graduate School of Medicine, Tohoku University, Japan

Rebecca A. Bader
Syracuse Biomaterials Institute, Syracuse University, USA

Nedžad Mulabegović, Jasna Kusturica, Maida Todić-Rakanović, Mirjana Mijanović, Fahir Bečić, Asija Začiragić, Selma Škrbo, Lejla Burnazović-Ristić, Aida Kulo and Svjetlana Loga-Zec
Medical Faculty University of Sarajevo Institute of Pharmacology, Clinical Pharmacology and Toxicology, Bosnia and Herzegovina

Aisha Siddiqah Ahmed
Karolinska Institutet, Sweden

Etsuo Chosa, Hiroaki Hamada and Toshiyuki Ohkura
Division of Orthopaedic Surgery, Department of Medicine of Sensory and Mortor Organs, Faculty of Medicine, University of Miyazaki, Japan

Theresa H. Page and Kim S. Midwood
Kennedy Institute of Rheumatology, Imperial College of Science, Technology and Medicine, London, UK

Sylvain G. Bourgoin, Chenqi Zhao and Maria J. Fernandes
Laval University, Canada

Katarina Bauerova, Silvester Poništ and Radomir Nosaľ
Institute of Experimental Pharmacology and Toxicology, Slovak Academy of Sciences, Slovakia

Maria Stančikova and Jozef Rovensky
National Institute of Rheumatic Diseases, Slovakia

Tomoyuki Nishizaki and Takeshi Kanno
Division of Bioinformation, Department of Physiology, Hyogo College of Medicine, Japan

Daniel J. Leong and Hui B. Sun
Department of Orthopaedic Surgery and Radiation Oncology, Oncophysics Research Institute, Albert Einstein College of Medicine/Montefiore Medical Center, New York, USA

Rebecca-Jane Law, David Markland, Peter Maddison and Jeanette M. Thom
School of Sport, Health and Exercise Sciences, Bangor University, Wales, United Kingdom

Andrew B. Lemmey
School of Sport, Health and Exercise Sciences, Bangor University, UK

Chenchen Wang
Tufts Medical Center/ Tufts University School of Medicine, USA